**7th** EDITION

# MEDICAL TERMINOLOGY
## FOR HEALTH PROFESSIONS

## Supplements At-a-Glance

| SUPPLEMENT: | WHAT IT IS: | WHAT'S IN IT: |
| --- | --- | --- |
| StudyWARE™ **StudyWARE** | Software program (DVD in the back of the book and online) | • Quizzes with immediate feedback<br>• Anatomy and pathology animations<br>• Image labeling<br>• Interactive games<br>• Crossword puzzles<br>• Word search<br>• Spelling bee |
| Workbook | Print | • Matching word parts<br>• Word construction<br>• Matching terms and definitions<br>• Word surgery<br>• Crossword puzzles |
| Premium Website | Online access | • StudyWARE™<br>• Slide presentations created in PowerPoint®<br>• Animations<br>• Mobile downloads with audio |
| Instructor Resources | CD-ROM | • Electronic Instructor's Manual files<br>• Electronic Testbank<br>• Slide presentations created in PowerPoint® with full-color art and animations |
| Instructor Companion Site | Online access | • Access the Instructor Resources online |
| CourseMate | | • CLe Book<br>• Textbook objectives<br>• Slide presentations created in PowerPoint®<br>• Quizzes<br>• Glossary<br>• Games<br>• Mobile downloads<br>• Animations<br>• Midterm and final exams<br>• Engagement Tracker |
| Learning Lab | | • Homework solution for mastering vocabulary with spelling, audio pronunciations, word building, and real-world applications |
| Audio CDs | Three Audio CDs | • Audio for 900 medical terms and definitions |
| WebTutor Advantage | Online access | • On Blackboard, WebCT, and Angel platforms (other platforms available upon request)<br>• Content and quizzes linked to each chapter<br>• Comprehensive glossary<br>• Animations<br>• StudyWARE™ interactive games<br>• Slide presentations created in PowerPoint®<br>• Discussion questions<br>• Mid-term and final exams |

# MEDICAL TERMINOLOGY
## FOR HEALTH PROFESSIONS

**7th EDITION**

Ann Ehrlich

Carol L. Schroeder

DELMAR
CENGAGE Learning

Australia • Brazil • Japan • Korea • Mexico • Singapore • Spain • United Kingdom • United States

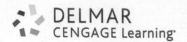
**DELMAR**
CENGAGE Learning·

*Medical Terminology for Health Professions,*
**Seventh Edition**
Ann Ehrlich and Carol L. Schroeder

Vice President, Careers and Computing:
Dave Garza

Director of Learning Solutions: Matthew Kane

Senior Acquisitions Editor: Matthew Seeley

Managing Editor: Marah Bellegarde

Senior Product Manager: Debra Myette-Flis

Editorial Assistant: Danielle Yannotti

Vice President, Marketing: Jennifer Baker

Marketing Director: Wendy Mapstone

Senior Marketing Manager: Kristin McNary

Associate Marketing Manager: Jonathan Sheehan

Production Director: Andrew Crouth

Content Project Manager: Thomas Heffernan

Senior Art Director: Jack Pendleton

Technology Project Manager: Patricia Allen

For product information and technology assistance, contact us at
**Cengage Learning Customer & Sales Support, 1-800-354-9706**
For permission to use material from this text or product,
submit all requests online at **www.cengage.com/permissions**.
Further permissions questions can be e-mailed to
**permissionrequest@cengage.com**

Library of Congress Control Number: 2011945075

ISBN-13: 978-1-111-54327-3

ISBN-10: 1-111-54327-5

**Delmar**
5 Maxwell Drive
Clifton Park, NY 12065-2919
USA

Cengage Learning is a leading provider of customized learning solutions with office locations around the globe, including Singapore, the United Kingdom, Australia, Mexico, Brazil, and Japan. Locate your local office at: **international.cengage.com/region**

Cengage Learning products are represented in Canada by Nelson Education, Ltd.

To learn more about Delmar, visit **www.cengage.com/delmar**

Purchase any of our products at your local college store or at our preferred online store **www.cengagebrain.com**

**Notice to the Reader**
Publisher does not warrant or guarantee any of the products described herein or perform any independent analysis in connection with any of the product information contained herein. Publisher does not assume, and expressly disclaims, any obligation to obtain and include information other than that provided to it by the manufacturer. The reader is expressly warned to consider and adopt all safety precautions that might be indicated by the activities described herein and to avoid all potential hazards. By following the instructions contained herein, the reader willingly assumes all risks in connection with such instructions. The publisher makes no representations or warranties of any kind, including but not limited to, the warranties of fitness for particular purpose or merchantability, nor are any such representations implied with respect to the material set forth herein, and the publisher takes no responsibility with respect to such material. The publisher shall not be liable for any special, consequential, or exemplary damages resulting, in whole or part, from the readers' use of, or reliance upon, this material.

Printed in the United States of America
1 2 3 4 5 6 7 16 15 14 13 12

# Contents

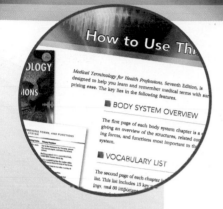

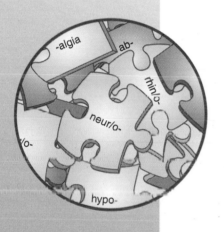

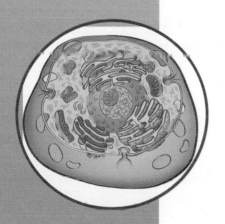

## Word Part Review                                56

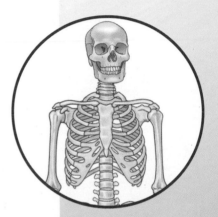

## Chapter 3: The Skeletal System                 63

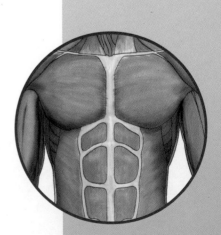

## Chapter 4: The Muscular System                 99

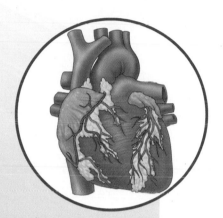

## Chapter 5: The Cardiovascular System          129

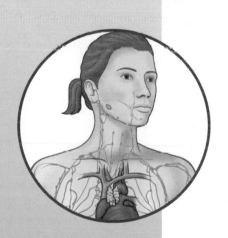

## Chapter 6: The Lymphatic and Immune Systems          169

## Chapter 7: The Respiratory System    204

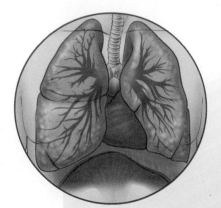

## Chapter 8: The Digestive System    237

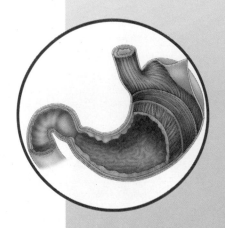

## Chapter 9: The Urinary System    274

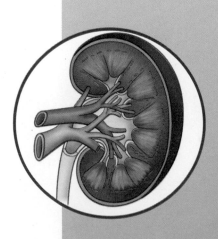

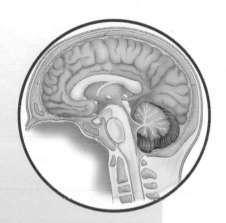

## Chapter 10: The Nervous System     305

## Chapter 11: Special Senses: The Eyes and Ears   344

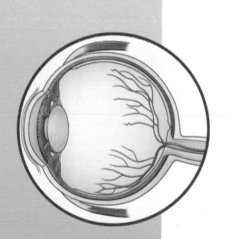

## Chapter 12: Skin: The Integumentary System    376

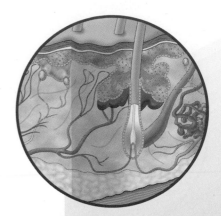

## Chapter 13: The Endocrine System    407

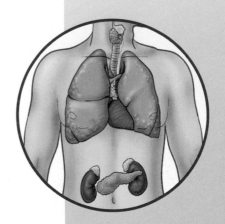

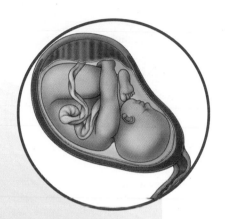

## Chapter 14: The Reproductive Systems          434

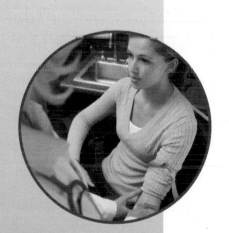

## Chapter 15: Diagnostic Procedures, Nuclear Medicine, and Pharmacology          471

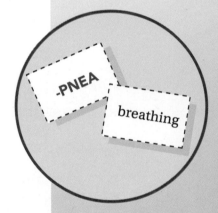

# Preface

## ■ TO THE LEARNER

Welcome to the world of medical terminology! Learning this special language is an important step in preparing for your career as a healthcare professional. Here's good news: Learning medical terms is much easier than learning a foreign language because you are already familiar with quite a few of the words, such as *appendicitis* and *tonsillectomy*. Understanding new words becomes easier with the discovery that many of these terms are made up of interchangeable word parts that are used in different combinations. Once you understand this, you'll be well on your way to translating even the most difficult medical terms, including words you have never seen before. You'll be amazed to see how quickly your vocabulary will grow!

This book and the accompanying learning materials are designed to make the process as simple as possible. Review the introductory sections at the beginning of the book, including "How to Use This Book" and "How to Use StudyWARE™" so you can find your way around easily. Once you become comfortable with the format, you'll discover you are learning faster than you ever imagined possible.

## CHAPTER ORGANIZATION

The text is designed to help you master medical terminology. It is organized into 15 chapters, the Word Part Review, the Comprehensive Medical Terminology Review, three appendices, an index, and removable Flashcards. To gain the most benefit from your use of this text, take advantage of the many features, including the "Learning Exercises" plus the "Human Touch" stories and discussion that are included at the end of each chapter.

**Primary terms** are the most important terms in a chapter. When first introduced, the term appears in boldface and, if appropriate, is followed by the "sounds-like pronunciation." Only primary terms are used as correct answers in the exercises and tests.

*Secondary terms* appear in *orange* italics. These terms, which are included to clarify the meaning of a primary term, are sometimes used as distracters, but not as correct answers, in exercises or tests.

Each chapter begins with a **vocabulary list** consisting of 15 word parts and 60 medical terms selected from among the primary terms in the chapter. These important words are pronounced in the StudyWARE™, as well as on the optional Audio CDs. Note: if your instructor is using the **Simplified Syllabus** version of this course, these are the terms that you will be expected to learn for all quizzes, tests, and exams.

### Introductory Chapters and Word Part Review

**Chapters 1 and 2** create the foundation that enables you to master the rest of the book. Chapter 1 introduces key word parts—the building blocks of most medical terms.

Chapter 2 introduces more word parts and provides an overview of basic terms used throughout the health field.

After studying these chapters, complete the **Word Part Review** that follows Chapter 2. These practice activities and the accompanying test will help you determine whether you've mastered the concept of these all-important building blocks. If you are having trouble here, it is important to put more effort into learning these basics.

## Body System Chapters

**Chapters 3 through 14** are organized by body system. Because each body system stands alone, you can study these chapters in any sequence. Each chapter begins with an overview of the structures and functions of that system so you can relate these to the specialists, pathology, diagnostics, and treatment procedures that follow.

**Chapter 15** introduces basic diagnostic procedures, examination positions, imaging techniques, laboratory tests, nuclear medicine, and pharmacology. It also includes a section on alternative and complementary medicines. This chapter can be studied at any point in the course.

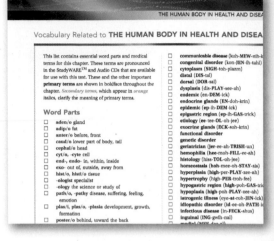

## Comprehensive Medical Terminology Review

This section, which follows Chapter 15, is designed to help you prepare for your final examination. It includes study tips, practice exercises, and a simulated final test; however, be aware that none of these questions are from the actual final test.

## Appendices

**Appendix A: Prefixes, Combining Forms, and Suffixes** is a convenient alphabetic reference for medical word parts. When you don't recognize a word part, you can look it up here.

**Appendix B: Abbreviations and Their Meanings** is an extensive list of commonly used abbreviations and their meanings. Abbreviations are important in medicine, and using them *accurately* is essential!

**Appendix C: Glossary of Pathology and Procedures** gives the definitions of all the primary terms in the text relating to diagnosis, pathology, and medical procedures.

## LEARNING SUPPLEMENTS

The following supplements are included with your textbook to provide even more help as you study.

- **Flashcards.** Improve your knowledge and test your mastery by using the flashcards provided in the last section of the book. Remove these perforated pages carefully and then separate the cards. Flashcards are an effective study aid for use even when you have only a small amount of time.

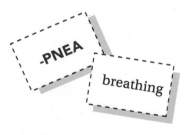

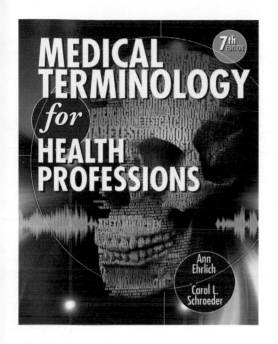

■ **StudyWARE™.** This interactive software packaged with the book, and available online, offers an exciting way to gain additional practice (while having fun) through exercises, game activities, and audio elements for each chapter. See "How to Use the StudyWare" on page xxv for details.

*The students who have used [StudyWARE™] show a significant lead in learning, retaining and understanding terminology as evidenced by 85% or greater on term tests and 80% or higher on the final spelling and terminology competencies. These students also are better documenters of patient treatment than those who did not utilize [StudyWARE™].*
—*Jane Dumas, Allied Health Department Chair*

Also available: StudyWARE™ CD-ROM Stand-alone to accompany Medical Terminology for Health Professions, Seventh Edition, ISBN: 1-1115-4334-8

## PREMIUM WEBSITE

A Premium Website is available to accompany the text that includes the StudyWARE™, slide presentations created in PowerPoint®, animations, and Mobile Downloads.

### Redeeming an Access Code:

1. Go To: www.CengageBrain.com
2. Enter The Access code in the Prepaid Code or Access Key field, REDEEM
3. REGISTER as a new user or LOG IN as an existing user if you already have an account with Cengage Learning or CengageBrain.com
4. SELECT **Go to MY Account**
5. OPEN the product from the My Account page

Also available:

■ Premium Website IAC to accompany *Medical Terminology for Health Professions,* Seventh Edition, ISBN 1-1115-4348-8

## ■ TO THE INSTRUCTOR

From the very first edition, *Medical Terminology for Health Professions* has been dedicated to breaking new ground that will make learning medical terminology faster and easier. In this seventh edition, the authors have maintained this standard of providing high-quality teaching materials for the mastery of medical terminology.

In the preparation of the seventh edition, all medical term definitions have been reviewed and updated as appropriate, and obsolete terms have been deleted. In addition, this latest edition of the text has an all-new art program, with original illustrations and contemporary photographs that will appeal to today's visual learner.

To help instructors make the transition from the sixth edition to the seventh, all major changes in terms and content can easily be accessed through the "Conversion Guide" found on the Instructor Resources CD-ROM.

## CHANGES TO THE SEVENTH EDITION

A detailed conversion guide that helps you make the change from the sixth to the seventh edition is included in the Instructor Resources. A brief summary of changes follows:

- The "Supplements At-a-Glance" feature briefly describes resource materials to accompany this textbook.
- Hundreds of new, full-color illustrations were added. There is also expanded use of photographs and multicultural images.
- Definitions for word parts were added to the vocabulary lists at the beginning of each chapter.
- Information was added in Chapter 1 on "Do Not Use" abbreviations.
- A section on complementary and alternative therapies was added to Chapter 15.
- Appendix C: Glossary of Pathology and Procedures is back by popular demand.
- A StudyWARE™ Connection feature was added to remind learners of animations, interactive games, and quizzes.
- A Mobile Downloads feature was added to direct learners to free online audio.
- A Workbook Practice feature was added.
- SOAP notes with study questions and answer keys were added to the Instructor's Manual.
- Word search games using the Simplified Syllabus terms were added to the StudyWARE and Instructor's Manual.

## USING THE SIMPLIFIED SYLLABUS

In response to the needs of instructors who face the challenge of teaching a "brief" medical terminology course, the authors have developed a program called the Simplified Syllabus. By using these specialized teaching materials, which are based on the 60 terms and 15 word parts from the vocabulary list for each chapter, you can hold your students responsible just for this key information. These materials have been expanded to include:

- A **Simplified Syllabus Computerized Test Bank** with questions using these key terms and word parts for each chapter, plus a midterm and final test
- A **Simplified Syllabus Workbook** with written questions plus, just for fun, a crossword puzzle and word search at the end of each chapter (Workbook ISBN 1-1115-4328-3)
- **Simplified Syllabus Activities** in the Instructor's Manual, which is part of the Instructor Resources CD-ROM and includes the new Word Search activity
- **Audio CDs** featuring all of the Simplified Syllabus terms pronounced and defined, which creates a flexible study aid for your students to use

# ■ SPECIAL RESOURCES TO ACCOMPANY THE BOOK

## AUDIO CDS

The Audio CDs include the pronunciation of the 60 terms from the vocabulary list for each chapter. After the pause, the word is pronounced again and then defined. These Audio CDs are a valuable, flexible, learning aid for use whenever and wherever the learner needs to study. Audio CDs, ISBN 978-1-1115-4332-7

## THE INSTRUCTOR RESOURCES

The Instructor Resources is a robust computerized tool for your instructional needs! A must-have for all instructors, this comprehensive and convenient CD-ROM contains the following:

■ **Textbook Teaching Resources** is an overview of the teaching resources featured in the text.

■ **Conversion Guide** helps you make the change from the sixth to the seventh edition of *Medical Terminology for Health Professions.*

■ **Textbook Learning Exercises Answer Keys** are included for your reference.

■ **Workbook Answer Keys** are also included.

■ **ExamView® Computerized Test Bank** contains two test banks of prepared questions: The **Standard Tests** include 100 questions per chapter plus a 50-question midterm test that covers Chapters 1 through 8, and a 100-question final test covering the entire text.

■ The **Simplified Syllabus** test bank includes 75 questions per chapter plus a 50-question midterm test that covers Chapters 1 through 8, and a 100-question final test covering the entire text. You can use these questions to create your own review materials or tests. This versatile program enables you to create your own tests and to write additional questions.

■ **Presentations Created in PowerPoint®**, including animations, are designed to aid you in planning your class presentations. If a learner misses a class, a printout of the slides for a lecture makes a helpful review page. To facilitate correcting Learning Exercises in class, the textbook Learning Exercises answer keys are included in the PowerPoint® slides. There are now also slides for the Personal Response Device Questions provided for each chapter.

■ The **Instructor's Manual** includes a wide variety of valuable resources to help you plan the course and implement activities by chapter. The availability of this manual in an electronic format increases its value as a teaching resource. This manual includes the following:

  ■ **Course Planning Tips**, including a sample 16-week syllabus and a sample course outline.

  ■ **Tips for New Teachers**, which includes practical ideas to help new teachers and their students have a successful experience.

  ■ The **Teaching Tools by Chapter** feature, which includes two 25-question chapter quizzes with answer keys, classroom activities, a crossword puzzle and answer, and a case study for each chapter. New to this edition are SOAP notes with questions and a word search game.

  ■ **Review Activities for Midterm and Final Tests.**
  Instructor Resources, ISBN 978-1-1115-4329-7

## INSTRUCTOR COMPANION SITE

An Instructor Companion Site is available that includes the Instructor Resources. To access the Instructor Companion Site, go to login.cengage.com/sso/.

## THE LEARNING LAB

Learning Lab is an online homework solution that maps to learning objectives in *Medical Terminology for Health Professions, Seventh Edition.* Interactive, scenario-based activities build students' medical vocabulary, strengthen word-building skills, and encourage an understanding of the importance of medical terminology as the basis of communication in the health care workplace, between health care professionals, and with patients. This simulated, immersive environment engages users with its real-life approach. The Learning Lab includes a pre-assessment, three learning activities, and a post-assessment organized around the chapters in this text. The post-assessment scores can be posted to the instructor grade book in any learning management system. The amount of time the student spends within the Learning Lab can also be tracked.

   IAC Learning Lab to Accompany *Medical Terminology for Health Professions*, 7th Edition, ISBN 978-1-1115-4342-6

## COURSEMATE

Medical Terminology CourseMate includes:

■ An interactive eBook, with highlighting, note taking, and search capabilities

■ Interactive learning tools including:

   ■ Quizzes

   ■ Flashcards

   ■ Animations

   ■ Mobile downloads

   ■ and more!

   Go to login.cengagebrain.com to access these resources, and look for this icon to find resources related to your text in Medical Terminology CourseMate.

   IAC CourseMate for *Medical Terminology for Health Professions*, 7th Edition, ISBN 978-1-1115-4339-6

## WEBTUTOR™ ADVANTAGE

Designed to complement the textbook, WebTUTOR™ is a content-rich, Web-based teaching and learning aid that reinforces and clarifies complex concepts. Animations enhance learning and retention of material. The WebCT™ and Blackboard™ platforms also provide rich communication tools to instructors and students, including a course calendar, chat, e-mail, and threaded discussions. WebTUTOR™ Advantage on WebCT™, ISBN 978-1-1115-4331-0

WebTUTOR™ Advantage on Blackboard™, ISBN 978-1-1115-4330-3
WebTUTOR™ Advantage on Angel, ISBN 978-1-1115-4349-5

## HEALTH SCIENCE GENERAL STUDIES CATALOG

Learn more about our health care solutions that increase retention and build critical thinking skills. Visit www.cengage.com/community/health_science.

# ■ ADDITIONAL RESOURCES

## DELMAR'S MEDICAL TERMINOLOGY STUDENT THEATER: AN INTERACTIVE VIDEO PROGRAM

Organized by body system, this CD-ROM is invaluable to learners trying to master the complex world of medical terminology. The program is designed for allied health and nursing students who are enrolled in medical terminology courses. A series of video clips leads learners through the various concepts, interspersing lectures with illustrations to emphasize key points. Quizzes and games allow learners to assess their understanding of the video content.
ISBN 978-1-4283-1863-2

## DELMAR LEARNING'S ANATOMY AND PHYSIOLOGY IMAGE LIBRARY CD-ROM, THIRD EDITION

This CD-ROM includes more than 1,050 graphic files. These files can be incorporated into a PowerPoint® or Microsoft® Word presentation, used directly from the CD-ROM in a classroom presentation, or used to make color transparencies. The Image Library is organized around body systems and medical specialties. The library includes various anatomy, physiology, and pathology graphics of different levels of complexity. Instructors can search and select the graphics that best apply to their teaching situation. This is an ideal resource to enhance your teaching presentation of medical terminology or anatomy and physiology.
ISBN 978-1-4180-3928-8

## COMPLETE MEDICAL TERMINOLOGY ONLINE COURSE

Designed as a stand-alone course, this eliminates the need for a separate book. Everything is online! Content is presented in four major sections: Study, Practice, Tests, and Reports. The Study section includes the content from the text, along with graphics, animations, and audio links. The Practice section includes exercises and games to reinforce learning. The Test section includes tests with a variety of question types for each chapter. A midterm and a final exam are also available. The Report section features learner reports and instructor reports.
Individual Course, ISBN 978-0-7668-2738-7
Educational Course, ISBN 978-0-7668-2737-0

## DELMAR'S MEDICAL TERMINOLOGY AUDIO LIBRARY

This extensive audio library of medical terminology includes three Audio CDs with more than 3,700 terms pronounced, and a software CD-ROM. The CD-ROM presents terms organized by body systems, medical specialty, and general medical term categories. The user can search for a specific term by typing in the term or key words, or click on a category to view an alphabetical list of all terms within the category. The user can hear the correct pronunciation of one term or listen to each term on the list pronounced automatically. Definitions can be viewed after hearing the pronunciation of terms.
Institutional Version, ISBN 978-1-4018-3223-0
Individual Version, ISBN 978-1-4018-3222-3

## DELMAR'S MEDICAL TERMINOLOGY CD-ROM INSTITUTIONAL VERSION

This is an exciting interactive reference, practice, and assessment tool designed to complement any medical terminology program. Features include the extensive use of multimedia—animations, video, graphics, and activities—to present terms and word-building features. Difficult functions, processes, and procedures are included, so learners can more effectively learn from a textbook.
ISBN 978-0-7668-0979-6

## DELMAR'S MEDICAL TERMINOLOGY FLASH! COMPUTERIZED FLASHCARDS

Learn and review more than 1,500 medical terms using this unique electronic flashcard program. Flash! is a computerized flashcard-type question-and-answer association program designed to help users learn correct spellings, definitions, and pronunciations. The use of graphics and audio clips make it a fun and easy way for users to learn and test their knowledge of medical terminology.
ISBN 978-0-7668-4320-2

## FUNDAMENTALS OF ANATOMY AND PHYSIOLOGY ONLINE COURSE

This fully developed online course introduces learners with little or no prior biology knowledge to the complex and exciting world of anatomy and physiology. The course is a complete interactive online learning solution. Chapter content is organized around body systems and focuses on how each system works together to promote homeostasis. Full-color art, 3-D anatomical animations, audio, and "bite-size" chunks of content fully engage the learner. Interactive games such as image labeling, concentration, and championship reinforce learning. Powerful customization tools allow administrators to individualize the course and assessment tools, while extensive tracking features allow administrators to monitor learner performance and progress.
Anatomy & Physiology Online—Academic Individual Access Code, ISBN 978-1-4180-0131-5
Anatomy & Physiology Online—Academic Institutional Access Code, ISBN 978-1-4180-0130-8

# Acknowledgements

Special thanks to Katrina Schroeder and Laura Ehrlich for their contributions to this edition of the text, and to the many reviewers who continue to be a valuable resource in guiding this book as it evolves. Their insights, comments, suggestions, and attention to detail were very important in creating this text.

Thanks also to the editorial and production staff of Delmar Learning for their very professional and extremely helpful assistance in making this revision possible, especially our editors, Deb Myette-Flis and Matthew Seeley. We would also like to thank Joanna Lundeen and the skilled medical illustrators of Dartmouth Publishing for their excellent work on the new art for this edition.

*Ann Ehrlich*
*Carol L. Schroeder*

## ◼ REVIEWERS

**Diana Alagna RN, RMA, CPT, AHI**
Medical Assistant Program Director
Branford Hall Career Institute
Southington, Connecticut

**Diane Roche Benson, CMA (AAMA), BSHCA, MSA, CFP, ASE, NSC-SCFAT, CDE, CMRS, CPC, AHA BLS-I, FA-I, PALS, ACLS, CAAM-I, CCT, NCI-I**
Wake Technical Community College
Raleigh, North Carolina
The University of Phoenix
Phoenix, Arizona
Johnston Community College
Smithfield, North Carolina

**Karla Knaussman Duran, AS, BS, MLS**
Instructor, Medical Terminology
Butler Community College
Andover, Kansas

**Anita Hazelwood, RHIA, FAHIMA**
Louisiana Health Systems/BORSF Professor in Health Care Administration
Health Information Management
Lafayette, Louisiana

**Norma Longoria, BS, COI**
Health and Medical Administrative Services Faculty
South Texas College
Nursing/Allied Health Division
McAllen, Texas

**Sharon F. Maiewski, MS, PA-C**
Assistant Professor
James Madison University
Physician Assistant Program
Harrisonburg, Virginia

**David Pintado, MD**
Instructor, Health Care Program
Corinthian Schools
Heald College
Concord, California

**Darlene Sirois Seay, RN, MSEd**
Assistant Professor
Practical Nursing
Piedmont Virginia Community College
Charlottesville, Virginia

**David Stump-Foughty**
MIBC Program Director
Medical Insurance Billing and Coding
Portland, Oregon

**Technical Reviewers**
**Karen R. Smith, RN, BSN**
Health Science Consultant
Kentucky Department of Education
Division of Career and Technical Education
Frankfort, Kentucky

**Kathy Pickrell, RN, MSN**
Associate Professor, Emerita
Nursing Department
Indiana State University, College of Nursing, Health, and Human Services
Terre Haute, Indiana

# How to Use This Book

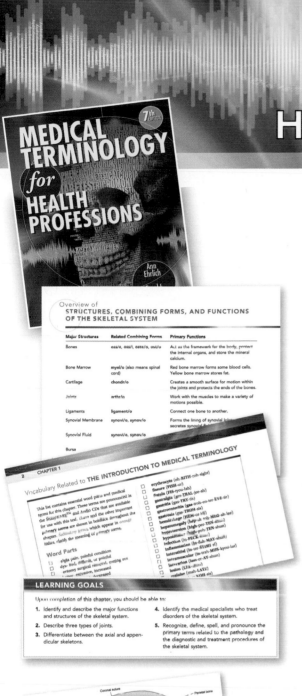

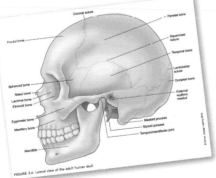

*Medical Terminology for Health Professions,* Seventh Edition, is designed to help you learn and remember medical terms with surprising ease. The key lies in the following features.

## ▮ BODY SYSTEM OVERVIEW

The first page of each body system chapter is a chart giving an overview of the structures, related combining forms, and functions most important to that system.

## ▮ VOCABULARY LIST

The second page of each chapter is a 75-item vocabulary list. This list includes 15 key word parts and their meanings, and 60 important terms for the chapter with their pronunciations. This immediately alerts you to the key terms in the chapter and acts as a review guide. Next to each term is a box so you can check off each term when you've learned it. The list includes the 60 terms pronounced in the StudyWARE™, which is included with the book and online, as well as on the optional Audio CDs.

## ▮ LEARNING GOALS

The beginning of each chapter lists learning goals to help you understand what is expected of you as you read the text and complete the exercises. These objectives are set off with a colored bar for easy identification.

## ▮ ALL-NEW ART PROGRAM

The all-new art program includes hundreds of photos and full-color illustrations that help clarify the text and contain important additional information. Review each illustration and read its caption carefully for easy and effective learning. There is also expanded use of photographs and multicultural images.

# "SOUNDS-LIKE" PRONUNCIATION SYSTEM

The sounds-like pronunciation system makes pronunciation easy by respelling the word with syllables you can understand—and say—at a glance. Simply pronounce the term just as it appears in parentheses, accenting the syllables as follows:

- **Primary** (strongest) **accent**: capital letters and bold type
- **Secondary accent**: lowercase letters and bold type

# WORD PARTS

Because word parts are so important to learning medical terminology, whenever a term made up of word parts is introduced, the definition is followed (in parentheses) by the word parts highlighted in **magenta** and defined.

# PRIMARY AND SECONDARY TERMS

- **Primary terms** are the most important medical words in a chapter. When first introduced, the term appears in **boldface** and, if appropriate, is followed by the sounds-like pronunciation. These are the words students need to concentrate on learning. Only primary terms are used as correct answers in the exercises and tests.
- *Secondary terms* appear in *orange* italics. These terms are included to clarify the meaning of a primary term. Although used as distracters in exercises, the secondary terms are not used as correct answers in exercises or tests.

# LEARNING EXERCISES

Each chapter includes 100 Learning Exercises in a variety of formats that require a one- or two-word written answer. Writing terms, rather than just circling a multiple-choice option, reinforces learning and provides practice in writing and spelling the terms.

# THE HUMAN TOUCH: CRITICAL THINKING EXERCISE

A real-life ministory and related critical thinking questions at the end of each chapter that involves patients and pathology helps you apply what you are learning to the real world. There are no right or wrong answers, but just questions to get you started thinking about and using the new terms you have learned.

## Cartilage

- **Cartilage** (**KAR**-tih-lidj) is the smooth, rubbery, blue-white connective tissue that acts as a shock absorber between bones. Cartilage, which is more elastic than bone, also makes up the flexible parts of the skeleton such as the outer ear and the tip of the nose.
- **Articular cartilage** (ar-**TICK**-you-lar **KAR**-tih-lidj) covers the surfaces of bones where they come together to form joints. This cartilage makes smooth joint movement possible and protects the ___ from rubbing against each other (Figures 3.1

- **Hemopoietic** (**hee**-moh-poy-**ET**-ick) means pertaining to the formation of blood cells (**hem/o** means blood, and **-poietic** means pertaining to formation). This term is also spelled *hematopoietic*.
- **Yellow bone marrow** functions as a fat storage area. It is composed chiefly of fat cells and is located in the medullary cavity of long bones.

**TABLE 3.1**
**Abbreviations Related to the Skeletal System**

| bone density testing = BDT | BDT = bone density testing |
| --- | --- |
| closed reduction = CR | CR = closed reduction |
| fracture = Fx | Fx = fracture |
| osteoarthritis = OA | OA = osteoarthritis |
| osteoporosis = OP | OP = osteoporosis |
| partial knee replacement = PKR | PKR = partial knee replacement |
| polymyalgia rheumatica = PMR | PMR = polymyalgia rheumatica |
| rheumatoid arthritis = RA | RA = rheumatoid arthritis |
| total hip arthroplasty = THA | THA = total hip arthroplasty |
| total knee arthroplasty = TKA | TKA = total knee arthroplasty |

**MATCHING WORD PARTS 1**

Write the correct answer in the middle column.

| Definition | Correct Answer | Possible Answers |
| --- | --- | --- |
| 3.1. hump | _____ | ankyl/o |
| 3.2. cartilage | _____ | |
| 3.3. crooked, bent, stiff | _____ | arthr/o |
| 3.4. joint | _____ | -um |
| 3.5. singular noun ending | _____ | kyph/o |
| | | chondr/l, chondr/o |

**MATCHING WORD PARTS 2**

Write the correct answer in t___ ___ column.

| Definition | | Possible Answers |
| --- | --- | --- |
| 3.6. cranium, skull | | |
| 3.7. rib | | |
| 3.8. setting free, loose | | |
| 3.9. spinal cord, bon | | |
| 3.10. to bind, tie tog | | |

**THE HUMAN TOUCH**
**Critical Thinking Exercise**

The following story and questions are designed to stimulate critical thinking through class discussion or as a brief essay response. There are no right or wrong answers to these questions.

Dr. Johnstone didn't like what he saw. The x-rays of Gladys Gwynn's hip showed a *fracture of the femoral neck and severe osteoporosis of the hip.* Mrs. Gwynn had been admitted to the orthopedic ward of Newton Hospital after a fall that morning at Sunny Meadows, an assisted-living facility. The accident had occurred when Sheri Smith, a new aide, lost her grip while helping Mrs. Gwynn in the shower.

A frail but alert and cheerful woman of 85, Mrs. Gwynn has *osteoarthritis* and *osteoporosis* that have forced her to rely on a walker. Although her finances were limited, she had been living at Sunny Meadows since her husband's death 1 year ago. Dr. Johnstone knew that she didn't have close relatives, and he did not think that she had signed a Health Care Power of Attorney designating someone to help with medical decisions like this.

A *total hip replacement* would be the logical treatment for a younger patient because it could restore some of her lost mobility. However, for a frail patient like Mrs. Gwynn, *internal fixation* of the fracture might be the treatment of choice. This would repair the break, but not improve her mobility.

Dr. Johnstone needs to make a decision soon, but he knows that Mrs. Gwynn is groggy from pain medication. With one more look at the x-ray, Dr. Johnstone sighed and walked toward Mrs. Gwynn's room.

**Suggested Discussion Topics**

1. Because of the pain medication, Gladys Gwynn may not be able to speak for herself. Since she has no relatives to help, is it appropriate for Dr. Johnstone to make the decision about surgery for her? Under the circumstances, is it possible that when Gladys moved into Sunny Meadows they had her sign a Health Care Power of Attorney to someone at the facility?

2. Because the accident happened when Sheri Smith was helping Mrs. Gwynn, do you think Sheri should be held responsible for the accident? Given that Sheri is an employee of Sunny Mea...

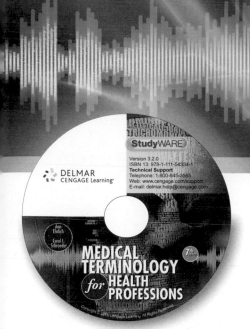

**StudyWARE™** to accompany
*Medical Terminology for Health Professions*, Seventh Edition

## SYSTEM REQUIREMENTS

Minimum System Requirements:

- Microsoft Windows XP w/SP 2, Windows Vista w/SP 1, Windows 7
- Mac OS X 10.4, 10.5, or 10.6
- Processor: Minimum required by Operating System
- Memory: Minimum required by Operating System
- Hard Drive Space: 540 MB
- Screen resolution: 1024 x 768 pixels
- CD-ROM drive
- Sound card and listening device required for audio features
- Flash Player 10. The Adobe Flash Player is free, and can be downloaded from www.adobe.com/products/flashplayer/

## WINDOWS SETUP INSTRUCTIONS

1. Insert disc into CD-ROM drive. The software installation should start automatically. If it does not, go to step 2.
2. From My Computer, double-click the icon for the CD drive.
3. Double-click the *setup.exe* file to start the program.

## MAC SETUP INSTRUCTIONS

1. Insert disc into CD-ROM drive.
2. Once the disc icon appears on your desktop, double click on it to open it.
3. Double-click the *StudyWARE* to start the program.

# TECHNICAL SUPPORT

Telephone: 1-800-648-7450

Monday-Friday

8:30 A.M.-6:30 P.M. EST

E-mail: delmar.help@cengage.com

StudyWare™ is a trademark used herein under license.

Microsoft® and Windows® are registered trademarks of the Microsoft Corporation.

Pentium® is a registered trademark of the Intel Corporation.

# GETTING STARTED

The StudyWARE™ software helps you learn material in *Medical Terminology for Health Professions,* Seventh Edition. As you study each chapter in the text, be sure to explore the activities in the corresponding chapter in the software. Use StudyWARE™ as your own private tutor.

Getting started is easy. Install the software by inserting the CD-ROM into your computer's CD-ROM drive and following the on-screen instructions. When you open the software, enter your first and last name so the software can store your quiz results. Then choose a chapter from the menu to take a quiz or explore one of the activities.

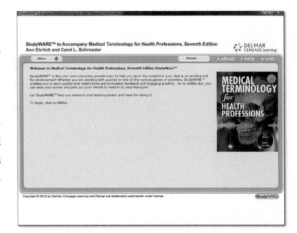

# MENUS

You can access the menus from wherever you are in the program. The menus include quizzes and other activities.

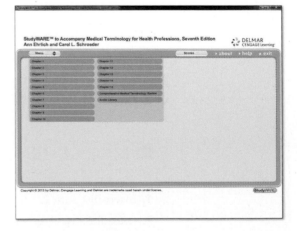

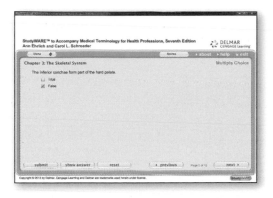

## QUIZZES

Quizzes include true/false, multiple-choice, fill-in-the-blank, and word-building questions. You can take the quizzes in both practice mode and quiz mode. Use practice mode to improve your mastery of the material. You have multiple tries to get the answers correct. Instant feedback tells you whether you're right or wrong and helps you learn quickly by explaining why an answer was correct or incorrect. Use quiz mode when you are ready to test yourself, and keep a record of your scores. In quiz mode, you have one try to get the answers right, but you can take each quiz as many times as you want.

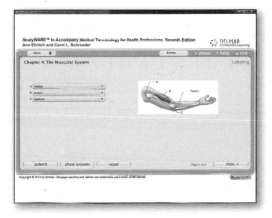

## SCORES

You can view your last scores for each quiz and print your results to hand in to your instructor.

## ACTIVITIES

Activities include image labeling, spelling bee, concentration, crossword and word search puzzles, and championship. Have fun while increasing your knowledge!

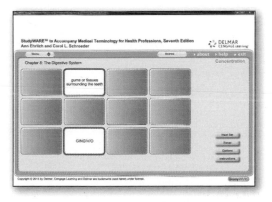

## AUDIO LIBRARY

The StudyWARE™ Audio Library is a reference that includes audio pronunciations and definitions for more than 900 medical terms! Use the audio library to practice pronunciation and review definitions for medical terms. You can browse terms by chapter or search by key word. Listen to pronunciations of the terms you select, or listen to an entire list of terms.

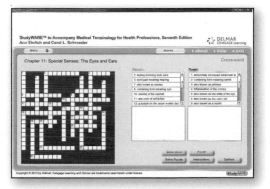

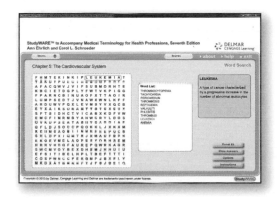

## ANIMATIONS

Animations expand your learning by helping you visualize concepts related to word-building, anatomy, physiology, and pathology.

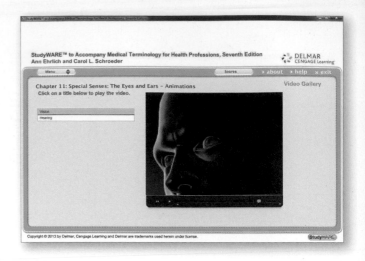

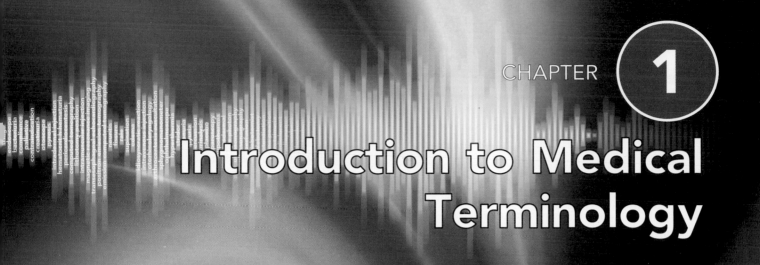

# Introduction to Medical Terminology

## Overview of
## INTRODUCTION TO MEDICAL TERMINOLOGY

| | |
|---|---|
| Primary Medical Terms | Primary terms enable you to prioritize terms in your study of medical terminology. These are the words that are shown in boldface. |
| Word Parts Are the Key | An introduction to medical word parts and how they are used to create complex medical terms. |
| Word Roots | The word parts that usually, but not always, indicate the part of the body involved. |
| Combining Form | A combining form is a word root that has had a vowel, usually the letter "o," added to the end. |
| Suffixes | The word part attached at the end of a word that usually, but not always, indicates the procedure, condition, disorder, or disease. |
| Prefixes | The word part attached at the beginning of a word that usually, but not always, indicates location, time, number, or status. |
| Determining Meanings on the Basis of Word Parts | Knowledge of word parts helps decipher medical terms. |
| Medical Dictionary Use | Guidelines to make the use of a medical dictionary easier. |
| Pronunciation | Use the easy-to-use "sounds-like" pronunciation system. |
| Spelling Is Always Important | A one-letter spelling error can change the entire meaning of a term. |
| Singular and Plural Endings | Unusual singular and plural endings used in medical terms. |
| Basic Medical Terms | Terms used to describe disease conditions. |
| Look-Alike, Sound-Alike Terms and Word Parts | Clarification of confusing terms and word parts that look or sound alike. |
| Using Abbreviations | Caution is always important when using abbreviations. |

## Vocabulary Related to **THE INTRODUCTION TO MEDICAL TERMINOLOGY**

This list contains essential word parts and medical terms for this chapter. These terms are pronounced in the StudyWARE™ and Audio CDs that are available for use with this text. These and the other important **primary terms** are shown in boldface throughout the chapter. *Secondary terms*, which appear in *orange* italics, clarify the meaning of primary terms.

### Word Parts

- ☐ **-algia** pain, painful condition
- ☐ **dys-** bad, difficult, or painful
- ☐ **-ectomy** surgical removal, cutting out
- ☐ **hyper-** excessive, increased
- ☐ **hypo-** deficient, decreased
- ☐ **-itis** inflammation
- ☐ **-osis** abnormal condition, disease
- ☐ **-ostomy** the surgical creation of an artificial opening to the body surface
- ☐ **-otomy** cutting, surgical incision
- ☐ **-plasty** surgical repair
- ☐ **-rrhage** bleeding, abnormal excessive fluid discharge
- ☐ **-rrhaphy** surgical suturing
- ☐ **-rrhea** flow or discharge
- ☐ **-rrhexis** rupture
- ☐ **-sclerosis** abnormal hardening

### Medical Terms

- ☐ **abdominocentesis** (ab-**dom**-ih-noh-sen-**TEE**-sis)
- ☐ **acronym** (**ACK**-roh-nim)
- ☐ **acute**
- ☐ **angiography** (**an**-jee-**OG**-rah-fee)
- ☐ **appendectomy** (**ap**-en-**DECK**-toh-mee)
- ☐ **arteriosclerosis** (ar-**tee**-ree-oh-skleh-**ROH**-sis)
- ☐ **arthralgia** (ar-**THRAL**-jee-ah)
- ☐ **colostomy** (koh-**LAHS**-toh-mee)
- ☐ **cyanosis** (**sigh**-ah-**NOH**-sis)
- ☐ **dermatologist** (**der**-mah-**TOL**-oh-jist)
- ☐ **diagnosis** (**dye**-ag-**NOH**-sis)
- ☐ **diarrhea** (**dye**-ah-**REE**-ah)
- ☐ **edema** (eh-**DEE**-mah)
- ☐ **endarterial** (**end**-ar-**TEE**-ree-al)
- ☐ **eponym** (**EP**-oh-nim)

- ☐ **erythrocyte** (eh-**RITH**-roh-sight)
- ☐ **fissure** (**FISH**-ur)
- ☐ **fistula** (**FIS**-tyou-lah)
- ☐ **gastralgia** (gas-**TRAL**-jee-ah)
- ☐ **gastritis** (gas-**TRY**-tis)
- ☐ **gastroenteritis** (**gas**-troh-en-ter-**EYE**-tis)
- ☐ **gastrosis** (gas-**TROH**-sis)
- ☐ **hemorrhage** (**HEM**-or-idj)
- ☐ **hepatomegaly** (**hep**-ah-toh-**MEG**-ah-lee)
- ☐ **hypertension** (**high**-per-**TEN**-shun)
- ☐ **hypotension** (**high**-poh-**TEN**-shun)
- ☐ **infection** (in-**FECK**-shun)
- ☐ **inflammation** (in-flah-**MAY**-shun)
- ☐ **interstitial** (**in**-ter-**STISH**-al)
- ☐ **intramuscular** (**in**-trah-**MUS**-kyou-lar)
- ☐ **laceration** (**lass**-er-**AY**-shun)
- ☐ **lesion** (**LEE**-zhun)
- ☐ **malaise** (mah-**LAYZ**)
- ☐ **mycosis** (my-**KOH**-sis)
- ☐ **myelopathy** (my-eh-**LOP**-ah-thee)
- ☐ **myopathy** (my-**OP**-ah-thee)
- ☐ **myorrhexis** (**my**-oh-**RECK**-sis)
- ☐ **natal** (**NAY**-tal)
- ☐ **neonatology** (**nee**-oh-nay-**TOL**-oh-jee)
- ☐ **neurorrhaphy** (new-**ROR**-ah-fee)
- ☐ **otorhinolaryngology** (**oh**-toh-**rye**-noh-**lar**-in-**GOL**-oh-jee)
- ☐ **palpation** (pal-**PAY**-shun)
- ☐ **palpitation** (**pal**-pih-**TAY**-shun)
- ☐ **pathology** (pah-**THOL**-oh-jee)
- ☐ **phalanges** (fah-**LAN**-jeez)
- ☐ **poliomyelitis** (**poh**-lee-oh-**my**-eh-**LYE**-tis)
- ☐ **prognosis** (prog-**NOH**-sis)
- ☐ **pyoderma** (**pye**-oh-**DER**-mah)
- ☐ **pyrosis** (pye-**ROH**-sis)
- ☐ **remission**
- ☐ **sign**
- ☐ **supination** (**soo**-pih-**NAY**-shun)
- ☐ **suppuration** (**sup**-you-**RAY**-shun)
- ☐ **supracostal** (**sue**-prah-**KOS**-tal)
- ☐ **symptom** (**SIMP**-tum)
- ☐ **syndrome** (**SIN**-drohm)
- ☐ **tonsillitis** (**ton**-sih-**LYE**-tis)
- ☐ **trauma** (**TRAW**-mah)
- ☐ **triage** (tree-**AHZH**)
- ☐ **viral** (**VYE**-ral)

## LEARNING GOALS

On completion of this chapter, you should be able to:

1. Identify the roles of the four types of word parts used in forming medical terms.

2. Use your knowledge of word parts to analyze unfamiliar medical terms.

3. Describe the steps in locating a term in a medical dictionary.

4. Define the commonly used word roots, combining forms, suffixes, and prefixes introduced in this chapter.

5. Use the "sounds-like" pronunciation system to correctly pronounce the primary terms introduced in this chapter.

6. Recognize the importance of spelling medical terms correctly.

7. State why caution is important when using abbreviations.

8. Recognize, define, spell, and correctly pronounce the primary terms introduced in this chapter.

## ◼ PRIMARY MEDICAL TERMS

In this book, you will be introduced to many medical terms; however, mastering them will be easier than you anticipate because this book has many features to make learning easier:

◼ **Primary terms** appear in boldface. Learning these terms should be your highest priority as only primary terms are used as correct answers in the Learning Exercises and tests.

◼ *Secondary terms* appear in *orange* italics. Some of these terms are the "also known as" names for conditions or procedures. Other secondary terms clarify words used in the definitions of primary terms.

## ◼ WORD PARTS ARE THE KEY

Learning medical terminology is much easier once you understand how word parts work together to form medical terms (Figure 1.1). This book includes many aids to help you continue reinforcing your word-building skills.

◼ The types of word parts and the rules for their use are explained in this chapter. Learn these rules and follow them.

◼ When a term is made up of recognizable word parts, those word parts and their meanings are included with the definition of that term. These word parts appear in **magenta**.

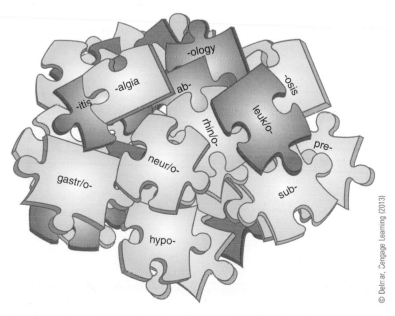

© Delmar, Cengage Learning (2013)

**FIGURE 1.1** Word parts (word roots, combining forms, suffixes, and prefixes) make up most medical terms.

- The Learning Exercises for each chapter include a "Challenge Word Building" section to help develop your skills in working with word parts.

- The Word Part Review follows Chapter 2. This section provides additional word part practice and enables you to evaluate your progress toward mastering the meaning of these word parts.

## The Four Types of Word Parts

The four types of word parts used to create medical terms are: **word roots**, **combining forms**, **suffixes**, and **prefixes**. Guidelines for their use are shown in Table 1.1.

1. A **word root** contains the basic meaning of the term. In medical terminology, this word part usually, *but not always*, indicates the involved body part. For example, the word root meaning stomach is **gastr**.

2. A **combining form** is a word root with a combining vowel added at the end. For example, the combining form meaning stomach is **gastr/o**. This form is used when a suffix beginning with a consonant is added. When a combining form appears alone, it is shown with a back slash (/) between the word root and the combining vowel.

3. A **suffix** usually, *but not always*, indicates the procedure, condition, disorder, or disease.

- A suffix always comes at the end of the word.

- You'll know a word part is a suffix when it is shown with a hyphen (-) preceding it. For example, the suffix **-itis** means inflammation.

4. A **prefix** usually, *but not always,* indicates location, time, number, or status.

- A prefix always comes at the beginning of a word.

## TABLE 1.1
## Word Part Guidelines

- A word root cannot stand alone. A suffix must always be added at the end of the word to complete the term.

- The rules for creating a combining form by adding a vowel apply when a suffix beginning with a consonant is added to a word root.

- When a prefix is added, it is *always* placed at the beginning of the word.

- You'll know a word part is a prefix when it is shown followed by a hyphen (-). For example, **hyper-** means excessive or increased.

## WORD ROOTS

Word roots act as the foundation for most medical terms. They usually, *but not always*, describe the part of the body that is involved (Figure 1.2). As shown in Table 1.2, some word roots indicate color.

**StudyWARE    CONNECTION**

Play an interactive game labeling word parts on your StudyWARE™.

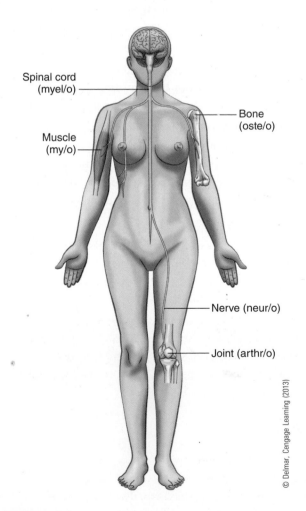

Spinal cord
(myel/o)

Bone
(oste/o)

Muscle
(my/o)

Nerve (neur/o)

Joint (arthr/o)

© Delmar, Cengage Learning (2013)

**FIGURE 1.2** Word roots, shown here as combining forms, usually indicate the involved body part.

## TABLE 1.2
## Word Roots and Combining Forms Indicating Color

| | |
|---|---|
| **cyan/o** means blue | **Cyanosis** (**sigh**-ah-**NOH**-sis) is blue discoloration of the skin caused by a lack of adequate oxygen in the blood (**cyan** means blue, and **-osis** means abnormal condition or disease). |
| **erythr/o** means red | An **erythrocyte** (eh-**RITH**-roh-sight) is a mature red blood cell (**erythr/o** means red, and **-cyte** means cell). |
| **leuk/o** means white | A **leukocyte** (**LOO**-koh-sight) is a white blood cell (**leuk/o** means white, and **-cyte** means cell). |
| **melan/o** means black | **Melanosis** (**mel**-ah-**NOH**-sis) is any condition of unusual deposits of black pigment in body tissues or organs (**melan** means black, and **-osis** means abnormal condition or disease). |
| **poli/o** means gray | **Poliomyelitis** (**poh**-lee-oh-**my**-eh-**LYE**-tis) is a viral infection of the gray matter of the spinal cord (**poli/o** means gray, **myel** means spinal cord, and **-itis** means inflammation). |

## Combining Forms Vowels

A combining form includes the vowel that has been added to the end of a word root. For example, **gastr/o** is the combining form of the word root for stomach. The letter *"o"* is the most commonly used combining vowel, and under certain conditions, this is added to make the resulting medical term easier to pronounce. The rules for the use of a combining vowel are:

- When two word roots are joined, a combining vowel is always added to the first word root. A combining vowel is used with the second word root *only if the suffix begins with a consonant.*

- For example, the term **gastroenteritis** combines two word roots with a suffix: when **gastr/o** (stomach) is joined with **enter/o** (small intestine), the combining vowel is used with **gastr/o**.

- The word root **enter** is joined to **–itis** *without a combining vowel* because this suffix begins with a vowel. **Gastroenteritis** (**gas**-troh-en-ter-**EYE**-tis) is an inflammation of the stomach and small intestine.

## ◼ SUFFIXES

A suffix is *always* added at the end of a word to complete that term. In medical terminology, suffixes usually, *but not always,* indicate a procedure, condition, disorder, or disease.

A combining vowel is used when the suffix begins with a consonant. For example, when **neur/o** (nerve) is joined with the suffix **-plasty** (surgical repair) or **-rrhaphy** (surgical suturing), the combining vowel "o" *is used* because **-plasty** and **-rrhaphy** both begin with a consonant.

- **Neuroplasty** (**NEW**-roh **plas**-tee) is the surgical repair of a nerve.

- **Neurorrhaphy** (new-**ROR**-ah-fee) is suturing together the ends of a severed nerve.

A combining vowel is *not* used when the suffix begins with a consonant. For example, the word root **tonsill** means tonsils. The suffix that is added to complete the term tells what is happening to the tonsils (Figure 1.3).

- **Tonsillitis** (**ton**-sih-**LYE**-tis) is an inflammation of the tonsils (**tonsill** means tonsils, and **-itis** means inflammation).

- A **tonsillectomy** (**ton**-sih-**LECK**-toh-mee) is the surgical removal of the tonsils (**tonsill** means tonsils, and **-ectomy** means surgical removal).

## Suffixes as Noun Endings

A *noun* is a word that is the name of a person, place, or thing. In medical terminology, some suffixes change the word root into a noun. For example, the **cranium** (**KRAY**-nee-um) is the portion of the skull that encloses the brain (**crani** means skull, and **-um** is a noun ending). Other suffixes complete the term by changing the word root into a noun. Suffixes that are commonly used as noun endings are shown in Table 1.3.

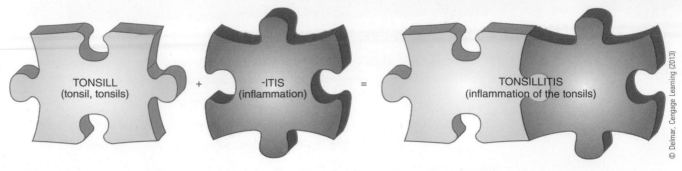

**FIGURE 1.3** The term *tonsillitis* is created by adding the suffix **-itis** to the word root **tonsill**.

## TABLE 1.3
### Suffixes as Noun Endings

| -a | -um | -y |
|---|---|---|
| -e | -us | |

## Suffixes Meaning "Pertaining To"

An *adjective* is a word that defines or describes a thing. In medical terminology, many suffixes meaning "pertaining to" are used to change the meaning of the word root into an adjective. For example, the term **cardiac** (**KAR**-dee-ack) is an adjective that means pertaining to the heart (**cardi** means heart, and **-ac** means pertaining to). Commonly used suffixes meaning "pertaining to" are shown in Table 1.4.

## TABLE 1.4
### Suffixes Meaning "Pertaining To"

| -ac | -eal | -ior |
|---|---|---|
| -al | -ical | -ory |
| -an | -ial | -ous |
| -ar | -ic | -tic |
| -ary | -ine | |

## Suffixes Meaning "Abnormal Condition"

In medical terminology, many suffixes, such as **-osis**, mean "abnormal condition or disease." For example, **gastrosis** (gas-**TROH**-sis) means any disease of the stomach (**gastr** means stomach, and **-osis** means abnormal condition or disease). Commonly used suffixes meaning "abnormal condition or disease" are shown in Table 1.5.

## TABLE 1.5
### Suffixes Meaning "Abnormal Condition"

| -ago | -iasis | -osis |
|---|---|---|
| -esis | -ion | |
| -ia | -ism | |

## Suffixes Related to Pathology

**Pathology** (pah-**THOL**-oh-jee) is the study of all aspects of diseases (**path** means disease, and **-ology** means study of). Suffixes related to pathology describe specific disease conditions.

- **-algia** means pain and suffering. **Gastralgia** (gas-**TRAL**-jee-ah), also known as a *stomachache*, means pain in the stomach (**gastr** means stomach, and **-algia** means pain).

- **-dynia** also means pain. **Gastrodynia** (gas-troh-**DIN**-ee-ah) also means pain in the stomach (**gastr/o** means stomach, and **-dynia** means pain). Although **-dynia** has the same meaning as **-algia**, it is not used as commonly. (Figure 1.4.)

- **-itis** means inflammation. **Gastritis** (gas-**TRY**-tis) is an inflammation of the stomach (**gastr** means stomach, and **-itis** means inflammation).

- **-megaly** means enlargement. **Hepatomegaly** (hep-ah-toh-**MEG**-ah-lee) is abnormal enlargement of the liver (**hepat/o** means liver, and **-megaly** means enlargement).

- **-malacia** means abnormal softening. **Arteriomalacia** (ar-**tee**-ree-oh-mah-**LAY**-shee-ah) is the abnormal

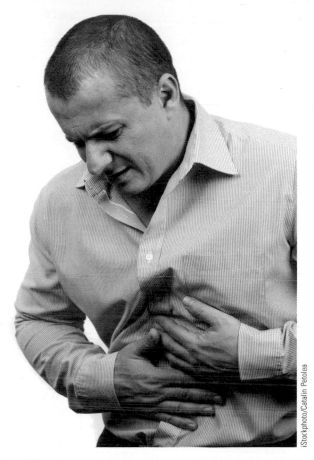

**FIGURE 1.4** *Gastrodynia* and *gastralgia* are both terms meaning stomach pain.

softening of the walls of an artery or arteries (**arteri/o** means artery, and -**malacia** means abnormal softening). Notice that -**malacia** is the opposite of -**sclerosis**.

- -**necrosis** means tissue death. **Arterionecrosis** (ar-tee-ree-oh-neh-**KROH**-sis) is the tissue death of an artery or arteries (**arteri/o** means artery, and -**necrosis** means tissue death).

- -**sclerosis** means abnormal hardening. **Arteriosclerosis** (ar-**tee**-ree-oh-skleh-**ROH**-sis) is the abnormal hardening of the walls of an artery or arteries (**arteri/o** means artery, and -**sclerosis** means abnormal hardening). Notice that -**sclerosis** is the opposite of -**malacia**.

- -**stenosis** means abnormal narrowing. **Arteriostenosis** (ar-**tee**-ree-oh-steh-**NOH**-sis) is the abnormal narrowing of an artery or arteries (**arteri/o** means artery, and -**stenosis** means abnormal narrowing).

## Suffixes Related to Procedures

Some suffixes identify the procedure that is performed on the body part identified by the word root.

- -**centesis** is a surgical puncture to remove fluid for diagnostic purposes or to remove excess fluid. **Abdominocentesis** (ab-**dom**-ih-noh-sen-**TEE**-sis) is the surgical puncture of the abdominal cavity to remove fluid (**abdomin/o** means abdomen, and -**centesis** means a surgical puncture to remove fluid).

- -**graphy** means the process of producing a picture or record. **Angiography** (an-jee-**OG**-rah-fee) is the process of producing a radiographic (x-ray) study of blood vessels after the injection of a contrast medium to make these blood vessels visible (**angi/o** means blood vessel, and -**graphy** means the process of recording).

- -**gram** means a picture or record. An **angiogram** (**AN**-jee-oh-**gram**) is the resulting film that is produced by angiography (**angi/o** means blood vessel, and -**gram** means a picture or record).

- -**plasty** means surgical repair. **Myoplasty** (**MY**-oh-**plas** tee) is the surgical repair of a muscle (**my/o** means muscle, and -**plasty** means surgical repair).

- -**scopy** means visual examination. **Arthroscopy** (ar-**THROS**-koh-pee) is the visual examination of the internal structure of a joint (**arthr/o** means joint, and -**scopy** means visual examination).

## The "Double R" Suffixes

Suffixes beginning with two *r*s, often referred to as the "double Rs," can be particularly confusing. They are grouped together here to help you understand the word parts and to remember the differences.

- -**rrhage** and -**rrhagia** mean bleeding; however, they are most often used to describe sudden, severe bleeding. A **hemorrhage** (**HEM**-or-idj) is the loss of a large amount of blood in a short time (**hem/o** means blood, and -**rrhage** means abnormal excessive fluid discharge). This term also means to bleed.

- -**rrhaphy** means surgical suturing to close a wound and includes the use of sutures, staples, or surgical glue. **Myorrhaphy** (my-**OR**-ah-fee) is the surgical suturing of a muscle wound (**my/o** means muscle, and -**rrhaphy** means surgical suturing).

- -**rrhea** means flow or discharge and refers to the flow of most body fluids. **Diarrhea** (dye-ah-**REE**-ah) is the frequent flow of loose or watery stools (**dia**- means through, and -**rrhea** means flow or discharge).

- -**rrhexis** means rupture. **Myorrhexis** (my-oh-**RECK**-sis) is the rupture of a muscle (**my/o** means muscle, and -**rrhexis** means rupture).

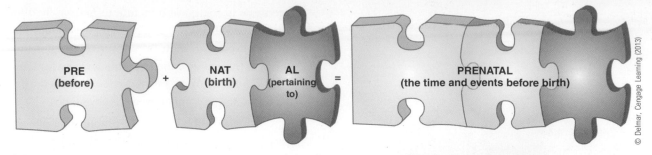

**FIGURE 1.5** The term *prenatal* is created by joining the suffix **-al** to the word root **nat** and then adding the prefix **pre-**.

## PREFIXES

A prefix is added to the beginning of a word to influence the meaning of that term. Prefixes usually, *but not always*, indicate location, time, or number. See Table 1.6 for a list of prefixes describing direction, quantity, size, and amount. The term **natal** (**NAY**-tal) means pertaining to birth (**nat** means birth, and **-al** means pertaining to). The following examples show how prefixes change the meaning of this term (Figures 1.5–1.8).

■ **Prenatal** (pre-**NAY**-tal) means the time and events before birth (**pre-** means before, **nat** means birth, and **-al** means pertaining to).

■ **Perinatal** (**pehr**-ih-**NAY**-tal) refers to the time and events surrounding birth (**peri-** means surrounding, **nat** means birth, and **-al** means pertaining to). This is the time just before, during, and just after birth.

■ **Postnatal** (pohst-**NAY**-tal) refers to the time and events after birth (**post-** means after, **nat** means birth, and **-al** means pertaining to).

## TABLE 1.6
### Prefixes Describing Direction, Quantity, Size, and Amount

| | |
|---|---|
| **ab-** away from, negative, absent | **ad-** toward, to, in the direction of |
| **dextr/o** right side | **sinistr/o** left side |
| **ex-** out of, outside, away from | **in-** in, into, not, without |
| **macro-** large, abnormal size, or long | **micr/o, micro-** small |
| **mega-, megal/o** large, great | **olig/o** scanty, few |
| **pre-** before | **post-** after, behind |

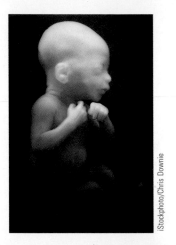

**FIGURE 1.6** The *prenatal* development of a fetus (baby).

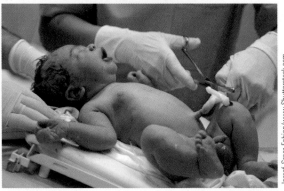

**FIGURE 1.7** A *perinatal* event of the umbilical cord being cut immediately after the baby is born.

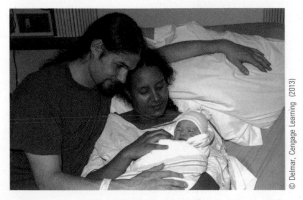

**FIGURE 1.8** A joyful *postnatal* moment as the parents bond with their new baby.

## TABLE 1.7
### Contrasting Prefixes

| | |
|---|---|
| **ab-** means away from.<br>**Abnormal** means not normal or away from normal. | **ad-** means toward or in the direction of.<br>**Addiction** means drawn toward or a strong dependence on a drug or substance. |
| **dys-** means bad, difficult, or painful.<br>**Dysfunctional** means an organ or body part that is not working properly. | **eu-** means good, normal, well, or easy.<br>**Eupnea** means easy or normal breathing. |
| **hyper-** means excessive or increased.<br>**Hypertension** is higher-than-normal blood pressure. | **hypo-** means deficient or decreased.<br>**Hypotension** is lower-than-normal blood pressure. |
| **inter-** means between or among.<br>**Interstitial** means between, but not within, the parts of a tissue. | **intra-** means within or inside.<br>**Intramuscular** means within the muscle. |
| **sub-** means under, less, or below.<br>**Subcostal** means below a rib or ribs. | **super-**, **supra-** mean above or excessive.<br>**Supracostal** means above or outside the ribs. |

## Contrasting and Confusing Prefixes

Some prefixes are confusing because they are similar in spelling, but opposite in meaning. The more common prefixes of this type are summarized in Table 1.7.

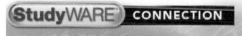

**StudyWARE CONNECTION**

Watch an animation on **How Word Parts Work Together** in the StudyWARE™.

## ■ DETERMINING MEANINGS ON THE BASIS OF WORD PARTS

Knowing the meaning of the word parts often makes it possible to figure out the definition of an unfamiliar medical term.

## Taking Terms Apart

To determine a word's meaning by looking at the component pieces, you must first separate it into word parts.

- Always start at the end of the word, with the suffix, and work toward the beginning.

- As you separate the word parts, identify the meaning of each. Identifying the meaning of each part should give you a definition of the term.

- Because some word parts have more than one meaning, it also is necessary to determine the context in which the term is being used. As used here, *context* means to determine which body system this term is referring to.

- If you have any doubt, use your medical dictionary to double-check your definition.

- Be aware that not all medical terms are made up of word parts.

## An Example to Take Apart

Look at the term **otorhinolaryngology** (**oh**-toh-**rye**-noh-**lar**-in-**GOL**-oh-jee) as shown in Figure 1.9. It is made up of two combining forms, a word root, and a suffix. This is how it looks when the word parts have been separated by working from the end to the beginning.

- The suffix **-ology** means the study of.

- The word root **laryng** means larynx or throat. The combining vowel *is not used* here, because the word root is joining a suffix that begins with a vowel.

- The combining form **rhin/o** means nose. The combining vowel *is used* here because the word root **rhin** is joining another word root.

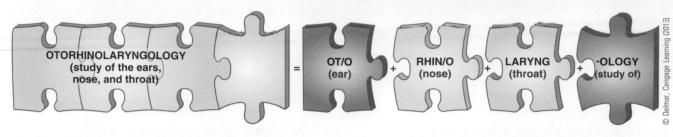

© Delmar, Cengage Learning (2013)

**FIGURE 1.9** To determine the meaning of a medical term, the word parts are separated working from the end of the word toward the beginning.

■ The combining form **ot/o** means ear. The combining vowel *is used* here because the word root **ot** is joining another word root.

■ Together they form *otorhinolaryngology*, which is the study of the ears, nose, and throat (**ot/o** means ear, **rhin/o** means nose, **laryng** means throat, and **-ology** means study of). Note: **Laryng/o** also means larynx and is discussed in Chapter 7.

■ Because this is such a long term, this specialty is frequently referred to as *ENT* (ears, nose, and throat).

■ A shortened version of this term is **otolaryngology** (**oh**-toh-**lar**-in-**GOL**-oh-jee), which is the study of the ears and larynx or throat (**ot/o** means ears, **laryng** means larynx, and **-ology** means study of).

**StudyWARE CONNECTION**

Watch the **Combining Word Roots** animation in the StudyWARE™.

## Guessing at Meanings

When you are able to guess at the meaning of a term on the basis of its word parts, you must always double-check for accuracy because some terms have more than one meaning. For example, look at the term **lithotomy** (lih-**THOT**-oh-mee):

■ On the basis of word parts, a **lithotomy** is a surgical incision for the removal of a stone (**lith** means stone, and **-otomy** means a surgical incision). This meaning is discussed further in Chapter 9.

■ However, **lithotomy** is also the name of an examination position in which the patient is lying on her back with her feet and legs raised and supported in stirrups. The term is used to describe this position because in the early days, this was the preferred position for lithotomy surgery. This term is discussed further in Chapter 15.

■ This type of possible confusion is one of the many reasons why a medical dictionary is an important medical terminology tool.

## ■ MEDICAL DICTIONARY USE

Learning to use a medical dictionary and other resources to find the definition of a term is an important part of mastering the correct use of medical terms. The following tips for dictionary use apply whether you are working with a traditional book-form dictionary or with electronic dictionary software, websites, or applications on your computer or handheld device.

### If You Know How to Spell the Word

When starting to work with an unfamiliar print dictionary, spend a few minutes reviewing its user guide, table of contents, and appendices. The time you spend reviewing now will be saved later when you are looking up unfamiliar terms.

■ On the basis of the first letter of the word, start in the appropriate section of the dictionary. Look at the top of the page for clues. The top left word is the first term on the page. The top right word is the last term on that page.

■ Next, look alphabetically for words that start with the first and second letters of the word you are researching. Continue looking through each letter until you find the term you are looking for.

■ When you think you have found it, check the spelling very carefully, letter by letter, working from left to right. Terms with similar spellings have very different meanings.

■ When you find the term, carefully check *all* of the definitions.

## If You Do Not Know How to Spell the Word

Listen carefully to the term, and write it down. If you cannot find the word on the basis of your spelling, start looking for alternative spellings based on the beginning sound as shown in Table 1.8. Note: All of these examples are in this textbook. However, you could practice looking them up in the dictionary!

## Look Under Categories

Most print dictionaries use categories such as *Diseases* and *Syndromes* to group disorders with these terms in their titles. For example:

■ *Venereal disease* would be found under *Disease, venereal*.

■ *Fetal alcohol syndrome* would be found under *Syndrome, fetal alcohol*.

■ When you come across such a term and cannot find it listed by the first word, the next step is to look under the appropriate category.

## Multiple-Word Terms

When you are looking for a term that includes more than one word, begin your search with the last term. If you do not find it there, move forward to the next word.

■ For example, *congestive heart failure* is sometimes listed under *heart failure, congestive*. This term is discussed in Chapter 5.

## Searching for Definitions on the Internet

Internet search engines are valuable resources in finding definitions and details about medical conditions and terms; however, it is important that you rely on a site, such as the National Institutes of Health (NIH) website (http://www.nih.gov), which is known to be a reputable information source.

■ For better results, an Internet search should include visits to at least two reputable sites. If there is a major difference in the definitions, go on to a third site. Sometimes a search engine will recommend a site that is not appropriate but appears because it paid to be listed.

■ Beware of suggested search terms. If you do not spell a term correctly, a website may guess what you were searching for. Make sure to double-check that the term you are defining is the intended term.

The same caution applies to medical dictionary applications on handheld devices. Make sure that the application comes from a reputable source, and always double-check that this definition is for the term that you intended to look up.

## TABLE 1.8
## Guidelines to Looking Up the Spelling of Unfamiliar Terms

| If it sounds like | It may begin with | Example |
|---|---|---|
| F | F | **flatus** (**FLAY**-tus) [see Chapter 8] |
|  | PH | **phlegm** (**FLEM**) [see Chapter 7] |
| J | G | **gingivitis** (**jin**-jih-**VYE**-tis) [see Chapter 8] |
|  | J | **jaundice** (**JAWN**-dis) [see Chapter 8] |
| K | C | **crepitus** (**KREP**-ih-tus) [see Chapter 3] |
|  | CH | **cholera** (**KOL**-er-ah) [see Chapter 8] |
|  | K | **kyphosis** (kye-**FOH**-sis) [see Chapter 3] |
|  | QU | **quadriplegia** (**kwad**-rih-**PLEE**-jee-ah) [see Chapter 4] |
| S | C | **cytology** (sigh-**TOL**-oh-jee) [see Chapter 2] |
|  | PS | **psychologist** (sigh-**KOL**-oh-jist) [see Chapter 10] |
|  | S | **serum** (**SEER**-um) [see Chapter 5] |
| Z | X | **xeroderma** (zee-roh-**DER**-mah) [see Chapter 12] |
|  | Z | **zygote** (**ZYE**-goht) [see Chapter 14] |

## PRONUNCIATION

A medical term is easier to understand and remember when you know how to pronounce it properly. To help you master the pronunciation of new terms, a commonly accepted pronunciation of that word appears in parentheses next to the term. Audio for the terms on the vocabulary list is available in the student StudyWARE™.

The sounds-like pronunciation system is used in this textbook. Here the word is respelled using normal English letters to create sounds that are familiar. To pronounce a new word, just say it as it is spelled in the parentheses.

■ The part of the word that receives the primary (most) emphasis when you say it is shown in uppercase boldface letters. For example, **edema** (eh-**DEE**-mah) is swelling caused by an abnormal accumulation of fluid in cells, tissues, or cavities of the body.

■ A part of the word that receives secondary (less) emphasis when you say it is shown in boldface lowercase letters. For example, **appendicitis** (ah-**pen**-dih-**SIGH**-tis) means an inflammation of the appendix (**appendic** means appendix, and -**itis** means inflammation).

### A Word of Caution

Frequently, there is more than one correct way to pronounce a medical term.

■ The pronunciation of many medical terms is based on their Greek, Latin, or other foreign origin. However, there is a trend toward pronouncing terms as they would sound in English.

■ The result is more than one "correct" pronunciation for a term. The text shows the most commonly accepted pronunciation.

■ If your instructor prefers an alternative pronunciation, follow the instructions you are given.

## SPELLING IS ALWAYS IMPORTANT

Accuracy in spelling medical terms is extremely important!

■ Changing just one or two letters can completely change the meaning of a word—and this difference literally could be a matter of life or death for the patient.

■ The section "Look-Alike, Sound-Alike Terms and Word Parts" later in this chapter will help you become aware of some terms and word parts that are frequently confused.

■ The spelling shown in this text is commonly accepted in the U.S. You may encounter alternative spellings used in England, Australia, and Canada.

## SINGULAR AND PLURAL ENDINGS

Many medical terms have Greek or Latin origins. As a result of these different origins, there are unusual rules for changing a singular word into a plural form. In addition, English endings have been adopted for some commonly used terms.

■ Table 1.9 provides guidelines to help you better understand how these plurals are formed.

■ Also, throughout the text, when a term with an unusual singular or plural form is introduced, both forms are included. For example, the **phalanges** (fah-**LAN**-jeez) are the bones of the fingers and toes (singular, *phalanx*) (Figure 1.10).

## BASIC MEDICAL TERMS TO DESCRIBE DISEASES

Some of the medical terms that are used to describe diseases and disease conditions can easily be confusing. Some of the more common terms of this type are described in Table 1.10. You will find that studying the groups of three as they are shown in the table makes it easier to master these terms.

## LOOK-ALIKE, SOUND-ALIKE TERMS AND WORD PARTS

This section highlights some frequently used terms and word parts that are confusing because they look and sound alike. However, their meanings are very different. It is important that you pay close attention to these terms and word parts as you encounter them in the text.

### arteri/o, ather/o, and arthr/o

■ **arteri/o** means artery. **Endarterial** (**end**-ar-**TEE**-ree-al) means pertaining to the interior or lining of an artery (**end-** means within, **arteri** means artery, and -**al** means pertaining to).

■ **ather/o** means plaque or fatty substance. An **atheroma** (**ath**-er-**OH**-mah) is a fatty deposit within the wall

## TABLE 1.9
## Guidelines to Unusual Plural Forms

| Guideline | Singular | Plural |
|---|---|---|
| If the singular term ends in the suffix **-a**, the plural is usually formed by changing the ending to **-ae**. | bursa vertebra | bursae vertebrae |
| If the singular term ends in the suffix **-ex** or **-ix**, the plural is usually formed by changing these endings to **-ices**. | appendix index | appendices indices |
| If the singular term ends in the suffix **-is**, the plural is usually formed by changing the ending to **-es**. | diagnosis metastasis | diagnoses metastases |
| If the singular term ends in the suffix **-itis**, the plural is usually formed by changing the **-is** ending to **-ides**. | arthritis meningitis | arthritides meningitides |
| If the singular term ends in the suffix **-nx**, the plural is usually formed by the **-x** ending to **-ges**. | phalanx meninx | phalanges meninges |
| If the singular term ends in the suffix **-on**, the plural is usually formed by changing the ending to **-a**. | criterion ganglion | criteria ganglia |
| If the singular term ends in the suffix **-um**, the plural usually is formed by changing the ending to **-a**. | diverticulum ovum | diverticula ova |
| If the singular term ends in the suffix **-us**, the plural is usually formed by changing the ending to **-i**. | alveolus malleolus | alveoli malleoli |

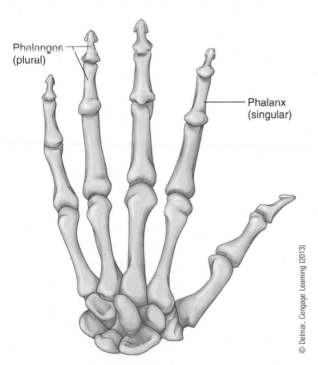

Phalanges (plural)

Phalanx (singular)

© Delmar, Cengage Learning (2013)

**FIGURE 1.10** Singular and plural endings. A phalanx is one finger or toe bone. Phalanges are more than one finger or toe bones.

of an artery (**ather** means fatty substance, and **-oma** means tumor).

- **arthr/o** means joint. **Arthralgia** (ar-**THRAL**-jee-ah) means pain in a joint or joints (**arthr** means joint, and **-algia** means pain).

## -ectomy, -ostomy, and -otomy

- **-ectomy** means surgical removal. An **appendectomy** (**ap**-en-**DECK**-toh-mee) is the surgical removal of the appendix (**append** means appendix, and **-ectomy** means surgical removal).

- **-ostomy** means the surgical creation of an artificial opening to the body surface. A **colostomy** (koh-**LAHS**-toh-mee) is the surgical creation of an artificial excretory opening between the colon and the body surface (**col** means colon, and **-ostomy** means the surgical creation of an artificial opening).

- **-otomy** means cutting or a surgical incision. A **colotomy** (koh-**LOT**-oh-mee) is a surgical incision into the colon (**col** means colon, and **-otomy** means a surgical incision).

**TABLE 1.10**

## Basic Medical Terms to Describe Disease Conditions

| | | |
|---|---|---|
| A **sign** is objective evidence of disease such as a fever. *Objective* means the sign can be evaluated or measured by the patient or others. | A **symptom** (**SIMP**-tum) is subjective evidence of a disease, such as pain or a headache. *Subjective* means that it can be evaluated or measured only by the patient. | A **syndrome** (**SIN**-drohm) is a set of the signs and symptoms that occur together as part of a specific disease process. |
| A **diagnosis** (dye-ag-**NOH**-sis) (DX) is the identification of a disease (plural, *diagnoses*). To *diagnose* is the process of reaching a diagnosis. | A **differential diagnosis** (D/DX), also known as a *rule out* (R/O) is an attempt to determine which one of several diseases can be causing the signs and symptoms that are present. | A **prognosis** (prog-**NOH**-sis) is a prediction of the probable course and outcome of a disorder (plural, *prognoses*). |
| An **acute** condition has a rapid onset, a severe course, and a relatively short duration. | A **chronic** condition is of long duration. Although such diseases can be controlled, they are rarely cured. | A **remission** is the temporary, partial, or complete disappearance of the symptoms of a disease without having achieved a cure. |
| A **disease** is a condition in which one or more body parts are not functioning normally. Some diseases are named for their signs and symptoms. For example, *chronic fatigue syndrome* (CFS) is a persistent overwhelming fatigue of unknown origin (see Chapter 4). | An **eponym** (**EP**-oh-nim) is a disease, structure, operation, or procedure named for the person who discovered or described it first. For example, *Alzheimer's disease* is named for German neurologist Alois Alzheimer (see Chapter 10). | An **acronym** (**ACK**-roh-nim) is a word formed from the initial letter of the major parts of a compound term. For example, the acronym **laser** stands for **l**ight **a**mplification by **s**timulated **e**mission of **r**adiation (see Chapter 12). |

## Fissure and *Fistula*

- A **fissure** (**FISH**-ur) is a groove or crack-like sore of the skin (see Chapter 12). This term also describes normal folds in the contours of the brain.

- A **fistula** (**FIS**-tyou-lah) is an abnormal passage, usually between two internal organs or leading from an organ to the surface of the body. A fistula may be due to surgery, injury, or the draining of an abscess.

## Ileum and *Ilium*

- The **ileum** (**ILL**-ee-um) is the last and longest portion of the small intestine. *Memory aid: ileum* is spelled with an *e* as in *intestine*.

- The **ilium** (**ILL**-ee-um) is part of the hip bone. *Memory aid: ilium* is spelled with an *i* as in *hip*. (Figure 1.11)

## Infection and *Inflammation*

- Although the suffix **-itis** means inflammation, it also is commonly used to indicate infection.

- An **infection** (in-**FECK**-shun) is the invasion of the body by a pathogenic (disease-producing) organism. The infection can remain localized (near the point of entry) or can be systemic (affecting the entire body). Signs and symptoms of infection include malaise, chills and fever, redness, heat and swelling, or exudate from a wound.

- **Malaise** (mah-**LAYZ**) is a feeling of general discomfort or uneasiness that is often the first indication of an infection or other disease.

- An **exudate** (**ECKS**-you-dayt) is fluid, such as pus, that leaks out of an infected wound.

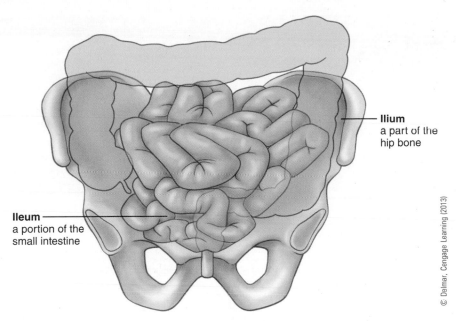

**Ilium**
a part of the
hip bone

**Ileum**
a portion of the
small intestine

© Delmar, Cengage Learning (2013)

**FIGURE 1.11** There is only one letter difference between *ileum* and *ilium*, but they are very different parts of the body.

■ **Inflammation** (in-flah-**MAY**-shun) is a localized response to an injury or to the destruction of tissues. The key indicators of inflammation are (1) *erythema* (redness), (2) *hyperthermia* (heat), (3) *edema* (swelling), and (4) *pain*. These are caused by extra blood flowing into the area as part of the healing process.

## Laceration and Lesion

■ A **laceration** (**lass**-er-**AY**-shun) is a torn or jagged wound or an accidental cut wound.

■ A **lesion** (**LEE**-zhun) is a pathologic change of the tissues due to disease or injury.

## Mucous and Mucus

■ The adjective **mucous** (**MYOU**-kus) describes the specialized membranes that line the body cavities.

■ The noun **mucus** (**MYOU**-kus) is the name of the fluid secreted by these mucous membranes.

## myc/o, myel/o, and my/o

■ **myc/o** means fungus. **Mycosis** (my-**KOH**-sis) describes any abnormal condition or disease caused by a fungus (**myc** means fungus, and **-osis** means abnormal condition or disease).

■ **myel/o** means bone marrow *or* spinal cord. The term **myelopathy** (my-eh-**LOP**-ah-thee) describes any pathologic change or disease in the spinal cord (**myel/o** means spinal cord or bone marrow, and **-pathy** means disease).

■ **my/o** means muscle. The term **myopathy** (my-**OP**-ah-thee) describes any pathologic change or disease of muscle tissue (**my/o** means muscle, and **-pathy** means disease).

## -ologist and -ology

■ **-ologist** means specialist. A **dermatologist** (**der**-mah-**TOL**-oh-jist) is a physician who specializes in diagnosing and treating disorders of the skin (**dermat** means skin, and **-ologist** means specialist).

■ **-ology** means the study of. **Neonatology** (**nee**-oh-nay-**TOL**-oh-jee) is the study of disorders of the newborn (**neo-** means new, **nat** means birth, and **-ology** means study of).

## Palpation and Palpitation

■ **Palpation** (pal-**PAY**-shun) is an examination technique in which the examiner's hands are used to feel the texture, size, consistency, and location of certain body parts.

■ **Palpitation** (pal-pih-**TAY**-shun) is a pounding or racing heart.

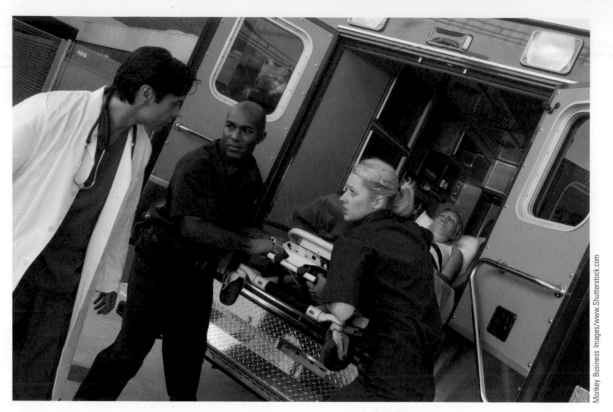

Monkey Business Images/www.Shutterstock.com

**FIGURE 1.12** Triage describes the process through which emergency personnel arriving on an accident scene identify which of the injured require care first and where they can be treated most effectively.

## pyel/o, py/o, and pyr/o

- **pyel/o** means renal pelvis, which is part of the kidney. **Pyelitis** (**pye**-eh-**LYE**-tis) is an inflammation of the renal pelvis (**pyel** means renal pelvis, and **-itis** means inflammation).

- **py/o** means pus. **Pyoderma (pye**-oh-**DER**-mah) is any acute, inflammatory, pus-forming bacterial skin infection such as impetigo (**py/o** means pus, and **-derma** means skin).

- **pyr/o** means fever or fire. **Pyrosis** (pye-**ROH**-sis), also known as *heartburn*, is discomfort due to the regurgitation of stomach acid upward into the esophagus (**pyr** means fever or fire, and **-osis** means abnormal condition or disease).

## Supination and Suppuration

- **Supination** (**soo**-pih-**NAY**-shun) is the act of rotating the arm so that the palm of the hand is forward or upward.

- **Suppuration** (**sup**-you-**RAY**-shun) is the formation or discharge of pus.

## Triage and Trauma

- **Triage** (tree-**AHZH**) is the medical screening of patients to determine their relative priority of need and the proper place of treatment. (Figure 1.12)

- **Trauma** (**TRAW**-mah) means wound or injury. These are the types of injuries that might occur in an accident, shooting, natural disaster, or fire.

## Viral and Virile

- **Viral** (**VYE**-ral) means pertaining to a virus (**vir** means virus or poison, and **-al** means pertaining to).

- **Virile** (**VIR**-ill) means having the nature, properties, or qualities of an adult male.

## ◼ USING ABBREVIATIONS

Abbreviations are frequently used as a shorthand way to record long and complex medical terms; Appendix B contains an alphabetized list of many of the more commonly used medical abbreviations.

- Abbreviations can also lead to confusion and errors! Therefore, it is important that you be very careful when using or interpreting an abbreviation.

- For example, the abbreviation *BE* means both "below elbow" (as in amputation) and "barium enema." Just imagine what a difference a mix-up here would make for the patient!

- Most clinical agencies have policies for accepted abbreviations. It is important to follow this list for the facility where you are working.

- If there is any question in your mind about which abbreviation to use, always follow this rule: ***When in doubt, spell it out***.

## TABLE 1.11
## Examples of Abbreviations Not to Be Used

| Abbreviation | Potential Problem |
| --- | --- |
| MS | can mean either morphine sulfate *or* magnesium sulfate |
| QD and QOD | mean daily and every other day, sometimes mistaken for each other |
| U | means unit, sometimes mistaken for 0 or 4 |

Some abbreviations should never be used (as decided by the *Joint Commission,* an organization founded in 1910 to standardize medical practices). See Table 1.11 for examples. The Joint Commission's latest standards are available at http://www.jointcommission.org. Many medical facilities have their own suggested "do not use" abbreviation list.

**StudyWARE CONNECTION**

For more practice and to test your mastery of this material, go to the StudyWARE™ to play interactive games and complete the quiz for this chapter.

## ☐ Workbook Practice

Go to your workbook, and complete the exercises for this chapter.

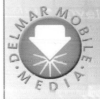

*Downloadable audio is available for selected medical terms in this chapter to enhance your learning of medical terminology.*

# LEARNING EXERCISES

## MATCHING WORD PARTS 1

Write the correct answer in the middle column.

| Definition | Correct Answer | Possible Answers |
|---|---|---|
| 1.1. bad, difficult, painful | _____ | -algia |
| 1.2. excessive, increased | _____ | dys- |
| 1.3. enlargement | *megaly* | -ectomy |
| 1.4. pain, suffering | *algia* | -megaly |
| 1.5. surgical removal | *ectomy* | hyper- |

## MATCHING WORD PARTS 2

Write the correct answer in the middle column.

| Definition | Correct Answer | Possible Answers |
|---|---|---|
| 1.6. abnormal condition or disease | _____ | hypo- |
| 1.7. abnormal softening | _____ | -itis |
| 1.8. deficient, decreased | _____ | -malacia |
| 1.9. inflammation | _____ | -necrosis |
| 1.10. tissue death | _____ | -osis |

## MATCHING WORD PARTS 3

Write the correct answer in the middle column.

| Definition | Correct Answer | Possible Answers |
|---|---|---|
| 1.11. bleeding, bursting forth | _____ | -ostomy |

| | | | |
|---|---|---|---|
| 1.12. | surgical creation of an artificial opening to the body surface | _____ | **-otomy** |
| 1.13. | surgical incision | _____ | **-plasty** |
| 1.14. | surgical repair | _____ | **-rrhage** |
| 1.15. | surgical suturing | _____ | **-rrhaphy** |

## MATCHING WORD PARTS 4

Write the correct answer in the middle column.

| | **Definition** | **Correct Answer** | **Possible Answers** |
|---|---|---|---|
| 1.16. | visual examination | _____ | **-rrhea** |
| 1.17. | rupture | _____ | **-rrhexis** |
| 1.18. | abnormal narrowing | _____ | **-sclerosis** |
| 1.19. | abnormal hardening | _____ | **-scopy** |
| 1.20. | flow or discharge | _____ | **-stenosis** |

## DEFINITIONS

Select the correct answer, and write it on the line provided.

1.21.   The term _____ describes any pathologic change or disease in the spinal cord.

   myelopathy          myopathy          pyelitis          pyrosis

1.22.   The medical term for higher-than-normal blood pressure is _____.

   hepatomegaly        hypertension      hypotension       supination

1.23.   The term _____ means pertaining to birth.

   natal               perinatal         postnatal         prenatal

1.24.   Pain is classified as a _____.

   diagnosis           sign              symptom           syndrome

1.25.   In the term *myopathy*, the suffix **-pathy** means _____.

   abnormal condition  disease           inflammation      swelling

## MATCHING TERMS AND DEFINITIONS 1

Write the correct answer in the middle column.

| Definition | Correct Answer | Possible Answers |
|---|---|---|
| 1.26.  white blood cell | _____ | acute |
| 1.27.  prediction of the probable course and outcome of a disorder | _____ | edema |
| 1.28.  swelling caused by an abnormal accumulation of fluid in cells, tissues, or cavities of the body | _____ | leukocyte |
| 1.29.  rapid onset | _____ | prognosis |
| 1.30.  turning the palm of the hand upward | _____ | supination |

## MATCHING TERMS AND DEFINITIONS 2

Write the correct answer in the middle column.

| Definition | Correct Answer | Possible Answers |
|---|---|---|
| 1.31.  examination procedure | _____ | laceration |
| 1.32.  fluid, such as pus, that leaks out of an infected wound | _____ | lesion |
| 1.33.  pathologic tissue change | _____ | palpitation |
| 1.34.  pounding heart | _____ | palpation |
| 1.35.  torn or jagged wound, or an accidental cut wound | _____ | exudate |

## WHICH WORD?

Select the correct answer, and write it on the line provided.

1.36.    The medical term _____ describes an inflammation of the stomach.

   gastritis            gastrosis

1.37.    The formation of pus is called _____.

   supination           suppuration

1.38.    The term meaning wound or injury is _____.

            trauma                      triage

1.39.    The term _____ means pertaining to a virus.

            viral                       virile

1.40.    A/an _____ is the surgical removal of the appendix.

            appendectomy         appendicitis

## SPELLING COUNTS

Find the misspelled word in each sentence. Then write that word, spelled correctly, on the line provided.

1.41.    A disease named for the person who discovered it is known as an

         enaponym. _____

1.42.    A localized response to injury or tissue destruction is called inflimmation. _____

1.43.    A fisure of the skin is a groove or crack-like sore of the skin. _____

1.44.    The medical term meaning suturing together the ends of a severed nerve is

         neurorraphy. _____

1.45.    The medical term meaning inflammation of the tonsils is tonsilitis. _____

## MATCHING TERMS

Write the correct answer in the middle column.

| Definition | Correct Answer | Possible Answers |
| --- | --- | --- |
| 1.46.  abnormal condition or disease of the stomach | _____ | syndrome |
| 1.47.  a set of signs and symptoms | _____ | gastralgia |
| 1.48.  rupture of a muscle | _____ | gastrosis |
| 1.49.  stomach pain | _____ | pyoderma |
| 1.50.  any acute, inflammatory, pus-forming bacterial skin infection | _____ | myorrhexis |

## TERM SELECTION

Select the correct answer, and write it on the line provided.

1.51.    The abnormal hardening of the walls of an artery or arteries is called _____.

        arteriosclerosis        arteriostenosis        arthrostenosis        atherosclerosis

1.52.    A fever is considered to be a _____.

        prognosis        sign        symptom        syndrome

1.53.    An inflammation of the stomach and small intestine is known as _____.

        gastralgia        gastroenteritis        gastritis        gastrosis

1.54.    The term meaning pain in a joint or joints is _____.

        arthralgia        arthritis        arthrocentesis        atherosclerosis

1.55.    A _____ is a physician who specializes in diagnosing and treating diseases and disorders of the skin.

        dermatologist        dermatology        neurologist        neurology

## SENTENCE COMPLETION

Write the correct term on the line provided.

1.56.    Lower-than-normal blood pressure is called _____.

1.57.    The process of recording a radiographic study of the blood vessels after the injection of a contrast medium is known as _____.

1.58.    The term meaning above or outside the ribs is _____.

1.59.    A/An _____ diagnosis is also known as a rule out.

1.60.    A/An _____ is an abnormal passage, usually between two internal organs or leading from an organ to the surface of the body.

## TRUE/FALSE

If the statement is true, write **True** on the line. If the statement is false, write **False** on the line.

1.61.    _____ An erythrocyte is commonly known as a red blood cell.

1.62.    _____ Arteriomalacia is abnormal hardening of blood vessels of the walls of an artery or arteries.

1.63. _____ A colostomy is the surgical creation of an artificial opening between the

colon and the body surface.

1.64. _____ Malaise is often the first symptom of inflammation.

1.65. _____ An infection is the invasion of the body by a disease-producing organism.

## WORD SURGERY

Divide each term into its component word parts. Write these word parts, in sequence, on the lines provided. When necessary, use a slash (/) to indicate a combining vowel. (You may not need all of the lines provided.)

1.66.   **Otorhinolaryngology** is the study of the ears, nose, and throat.

_____    _____    _____    _____

1.67.   The term **mycosis** means any abnormal condition or disease caused by a fungus.

_____    _____    _____    _____

1.68.   **Poliomyelitis** is a viral infection of the gray matter of the spinal cord.

_____    _____    _____    _____

1.69.   **Neonatology** is the study of disorders of the newborn.

_____    _____    _____    _____

1.70.   The term **endarterial** means pertaining to the interior or lining of an artery.

_____    _____    _____    _____

## CLINICAL CONDITIONS

Write the correct answer on the line provided.

1.71.   Miguel required a/an _____ injection. This term means that the medication was

placed directly within the muscle.

1.72.   Mrs. Tillson underwent _____ to remove excess fluid from her abdomen.

1.73.   The term *laser* is a/an _____. This means that it is a word formed from the initial

letters of the major parts of a compound term.

1.74.   In an accident, Felipe Valladares broke several bones in his fingers. The medical term for these injuries is

fractured _____.

1.75. In case of a major disaster Cheng Lee, who is a trained paramedic, helps perform

_____. This is the screening of patients to determine their relative priority of need

and the proper place of treatment.

1.76. Gina's physician ordered laboratory tests that would enable him to establish a differential

_____ to identify the cause of her signs and symptoms.

1.77. Jennifer plans to go to graduate school so she can specialize in _____. This

specialty is concerned with the study of all aspects of diseases.

1.78. John Randolph's cancer went into _____. Although this is not a cure, his

symptoms disappeared and he felt much better.

1.79. Mr. Jankowski describes that uncomfortable feeling as heartburn. The medical term for this condition

is _____.

1.80. Phyllis was having great fun traveling until she ate some contaminated food and developed

_____. She felt miserable and needed to stay in her hotel because of the

frequent flow of loose or watery stools.

## WHICH IS THE CORRECT MEDICAL TERM?

Select the correct answer, and write it on the line provided.

1.81. The term _____ describes the surgical repair of a nerve.

neuralgia          neurorrhaphy          neurology          neuroplasty

1.82. The term _____ means loss of a large amount of blood in a short time.

diarrhea          hemorrhage          hepatorrhagia          otorrhagia

1.83. The term _____ means the tissue death of an artery or arteries.

arteriomalacia          arterionecrosis          arteriosclerosis          arteriostenosis

1.84. The term _____ means between, but not within, the parts of a tissue.

interstitial          intrastitial          intermuscular          intramuscular

1.85. The term _____ means enlargement of the liver.

hepatitis          hepatomegaly          nephromegaly          nephritis

## CHALLENGE WORD BUILDING

These terms are *not* found in this chapter; however, they are made up of the following familiar word parts. If you need help in creating the term, refer to your medical dictionary.

| | | |
|---|---|---|
| **neo-** = new | **arteri/o** = artery | **-algia** = pain and suffering |
| | **arthr/o** = joint | **-itis** = inflammation |
| | **cardi/o** = heart | **-ologist** = specialist |
| | **nat/o** = birth | **-otomy** = a surgical incision |
| | **neur/o** = nerve | **-rrhea** = flow or discharge |
| | **rhin/o** = nose | **-scopy** = visual examination |

1.86.   A medical specialist concerned with the diagnosis and treatment of heart disease is a/

an _____.

1.87.   The term meaning a runny nose is _____.

1.88.   The term meaning the inflammation of a joint or joints is _____.

1.89.   A medical specialist in disorders of the newborn is a/an _____.

1.90.   The term meaning a surgical incision into a nerve is a/an _____.

1.91.   The term meaning inflammation of the heart is _____.

1.92.   The term meaning pain in the nose is _____.

1.93.   The term meaning pain in a nerve or nerves is _____.

1.94.   The term meaning a surgical incision into the heart is a/an _____.

1.95.   The term meaning an inflammation of the nose is _____.

## LABELING EXERCISES

1.96.  The combining form meaning spinal cord is

_____.

1.97.  The combining form meaning muscle is

_____.

1.98.  The combining form meaning bone is

_____.

1.99.  The combining form meaning nerve is

_____.

1.100.  The combining form meaning joint is

_____.

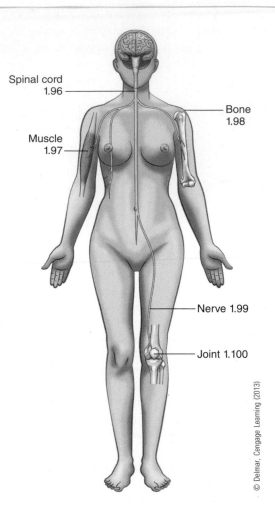

Spinal cord
1.96

Bone
1.98

Muscle
1.97

Nerve 1.99

Joint 1.100

© Delmar, Cengage Learning (2013)

## THE HUMAN TOUCH

# Critical Thinking Exercise

The following story and questions are designed to stimulate critical thinking through class discussion or as a brief essay response. There are no right or wrong answers to these questions.

*Baylie Hutchins sits at her kitchen table, highlighter in hand, with her medical terminology book opened to the first chapter. Her 2-year-old son, Mathias, plays with a box of animal crackers in his high chair, some even finding his mouth. "Arteri/o, ather/o, and arthr/o," she mutters, lips moving to shape unfamiliar sounds. "They're too much alike, and they mean totally different things." Mathias sneezes loudly, and spots of animal cracker rain on the page, punctuating her frustration.*

*"Great job, Thias," she says wiping the text with her finger. "I planned on using the highlighter to mark with, not your lunch." Mathias giggles and peeks through the tunnel made by one small hand.*

*"Mucous and mucus," she reads aloud, each sounding the same. Then she remembers her teacher's tip for remembering the difference, "The long word is the membrane, and the short one is the secretion."*

*Mathias picks up an animal cracker and excitedly shouts, "Tiger, Mommy! Tiger!" "That's right, Thias. Good job!"*

*Turning back to the page she stares at the red word parts -rrhagia, -rrhaphy, -rrhea, and -rrhexis. Stumbling over the pronunciations, Baylie closes her eyes and tries to silence the voices in her head. "You can't do anything right," her ex-husband says. "Couldn't finish if your life depended on it," her mother's voice snaps.*

*Baylie keeps at it, "Rhin/o means nose," as she highlights those three words, "and a rhinoceros has a big horn on his nose."*

*"Rhino!" Matthias shouts, holding up an animal cracker. Baylie laughs. We both have new things to learn, she realizes. And we can do it!*

## Suggested Discussion Topics

1.  Baylie needs to learn medical terminology because she wants a career in the medical field. What study habits would help Baylie accomplish this task?

2.  A support group could help empower Baylie to accomplish her goals. What people would you suggest for this group and why?

3.  How can this textbook and other resource materials help her, and you, learn medical terminology?

4.  Discuss strategies that the instructor could use and has already used to help Baylie improve her terminology skills.

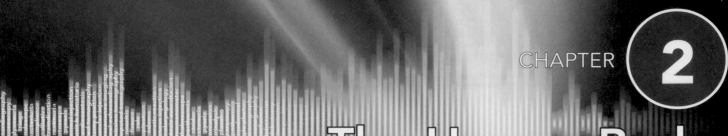

# The Human Body in Health and Disease

## Overview of
## THE HUMAN BODY IN HEALTH AND DISEASE

| | |
|---|---|
| Anatomic Reference Systems | Terms used to describe the location of body planes, directions, and cavities. |
| Structures of the Body | The cells, tissues, and glands that form the body systems that work together to enable the body to function properly. |
| Genetics | The genetic components that transfer characteristics from parents to their children. |
| Tissues | A group of similarly specialized cells that work together to perform specific functions. |
| Glands | A group of specialized cells that is capable of producing secretions. |
| Body Systems and Related Organs | Organs are somewhat independent parts of the body that perform specific functions. Organs with related functions are organized into body systems. |
| Pathology | The study of the nature and cause of disease that involve changes in structure and function. |

## Vocabulary Related to **THE HUMAN BODY IN HEALTH AND DISEASE**

This list contains essential word parts and medical terms for this chapter. These terms are pronounced in the StudyWARE™ and Audio CDs that are available for use with this text. These and the other important **primary terms** are shown in boldface throughout the chapter. *Secondary terms*, which appear in *orange* italics, clarify the meaning of primary terms.

### Word Parts

- [ ] **aden/o** gland
- [ ] **adip/o** fat
- [ ] **anter/o** before, front
- [ ] **caud/o** lower part of body, tail
- [ ] **cephal/o** head
- [ ] **cyt/o, -cyte** cell
- [ ] **end-, endo-** in, within, inside
- [ ] **exo-** out of, outside, away from
- [ ] **hist/o, histi/o** tissue
- [ ] **-ologist** specialist
- [ ] **-ology** the science or study of
- [ ] **path/o, -pathy** disease, suffering, feeling, emotion
- [ ] **plas/i, plas/o, -plasia** development, growth, formation
- [ ] **poster/o** behind, toward the back
- [ ] **-stasis, -static** control, maintenance of a constant level

### Medical Terms

- [ ] **abdominal cavity** (ab-**DOM**-ih-nal)
- [ ] **adenectomy** (ad-eh-**NECK**-toh-mee)
- [ ] **adenocarcinoma** (ad-eh-noh-**kar**-sih-**NOH**-mah)
- [ ] **adenoma** (ad-eh-**NOH**-mah)
- [ ] **adenomalacia** (ad-eh-noh-mah-**LAY**-shee-ah)
- [ ] **adenosclerosis** (ad-eh-noh-skleh-**ROH**-sis)
- [ ] **anaplasia** (an-ah-**PLAY**-zee-ah)
- [ ] **anatomy** (ah-**NAT**-oh-mee)
- [ ] **anomaly** (ah-**NOM**-ah-lee)
- [ ] **anterior** (an-**TEER**-ee-or)
- [ ] **aplasia** (ah-**PLAY**-zee-ah)
- [ ] **bloodborne transmission**
- [ ] **caudal** (**KAW**-dal)
- [ ] **cephalic** (seh-**FAL**-ick)
- [ ] **chromosomes** (**KROH**-moh-sohmes)

- [ ] **communicable disease** (kuh-**MEW**-nih-kuh-bul)
- [ ] **congenital disorder** (kon-**JEN**-ih-tahl)
- [ ] **cytoplasm** (**SIGH**-toh-plazm)
- [ ] **distal** (**DIS**-tal)
- [ ] **dorsal** (**DOR**-sal)
- [ ] **dysplasia** (dis-**PLAY**-see-ah)
- [ ] **endemic** (en-**DEM**-ick)
- [ ] **endocrine glands** (**EN**-doh-krin)
- [ ] **epidemic** (ep-ih-**DEM**-ick)
- [ ] **epigastric region** (ep-ih-**GAS**-trick)
- [ ] **etiology** (ee-tee-**OL**-oh-jee)
- [ ] **exocrine glands** (**ECK**-soh-krin)
- [ ] **functional disorder**
- [ ] **genetic disorder**
- [ ] **geriatrician** (jer-ee-ah-**TRISH**-un)
- [ ] **hemophilia** (hee-moh-**FILL**-ee-ah)
- [ ] **histology** (hiss-**TOL**-oh-jee)
- [ ] **homeostasis** (hoh-mee-oh-**STAY**-sis)
- [ ] **hyperplasia** (high-per-**PLAY**-zee-ah)
- [ ] **hypertrophy** (high-**PER**-troh-fee)
- [ ] **hypogastric region** (high-poh-**GAS**-trick)
- [ ] **hypoplasia** (high-poh-**PLAY**-zee-ah)
- [ ] **iatrogenic illness** (eye-at-roh-**JEN**-ick)
- [ ] **idiopathic disorder** (id-ee-oh-**PATII**-ick)
- [ ] **infectious disease** (in-**FECK**-shus)
- [ ] **inguinal** (**ING**-gwih-nal)
- [ ] **medial** (**MEE**-dee-al)
- [ ] **mesentery** (**MESS**-en-**terr**-ee)
- [ ] **midsagittal plane** (mid-**SADJ**-ih-tal)
- [ ] **nosocomial infection** (nos-oh-**KOH**-mee-al in-**FECK**-shun)
- [ ] **pandemic** (pan-**DEM**-ick)
- [ ] **pelvic cavity** (**PEL**-vick)
- [ ] **peritoneum** (pehr-ih-toh-**NEE**-um)
- [ ] **peritonitis** (pehr-ih-toh-**NIGH**-tis)
- [ ] **phenylketonuria** (fen-il-**kee**-toh-**NEW**-ree-ah)
- [ ] **physiology** (fiz-ee-**OL**-oh-jee)
- [ ] **posterior** (pos-**TEER**-ee-or)
- [ ] **proximal** (**PROCK**-sih-mal)
- [ ] **retroperitoneal** (ret-roh-**pehr**-ih-toh-**NEE**-al)
- [ ] **stem cells**
- [ ] **thoracic cavity** (thoh-**RAS**-ick)
- [ ] **transverse plane** (trans-**VERSE**)
- [ ] **umbilicus** (um-**BILL**-ih-kus)
- [ ] **vector-borne transmission**
- [ ] **ventral** (**VEN**-tral)

## LEARNING GOALS

On completion of this chapter, you should be able to:

1. Define anatomy and physiology and the uses of anatomic reference systems to identify the anatomic position plus body planes, directions, and cavities.

2. Recognize, define, spell, and pronounce the primary terms related to cells and genetics.

3. Recognize, define, spell, and pronounce the primary terms related to the structure, function, pathology, and procedures of tissues and glands.

4. Identify the major organs and functions of the body systems.

5. Recognize, define, spell, and pronounce the primary terms used to describe pathology, the modes of transmission, and the types of diseases.

## ■ ANATOMIC REFERENCE SYSTEMS

**Anatomic reference systems** are used to describe the locations of the structural units of the body. The simplest anatomic reference is the one we learn in childhood: our right hand is on the right, and our left hand on the left.

In medical terminology, there are several additional ways to describe the location of different body parts. These anatomical reference systems include:

■ Body planes

■ Body directions

■ Body cavities

■ Structural units

When body parts work together to perform a related function, they are grouped together and are known as a body system.

### Anatomy and Physiology Defined

■ **Anatomy** (ah-**NAT**-oh-mee) is the study of the structures of the body.

■ **Physiology** (**fiz**-ee-**OL**-oh-jee) is the study of the functions of the structures of the body (**physi** means nature or physical, and **-ology** means study of).

### The Anatomic Position

The **anatomic position** describes the body standing in the standard position. This includes:

■ Standing up straight so that the body is erect and facing forward

■ Holding the arms at the sides with the hands turned so that the palms face toward the front.

## The Body Planes

**Body planes** are imaginary vertical and horizontal lines used to divide the body into sections for descriptive purposes (Figure 2.1). These planes are aligned to a body standing in the anatomic position.

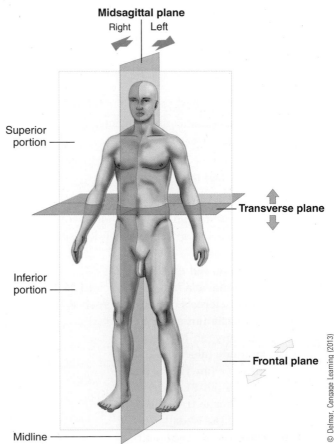

**Midsagittal plane**
Right | Left

Superior portion

Transverse plane

Inferior portion

Frontal plane

Midline

© Delmar, Cengage Learning (2013)

**FIGURE 2.1** Body planes: the midsagittal plane divides the body into equal left and right halves. The transverse plane divides the body into superior (upper) and inferior (lower) portions. The frontal plane divides the body into anterior (front) and posterior (back) portions.

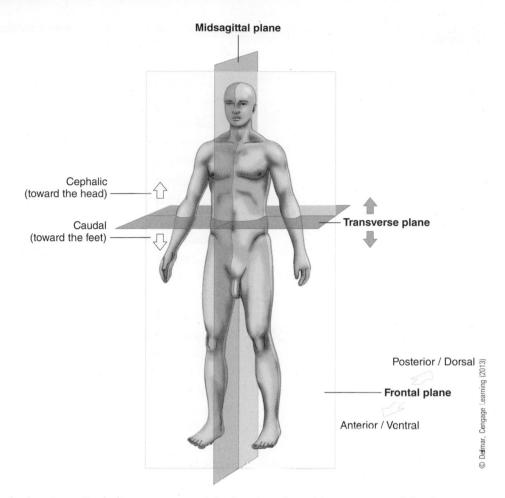

Midsagittal plane

Cephalic
(toward the head)

Caudal
(toward the feet)

Transverse plane

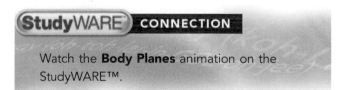

Posterior / Dorsal

**Frontal plane**

Anterior / Ventral

© Delmar, Cengage Learning (2013)

**FIGURE 2.2** Body directions: Cephalic means toward the head, and caudal means toward the feet. Anterior means toward the front, and the front of the body is known as the ventral surface. Posterior means toward the back, and the back of the body is known as the dorsal surface.

## The Vertical Planes

A **vertical plane** is an up-and-down plane that is a right angle to the horizon.

- A **sagittal plane** (**SADJ**-ih-tal) is a vertical plane that divides the body into *unequal* left and right portions.

- The **midsagittal plane** (mid-**SADJ**-ih-tal), also known as the *midline*, is the sagittal plane that divides the body into *equal* left and right halves (Figure 2.1).

- A **frontal plane** is a vertical plane that divides the body into anterior (front) and posterior (back) portions. Also known as the *coronal plane*, it is located at right angles to the sagittal plane (Figure 2.1).

## The Horizontal Plane

A **horizontal plane** is a flat crosswise plane, such as the horizon.

- A **transverse plane** (trans-**VERSE**) is a horizontal plane that divides the body into superior (upper) and

inferior (lower) portions. A transverse plane can be at the waist or at any other level across the body (Figure 2.1).

**StudyWARE  CONNECTION**

Watch the **Body Planes** animation on the StudyWARE™.

## Body Direction Terms

The relative location of sections of the body or of an organ can be described through the use of pairs of contrasting body direction terms. These terms are illustrated in Figures 2.2 and 2.3.

- **Ventral** (**VEN**-tral) refers to the front, or belly side, of the organ or body (**ventr** means belly side of the body, and **-al** means pertaining to). Ventral is the opposite of *dorsal*.

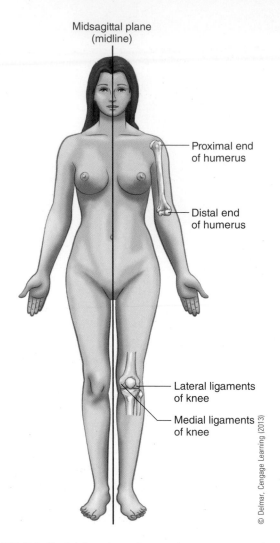

Midsagittal plane
(midline)

Proximal end
of humerus

Distal end
of humerus

Lateral ligaments
of knee

Medial ligaments
of knee

© Delmar, Cengage Learning (2013)

**FIGURE 2.3** Body directions: Proximal means situated nearest the midline, and distal means situated farthest from the midline. Medial means toward or nearer the midline, and lateral means toward the side and away from the midline.

- **Dorsal** (**DOR**-sal) refers to the back of the organ or body (**dors** means back of the body, and **-al** means pertaining to). Dorsal is the opposite of *ventral*.

- **Anterior** (an-**TEER**-ee-or) means situated in the front. It also means on the front or forward part of an organ (**anter** means front or before, and **-ior** means pertaining to). For example, the stomach is located anterior to (in front of) the pancreas. *Anterior* is also used in reference to the ventral surface of the body. *Anterior* is the opposite of *posterior*.

- **Posterior** (pos-**TEER**-ee-or) means situated in the back. It also means on the back part of an organ (**poster** means back or toward the back, and **-ior** means pertaining to). For example, the pancreas is located posterior to (behind) the stomach. The term *posterior* is also used

in reference to the dorsal surface of the body. *Posterior* is the opposite of *anterior*.

- **Superior** means uppermost, above, or toward the head. For example, the lungs are located superior to (above) the diaphragm. *Superior* is the opposite of *inferior*.

- **Inferior** means lowermost, below, or toward the feet. For example, the stomach is located inferior to (below) the diaphragm. *Inferior* is the opposite of *superior*.

- **Cephalic** (seh-**FAL**-ick) means toward the head (**cephal** means head, and **-ic** means pertaining to). *Cephalic* is the opposite of *caudal*.

- **Caudal** (**KAW**-dal) means toward the lower part of the body (**caud** means tail or lower part of the body, and **-al** means pertaining to). *Caudal* is the opposite of *cephalic*.

- **Proximal** (**PROCK**-sih-mal) means situated nearest the midline or beginning of a body structure. For example, the proximal end of the humerus (bone of the upper arm) forms part of the shoulder. *Proximal* is the opposite of *distal*.

- **Distal** (**DIS**-tal) means situated farthest from the midline or beginning of a body structure. For example, the distal end of the humerus forms part of the elbow (Figure 2.3). *Distal* is the opposite of *proximal*.

- **Medial** (**MEE**-dee-al) means the direction toward, or nearer, the midline. For example, the medial ligament of the knee is near the inner surface of the leg (Figure 2.3). *Medial* is the opposite of *lateral*.

- **Lateral** means the direction toward, or nearer, the side of the body, away from the midline. For example, the lateral ligament of the knee is near the side of the leg. *Lateral* is the opposite of *medial*. *Bilateral* means relating to, or having, two sides.

## Major Body Cavities

The two major **body cavities**, which are the dorsal (back) and the ventral (front) cavities, are spaces within the body that contain and protect internal organs (Figure 2.4).

### *The Dorsal Cavity*

The **dorsal cavity**, which is located along the back of the body and head, contains organs of the nervous system that coordinate body functions and is divided into two portions:

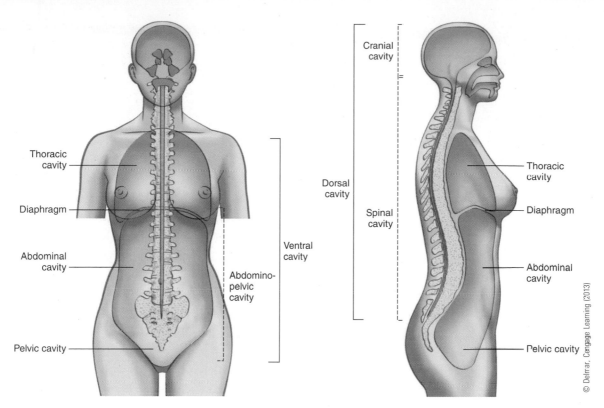

**FIGURE 2.4** The major body cavities.

■ The **cranial cavity**, which is located within the skull, surrounds and protects the brain. *Cranial* means pertaining to the skull.

■ The **spinal cavity**, which is located within the spinal column, surrounds and protects the spinal cord.

## The Ventral Cavity

The **ventral cavity**, which is located along the front of the body, contains the body organs that sustain homeostasis. **Homeostasis** (hoh-mee-oh-**STAY**-sis) is the processes through which the body maintains a constant internal environment (**home/o** means constant, and **-stasis** means control). The ventral cavity is divided into the following portions:

■ The **thoracic cavity** (thoh-**RAS**-ick), also known as the *chest cavity* or *thorax*, surrounds and protects the heart and the lungs. The *diaphragm* is a muscle that separates the thoracic and abdominal cavities.

■ The **abdominal cavity** (ab-**DOM**-ih-nal) contains primarily the major organs of digestion. This cavity is frequently referred to simply as the **abdomen** (**AB**-doh-men).

■ The **pelvic cavity** (**PEL**-vick) is the space formed by the hip bones and contains primarily the organs of the reproductive and excretory systems.

There is no physical division between the abdominal and pelvic cavities. The term **abdominopelvic cavity** (ab-**dom**-ih-noh-**PEL**-vick) refers to these two cavities as a single unit (**abdomin/o** means abdomen, **pelv** means pelvis, and **-ic** means pertaining to).

The term **inguinal** (**ING**-gwih-nal), which means relating to the groin, refers to the entire lower area of the abdomen. This includes the *groin*, which is the crease at the junction of the trunk with the upper end of the thigh.

## Regions of the Thorax and Abdomen

**Regions of the thorax and abdomen** are a descriptive system that divides the abdomen and lower portion of the thorax into nine parts (Figure 2.5). These parts are:

■ The **right and left hypochondriac regions** (high-poh-**KON**-dree-ack) are covered by the lower ribs (**hypo-** means below, **chondr/i** means cartilage, and **-ac** means pertaining to). As used here, the term *hypochondriac* means below the ribs. This term also describes an individual with an abnormal concern about his or her health.

■ The **epigastric region** (ep-ih-**GAS**-trick) is located above the stomach (**epi-** means above, **gastr** means stomach, and **-ic** means pertaining to).

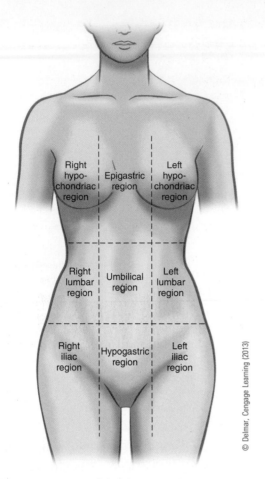

© Delmar, Cengage Learning (2013)

**FIGURE 2.5** Regions of the thorax and abdomen.

- The **right and left lumbar regions** (**LUM**-bar) are located near the inward curve of the spine (**lumb** means lower back, and **-ar** means pertaining to). The term *lumbar* describes the part of the back between the ribs and the pelvis.

- The **umbilical region** (um-**BILL**-ih-kal) surrounds the **umbilicus** (um-**BILL**-ih-kus), which is commonly known as the *belly button* or *navel*. This pit in the center of the abdominal wall marks the point where the umbilical cord was attached before birth.

- The **right and left iliac regions** (**ILL**-ee-ack) are located over the hip bones (**ili** means hip bone, and **-ac** means pertaining to).

- The **hypogastric region** (**high**-poh-**GAS**-trick) is located below the stomach (**hypo-** means below, **gastr** means stomach, and **-ic** means pertaining to).

## Quadrants of the Abdomen

Describing where an abdominal organ or pain is located is made easier by dividing the abdomen into four

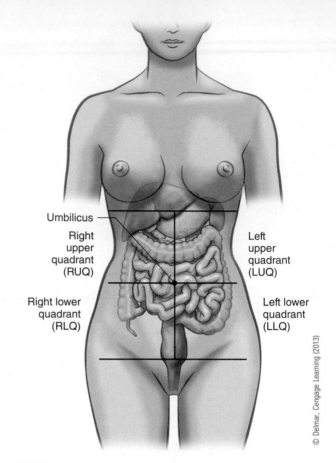

© Delmar, Cengage Learning (2013)

**FIGURE 2.6** Division of the abdomen into quadrants.

imaginary quadrants. The term **quadrant** means divided into four. As shown in Figure 2.6 the quadrants of the abdomen are:

- Right upper quadrant (RUQ)
- Left upper quadrant (LUQ)
- Right lower quadrant (RLQ)
- Left lower quadrant (LLQ)

## The Peritoneum

The **peritoneum** (**pehr**-ih-toh-**NEE**-um) is a multilayered membrane that protects and holds the organs in place within the abdominal cavity. A *membrane* is a thin layer of tissue that covers a surface, lines a cavity, or divides a space or organ.

- The **parietal peritoneum** (pah-**RYE**-eh-tal **pehr**-ih-toh-**NEE**-um) is the outer layer of the peritoneum that lines the interior of the abdominal wall. *Parietal* means cavity wall.

- The **mesentery** (**MESS**-en-**terr**-ee) is a fused double layer of the parietal peritoneum that attaches parts of the intestine to the interior abdominal wall.

- The **visceral peritoneum** (**VIS**-er-al **pehr**-ih-toh-**NEE**-um) is the inner layer of the peritoneum that surrounds the organs of the abdominal cavity. *Visceral* means relating to the internal organs.

   **Retroperitoneal** (**ret**-roh-**pehr**-ih-toh-**NEE**-al) means located behind the peritoneum (**retro-** means behind, **periton** means peritoneum, and **-eal** means pertaining to). For example, the location of the kidneys is retroperitoneal with one on each side of the spinal column. **Peritonitis** (**pehr**-ih-toh-**NIGH**-tis) is inflammation of the peritoneum.

## STRUCTURES OF THE BODY

The body is made up of increasingly larger and more complex structural units. From smallest to largest, these are cells, tissues, organs, and the body systems (Figure 2.7). Working together, these structures form the complete body and enable it to function properly.

## CELLS

**Cells** are the basic structural and functional units of the body. Cells are specialized and grouped together to form tissues and organs.

- **Cytology** (sigh-**TOL**-oh-jee) is the study of the anatomy, physiology, pathology, and chemistry of the cell (**cyt** means cell, and **-ology** means study of).
- A **cytologist** (sigh-**TOL**-oh-jist) is a specialist in the study and analysis of cells (**cyt** means cell, and **-ologist** means specialist).

## The Structure of Cells

- The **cell membrane** (**MEM**-brain) is the tissue that surrounds and protects the contents of the cell by separating them from its external environment (Figure 2.8).
- **Cytoplasm** (**SIGH**-toh-plazm) is the material within the cell membrane that is *not* part of the nucleus (**cyt/o** means cell, and **-plasm** means formative material of cells).
- The **nucleus** (**NEW**-klee-us), which is surrounded by the nuclear membrane, is a structure within the cell. It has two important functions: it controls the activities of the cell, and it helps the cell divide.

## Stem Cells

Stem cells differ from other kinds of cells in the body because of two characteristics:

- **Stem cells** are unspecialized cells that are able to renew themselves for long periods of time by cell

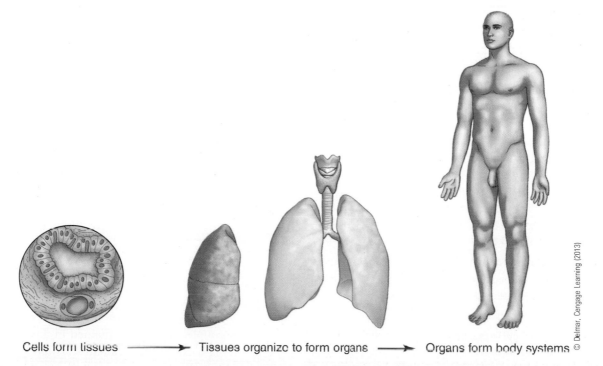

Cells form tissues ⟶ Tissues organize to form organs ⟶ Organs form body systems    © Delmar, Cengage Learning (2013)

**FIGURE 2.7** The human body is highly organized, from the single cell to the total organism.

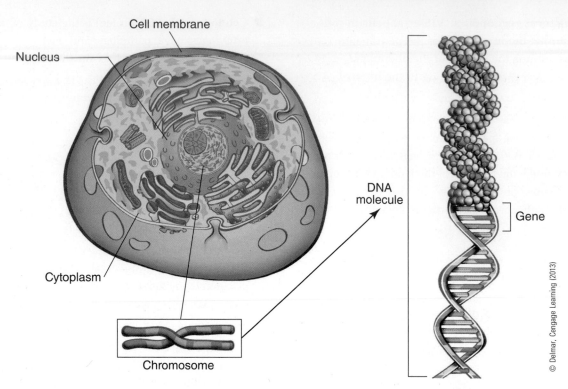

Cell membrane

Nucleus

Cytoplasm

Chromosome

DNA molecule

Gene

© Delmar, Cengage Learning (2013)

**FIGURE 2.8**  A basic cell and DNA molecule.

division. This is in contrast to other types of cells that have a specialized role and die after a determined life span.

■ Under certain conditions stem cells can be transformed into cells with special functions such as the cells of the heart muscle that make the heartbeat possible or the specialized cells of the pancreas that are capable of producing insulin.

## Adult Stem Cells

**Adult stem cells**, also known as *somatic stem cells*, are undifferentiated cells found among differentiated cells in a tissue or organ. Normally the primary role of these cells is to maintain and repair the tissue in which they are found. The term *undifferentiated* means not having a specialized function or structure. In contrast the term *differentiated* means having a specialized function or structure.

Stem cells potentially have many therapeutic uses, including being transplanted from one individual to another. Cells for this purpose are harvested from the *hemopoietic* (blood forming) tissue of the donor's bone marrow. However, unless there is an excellent match between the donor and recipient, there is the possibility of rejection known as *graft-versus-host disease*.

## Embryonic Stem Cells

**Embryonic stem cells** are undifferentiated cells that are unlike any specific adult cell; however, they have the important ability to form *any* adult cell.

■ These cells can proliferate (grow rapidly) indefinitely in a laboratory and could therefore potentially provide a source for adult muscle, liver, bone, or blood cells.

■ Because these cells are more primitive than adult stem cells, an embryonic stem cell transplant does not require as perfect a match between the patient and donor as the transplantation of adult stem cells.

■ Embryonic stem cells come from the *cord blood* found in the umbilical cord and placenta of a newborn infant. Embryonic stem cells from cord blood can be harvested at the time of birth without danger to mother or child. These cells are kept frozen until needed for treatment purposes.

■ Embryonic stem cells can also be obtained from surplus embryos produced by in vitro (test tube) fertilization. With the informed consent of the donor couple, stem cells obtained in this manner are being used for medical and scientific research.

# GENETICS

A **gene** is a fundamental physical and functional unit of heredity. Genes control hereditary disorders and all physical traits such as hair, skin, and eye color.

**Genetics** is the study of how genes are transferred from parents to their children and the role of genes in health and disease (**gene** means producing, and **-tics** means pertaining to). A specialist in this field is known as a **geneticist** (jeh-**NET**-ih-sist).

## Dominant and Recessive Genes

Each newly formed individual receives two genes of each genetic trait: one from the father and one from the mother.

- When a **dominant gene** is inherited from either parent, the offspring *will* inherit that genetic condition or characteristic. For example, freckles are a physical trait that is transmitted by a dominant gene. So, too, is the hereditary disorder Huntington's disease.

- When the same **recessive gene** is inherited from both parents, the offspring *will have* that condition. For example, *sickle cell anemia* is a group of inherited red blood cell disorders that are transmitted by a recessive gene. When this gene is transmitted by both parents, the child *will have* sickle cell anemia.

- When a **recessive gene** is inherited from only one parent, and a normal gene is inherited from the other parent, the offspring *will not have* the condition. Although this child will not develop sickle cell anemia, he or she will have the *sickle cell anemia trait*. People with this trait can transmit the sickle cell gene to their offspring.

## The Human Genome

A **genome** (**JEE**-nohm) is the complete set of genetic information of an organism. The Human Genome Project studied this genetic code for individual people and found that it is more than 99 percent identical among humans throughout the world. The first complete mapping of the *human genome*, which took 13 years to complete, was published in 2003.

Having access to this data is a very important step in studying the use of genetics in health and science. Scientists have begun to take the next step: attempting to understand the proteins encoded by the sequence of the 30,000 genes.

## Chromosomes

**Chromosomes** (**KROH**-moh-sohmes) are the genetic structures located within the nucleus of each cell (Figure 2.8). These chromosomes are made up of the DNA molecules containing the body's genes. Packaging genetic information into chromosomes helps a cell keep a large amount of genetic information neat, organized, and compact. Each chromosome contains about 100,000 genes.

- A *somatic cell* is any cell in the body except the gametes (sex cells). *Somatic* means pertaining to the body in general. Somatic cells contain 46 chromosomes arranged into 23 pairs. There are 22 identical pairs of chromosomes, plus another pair. In a typical female, this remaining pair consists of XX chromosomes. In a typical male, this pair consists of an XY chromosome pair. This chromosome pair determines the sex of the individual.

- A *sex cell* (sperm or egg), also known as a *gamete*, is the only type of cell that *does not* contain 46 chromosomes. Instead, each ovum (egg) or sperm has 23 single chromosomes. In a female, one of these will be an X chromosome. In a male, one of these will be either an X or a Y chromosome. When a sperm and ovum join, the newly formed offspring receives 23 chromosomes from each parent, for a total of 46.

- It is the X or Y chromosome from the father that determines the gender of the child.

- A defect in chromosomes can lead to birth defects. For example, individuals with Down syndrome have 47 chromosomes instead of the usual 46.

## DNA

The basic structure of the **DNA** molecule, which is located on the pairs of chromosomes in the nucleus of each cell, is the same for all living organisms. Human DNA contains thousands of genes that provide the information essential for heredity, determining physical appearance, disease risks, and other traits (Figure 2.8).

- DNA is packaged in a chromosome as two spiraling strands that twist together to form a double helix. A *helix* is a shape twisted like a spiral staircase. A *double helix* consists of two of these strands twisted together.

- DNA, which is an abbreviation for *deoxyribonucleic acid*, is found in the nucleus of all types of cells except erythrocytes (red blood cells). The difference here is due to the fact that erythrocytes do not have a nucleus.

- The DNA for each individual is different, and no two DNA patterns are exactly the same. The only exception to this rule is identical twins, which are formed from one fertilized egg that divides. Although their DNA is identical, these twins do develop characteristics that make each of them unique, such as fingerprints.

- A very small sample of DNA, such as from human hair or tissue, can be used to identify individuals in instances such as criminal investigations, paternity suits, or genealogy research.

## Genetic Mutation

A **genetic mutation** is a change of the sequence of a DNA molecule. Potential causes of genetic mutation include exposure to radiation or environmental pollution.

- A *somatic cell mutation* is a change within the cells of the body. These changes affect the individual but *cannot* be transmitted to the next generation.

- A *gametic cell mutation* is a change within the genes in a gamete (sex cell) that *can* be transmitted by a parent to his or her children.

- *Genetic engineering* is the manipulating or splicing of genes for scientific or medical purposes. The production of human insulin from modified bacteria is an example of one result of genetic engineering.

## Genetic Disorders

A **genetic disorder**, also known as a *hereditary disorder*, is a pathological condition caused by an absent or defective gene. Some genetic disorders are obvious at birth. Others may manifest (become evident) at any time in life. The following are examples of genetic disorders:

- **Cystic fibrosis** (CF), a genetic disorder that is present at birth and affects both the respiratory and digestive systems (See Chapter 7).

- **Down syndrome** (DS), a genetic variation that is associated with a characteristic facial appearance, learning disabilities, and physical abnormalities such as heart valve disease (Figure 2.9).

- **Hemophilia** (**hee**-moh-**FILL**-ee-ah), a group of hereditary bleeding disorders in which a blood-clotting factor is missing. This blood coagulation disorder is

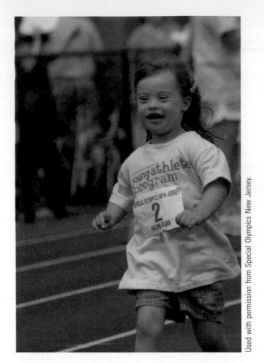

Used with permission from Special Olympics New Jersey.

**FIGURE 2.9** Down syndrome is a genetic disorder that causes learning disabilities, developmental delays, and a characteristic facial appearance.

characterized by spontaneous hemorrhages or severe bleeding following an injury.

- **Huntington's disease** (HD), a genetic disorder that is passed from parent to child. Each child of a parent with the gene for Huntington's disease has a 50-50 chance of inheriting this defective gene. This condition causes nerve degeneration with symptoms that most often appear in midlife. (*Degeneration* means worsening condition.) This damage eventually results in uncontrolled movements and the loss of some mental abilities.

- **Muscular dystrophy** (**DIS**-troh-fee), a group of genetic diseases that are characterized by progressive weakness and degeneration of the skeletal muscles that control movement.

- **Phenylketonuria** (**fen**-il-**kee**-toh-**NEW**-ree-ah), a genetic disorder in which the essential digestive enzyme *phenylalanine hydroxylase* is missing. This is commonly known as *PKU*. PKU can be detected by a blood test performed on infants at birth. With careful dietary supervision, children born with PKU can lead normal lives. Without early detection and treatment, PKU causes severe mental retardation.

■ **Tay-Sachs disease** (**TAY SAKS**), a fatal genetic disorder in which harmful quantities of a fatty substance buildup in tissues and nerve cells in the brain. Both parents must carry the mutated gene to have an affected child. The most common form of the disease affects babies who appear healthy at birth and seem to develop normally for the first few months. Development then slows, and a relentless deterioration of mental and physical abilities results in progressive blindness, paralysis, and early death.

# ■ TISSUES

A **tissue** is a group or layer of similarly specialized cells that join together to perform certain specific functions. **Histology** (hiss-**TOL**-oh-jee) is the study of the structure, composition, and function of tissues (**hist** means tissue, and **-ology** means a study of). A **histologist** (hiss-**TOL**-oh-jist) is a specialist in the study of the organization of tissues at all levels (**hist** means tissue, and **-ologist** means specialist). The four main types of tissue are:

■ Epithelial tissues

■ Connective tissues

■ Muscle tissue

■ Nerve tissue

## Epithelial Tissues

**Epithelial tissues** (**ep**-ih-**THEE**-lee-al) form a protective covering for all of the internal and external surfaces of the body. These tissues also form glands.

■ **Epithelium** (**ep**-ih-**THEE**-lee-um) is the specialized epithelial tissue that forms the epidermis of the skin and the surface layer of mucous membranes (see Chapter 12).

■ **Endothelium** (**en**-doh-**THEE**-lee-um) is the specialized epithelial tissue that lines the blood and lymph vessels, body cavities, glands, and organs.

## Connective Tissues

**Connective tissues** support and connect organs and other body tissues. The four kinds of connective tissue are:

■ **Dense connective tissues**, such as bone and cartilage, form the joints and framework of the body.

■ **Adipose tissue**, also known as *fat*, provides protective padding, insulation, and support (**adip** means fat, and **-ose** means pertaining to).

■ **Loose connective tissue** surrounds various organs and supports both nerve cells and blood vessels.

■ **Liquid connective tissues**, which are blood and lymph, transport nutrients and waste products throughout the body.

## Muscle Tissue

**Muscle tissue** contains cells with the specialized ability to contract and relax.

## Nerve Tissue

**Nerve tissue** contains cells with the specialized ability to react to stimuli and to conduct electrical impulses.

## Pathology of Tissue Formation

Disorders of the tissues, which are frequently due to unknown causes, can occur before birth as the tissues are forming or appear later in life.

### Incomplete Tissue Formation

■ **Aplasia** (ah-**PLAY**-zee-ah) is the defective development, or the congenital absence, of an organ or tissue (**a-** means without, and **-plasia** means formation). Compare aplasia with *hypoplasia*.

■ **Hypoplasia** (high-poh-**PLAY**-zee-ah) is the incomplete development of an organ or tissue usually due to a deficiency in the number of cells (**hypo-** means deficient, and **-plasia** means formation). Compare hypoplasia with *aplasia*.

### Abnormal Tissue Formation

■ **Anaplasia** (an-ah-**PLAY**-zee-ah) is a change in the structure of cells and in their orientation to each other (**ana-** means backward, and **-plasia** means formation). This abnormal cell development is characteristic of tumor formation in cancers. Contrast anaplasia with *hypertrophy*.

■ **Dysplasia** (dis-**PLAY**-see-ah) is the abnormal development or growth of cells, tissues, or organs (**dys-** means bad, and **-plasia** means formation).

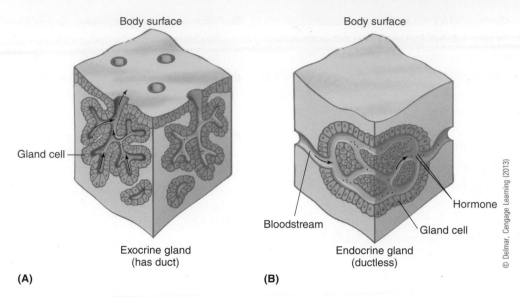

Body surface

Gland cell

Exocrine gland
(has duct)

**(A)**

Body surface

Hormone

Bloodstream

Gland cell

Endocrine gland
(ductless)

**(B)**

© Delmar, Cengage Learning (2013)

**FIGURE 2.10** A. Exocrine glands secrete their chemical substances into ducts that lead either to other organs or out of the body. B. Endocrine glands pour their secretions directly into the bloodstream.

■ **Hyperplasia** (**high**-per-**PLAY**-zee-ah) is the enlargement of an organ or tissue because of an abnormal increase in the number of cells in the tissues (**hyper-** means excessive, and **-plasia** means formation). Contrast hyperplasia with *hypertrophy*.

■ **Hypertrophy** (high-**PER**-troh-fee) is a general increase in the bulk of a body part or organ that is due to an increase in the size, but not in the number, of cells in the tissues (**hyper-** means excessive, and **-trophy** means development). This enlargement is not due to tumor formation. Contrast hypertrophy with *anaplasia* and *hyperplasia*.

## ▮ GLANDS

A **gland** is a group of specialized epithelial cells that are capable of producing secretions. A *secretion* is the substance produced by a gland. The two major types of glands are (Figure 2.10):

■ **Exocrine glands** (**ECK**-soh-krin) secrete chemical substances into ducts that lead either to other organs or out of the body, such as sweat glands (**exo-** means out of, and **-crine** means to secrete) (See Chapter 12).

■ **Endocrine glands** (**EN**-doh-krin), which produce hormones, do not have ducts (**endo-** means within, and **-crine** means to secrete). These hormones are secreted directly into the bloodstream, and are then transported to organs and structures throughout the body (See Chapter 13).

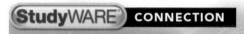

**StudyWARE** **CONNECTION**

Watch the **Exocrine and Endocrine Glands** animation on the StudyWARE™.

## Pathology and Procedures of the Glands

■ **Adenitis** (**ad**-eh-**NIGH**-tis) is the inflammation of a gland (**aden** means gland, and **-itis** means inflammation).

■ An **adenocarcinoma** (**ad**-eh-noh-**kar**-sih-**NOH**-mah) is a malignant tumor that originates in glandular tissue (**aden/o** means gland, **carcin** means cancerous, and **-oma** means tumor). *Malignant* means harmful, capable of spreading, and potentially life threatening.

■ An **adenoma** (**ad**-eh-**NOH**-mah) is a benign tumor that arises in or resembles glandular tissue (**aden** means gland, and **-oma** means tumor). *Benign* means not life threatening.

■ **Adenomalacia** (**ad**-eh-noh-mah-**LAY**-shee-ah) is the abnormal softening of a gland (**aden/o** means gland, and **-malacia** means abnormal softening). *Adenomalacia* is the opposite of *adenosclerosis*.

- **Adenosis** (ad-eh-**NOH**-sis) is any disease or condition of a gland (**aden** means gland, and **-osis** means an abnormal condition or disease).

- **Adenosclerosis** (ad-eh-noh-skleh-**ROH**-sis) is the abnormal hardening of a gland (**aden/o** means gland, and **-sclerosis** means abnormal hardening). *Adenosclerosis* is the opposite of *adenomalacia*.

- An **adenectomy** (ad-eh-**NECK**-toh-mee) is the surgical removal of a gland (**aden** means gland, and **-ectomy** means surgical removal).

## BODY SYSTEMS AND RELATED ORGANS

A body **organ** is a somewhat independent part of the body that performs a specific function. For purposes of description, the related tissues and organs are described as being organized into *body systems* with specialized functions. These body systems are explained in Table 2.1.

## PATHOLOGY

**Pathology** (pah-**THOL**-oh-jee) is the study of disease: the nature and cause as well as the produced changes in structure and function. *Pathology* also means a condition produced by disease. The word root (combining form) **path/o** and the suffix **-pathy** mean disease; however, they also mean suffering, feeling, and emotion.

- A **pathologist** (pah-**THOL**-oh-jist) specializes in the laboratory analysis of tissue samples to confirm or establish a diagnosis (**path** means disease, and **-ologist** means specialist). These tissue specimens can be removed in biopsies, during operations, or in post-mortem examinations.

- **Etiology** (ee-tee-**OL**-oh-jee) is the study of the causes of diseases (**eti-** means cause, and **-ology** means study of).

### Disease Transmission

A **pathogen** is a disease-producing microorganism such as a virus. *Transmission* is the spread of a disease. *Contamination* means that a pathogen is possibly present. Contamination occurs through a lack of proper hygiene standards or by failure to take appropriate infection control precautions.

- A **communicable disease** (kuh-**MEW**-nih-kuh-bul), also known as a *contagious disease*, is any condition that is transmitted from one person to another either by direct or by indirect contact with contaminated objects. *Communicable* means capable of being transmitted.

- **Indirect contact transmission** refers to situations in which a susceptible person is infected by contact with a contaminated surface.

- **Bloodborne transmission** is the spread of a disease through contact with blood or other body fluids that are contaminated with blood. Examples include human immunodeficiency virus (HIV), hepatitis B, and most sexually transmitted diseases (STDs).

- **Airborne transmission** occurs through contact with contaminated respiratory droplets spread by a cough or sneeze. Examples include tuberculosis, flu, colds, and measles.

- **Food-borne and waterborne transmission**, also known as *fecal-oral transmission*, is caused by eating or drinking contaminated food or water that has not been properly treated to remove contamination or kill any pathogens present.

- **Vector-borne transmission** is the spread of certain disease due to the bite of a vector. As used here, the term *vector* describes insects or animals such as flies, mites, fleas, ticks, rats, and dogs that are capable of transmitting a disease. Mosquitoes are the most common vectors, and the diseases they transmit include malaria and West Nile virus.

### Outbreaks of Diseases

An **epidemiologist** (ep-ih-**dee**-mee-**OL**-oh-jist) is a specialist in the study of outbreaks of disease within a population group (**epi-** means above, **dem/i** means population, and **-ologist** means specialist).

- **Endemic** (en-**DEM**-ick) refers to the ongoing presence of a disease within a population, group, or area (**en-** means within, **dem** means population, and **-ic** means pertaining to). For example, the common cold is endemic because it is always present within the general population.

- An **epidemic** (ep-ih-**DEM**-ick) is a sudden and widespread outbreak of a disease within a specific population group or area (**epi-** means above, **dem** means population, and **-ic** means pertaining to). For example, a sudden widespread outbreak of measles is an epidemic.

**TABLE 2.1**

Major Body Systems

| Body System | Major Structures | Major Functions |
| --- | --- | --- |
| Skeletal System (Chapter 3) | bones, joints, and cartilage | Supports and shapes the body. Protects the internal organs. Forms some blood cells and stores minerals. |
| Muscular System (Chapter 4) | muscles, fascia, and tendons | Holds the body erect. Makes movement possible. Moves body fluids and generates body heat. |
| Cardiovascular System (Chapter 5) | heart, arteries, veins, capillaries, and blood | Blood circulates throughout the body to transport oxygen and nutrients to cells, and to carry waste products to the kidneys where waste is removed by filtration. |
| Lymphatic System (Chapter 6) | lymph, lymphatic vessels, and lymph nodes | Removes and transports waste products from the fluid between the cells. Destroys harmful substances such as pathogens and cancer cells in the lymph nodes. Returns the filtered lymph to the bloodstream where it becomes plasma again. |
| Immune System (Chapter 6) | tonsils, spleen, thymus, skin, and specialized blood cells | Defends the body against invading pathogens and allergens. |
| Respiratory System (Chapter 7) | nose, pharynx, trachea, larynx, and lungs | Brings oxygen into the body for transportation to the cells. Removes carbon dioxide and some water waste from the body. |
| Digestive System (Chapter 8) | mouth, esophagus, stomach, small intestine, large intestine, liver, and pancreas | Digests ingested food so it can be absorbed into the bloodstream. Eliminates solid waste. |
| Urinary System (Chapter 9) | kidneys, ureters, urinary bladder, and urethra | Filters blood to remove waste. Maintains the electrolyte and fluid balance within the body. |
| Nervous System (Chapter 10) | nerves, brain, and spinal cord | Coordinates the reception of stimuli. Transmits messages throughout the body. |
| Special Senses (Chapter 11) | eyes and ears | Receive visual and auditory information, and transmit it to the brain. |
| Integumentary System (Chapter 12) | skin, sebaceous glands, and sweat glands | Protects the body against invasion by bacteria. Aids in regulating the body temperature and water content. |
| Endocrine System (Chapter 13) | adrenal glands, gonads, pancreas, parathyroids, pineal, pituitary, thymus, and thyroid | Integrates all body functions. |
| Reproductive Systems (Chapter 14) | *Male:* penis and testicles; *Female:* ovaries, uterus, and vagina | Produces new life. |

■ **Pandemic** (pan-**DEM**-ick) refers to an outbreak of a disease occurring over a large geographic area, possibly worldwide (**pan-** means entire, **dem** means population, and **-ic** means pertaining to). For example, the worldwide spread of acquired immunodeficiency syndrome (AIDS) is pandemic.

## Types of Diseases

■ A **functional disorder** produces symptoms for which no physiological or anatomical cause can be identified. For example, a panic attack is a functional disorder (see Chapter 10).

■ An **iatrogenic illness** (eye-**at**-roh-**JEN**-ick) is an unfavorable response due to prescribed medical treatment. For example, severe burns resulting from radiation therapy are iatrogenic.

■ An **idiopathic disorder** (id-ee-oh-**PATH**-ick) is an illness without known cause (**idi/o** means peculiar to the individual, **path** means disease, and **-ic** means pertaining to). *Idiopathic* means without known cause.

■ An **infectious disease** (in-**FECK**-shus) is an illness caused by living pathogenic organisms such as bacteria and viruses (see Chapter 6).

■ A **nosocomial infection** (**nos**-oh-**KOH**-mee-al in-**FECK**-shun) is a disease acquired in a hospital or clinical setting. For example, MRSA infections are often spread in hospitals (see Chapter 6). *Nosocomial* comes from the Greek word for hospital.

■ An **organic disorder** (or-**GAN**-ick) produces symptoms caused by detectable physical changes in the body. For example, chickenpox, which has a characteristic rash, is an organic disorder caused by a virus (see Chapter 6).

## Congenital Disorders

A **congenital disorder** (kon-**JEN**-ih-tahl) is an abnormal condition that exists at the time of birth. *Congenital* means existing at birth. These conditions can be caused by a developmental disorder before birth, prenatal influences, premature birth, or injuries during the birth process.

## Developmental Disorders

A **developmental disorder**, also known as a *birth defect*, can result in an anomaly or malformation such as the absence of a limb or the presence of an extra toe. An **anomaly** (ah-**NOM**-ah-lee) is a deviation from what is regarded as normal.

■ The term **atresia** (at-**TREE**-zee-ah) describes the congenital absence of a normal body opening or the failure of a structure to be tubular. For example, anal atresia is the congenital absence of the opening at the bottom end of the anus; pulmonary atresia is the absence of a pulmonary valve.

### Prenatal Influences

**Prenatal influences** are the mother's health, behavior, and the prenatal medical care she does or does not receive before delivery.

■ An example of a problem with the mother's health is a *rubella* infection (see Chapter 6). Birth defects often develop if a pregnant woman contracts this viral infection early in her pregnancy.

■ An example of a problem caused by the mother's behavior is **fetal alcohol syndrome** (FAS), which is caused by the mother's consumption of alcohol during the pregnancy. This resulting condition of the baby is characterized by physical and behavioral traits, including growth abnormalities, mental retardation, brain damage, and socialization difficulties.

■ Examples of problems caused by lack of adequate prenatal medical care are premature delivery or a low birth-weight baby.

### Premature Birth and Birth Injuries

■ *Premature birth*, which is a birth that occurs earlier than 37 weeks of development, can cause serious health problems because the baby's body systems have not had time to form completely. Breathing difficulties and heart problems are common in premature babies.

■ *Birth injuries* are congenital disorders that were not present before the events surrounding the time of birth. For example, *cerebral palsy*, which is the result of brain damage, can be caused by premature birth or inadequate oxygen to the brain during the birth process.

## ■ AGING AND DEATH

Aging is the normal progression of the life cycle that will eventually end in death. During the latter portion of life, individuals become increasingly at higher risk of developing health problems that are chronic or eventually fatal. As the average life span is becoming longer, a larger

56
↓
63

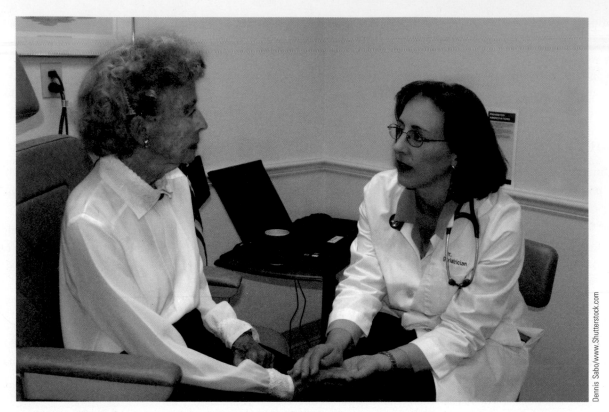

**FIGURE 2.11** A geriatrician specializes in problems related to aging, and in the diagnosis, treatment, and prevention of disease in older people.

portion of the population are affected by such disorders related to aging.

- The study of the medical problems and care of older people is known as **geriatrics** (jer-ee-**AT**-ricks) or as *gerontology*.

- *Postmortem* means after death. A postmortem examination is also known as an **autopsy** (**AW**-top-see).

## GENERAL MEDICAL SPECIALTIES RELATING TO HEALTH AND DISEASE

Physicians caring for the well-being of patients during their lifetime include the following specialists:

- A **general practitioner** (GP), or *family practice physician*, provides ongoing care for patients of all ages.

- An **internist** is a physician who specializes in diagnosing and treating diseases and disorders of the internal organs and related body systems.

- A **pediatrician** (**pee**-dee-ah-**TRISH**-un) is a physician who specializes in diagnosing, treating, and preventing disorders and diseases of infants and children. This specialty is known as *pediatrics*.

- A **geriatrician** (**jer**-ee-ah-**TRISH**-un), or *gerontologist*, is a physician who specializes in the care of older people (Figure 2.11).

- A **hospitalist** focuses on the general medical care of hospitalized patients.

## ABBREVIATIONS RELATED TO THE HUMAN BODY IN HEALTH AND DISEASE

Table 2.2 presents an overview of the abbreviations related to the terms introduced in this chapter. Note: To avoid errors or confusion, always be cautious when using abbreviations.

## TABLE 2.2
## Abbreviations Related to the Human Body in Health and Disease

| | |
|---|---|
| **anatomy and physiology** = A & P | **A & P** = anatomy and physiology |
| **communicable disease** = CD | **CD** = communicable disease |
| **chromosome** = CH, chr | **CH, chr** = chromosome |
| **deoxyribonucleic acid** = DNA | **DNA** = deoxyribonucleic acid |
| **epidemic** = epid | **epid** = epidemic |
| **general practitioner** = GP | **GP** = general practitioner |
| **Huntington's disease** = HD | **HD** = Huntington's disease |
| **left lower quadrant** = LLQ | **LLQ** = left lower quadrant |
| **left upper quadrant** = LUQ | **LUQ** = left upper quadrant |
| **phenylketonuria** = PKU | **PKU** = phenylketonuria |
| **right lower quadrant** = RLQ | **RLQ** = right lower quadrant |
| **right upper quadrant** = RUQ | **RUQ** = right upper quadrant |

**StudyWARE** CONNECTION

For more practice and to test your mastery of this material, go to the StudyWARE™ to play interactive games and complete the quiz for this chapter.

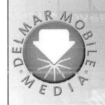

*Downloadable audio is available for selected medical terms in this chapter to enhance your learning of medical terminology.*

## ☐ Workbook Practice

Go to your workbook and complete the exercises for this chapter.

# LEARNING EXERCISES

## MATCHING WORD PARTS 1

Write the correct answer in the middle column.

| Definition | Correct Answer | Possible Answers |
|---|---|---|
| 2.1.   fat | _____ | **aden/o** |
| 2.2.   front | _____ | **adip/o** |
| 2.3.   gland | _____ | **anter/o** |
| 2.4.   specialist | _____ | **-ologist** |
| 2.5.   study of | _____ | **-ology** |

## MATCHING WORD PARTS 2

Write the correct answer in the middle column.

| Definition | Correct Answer | Possible Answers |
|---|---|---|
| 2.6.   cell | _____ | **caud/o** |
| 2.7.   head | _____ | **cephal/o** |
| 2.8.   lower part of the body | _____ | **cyt/o** |
| 2.9.   out of | _____ | **endo-** |
| 2.10.   within | _____ | **exo-** |

## MATCHING WORD PARTS 3

Write the correct answer in the middle column.

| Definition | Correct Answer | Possible Answers |
|---|---|---|
| 2.11.   back | _____ | **hist/o** |
| 2.12.   control | _____ | **path/o** |

2.13.   disease, suffering, emotion          _____          **-plasia**

2.14.   formation                            _____          **poster/o**

2.15.   tissue                               _____          **-stasis**

## DEFINITIONS

Select the correct answer, and write it on the line provided.

2.16.   A/An _*nosocomial*_ is acquired in a hospital setting.

      iatrogenic illness        idiopathic disorder        (nosocomial infection)        organic disorder

2.17.   When a _____ is inherited from only one parent, the offspring will have that genetic condition or characteristic.

      dominant gene          (genome)          recessive gene          recessive trait

2.18.   The _____ contains the major organs of digestion.

      abdominal cavity          cranial cavity          (dorsal cavity)          pelvic cavity

2.19.   The term _*Proximal*_ means the direction toward or nearer the midline.

      distal          lateral          medial          proximal

2.20.   The primary role of the undifferentiated _____ cells is to maintain and repair the tissue in which they are found.

      (adult stem)          cord blood          embryonic stem          hemopoietic

2.21.   The genetic disorder in which an essential digestive enzyme is missing is known as _____.

      Down syndrome          Huntington's disease          (phenylketonuria)          Tay-Sachs disease

2.22.   The inflammation of a gland is known as _*adenitis*_.

      adenectomy          adenitis          adenoma          adenosis

2.23.   The _____ is the outer layer of the peritoneum that lines the interior of the abdominal wall.

      mesentery          (parietal peritoneum)          retroperitoneum          visceral peritoneum

2.24. A _____ is a fundamental physical and functional unit of heredity.

cell          gamete          gene          genome

2.25. The study of the structure, composition, and function of tissues is known as _____.

anatomy          cytology          histology          physiology

## MATCHING REGIONS OF THE THORAX AND ABDOMEN

Write the correct answer in the middle column.

| Definition | Correct Answer | Possible Answers |
|---|---|---|
| 2.26. above the stomach | _____ | epigastric region |
| 2.27. belly button area | _____ | hypochondriac region |
| 2.28. below the ribs | _____ | hypogastric region |
| 2.29. below the stomach | _____ | iliac region |
| 2.30. hip bone area | _____ | umbilical region |

## WHICH WORD?

Select the correct answer, and write it on the line provided.

2.31. The term _____ refers to the entire lower area of the abdomen.

inguinal          umbilicus

2.32. The study of how genes are transferred from parents to their children and the role of genes in health and disease is known as _____.

cytology          genetics

2.33. A specialist in the study of the outbreaks of disease is a/an _____.

epidemiologist          pathologist

2.34. The _____ secrete chemical substances into ducts.

endocrine glands          exocrine glands

2.35. The location of the stomach is _____ to the diaphragm.

inferior          superior

## SPELLING COUNTS

Find the misspelled word in each sentence. Then write that word, spelled correctly, on the line provided.

2.36.    The mesantry is a fused double layer of the parietal peritoneum. _____

2.37.    Hemaphilia is a group of hereditary bleeding disorders in which a blood-clotting factor is

missing. _____

2.38.    Hypretrophy is a general increase in the bulk of a body part or organ due to an increase in the size, but

not in the number, of cells in the tissues. _____

2.39.    The protective covering for all of the internal and external surfaces of the body is formed by epithealial

tissues. _____

2.40.    An abnomolly is any deviation from what is regarded as normal. _____

## ABBREVIATION IDENTIFICATION

Write the correct terms for the abbreviations on the lines provided.

2.41.    **HD**    _____

2.42.    **CD**    _____

2.43.    **GP**    _____

2.44.    **LUQ**    _____

2.45.    **CH**    _____

## TERM SELECTION

Select the correct answer, and write it on the line provided.

2.46.    The term meaning situated nearest the midline or beginning of a body structure

is _____.

distal            lateral            medial            proximal

2.47.    The term meaning situated in the back is _____.

anterior        posterior        superior        ventral

2.48.    The body is divided into anterior and posterior portions by the _____ plane.

frontal        horizontal        sagittal        transverse

2.49.   The body is divided into equal vertical left and right halves by the _____ plane.

        coronal          midsagittal          sagittal          transverse

2.50.   Part of the elbow is formed by the _____ end of the humerus.

        distal          lateral          medial          proximal

## SENTENCE COMPLETION

Write the correct term or terms on the lines provided.

2.51.   _____ is a genetic variation that is associated with characteristic facial appearance,

learning disabilities, and physical abnormalities such as heart valve disease.

2.52.   The study of the functions of the structures of the body is known as _____.

2.53.   The heart and the lungs are surrounded and protected by the _____ cavity.

2.54.   An unfavorable response to prescribed medical treatment, such as severe burns resulting from radiation

therapy, is known as a/an _____ illness.

2.55.   The genetic structures located within the nucleus of each cell are known as _____.

These structures are made up of the DNA molecules containing the body's genes.

## WORD SURGERY

Divide each term into its component word parts. Write these word parts, in sequence, on the lines provided. When necessary use a slash (/) to indicate a combining vowel. (You may not need all of the lines provided.)

2.56.   An **adenectomy** is the surgical removal of a gland.

    aden/ec _____     tomy _____     _____     _____

2.57.   Hormones are secreted directly into the bloodstream by the **endocrine** glands.

    endo _____     crine _____     _____     _____

2.58.   A **histologist** is a specialist in the study of the organization of tissues at all levels.

    Histo _____     lo/gist _____     _____     _____

2.59.   The term **retroperitoneal** means located behind the peritoneum.

    retro _____     perito _____     neal _____     _____

2.60.   A **pathologist** specializes in the laboratory analysis of tissue samples to confirm or establish a diagnosis.

_____      _____      _____      _____

2.61.   The study of the causes of diseases is known as **etiology**.

_____      _____      _____      _____

2.62.   The term **homeostasis** refers to the processes through which the body maintains a constant internal

environment.

_____      _____      _____      _____

2.63.   A **pandemic** is an outbreak of a disease occurring over a large geographic area, possibly worldwide.

_____      _____      _____      _____

2.64.   The **epigastric** region is located above the stomach.

_____      _____      _____      _____

2.65.   An **idiopathic** disorder is an illness without known cause.

_____      _____      _____      _____

## CLINICAL CONDITIONS

Write the correct answer on the line provided.

2.66.   Mr. Tseng died of cholera during a sudden and widespread outbreak of this disease in his village. Such

an outbreak is described as being a/an _____.

2.67.   Brenda Farmer's doctor could not find any physical changes to explain her symptoms. The doctor refers

to this as a/an _____ disorder.

2.68.   Gerald Carlson was infected with hepatitis B through _____ transmission.

2.69.   To become a specialist in the study and analysis of cells, Lee Wong signed up for courses

in _____.

2.70.   Malaria and West Nile virus are spread by mosquitoes. This is known as _____

transmission.

2.71.   Jose Ortega complained of pain in the lower right area of his abdomen. Using the system that divides the

abdomen into four sections, his doctor recorded the pain as being in the lower

right _____.

2.72. Ralph Jenkins was very sick after drinking contaminated water during a camping trip. His doctor says that

he contracted the illness through _____ transmission.

2.73. Tracy Ames has a bladder inflammation. This organ of the urinary system is located in

the _____ cavity.

2.74. Mrs. Reynolds was diagnosed as having inflammation of the peritoneum. The medical term for this condition is _____.

2.75. Ashley Goldberg is fascinated by genetics. She wants to specialize in this field and is studying to become

a/an _____.

## WHICH IS THE CORRECT MEDICAL TERM?

Select the correct answer, and write it on the line provided.

2.76. Debbie Sanchez fell against a rock and injured her left hip and upper leg. This area is known as the

left _____ region.

| hypochondriac | iliac | lumbar | umbilical |

2.77. A _____ is the complete set of genetic information of an organism.

| cell | gamete | gene | genome |

2.78. An _____ is a malignant tumor that originates in glandular tissue.

| adenocarcinoma | adenitis | adenoma | adenosis |

2.79. Nerve cells and blood vessels are surrounded and supported by _____ connective

tissue.

| adipose | epithelial | liquid | loose |

2.80. A mother's consumption of alcohol during pregnancy can cause _____.

| cerebral palsy | Down syndrome | fetal alcohol syndrome | genetic disorders |

## CHALLENGE WORD BUILDING

These terms are *not* found in this chapter; however, they are made up of the following familiar word parts. If you need help in creating the term, refer to your medical dictionary.

| | |
|---|---|
| **gastr/o** | **my/o** |
| **laryng/o** | **nephr/o** |
| **neur/o** | **-itis** |
| **-algia** | **-osis** |
| **-ectomy** | **-plasty** |

2.81.    The term meaning the surgical repair of a muscle is ___*neuroplasty*___.

2.82.    The term meaning muscle pain is ___*neuroitis*___.

2.83.    The term meaning an abnormal condition of the stomach is ___*gastroitis*___.

2.84.    The term meaning inflammation of the larynx is ___*laryngosis*___.

2.85.    The term meaning the surgical removal of part of a muscle is a/an ___*neuroplasty*___.

2.86.    The term meaning pain in the stomach is ___*gastritis*___.

2.87.    The term meaning surgical removal of the larynx is ___*laryngectomy*___.

2.88.    The term meaning an abnormal condition of the kidney is ___*nephrosis*___.

2.89.    The medical term meaning surgical repair of a nerve is ___*neuroplasty*___.

2.90.    The term meaning inflammation of the kidney is ___*nephritides*___.

## LABELING EXERCISES

Identify the numbered items in the accompanying figures.

2.91. This is the right

_____ region.

2.92. This is the _____

region.

2.93. This is the _____

region.

2.94. This is the left _____

region.

2.95. This is the left _____

region.

2.96. This is the _____

plane, which is also known as the midline.

2.97. This is the _____

surface, which is also known as the ventral

surface.

2.98. This arrow is pointing in a/

an _____ direction.

2.99. This is the _____

surface, which is also known as the dorsal

surface.

2.100. This is the _____ plane,

which is a horizontal plane.

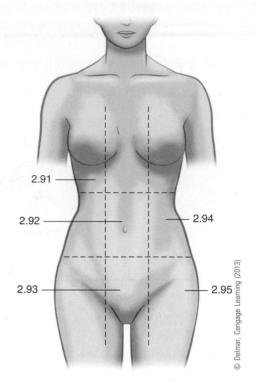

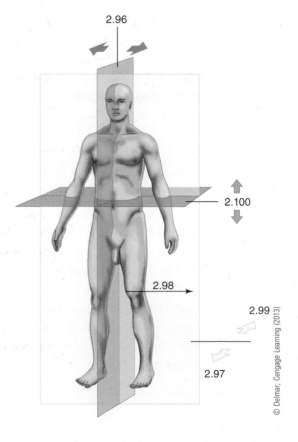

## THE HUMAN TOUCH
# Critical Thinking Exercise

The following story and questions are designed to stimulate critical thinking through class discussion or as a brief essay response. There are no right or wrong answers to these questions.

*The sign in the fifth-floor restroom read, "Dirty hands spread disease. Always use soap." Dave rinsed his hands with water, quickly ran his fingers through his hair, and then rushed into the hallway, already late for biology class.*

*There was an overwhelming smell as he entered the classroom, and he could immediately tell why: on each counter was sitting the day's project, a fetal pig. "Do these things have to stink?" he asked his teacher. "Well, Dave, if they didn't 'stink' of the formaldehyde, they would be rotting and could be spreading diseases. Now let's get started," the teacher said. At the end of class period, they were told, "Be sure to wash your hands thoroughly before leaving this classroom."*

*This reminded Dave of the lectures they had earlier in the semester about diseases caused by pathogens and how these diseases are spread. As he looked around the classroom, Dave was aware of the other students. Most were gathering up their books to go directly to lunch without washing their hands, Gail and Susan were sharing a bottle of water, Beth was rubbing her eyes, and Jim was coughing without covering his mouth! Suddenly, Dave had a mental image of pathogens everywhere: lying on hands and countertops, floating in the air—and all of these pathogens were looking for someone to infect! Dave shook his head to get rid of this mental image. Then he went to the sink and carefully washed his hands again—this time with soap.*

## Suggested Discussion Topics

1. Identify and discuss the examples of the potential disease transmission methods that are included in Dave's story, and describe what should have been done to eliminate these risks.

2. Describe how bloodborne, airborne, and food-borne diseases are transmitted, and give an example of each type of transmission.

3. Discuss what might happen in a school if a cafeteria worker has a food-borne disease and after a trip to the lavatory did not wash his or her hands. Instead, the worker went right back to work without putting on gloves—preparing salads and putting out fresh fruit for lunch.

4. When treating a bloody wound, the caregiver is required to wear protective gloves. Discuss the possible reasons for this. Is this step taken to protect the patient against diseases on the caregiver's hands? Is this step required to protect the caregiver from a bloodborne disease that the patient might have?

The first two chapters of your textbook have introduced you to many word parts. In the next 13 chapters, you will learn about the body systems. You will find that mastering this information is much easier if you have already learned *at least some* of the word parts you met in the first two chapters.

This special **Word Part Review** is designed to reinforce your knowledge of these word parts and to confirm your mastery of them. To assist you with learning these word parts, this section is divided into two parts:

■ The first part is **Word Part Practice.** It consists of 50 questions to provide practice in the use of the word parts you were introduced to in Chapters 1 and 2. It also provides opportunities to work with the use of combining vowels and word parts. If you are not certain of an answer, look it up in your textbook.

■ The second part is a **Post-Test.** It includes 50 questions designed to enable you to evaluate your mastery of these word parts. Try to answer these questions without looking up the answers in Chapters 1 and 2.

**If you are having problems in this section, ask your instructor for help NOW!**

## ■ WORD PART PRACTICE SESSION

This is a practice session and you can go back into Chapters 1 and 2 to find the answers. This is a good idea because it gives you more experience in working with the terms and word parts found in these chapters.

## Matching Word Roots and Their Meanings

Enter the correct **word root** in the middle column.

| | Definition | Correct Answer | Possible Answer |
|---|---|---|---|
| WP.1. | joint | *arthr* | **melan** |
| WP.2. | skull | *crani* | **gastr** |
| WP.3. | red | *erythr* | **erythr** |
| WP.4. | stomach | *gastr* | **crani** |
| WP.5. | black | *melan* | **arthr** |

## Matching Combining Forms and Their Meanings

Enter the correct **combining forms** in the middle column.

| Definition | Correct Answer | Possible Answer |
|---|---|---|
| WP.6. nose | rhin/o | aden/o |
| WP.7. liver | hepato | cardi/o |
| WP.8. gland | aden/o | hepat/o |
| WP.9. heart | cardio | ot/o |
| WP.10. ear | ot/o | rhin/o |

## Matching Prefixes and Their Meanings

Enter the correct **prefix** in the middle column.

| Definition | Correct Answer | Prefix |
|---|---|---|
| WP.11. bad, difficult | dys | intra- |
| WP.12. between, among | inter | hypo- |
| WP.13. excessive, increased | hyper | hyper- |
| WP.14. within, inside | intra | inter- |
| WP.15. deficient, decreased | hypo | dys- |

## Matching Suffixes and Their Meanings

Enter the correct **suffix** in the middle column.

| Definition | Correct Answer | Suffix |
|---|---|---|
| WP.16. abnormal condition | osis | -megaly |
| WP.17. bleeding | rrhagia | -ologist |
| WP.18. enlargement | megaly | -osis |
| WP.19. surgical repair | plasty | -plasty |
| WP.20. specialist | ologist | -rrhagia |

## Matching Suffixes and Their Meanings

Enter the correct **suffix** in the middle column.

| Definition | Correct Answer | Word Part |
|---|---|---|
| WP.21. inflammation | *itis* | **-algia** |
| WP.22. pain, suffering | *algia* | **-centesis** |
| WP.23. process of producing a picture or record | *graphy* | **-ectomy** |
| WP.24. surgical puncture to remove fluid | *ectomy* | **-itis** |
| WP.25. surgical removal | *centesis* | **-graphy** |

## Matching Suffixes and Their Meanings

Enter the correct **suffix** in the middle column.

| Definition | Correct Answer | Suffix |
|---|---|---|
| WP.26. abnormal flow, discharge | *rrhea* | **-oma** |
| WP.27. abnormal narrowing | | **-rrhaphy** |
| WP.28. tumor | | **-rrhea** |
| WP.29. rupture | | **-rrhexis** |
| WP.30. to suture | | **-stenosis** |

## Word Building

Write the word you create on the line provided.

WP.31. The term _Rhinoplasty_ means the surgical repair of the nose (**rhin/o** means nose).

WP.32. The term _nephrectomy_ means the surgical removal of a kidney (**nephr/o** means kidney).

WP.33. The term _otitis_ means inflammation of the ear (**ot/o** means ear).

WP.34. The term _hematology_ means the study of disorders of the blood (**hemat/o** means blood).

WP.35. The term _hepatitis_ means inflammation of the liver (**hepat/o** means liver).

WP.36. The term _arthroscopy_ means the visual examination of the interior of a joint (**arthr/o** means joint).

WP.37. The term _appendicitis_ means an inflammation of the appendix (**appendic** means appendix).

WP.38. The term _colotomy_ means a surgical incision into the colon (**col/o** means colon).

WP.39. The term _Physiology_ means the study of the functions of the structures of the body (**physi** means nature or physical).

WP.40. The term _electrocardiogram_ (ECG) means a record or picture of the electrical activity of the heart (**electr/o** means electric, and **cardi/o** means heart).

## True/False

If the word part definition is accurate, write **True** on the line. If the definition is not accurate, write **False** on the line.

WP.41. _____F_____ **myc/o** means mucous. *mucus*

WP.42. _____T_____ **peri-** means surrounding.

WP.43. _____F_____ **hypo-** means increased.

WP.44. _____T_____ **ather/o** means plaque or fatty substance.

WP.45. _____T_____ **-graphy** means the process of producing a picture or record.

WP.46. _____F_____ **pyel/o** means pus.

WP.47. _____T_____ **-ostomy** means the surgical creation of an artificial opening to the body surface.

WP.48. _____F_____ **hist** means tissue.

WP.49. _____F_____ **-centesis** means to see or a visual examination.

WP.50. _____T_____ **-cyte** means cell.

## Word Part Post-Test

Answer these questions without looking them up in Chapters 1 and 2. If you have trouble, you should arrange to get extra help or practice more in working with word parts.

Write the word part on the line provided.

PT.1.  The **suffix** meaning surgical removal is _ectomy_.

PT.2.  The **prefix** meaning under, less, or below is _sub_.

PT.3.    The **suffix** meaning surgical repair is _plasty_.

PT.4.    The **combining form** meaning fungus is _Myco_.

PT.5.    The **combining form** meaning joint is _arthr/o_.

PT.6.    The **combining form** meaning muscle is _Myo_.

PT.7.    The **prefix** meaning between or among is _enter_.

PT.8.    The **combining form** meaning bone marrow *or* spinal cord is _Myel/o_.

PT.9.    The **suffix** meaning a visual examination is _scopy_.

PT.10.   The **suffix** meaning the study of is _Logy_.

## Matching Word Parts 1

**Matching Suffixes and Prefixes with Their Meanings.**

Enter the correct **word part** in the middle column.

| Definition | Correct Answer | Possible Answer |
|---|---|---|
| PT.11.  tumor | _____ | **arteri/o** |
| PT.12.  surgical suturing | _____ | **-oma** |
| PT.13.  surrounding | _____ | **peri-** |
| PT.14.  rupture | _____ | **-rrhaphy** |
| PT.15.  artery | _____ | **-rrhexis** |

## Matching Word Parts 2

**Matching Suffixes and Prefixes with Their Meanings.**

Enter the correct **word part** in the middle column.

| Definition | Correct Answer | Possible Answer |
|---|---|---|
| PT.16.  abnormal hardening | _____ | **dys-** |
| PT.17.  bad, difficult, painful | _____ | **-itis** |
| PT.18.  inflammation | _____ | **-ostomy** |
| PT.19.  surgical creation of an artificial opening | _____ | **-osis** |
| PT.20.  abnormal condition or disease | _____ | **-sclerosis** |

## True/False

If the statement is accurate, write **True** on the line. If the statement is not correct, write **False** on the line.

PT.21. _____ T _____ The combining form **hem/o** means blood.

PT.22. _____ T _____ The suffix **-algia** means pain.

PT.23. _____ T _____ The combining form **oste/o** means bone.

PT.24. _____ F _____ The prefix **hyper-** means deficient or decreased.

PT.25. _____ T _____ The combining form **rhin/o** means nose.

## Word Surgery

Use your knowledge of word parts to identify the parts of these terms. Write the word parts, in sequence, on the lines provided.  When necessary, use a slash (/) to indicate a combining vowel.

PT.26. The term meaning the surgical repair of a nerve is **neuroplasty**. This word is made up of the word

parts _____neur/o_____ and _____plasty_____

PT.27. The term describing any pathological change or disease in the spinal cord is **myelopathy**. This term is

made up of the word parts _____myel_____ and _____pathy_____.

PT.28. The medical condition **pyrosis** is commonly known as heartburn. This term is made up of the word

parts _____pyr_____ and _____sis_____.

PT.29. The **endocrine** glands produce hormones, but do not have ducts. This term is made up of the word

parts _____end_____ and _____crine_____.

PT.30. The term meaning a mature red blood cell is **erythrocyte**. This term is made up of the word

parts _____erythro_____ and _____cyte_____.

## Word Building

Write the word you created on the line provided.

### Regarding Nerves (neur/o means nerve)

PT.31. A surgical incision into a nerve is a/an _____Neurotomy_____.

PT.32. The study of the nervous system is known as _____Neuroscience_____.

PT.33. The surgical repair of a nerve or nerves is a/an _____Neuroplasty_____.

PT.34. The term meaning to suture the ends of a severed nerve is _neurorrhaphy_.

PT.35. Abnormal softening of the nerves is called _neuromalacia_

PT.36. A specialist in diagnosing and treating disorders of the nervous system is a/an _Neurologist_

PT.37. The term meaning inflammation of a nerve or nerves is _Neuritis_.

**Relating to Blood Vessels (angi/o means relating to the blood vessels)**

PT.38. The death of the walls of blood vessels is _Atherosclerosis_

PT.39. The abnormal hardening of the walls of blood vessels is _atherosclerosis_ ?

PT.40. The abnormal narrowing of a blood vessel is _stenosis_.

PT.41. The surgical removal of a blood vessel is a/an _Arteriectomy_

PT.42. The process of recording a picture of blood vessels is called _Angiography_

## Missing Words

Write the missing word on the line provided.

PT.43. The surgical repair of an artery is a/an _arterectomy_ (**arteri/o** means artery).

PT.44. The medical term meaning inflammation of the larynx is _larynxitis_ (**laryng/o** means larynx).

PT.45. The surgical removal of all or part of the colon is a/an _Colectomy_ (**col/o** means colon).

PT.46. The abnormal softening of muscle tissue is _myomalacia_ (**my/o** means muscle).

PT.47. The term meaning any abnormal condition of the stomach is _gastrosis_ (**gastr/o** means stomach).

PT.48. The term meaning the study of the heart is _Cardiology_ (**cardi/o** means heart).

PT.49. The term meaning inflammation of the colon is _colonitis_ (**col/o** means colon).

PT.50. The term meaning a surgical incision into a vein is _phlebotomy_ (**phleb/o** means vein).

# The Skeletal System

Overview of
## STRUCTURES, COMBINING FORMS, AND FUNCTIONS OF THE SKELETAL SYSTEM

| Major Structures | Related Combining Forms | Primary Functions |
| --- | --- | --- |
| Bones | **oss/e, oss/i, oste/o, ost/o** | Act as the framework for the body, protect the internal organs, and store the mineral calcium. |
| Bone Marrow | **myel/o** (also means spinal cord) | Red bone marrow forms some blood cells. Yellow bone marrow stores fat. |
| Cartilage | **chondr/o** | Creates a smooth surface for motion within the joints and protects the ends of the bones. |
| Joints | **arthr/o** | Work with the muscles to make a variety of motions possible. |
| Ligaments | **ligament/o** | Connect one bone to another. |
| Synovial Membrane | **synovi/o, synov/o** | Forms the lining of synovial joints and secretes synovial fluid. |
| Synovial Fluid | **synovi/o, synov/o** | Lubricant that makes smooth joint movements possible. |
| Bursa | **burs/o** | Cushions areas subject to friction during movement. |

## Vocabulary Related to **THE SKELETAL SYSTEM**

This list contains essential word parts and medical terms for this chapter. These terms are pronounced in the StudyWARE™ and Audio CDs that are available for use with this text. These and the other important **primary terms** are shown in boldface throughout the chapter. *Secondary terms*, which appear in *orange* italics, clarify the meaning of primary terms.

### Word Parts

- [ ] **ankyl/o** crooked, bent, stiff
- [ ] **arthr/o** joint
- [ ] **chondr/i, chondr/o** cartilage
- [ ] **cost/o** rib
- [ ] **crani/o** skull
- [ ] **-desis** to bind, tie together
- [ ] **kyph/o** bent, hump
- [ ] **lord/o** curve, swayback, bent
- [ ] **-lysis** loosening or setting free
- [ ] **myel/o** spinal cord, bone marrow
- [ ] **oss/e, oss/i, ost/o, oste/o** bone
- [ ] **scoli/o** curved, bent
- [ ] **spondyl/o** vertebrae, vertebral column, backbone
- [ ] **synovi/o, synov/o** synovial membrane, synovial fluid
- [ ] **-um** singular noun ending

### Medical Terms

- [ ] **acetabulum** (**ass**-eh-**TAB**-you-lum)
- [ ] **allogenic** (**al**-oh-**JEN**-ick)
- [ ] **ankylosing spondylitis** (**ang**-kih-**LOH**-sing spon-dih-**LYE**-tis)
- [ ] **arthrodesis** (**ar**-throh-**DEE**-sis)
- [ ] **arthrolysis** (ar-**THROL**-ih-sis)
- [ ] **arthroscopy** (ar-**THROS**-koh-pee)
- [ ] **autologous** (aw-**TOL**-uh-guss)
- [ ] **chondroma** (kon-**DROH**-mah)
- [ ] **chondromalacia** (**kon**-droh-mah-**LAY**-shee-ah)
- [ ] **comminuted fracture** (**KOM**-ih-**newt**-ed)
- [ ] **compression fracture**
- [ ] **costochondritis** (**kos**-toh-kon-**DRIGH**-tis)
- [ ] **craniostenosis** (**kray**-nee-oh-steh-**NOH**-sis)
- [ ] **crepitation** (**krep**-ih-**TAY**-shun)
- [ ] **dual x-ray absorptiometry** (ab-**sorp**-shee-**OM**-eh-tree)
- [ ] **fibrous dysplasia** (dis-**PLAY**-see-ah)
- [ ] **hallux valgus** (**HAL**-ucks **VAL**-guss)

- [ ] **hemarthrosis** (**hem**-ar-**THROH**-sis)
- [ ] **hemopoietic** (**hee**-moh-poy-**ET**-ick)
- [ ] **internal fixation**
- [ ] **juvenile rheumatoid arthritis** (**ROO**-mah-toyd ar-**THRIGH**-tis)
- [ ] **kyphosis** (kye-**FOH**-sis)
- [ ] **laminectomy** (**lam**-ih-**NECK**-toh-mee)
- [ ] **lordosis** (lor-**DOH**-sis)
- [ ] **lumbago** (lum-**BAY**-goh)
- [ ] **malleolus** (mal-**LEE**-oh-lus)
- [ ] **manubrium** (mah-**NEW**-bree-um)
- [ ] **metacarpals** (met-ah-**KAR**-palz)
- [ ] **metatarsals** (met-ah-**TAHR**-salz)
- [ ] **myeloma** (my-eh-**LOH**-mah)
- [ ] **open fracture**
- [ ] **orthopedic surgeon** (**or**-thoh-**PEE**-dick)
- [ ] **orthotic** (or-**THOT**-ick)
- [ ] **osteitis** (**oss**-tee-**EYE**-tis)
- [ ] **osteoarthritis** (**oss**-tee-oh-ar-**THRIGH**-tis)
- [ ] **osteochondroma** (**oss**-tee-oh-kon-**DROH**-mah)
- [ ] **osteoclasis** (**oss**-tee-**OCK**-lah-sis)
- [ ] **osteomalacia** (**oss**-tee-oh-mah-**LAY**-shee-ah)
- [ ] **osteomyelitis** (**oss**-tee-oh-**my**-eh-**LYE**-tis)
- [ ] **osteonecrosis** (**oss**-tee-oh-neh-**KROH**-sis)
- [ ] **osteopenia** (**oss**-tee-oh-**PEE**-nee-ah)
- [ ] **osteoporosis** (**oss**-tee-oh-poh-**ROH**-sis)
- [ ] **osteoporotic hip fracture** (**oss**-tee-oh-pah-**ROT**-ick)
- [ ] **osteorrhaphy** (**oss**-tee-**OR**-ah-fee)
- [ ] **Paget's disease** (**PAJ**-its)
- [ ] **pathologic fracture**
- [ ] **percutaneous vertebroplasty** (**per**-kyou-**TAY**-nee-us **VER**-tee-broh-**plas**-tee)
- [ ] **periostitis** (**pehr**-ee-oss-**TYE**-tis)
- [ ] **podiatrist** (poh-**DYE**-ah-trist)
- [ ] **prosthesis** (pros-**THEE**-sis)
- [ ] **rheumatoid arthritis** (**ROO**-mah-toyd ar-**THRIGH**-tis)
- [ ] **rickets** (**RICK**-ets)
- [ ] **scoliosis** (**skoh**-lee-**OH**-sis)
- [ ] **spina bifida** (**SPY**-nah **BIF**-ih-dah)
- [ ] **spiral fracture**
- [ ] **spondylolisthesis** (**spon**-dih-loh-liss-**THEE**-sis)
- [ ] **spondylosis** (**spon**-dih-**LOH**-sis)
- [ ] **subluxation** (**sub**-luck-**SAY**-shun)
- [ ] **synovectomy** (**sin**-oh-**VECK**-toh-mee)
- [ ] **vertebrae** (**VER**-teh-bray)

## LEARNING GOALS

On completion of this chapter, you should be able to:

1. Identify and describe the major functions and structures of the skeletal system.

2. Describe three types of joints.

3. Differentiate between the axial and appendicular skeletons.

4. Identify the medical specialists who treat disorders of the skeletal system.

5. Recognize, define, spell, and pronounce the primary terms related to the pathology and the diagnostic and treatment procedures of the skeletal system.

# ■ STRUCTURES AND FUNCTIONS OF THE SKELETAL SYSTEM

The skeletal system consists of the bones, bone marrow, cartilage, joints, ligaments, synovial membrane, synovial fluid, and bursa. This body system has many important functions:

- Bones act as the framework of the body.

- Bones support and protect the internal organs.

- Joints work in conjunction with muscles, ligaments, and tendons, making possible the wide variety of body movements. (Muscles and tendons are discussed in Chapter 4.)

- Calcium, which is required for normal nerve and muscle function, is stored in bones.

- Red bone marrow, which has an important function in the formation of blood cells, is located within spongy bone.

## The Formation of Bones

A baby's skeleton begins as fragile membranes and cartilage, but after three months it starts turning into bone in a process called **ossification** (**oss**-us-fih-**KAY**-shun), which continues through adolescence.

Even after growth is completed, this process of new bone formation continues as *osteoclasts* break down old or damaged bone and *osteoblasts* help rebuild the bone. Ossification repairs the minor damage to the skeletal system that occurs during normal activity and also repairs bones after injuries such as fractures.

# ■ THE STRUCTURE OF BONES

Bone is the form of connective tissue that is the second hardest tissue in the human body. Only dental enamel is harder than bone.

## The Tissues of Bone

Although it is a dense and rigid tissue, bone is also capable of growth, healing, and reshaping itself (Figure 3.1).

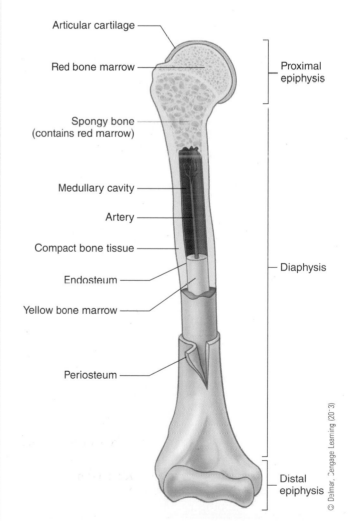

Articular cartilage

Red bone marrow

Spongy bone (contains red marrow)

Medullary cavity

Artery

Compact bone tissue

Endosteum

Yellow bone marrow

Periosteum

Proximal epiphysis

Diaphysis

Distal epiphysis

© Dalmar, Cengage Learning (2013)

**FIGURE 3.1** Anatomic features of a typical long bone.

- **Periosteum** (**pehr**-ee-**OSS**-tee-um) is the tough, fibrous tissue that forms the outermost covering of bone (**peri-** means surrounding, **oste** means bone, and **-um** is a noun ending).

- **Compact bone**, also known as *cortical bone*, is the dense, hard, and very strong bone that forms the protective outer layer of bones.

- **Spongy bone**, also known as *cancellous bone*, is lighter and not as strong as compact bone. This type of bone is commonly found in the ends and inner portions of long bones such as the femur. Red bone marrow is located within this spongy bone.

- The **medullary cavity** (**MED**-you-**lehr**-ee) is the central cavity located in the shaft of long bones where it is surrounded by compact bone. It is here that red and yellow bone marrow are stored. *Medullary* means pertaining to the inner section.

- The **endosteum** (en-**DOS**-tee-um) is the tissue that lines the medullary cavity (**end-** means within, **oste** means bone, and **-um** is a noun ending).

## Bone Marrow

- **Red bone marrow**, which is located within the spongy bone, is a hemopoietic tissue that manufactures red blood cells, hemoglobin, white blood cells, and thrombocytes. These types of cells are discussed in Chapter 5.

- **Hemopoietic** (**hee**-moh-poy-**ET**-ick) means pertaining to the formation of blood cells (**hem/o** means blood, and **-poietic** means pertaining to formation). This term is also spelled *hematopoietic*.

- **Yellow bone marrow** functions as a fat storage area. It is composed chiefly of fat cells and is located in the medullary cavity of long bones.

## Cartilage

- **Cartilage** (**KAR**-tih-lidj) is the smooth, rubbery, blue-white connective tissue that acts as a shock absorber between bones. Cartilage, which is more elastic than bone, also makes up the flexible parts of the skeleton such as the outer ear and the tip of the nose.

- **Articular cartilage** (ar-**TICK**-you-lar **KAR**-tih-lidj) covers the surfaces of bones where they come together to form joints. This cartilage makes smooth joint movement possible and protects the bones from rubbing against each other (Figures 3.1 and 3.3).

- The **meniscus** (meh-**NIS**-kus) is the curved fibrous cartilage found in some joints, such as the knee and the temporomandibular joint of the jaw (Figure 3.3).

## Anatomic Landmarks of Bones

- The **diaphysis** (dye-**AF**-ih-sis) is the shaft of a long bone (Figure 3.1).

- The **epiphyses** (ep-**PIF**-ih-seez) are the wider ends of long bones such as the femurs of the legs (singular *epiphysis*). Each epiphysis is covered with articular cartilage to protect it. The *proximal epiphysis* is the end of the bone located nearest to the midline of the body. The *distal epiphysis* is the end of the bone located farthest away from the midline of the body.

- A **foramen** (foh-**RAY**-men) is an opening in a bone through which blood vessels, nerves, and ligaments pass (plural, *foramina*). For example, the spinal cord passes through the *foramen magnum* of the occipital bone at the base of the skull.

- A **process** is a normal projection on the surface of a bone that most commonly serves as an attachment for a muscle or tendon For example, the *mastoid process* is the bony projection located on temporal bones just behind the ears (Figure 3.6).

# ■ JOINTS

**Joints**, which are also known as *articulations*, are the place of union between two or more bones. Joints are classified either according to their construction or based on the degree of movement they allow.

## Fibrous Joints

**Fibrous joints**, consisting of inflexible layers of dense connective tissue, hold the bones tightly together. In adults these joints, which are also known as *sutures*, do not allow any movement (Figure 3.6). In newborns and very young children, some fibrous joints are movable before they have solidified.

- The **fontanelles** (**fon**-tah-**NELLS**), also known as the *soft spots*, are normally present on the skull of a newborn. These flexible soft spots facilitate the passage of the infant through the birth canal. They also allow for the growth of the skull during the first year. As the child matures, and the sutures close, the fontanelles gradually harden.

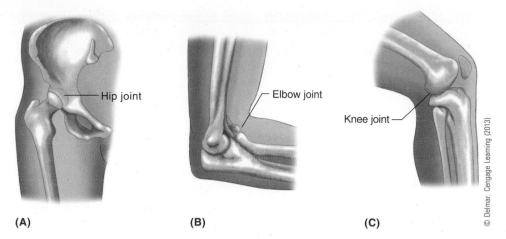

**FIGURE 3.2** Examples of *synovial joints*. (A) Ball-and-socket joint of the hip. (B) Hinge joint of the elbow. (C) Hinge joint of the knee.

## Cartilaginous Joints

**Cartilaginous joints** (**kar**-tih-**LADJ**-ih-nus) allow only slight movement and consist of bones connected entirely by cartilage. For example:

- Where the ribs connect to the sternum (breast bone), shown in Figure 3.8, these joints allow movement during breathing.

- The **pubic symphysis** (**PEW**-bick **SIM**-fih-sis) allows some movement to facilitate childbirth. This joint is located between the pubic bones in the anterior (front) of the pelvis as shown in Figure 3.12.

## Synovial Joints

A **synovial joint** (sih-**NOH**-vee-al) is created where two bones articulate to permit a variety of motions. As used here, the term *articulate* means to come together. These joints are also described based on their type of motion (Figure 3.2).

- *Ball-and-socket joints*, such as the hips and shoulders, allow a wide range of movement in many directions (Figure 3.2A).

- *Hinge joints*, such as the knees and elbows, are synovial joints that allow movement primarily in one direction or plane (Figure 3.2B and 3.2C).

### Components of Synovial Joints

Synovial joints consist of several components that make complex movements possible (Figure 3.3).

- The **synovial capsule** is the outermost layer of strong fibrous tissue that resembles a sleeve as it surrounds the joint.

- The **synovial membrane** lines the capsule and secretes synovial fluid.

- **Synovial fluid**, which flows within the synovial cavity, acts as a lubricant to make the smooth movement of the joint possible.

- **Ligaments** (**LIG**-ah-mentz) are bands of fibrous tissue that form joints by connecting one bone to another bone or by joining a bone to cartilage. Complex hinge joints, such as the knee as shown in Figures 3.2 and 3.3, are made up of a series of ligaments that permit movement in different directions.

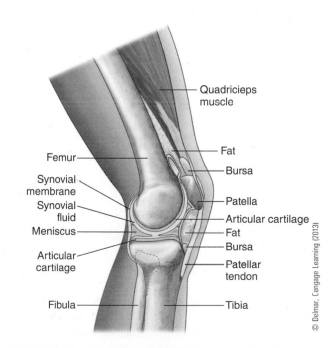

**FIGURE 3.3** A lateral view of the knee showing the structures of a *synovial joint* and *bursa*.

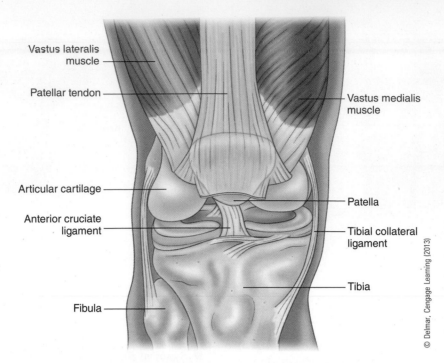

Vastus lateralis
muscle

Patellar tendon

Vastus medialis
muscle

Articular cartilage

Patella

Anterior cruciate
ligament

Tibial collateral
ligament

Tibia

Fibula

© Delmar, Cengage Learning (2013)

**FIGURE 3.4** Major ligaments of the knee. This anterior view of the knee shows the complex system of ligaments that make its movements possible.

■ A **bursa** (**BER**-sah) is a fibrous sac that acts as a cushion to ease movement in areas that are subject to friction, such as in the shoulder, elbow, and knee joints where a tendon passes over a bone (plural, *bursae*).

## ■ THE SKELETON

The typical adult human skeleton consists of approximately 206 bones, as shown in Figure 3.5. Depending upon the age of the individual, the exact number of bones ranges from 206 to 350. For descriptive purposes, the skeleton is divided into the axial and appendicular skeletal systems.

### Axial Skeleton

The **axial skeleton** protects the major organs of the nervous, respiratory, and circulatory systems. In the human, the axial skeleton consists of the 80 bones of the head and body that are organized into five parts. These are (1) the bones of the skull, (2) the ossicles (bones) of the middle ear, (3) the hyoid bone, located on the throat between the chin and the thyroid, (4) the rib cage, and (5) the vertebral column.

### Appendicular Skeleton

The **appendicular skeleton** makes body movement possible and also protects the organs of digestion, excretion, and reproduction. In the human, the appendicular skeleton consists of 126 bones that are organized into: (1) the

*upper extremities* (shoulders, arms, forearms, wrists, and hands) and (2) the *lower extremities* (hips, thighs, legs, ankles, and feet).

An *appendage* is anything that is attached to a major part of the body and the term *appendicular* means referring to an appendage. An *extremity* is the terminal end of a body part such as an arm or leg.

## Bones of the Skull

The **skull** consists of the 8 bones that form the cranium, 14 bones that form the face, and 6 bones in the middle ear. As you study the following bones of the skull, refer to Figures 3.6 and 3.7.

### The Bones of the Cranium

The **cranium** (**KRAY**-nee-um), which is made up of the following eight bones, is that portion of the skull that encloses and protects the brain (**crani** means skull, and **-um** is a noun ending). These cranial bones are joined by jagged fibrous joints that are often referred to as **sutures.**

■ The **frontal bone** is the anterior portion of the cranium that forms the forehead. This bone houses the frontal sinuses and forms the roof of the ethmoid sinuses, the nose and part of the socket that protects the eyeball.

■ The **parietal bones** (pah-**RYE**-eh-tal) are two of the largest bones of the skull. Together they form most of the roof and upper sides of the cranium.

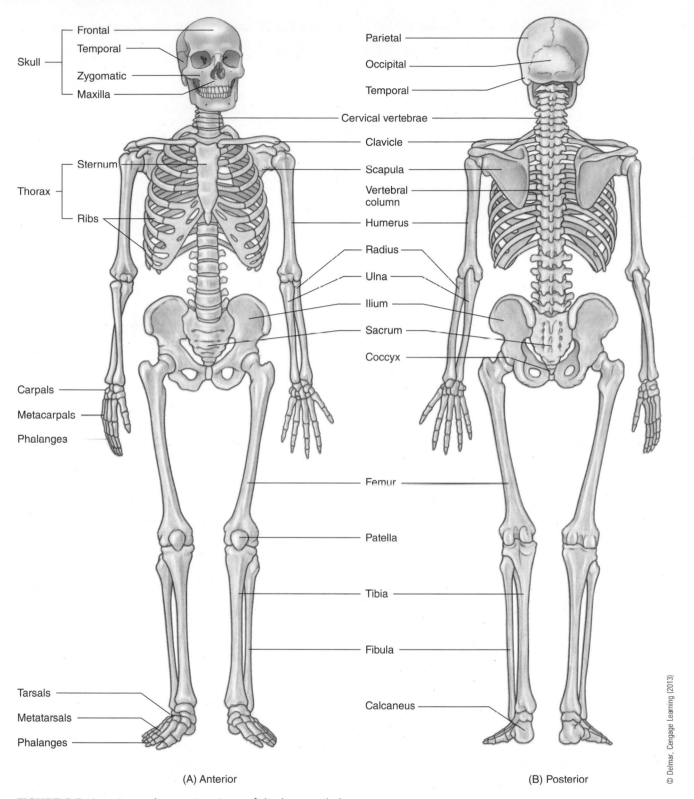

**FIGURE 3.5** Anterior and posterior views of the human skeleton.

- The **occipital bone** (ock-**SIP**-ih-tal) forms the back part of the skull and the base of the cranium.
- The two **temporal bones** form the sides and base of the cranium.

- The **external auditory meatus** (mee-**AY**-tus) is the opening of the external auditory canal of the outer ear. This canal is located within the temporal bone on each side of the skull. A *meatus* is the external opening of a canal.

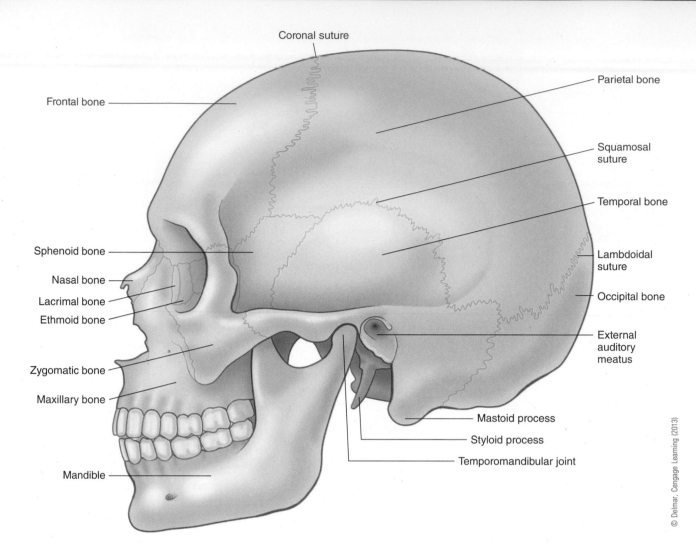

**FIGURE 3.6** Lateral view of the adult human skull.

- The **sphenoid bone** (**SFEE**-noid) is an irregular, wedge-shaped bone at the base of the skull. This bone makes contact with all of the other cranial bones and helps form the base of the cranium, the sides of the skull, and the floors and sides of the eye sockets.

- The **ethmoid bone** (**ETH**-moid) is light, spongy bone located at the roof and sides of the nose. Here it separates the nasal cavity from the brain, and it also forms a portion of each orbit. An *orbit* is the bony socket that surrounds and protects each eyeball.

### The Auditory Ossicles

The **auditory ossicles** (**OSS**-ih-kulz) are the three tiny bones located in each middle ear. These bones, known as the *malleus*, *incus*, and *stapes*, are discussed in Chapter 11.

### The Bones of the Face

- The face is made up of the following 14 bones. Some of these bones contain air-filled cavities known as

sinuses. Among the purposes of these sinuses is to lighten the weight of the skull. (These sinuses are discussed in Chapter 7.)

- The two **nasal bones** form the upper part of the bridge of the nose.

- The two **zygomatic bones** (**zye**-goh-**MAT**-ick), also known as the *cheekbones*, articulate with the frontal bone that makes up the forehead. The term *articulate* means to join together with.

- The two **maxillary bones** (**MACK**-sih-**ler**-ee) form most of the upper jaw (singular, *maxilla*). These bones are also known as the *maxillae.*

- The two **palatine bones** (**PAL**-ah-tine) form the anterior (front) part of the hard palate of the mouth and the floor of the nose.

- The two **lacrimal bones** (**LACK**-rih-mal) make up part of the orbit (socket of the eye) at the inner angle.

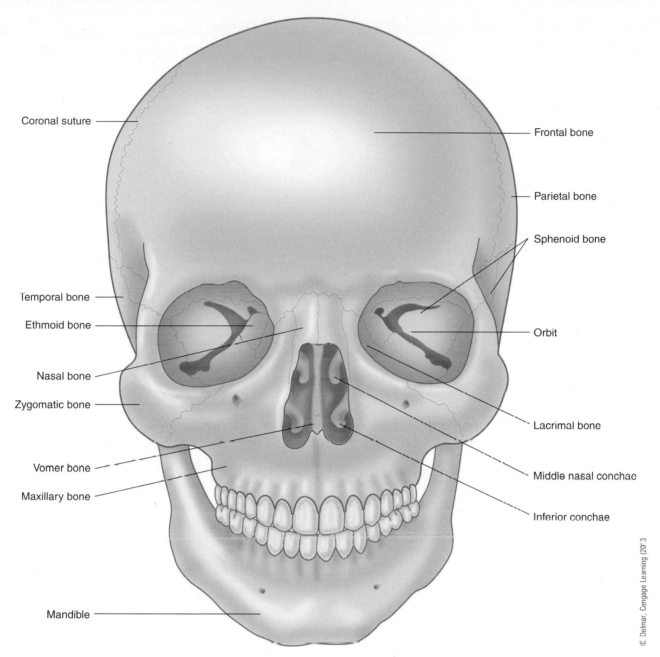

Coronal suture

Frontal bone

Parietal bone

Sphenoid bone

Temporal bone

Ethmoid bone

Orbit

Nasal bone

Zygomatic bone

Lacrimal bone

Vomer bone

Middle nasal conchae

Maxillary bone

Inferior conchae

Mandible

© Delmar, Cengage Learning (2013)

**FIGURE 3.7** Anterior view of the adult human skull.

- The two **inferior conchae** (**KONG** kee *or* **KONG**-kay) are the thin, scroll-like bones that form part of the interior of the nose (singular, *concha*).

- The **vomer bone** (**VOH**-mer) forms the base for the nasal septum. The *nasal septum* is the cartilage wall that divides the two nasal cavities.

- The **mandible** (**MAN**-dih-bul), also known as the *jawbone*, is the only movable bone of the skull. The mandible is attached to the skull at the **temporo-mandibular joint** (**tem**-poh-roh-man-**DIB**-you-lar), which is commonly known as the *TMJ* (Figure 3.6).

## Thoracic Cavity

The **thoracic cavity** (thoh-**RAS**-ick), also known as the *rib cage*, is the bony structure that protects the heart and lungs. It consists of the ribs, sternum, and upper portion of the spinal column extending from the neck to the diaphragm, but not including the arms.

### The Ribs

The 12 pairs of **ribs**, which are also known as *costals*, attach posteriorly to the thoracic vertebrae (**cost** means rib, and -**al** means pertaining to) (Figure 3.8).

- The first seven pairs of ribs are called *true ribs*, and they attach anteriorly to the sternum.
- The next three pairs of ribs are called *false ribs*, and they attach anteriorly to cartilage that connects them to the sternum.
- The last two pairs of ribs are called *floating ribs*, because they are only attached posteriorly to the vertebrae but are not attached anteriorly.

## The Sternum

The **sternum** (**STER**-num), which is also known as the *breast bone*, is a flat, dagger-shaped bone located in the middle of the chest. By joining with the ribs, it forms the front of the rib cage. This is divided into three parts (Figure 3.8).

- The **manubrium** (mah-**NEW**-bree-um) is the bony structure that forms the upper portion of the sternum.
- The **body of the sternum** is the bony structure that forms the middle portion of the sternum.
- The **xiphoid process** (**ZIF**-oid) is the structure made of cartilage that forms the lower portion of the sternum.

## The Shoulders

The shoulders form the **pectoral girdle** (**PECK**-toh-rahl), which supports the arms and hands. This is also known as the *shoulder girdle*. As used here, the term *girdle* refers to a structure that encircles the body. As you study the bones of the shoulder, refer to Figures 3.5 and 3.8.

- The **clavicle** (**KLAV**-ih-kul), also known as the *collar bone*, is a slender bone that connects the manubrium of the sternum to the scapula.
- The **scapula** (**SKAP**-you-lah) is also known as the *shoulder blade* (plural, *scapulae*).
- The **acromion** (ah-**KROH**-mee-on) is an extension of the scapula that forms the high point of the shoulder.

## The Arms

As you study the bones of the arms, refer to Figures 3.5 and 3.8.

- The **humerus** (**HEW**-mer-us) is the bone of the upper arm (plural, *humeri*).
- The **radius** (**RAY**-dee-us) is the smaller and shorter bone in the forearm. The radius runs up the thumb side of the forearm (plural, *radius bones*).

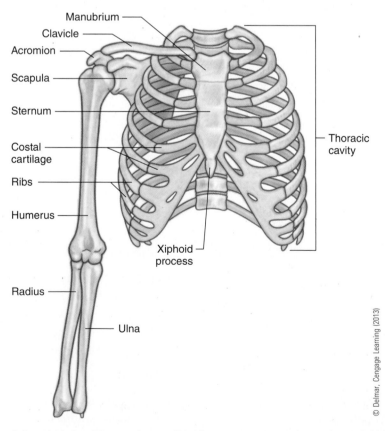

**FIGURE 3.8** Anterior view of the ribs, shoulder, and arm. (Cartilaginous structures are shown in blue.)

© Delmar, Cengage Learning (2013)

- The **ulna** (**ULL**-nah) is the larger and longer bone of the forearm (plural, *ulnae*). The proximal end of the ulna articulates with the distal end of the humerus to form the elbow joint.

- The **olecranon process** (oh-**LEK**-rah-non), commonly known as the *funny bone*, is a large projection on the upper end of the ulna. This forms the point of the elbow and exposes a nerve that tingles when struck.

## The Wrists, Hands, and Fingers

As you study these bones, refer to Figure 3.9.

- The eight **carpals** (**KAR**-palz) are the bones that form the wrist (singular, *carpal*). These bones form a narrow bony passage known as the *carpal tunnel*. The median nerve and the tendons of the fingers pass through this tunnel to reach the hand. *Carpal tunnel syndrome* is described in Chapter 4.

- The **metacarpals** (met-ah-**KAR**-palz) are the five bones that form the palms of the hand.

- The **phalanges** (fah-**LAN**-jeez) are the 14 bones of the fingers (singular, *phalanx*). The bones of the toes are also known as phalanges.

- Each of the four fingers has three bones. These are the distal (outermost), middle, and proximal (nearest the hand) phalanges.

- The thumb has two bones. These are the distal and proximal phalanges.

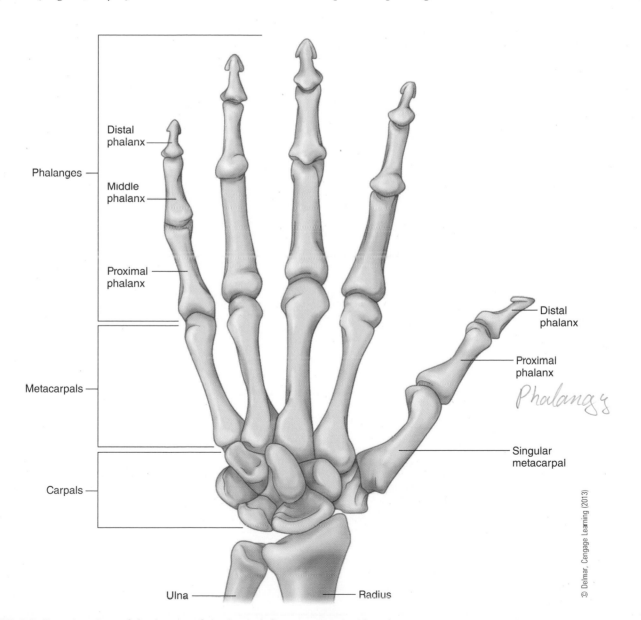

**FIGURE 3.9** Superior view of the bones of the lower left arm, wrist, and hand.

© Delmar, Cengage Learning (2013)

# The Spinal Column

The **spinal column,** which is also known as the *vertebral column*, protects the spinal cord and supports the head and body. The spinal column consists of 26 **vertebrae** (**VER**-teh-bray). Each of these bony units is known as a **vertebra** (**VER**-teh-bruh), and the term *vertebral* means pertaining to the vertebrae.

## The Structures of Vertebrae

As you study the structures of a vertebra, refer to Figure 3.10.

■ The anterior portion of the vertebra is solid to provide strength and is known as the *body of the vertebra.*

■ The posterior portion of a vertebra is known as the **lamina** (**LAM**-ih-nah) (plural, *laminae*). The transverse and spinous processes extend from this area and serve as attachments for muscles and tendons.

■ The *vertebral foramen* is the opening in the middle of the vertebra. This opening allows the spinal cord to pass through and to protect the spinal cord.

## Intervertebral Disks

**Intervertebral disks** (in-ter-**VER**-teh-bral), which are made of cartilage, separate and cushion the vertebrae from each other. They also act as shock absorbers and allow for movement of the spinal column (Figure 3.18A).

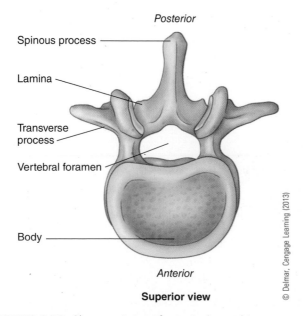

**FIGURE 3.10** Characteristics of a typical vertebra.

# The Types of Vertebrae

As you study the types of vertebrae, refer to Figure 3.11A & B.

■ The **cervical vertebrae** (**SER**-vih-kal) are the first set of 7 vertebrae, and they form the neck. The term *cervical* means pertaining to the neck, and these vertebrae are also known as **C1** through **C7**.

■ The **thoracic vertebrae** (thoh-**RASS**-ick), known as **T1** through **T12**, are the second set of 12 vertebrae.

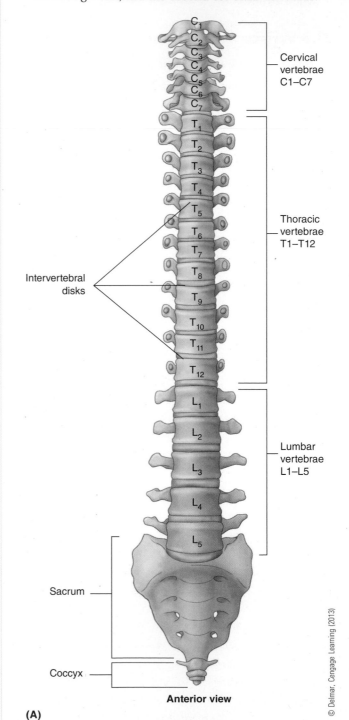

**(A)**

**FIGURE 3.11A** Anterior view of the vertebral column.

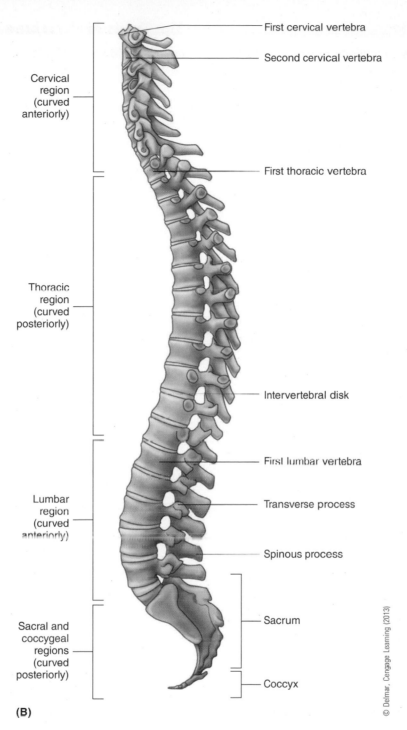

Cervical region (curved anteriorly)

Thoracic region (curved posteriorly)

Lumbar region (curved anteriorly)

Sacral and coccygeal regions (curved posteriorly)

First cervical vertebra

Second cervical vertebra

First thoracic vertebra

Intervertebral disk

First lumbar vertebra

Transverse process

Spinous process

Sacrum

Coccyx

© Delmar, Cengage Learning (2013)

**(B)**

**FIGURE 3.11B** Lateral view of the vertebral column.

Each of these vertebra has a pair of ribs attached to it, and together they form the outward curve of the spine. *Thoracic* means pertaining to the thoracic cavity.

- The **lumbar vertebrae** (**LUM**-bar), known as **L1** through **L5**, make up the third set of 5 vertebrae, and together they form the inward curve of the lower spine. These are the largest and strongest of the vertebrae, and they bear most of the body's weight. *Lumbar* means relating to the part of the back and sides between the ribs and the pelvis.

The remaining two vertebrae are the sacrum and the coccyx. As you study these structures, refer to Figure 3.11.

- The **sacrum** (**SAY**-krum) is the slightly curved, triangular-shaped bone near the base of the spine that forms the lower portion of the back. At birth, the sacrum is composed of five separate bones; however in the young child, they fuse together to form a single bone.

- The **coccyx** (**KOCK**-sicks), which is also known as the *tailbone*, forms the end of the spine and is actually made up of four small vertebrae that are fused together.

## The Pelvic Girdle

The **pelvic girdle** protects internal organs and supports the lower extremities. It is commonly known as the *pelvis* or *hips*. The pelvis is a cup-shaped ring of bone at the lower end of the trunk, and it consists of the *ilium*, *ischium*, and *pubis* (Figures 3.12 and 3.14).

- The **ilium** (**ILL**-ee-um) is the broad blade-shaped bone that forms the back and sides of the pubic bone.

- The **sacroiliac** (**say**-kroh-**ILL**-ee-ack) is the slightly movable articulation between the sacrum and posterior portion of the ilium (**sacr/o** means sacrum, **ili** means ilium, and **-ac** means pertaining to).

- The **ischium** (**ISS**-kee-um), which forms the lower posterior portion of the pubic bone, bears the weight of the body when sitting.

- The **pubis** (**PEW**-bis), which forms the anterior portion of the pubic bone, is located just below the urinary bladder.

- At birth the *ilium*, *ischium*, and *pubis* are three separate bones. As the child matures, these bones fuse to form the left and right **pubic bones**, which are held securely together by the pubic symphysis.

- The **pubic symphysis** is the cartilaginous joint that unites the left and right pubic bones. A *cartilaginous joint* allows slight movement between bones.

- The **acetabulum** (**ass**-eh-**TAB**-you-lum), also known as the *hip socket*, is the large circular cavity in each side of the pelvis that articulates with the head of the femur to form the hip joint (Figures 3.12 and 3.14).

## The Legs and Knees

As you study these bones, refer to Figures 3.13 and 3.14.

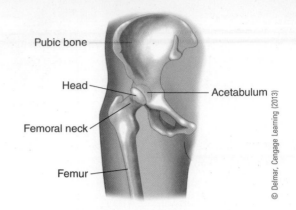

**FIGURE 3.13** Structures of the proximal end of the femur and the acetabulum (hip socket).

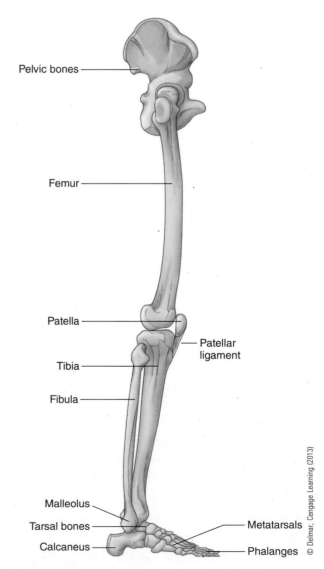

**FIGURE 3.14** Lateral view of bones of the lower extremity.

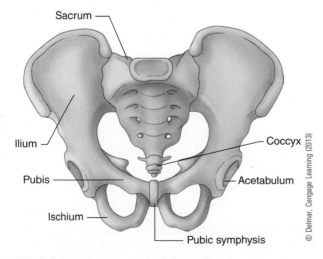

**FIGURE 3.12** Anterior view of the pelvis.

### The Femurs

- The **femurs** (**FEE**-murz) are the largest bones in the body. *Femoral* means pertaining to the femur.
- These bones are also known as *thigh bones.*
- The *head of the femur* articulates with the acetabulum (hip socket).
- The *femoral neck* is the narrow area just below the head of the femur.

### The Knees

- The **patella** (pah-**TEL**-ah), also known as the *kneecap*, is the bony anterior portion of the knee.
- The term **popliteal** (pop-**LIT**-ee-al) describes the posterior space behind the knee where the ligaments, vessels, and muscles related to this joint are located.
- The **cruciate ligaments** (**KROO**-shee-ayt), which are shown in Figure 3.4, make possible the movements of the knee. These are known as the *anterior* and *posterior cruciate ligaments* because they are shaped like a cross.

### The Lower Legs

The lower leg is made up of the *tibia* and the *fibula* (Figure 3.14).

- The **tibia** (**TIB**-ee-ah), also known as the *shinbone*, is the larger anterior weight-bearing bone of the lower leg.
- The **fibula** (**FIB**-you-lah) is the smaller of the two bones of the lower leg.

### The Ankles

- The **ankles** are the joints that connect the lower leg and foot and make the necessary movements possible.
- Each ankle is made up of seven short **tarsal** (**TAHR**-sal) bones. These bones are similar to the bones of the wrists; however, they are much larger in size (Figure 3.15).
- The **malleolus** (mal-**LEE**-oh-lus) is a rounded bony projection on the tibia and fibula on the sides of each ankle joint (plural, *malleoli*).
- The **talus** (**TAY**-luss) is the ankle bone that articulates with the tibia and fibula (Figures 3.15 and 3.17).
- The **calcaneus** (kal-**KAY**-nee-uss), also known as the *heel bone*, is the largest of the tarsal bones (Figures 3.14 and 3.15).

### The Feet and Toes

The feet and toes are made up of the following bones as shown in Figure 3.15.

- The five **metatarsals** (met-ah-**TAHR**-salz) form that part of the foot to which the toes are attached.
- The **phalanges** are the bones of the toes. The great toe has two phalanges. Each of the other toes has three phalanges. The bones of the fingers are also called phalanges.

## ▪ MEDICAL SPECIALTIES RELATED TO THE SKELETAL SYSTEM

- A **chiropractor** (**KYE**-roh-**prack**-tor) holds a Doctor of Chiropractic (DC) degree and specializes in the manipulative treatment of disorders originating from misalignment of the spine. *Manipulative treatment* involves manually adjusting the positions of the bones.
- An **orthopedic surgeon** (or-thoh-**PEE**-dick), also known as an *orthopedist*, is a physician who specializes in diagnosing and treating diseases and disorders involving the bones, joints, and muscles.
- An **osteopath** (**oss**-tee-oh-**PATH**) holds a Doctor of Osteopathy (DO) degree and uses traditional forms of medical treatment in addition to specializing in treating health problems by spinal manipulation (**oste/o** means bone, and **-path** means disease). This type of medical practice is known as *osteopathy*; however, that term is also used to mean any bone disease.
- A **podiatrist** (poh-**DYE**-ah-trist) holds a Doctor of Podiatry (DP) or Doctor of Podiatric Medicine (DPM) degree and specializes in diagnosing and treating disorders of the foot (**pod** mean foot, and **-iatrist** means specialist).
- A **rheumatologist** (roo-mah-**TOL**-oh-jist) is a physician who specializes in the diagnosis and treatment of arthritis and disorders such as osteoporosis, fibromyalgia, and tendinitis that are characterized by inflammation in the joints and connective tissues.

## ▪ PATHOLOGY OF THE SKELETAL SYSTEM

### Joints

- **Ankylosis** (**ang**-kih-**LOH**-sis) is the loss or absence of mobility in a joint due to disease, injury, or a surgical procedure (**ankyl** means crooked, bent, or stiff, and

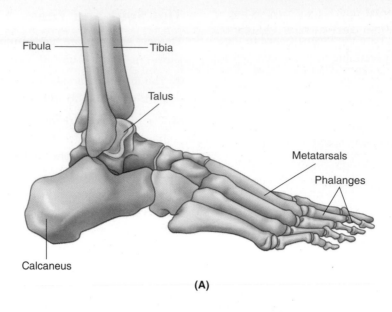

**(A)**

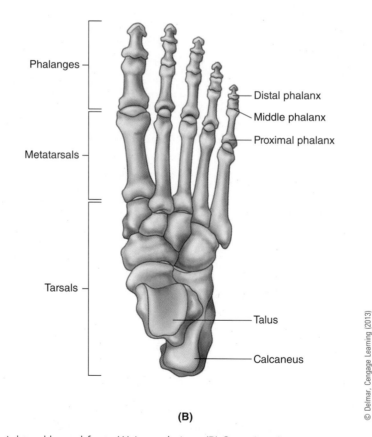

**(B)**

**FIGURE 3.15** Bones of the right ankle and foot. (A) Lateral view. (B) Superior view.

© Delmar, Cengage Learning (2013)

-**osis** means abnormal condition or disease). *Mobility* means being capable of movement.

■ **Arthrosclerosis** (**ar**-throh-skleh-**ROH**-sis) is stiffness of the joints, especially in the elderly (**arthr/o** means joint, and -**sclerosis** means abnormal hardening).

■ **Bursitis** (ber-**SIGH**-tis) is an inflammation of a bursa (**burs** means bursa, and -**itis** means inflammation).

■ **Chondromalacia** (**kon**-droh-mah-**LAY**-shee-ah) is the abnormal softening of cartilage (**chondr/o** means cartilage, and -**malacia** means abnormal softening).

- A **chondroma** (kon-**DROH**-mah) is a slow-growing benign tumor derived from cartilage cells (**chondr** means cartilage, and **-oma** means tumor).

- **Costochondritis** (**kos**-toh-kon-**DRIGH**-tis) is an inflammation of the cartilage that connects a rib to the sternum (**cost/o** means rib, **chondr** means cartilage, and **-itis** means inflammation).

- **Hallux valgus** (**HAL**-ucks **VAL**-guss), also known as a *bunion*, is an abnormal enlargement of the joint at the base of the great toe (*hallux* means big toe, and *valgus* means bent).

- **Hemarthrosis** (hem-ar-**THROH**-sis) is blood within a joint (**hem** means blood, **arthr** means joint, and **-osis** means abnormal condition or disease). This condition is frequently due to a joint injury. It also can occur spontaneously in patients taking blood-thinning medications or those having a blood clotting disorder such as hemophilia (see Chapters 2 and 5).

- **Polymyalgia rheumatica** (PMR) (pol-ee-my-**AL**-jah roo-**MA**-tih-kah) is a geriatric inflammatory disorder of the muscles and joints characterized by pain and stiffness in the neck, shoulders, upper arms, and hips and thighs (**poly-** means many, **my** means muscle, and **–algia** means pain). *Rheumatica* is the Latin word for *rheumatism*, an obsolete term for arthritis and other disorders causing pain in the joints and supporting tissue.

- A *sprain* occurs when a ligament that connects bones to a joint is wrenched or torn (see Chapter 4).

- **Synovitis** (sin-oh-**VYE**-tiss) is inflammation of the synovial membrane that results in swelling and pain of the affected joint (**synov** means synovial membrane, and **-itis** means inflammation). This condition can be caused by arthritis, trauma, infection, or irritation produced by damaged cartilage.

## Dislocation

- **Dislocation**, also known as *luxation* (luck-**SAY**-shun), is the total displacement of a bone from its joint (Figure 3.16).

- **Subluxation** (**sub**-luck-**SAY**-shun) is the partial displacement of a bone from its joint.

## Arthritis

**Arthritis** (ar-**THRIGH**-tis) is an inflammatory condition of one or more joints (**arthr** means joint, and **-itis** means inflammation). There are more than 100 types of arthritis with many different causes. Some of the more common types of arthritis follow.

## Osteoarthritis

**Osteoarthritis** (OA) (oss-tee-oh-ar-**THRIGH**-tis), also known as *wear-and-tear arthritis*, is most commonly associated with aging (**oste/o** means bone, **arthr** means joint, and **-itis** means inflammation) (Figure 3.17).

- OA is known as a *degenerative joint disease* because it is characterized by the wearing away of the articular cartilage within the joints. *Degenerative* means the breaking down or impairment of a body part.

- It is also characterized by hypertrophy of bone and the formation of **osteophytes** (**OSS**-tee-oh-fites), also known as bone spurs.

  **Spondylosis** (**spon**-dih-**LOH**-sis) is also known as *spinal osteoarthritis*. This degenerative disorder can cause the loss of normal spinal structure and function (**spondyl** means vertebrae, and **-osis** means abnormal condition or disease).

## Gouty Arthritis

**Gouty arthritis** (**GOW**-tee ar-**THRIGH**-tis), also known as *gout*, is a type of arthritis characterized by deposits of uric

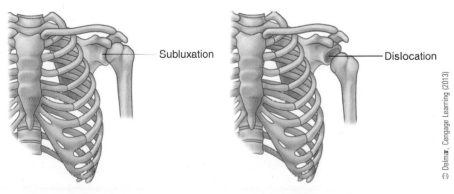

**FIGURE 3.16** *Subluxation* and *dislocation* shown on an anterior view of the left shoulder.

Subluxation

Dislocation

© Delmar, Cengage Learning (2013)

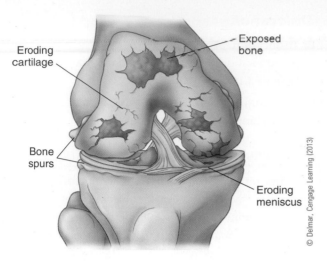

**FIGURE 3.17** Damage to the knee joint caused by *osteoarthritis*.

acid in the joints. *Uric acid* is a by-product that is normally excreted by the kidneys. Gout develops when excess uric acid, which is present in the blood, forms crystals in the joints of the feet and legs.

## Rheumatoid Arthritis

**Rheumatoid arthritis** (**ROO**-mah-toyd ar-**THRIGH**-tis), commonly known as *RA*, is a chronic autoimmune disorder in which the joints and some organs of other body systems are attacked. *Autoimmune disorders* are described in Chapter 6.

- As RA progressively attacks the synovial membranes, they become inflamed and thickened so that the joints are increasingly swollen, painful, and immobile.

## Ankylosing Spondylitis

**Ankylosing spondylitis** (**ang**-kih-**LOH**-sing **spon** dih-**LYE**-tis) is a form of rheumatoid arthritis that primarily causes inflammation of the joints between the vertebrae. *Ankylosing* means the progressive stiffening of a joint or joints, and *spondylitis* means inflammation of the vertebrae.

## Juvenile Rheumatoid Arthritis

**Juvenile rheumatoid arthritis** is an autoimmune disorder that affects children ages 16 years or less with symptoms that include stiffness, pain, joint swelling, skin rash, fever, slowed growth, and fatigue.

## The Spinal Column

- A **herniated disk** (**HER**-nee-**ayt**-ed), also known as a *slipped* or *ruptured disk*, is the breaking apart of an intervertebral disk that results in pressure on spinal nerve roots (Figure 3.18B).

- **Lumbago** (lum-**BAY**-goh), also known as *low back pain*, is pain of the lumbar region of the spine (**lumb** means lumbar, and **-ago** means diseased condition).

- **Spondylolisthesis** (**spon**-dih-loh-liss-**THEE**-sis) is the forward slipping movement of the body of one of the lower lumbar vertebrae on the vertebra or sacrum below it (**spondyl/o** means vertebrae, and **-listhesis** means slipping).

- **Spina bifida** (**SPY**-nah **BIF**-ih-dah) is a congenital defect that occurs during early pregnancy when the spinal canal fails to close completely around the spinal

*Hernia abnound*

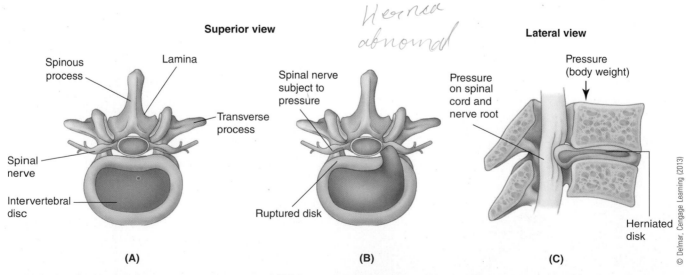

**FIGURE 3.18** (A) Superior view of a normal intervertebral disk. (B) Superior and (C) lateral views of a ruptured disk causing pressure on a spinal nerve.

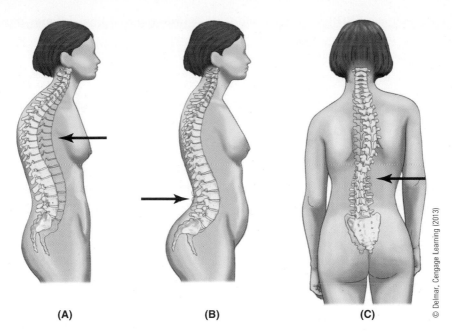

**FIGURE 3.19** Abnormal curvatures of the spine. (A) *Kyphosis*. (B) *Lordosis*. (C) *Scoliosis*. (Normal curvatures are shown in shadow.)

cord to protect it. *Spina* means pertaining to the spine. *Bifida* means split. Some cases of spina bifida are due to a lack of the nutrient folic acid during the early stages of pregnancy.

## Curvatures of the Spine

■ **Kyphosis** (kye-**FOH**-sis) is an abnormal increase in the outward curvature of the thoracic spine as viewed from the side (**kyph** means hump, and -**osis** means abnormal condition or disease). This condition, also known as *humpback* or *dowager's hump*, is frequently associated with aging (Figure 3.19A).

■ **Lordosis** (lor-**DOH**-sis) is an abnormal increase in the forward curvature of the lumbar spine (**lord** means bent backward, and -**osis** means abnormal condition or disease). This condition is also known as *swayback* (Figure 3.19B).

■ **Scoliosis** (skoh-lee-**OH**-sis) is an abnormal lateral (sideways) curvature of the spine (**scoli** means curved, and -**osis** means abnormal condition or disease) (Figure 3.19C).

**StudyWARE   CONNECTION**

View the **Curvatures of the Spine** animation in the StudyWARE™.

## Bones

■ **Craniostenosis** (**kray**-nee-oh-steh-**NOH**-sis) is a malformation of the skull due to the premature closure of the cranial sutures (**crani/o** means skull, and -**stenosis** means abnormal narrowing).

■ **Fibrous dysplasia** (dis-**PLAY**-see-ah) is a bone disorder of unknown cause that destroys normal bone structure and replaces it with fibrous (scarlike) tissue. This leads to uneven growth, brittleness, and deformity of the affected bones.

■ **Ostealgia** (**oss**-tee-**AL**-jee-ah), also known as *osteodynia*, means pain in a bone (**oste** means bone, and -**algia** means pain).

■ **Osteitis** (**oss**-tee-**EYE**-tis), also spelled *ostitis*, is an inflammation of a bone (**oste** means bone, and -**itis** means inflammation).

■ **Osteomalacia** (**oss**-tee-oh-mah-**LAY**-shee-ah), also known as *adult rickets*, is abnormal softening of bones in adults (**oste/o** means bone, and -**malacia** means abnormal softening). This condition is usually caused by a deficiency of vitamin D, calcium, and/or phosphate. Compare with *rickets*, below.

■ **Osteomyelitis** (**oss**-tee-oh-**my**-eh-**LYE**-tis) is an inflammation of the bone marrow and adjacent bone (**oste/o** means bone, **myel** means bone marrow, and -**itis** means inflammation). The bacterial infection that causes osteomyelitis often originates in another part of the body and spreads to the bone via the blood.

- **Osteonecrosis** (oss-tee-oh-neh-**KROH**-sis) is the death of bone tissue due to insufficient blood supply (**oste/o** means bone, and **-necrosis** means tissue death).

- **Paget's disease** (**PAJ**-its), also known as *osteitis deformans*, is a bone disease of unknown cause. This condition is characterized by the excessive breakdown of bone tissue, followed by abnormal bone formation. The new bone is structurally enlarged, but weakened and filled with new blood vessels.

- **Periostitis** (pehr-ee-oss-**TYE**-tis) is an inflammation of the periosteum (**peri-** means surrounding, **ost** means bone, and **-itis** means inflammation). This condition is often associated with shin splints, which are discussed in Chapter 4.

- **Rickets** (**RICK**-ets), also known as *infantile osteomalacia*, is a deficiency disease occurring in children. This condition, which is characterized by defective bone growth, results from a vitamin D deficiency that is sometimes due to insufficient exposure to sunlight.

- **Short stature**, formerly known as *dwarfism*, is a condition resulting from the failure of the bones of the limbs to grow to an appropriate length compared to the size of the head and trunk. The average adult height is no more than 4 feet 10 inches, and these individuals now prefer to be referred to as *little people*.

- The term **talipes** (**TAL**-ih-peez), which is also known as *clubfoot*, describes any congenital deformity of the foot involving the talus (ankle bones).

## Bone Tumors

- **Primary bone cancer** is a relatively rare malignant tumor that originates in a bone. *Malignant* means becoming progressively worse and life-threatening. As an example, *Ewing's sarcoma* is a tumor that occurs in the bones of the upper arm, legs, pelvis, or rib. The peak incidence for the development of this condition is between ages 10 and 20 years.

- The term **secondary bone cancer** describes tumors that have metastasized (spread) to bones from other organs such as the breasts and lungs. Additional malignancies, sarcomas, and tumors are discussed in Chapter 6.

- A **myeloma** (my-eh-**LOH**-mah) is a type of cancer that occurs in blood-making cells found in the red bone marrow (**myel** means bone marrow, and **-oma** means tumor). This condition can cause pathologic fractures and is often fatal.

- An **osteochondroma** (oss-tee-oh-kon-**DROH**-mah) is a benign bony projection covered with cartilage

*non cancer*

(**oste/o** means bone, **chondr** means cartilage, and **-oma** means tumor). *Benign* means something that is not life-threatening and does not recur. This type of tumor is also known as an *exostosis* (plural, *exostoses*).

## Osteoporosis and Osteopenia Compared

**Osteoporosis** (oss-tee-oh-poh-**ROH**-sis) (OP) is a marked loss of bone density and an increase in bone porosity that is frequently associated with aging (**oste/o** means bone, **por** means small opening, and **-osis** means abnormal condition or disease).

**Osteopenia** (oss-tee-oh-**PEE**-nee-ah) is thinner-than-average bone density (**oste/o** means bone, and **-penia** means deficiency). This term is used to describe the condition of someone who does not yet have osteoporosis, but is at risk for developing it.

## Osteoporosis-Related Fractures

Osteoporosis is primarily responsible for three types of fractures:

- A **compression fracture**, also known as a *vertebral crush fracture*, occurs when the bone is pressed together (compressed) on itself. These fractures are sometimes caused by the spontaneous collapse of weakened vertebrae or can be due to an injury. This results in pain, loss of height, and development of the spinal curvature known as *dowager's hump*.

- A **Colles' fracture**, which is named for the Irish surgeon Abraham Colles, is also known as a *fractured wrist*. This fracture occurs at the lower end of the radius when a person tries to stop a fall by landing on his or her hands. The impact of this fall causes the bone weakened by osteoporosis to break (Figure 3.20).

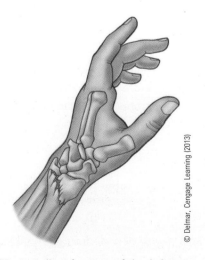

© Delmar, Cengage Learning (2013)

**FIGURE 3.20** A *Colles' fracture* of the left wrist.

■ An **osteoporotic hip fracture** (**oss**-tee-oh-pah-**ROT**-ick), also known as a *broken hip*, is usually caused by weakening of the bones due to osteoporosis and can occur either spontaneously or as the result of a fall. Complications from these fractures can result in the loss of function, mobility, independence, or death. *Osteoporotic* means pertaining to or caused by the porous condition of bones.

## Fractures

A **fracture**, which is a *broken bone*, is described in terms of its complexity. As you study this section, follow Figure 3.21.

■ A **closed fracture**, also known as a *simple fracture* or a *complete fracture*, is one in which the bone is broken, but there is no open wound in the skin (see also Figure 3.22).

■ An **open fracture**, also known as a *compound fracture*, is one in which the bone is broken and there is an open wound in the skin.

■ A **comminuted fracture** (**KOM**-ih-**newt**-ed) is one in which the bone is splintered or crushed. Comminuted means crushed into small pieces.

■ A **greenstick fracture**, or *incomplete fracture*, is one in which the bone is bent and only partially broken. This type of fracture occurs primarily in children.

■ An **oblique fracture** occurs at an angle across the bone.

■ A **pathologic fracture** occurs when a weakened bone breaks under normal strain. This is due to bones being

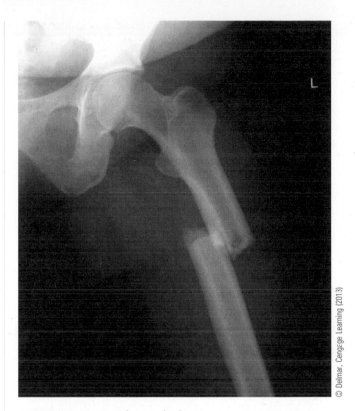

weakened by osteoporosis or a disease process such as cancer.

■ A **spiral fracture** is a fracture in which the bone has been twisted apart. This type of fracture occurs as the result of a severe twisting motion such as in a sports injury.

■ A **stress fracture**, which is an overuse injury, is a small crack in the bone that often develops from chronic,

**FIGURE 3.22** A radiograph showing an anteroposterior (AP) view of a closed fracture of the femur.

© Delmar, Cengage Learning (2013)

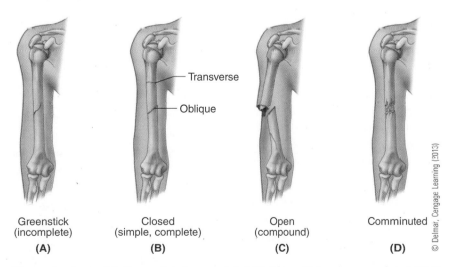

Greenstick
(incomplete)
**(A)**

Closed
(simple, complete)
**(B)**

Open
(compound)
**(C)**

Comminuted

**(D)**

Transverse

Oblique

© Delmar, Cengage Learning (2013)

**FIGURE 3.21** Types of bone fractures. (A) Greenstick (incomplete) (B) Closed (simple, complete) (C) Open (compound) (D) Comminuted

excessive impact. Additional overuse and sports injuries are discussed in Chapter 4.

- A **transverse fracture** occurs straight across the bone.

## Additional Terms Associated with Fractures

- A **fat embolus** (**EM**-boh-lus) can form when a long bone is fractured and fat cells from yellow bone marrow are released into the blood. An *embolus* is any foreign matter circulating in the blood that can become lodged and block the blood vessel.

- **Crepitation** (**krep**-ih-**TAY**-shun), also known as *crepitus*, is the grating sound heard when the ends of a broken bone move together. This term also describes the crackling sound heard in lungs affected with pneumonia and the clicking sound heard in the movements of some joints.

- As the bone heals, a **callus** (**KAL**-us) forms as a bulging deposit around the area of the break. This tissue eventually becomes bone. A *callus* is also a thickening of the skin caused by repeated rubbing.

## ■ DIAGNOSTIC PROCEDURES OF THE SKELETAL SYSTEM

- A **radiograph**, also known as an *x-ray*, is the use of x-radiation to visualize bone fractures and other abnormalities (Figure 3.22).

- **Arthroscopy** (ar-**THROS**-koh-pee) is the visual examination of the internal structure of a joint (**arthr/o** means joint, and **-scopy** means visual examination) using an *arthroscope*.

- A **bone marrow biopsy** is a diagnostic test that may be necessary after abnormal types or numbers of red or white blood cells are found in a complete blood count test.

- *Bone marrow aspiration* is the use of a syringe to withdraw the liquid bone marrow. This procedure is used to obtain tissue for diagnostic purposes or to collect bone marrow for medical procedures such as stem cell transplantation.

- **Magnetic resonance imaging** (MRI) is used to image soft tissue structures such as the interior of complex joints. It is not the most effective method of imaging hard tissues such as bone.

- *Bone scans* and *arthrocentesis*, which are additional diagnostic procedures, are discussed in Chapter 15.

## Bone Density Testing

**Bone density testing** (BDT) is used to determine losses or changes in bone density. These tests are used to diagnose conditions such as osteoporosis, osteomalacia, osteopenia, and Paget's disease.

- **Ultrasonic bone density testing** is a screening test for osteoporosis or other conditions that cause a loss of bone mass. In this procedure, sound waves are used to take measurements of the calcaneus (heel) bone. If the results indicate risks, more definitive testing is indicated.

- **Dual x-ray absorptiometry** (ab-**sorp**-shee-**OM**-eh-tree) is a low-exposure radiographic measurement of the spine and hips to measure bone density. This test produces more accurate results than ultrasonic bone density testing.

## ■ TREATMENT PROCEDURES OF THE SKELETAL SYSTEM

### Bone Marrow Transplants

A **bone marrow transplant** (BMT) is used to treat certain types of cancers, such as leukemia and lymphomas, which affect bone marrow. Leukemia is discussed in Chapter 5, and lymphomas are discussed in Chapter 6.

- In this treatment, initially both the cancer cells and the patient's bone marrow are destroyed with high-intensity radiation and chemotherapy.

- Next, healthy bone marrow stem cells are transfused into the recipient's blood. These cells migrate to the spongy bone, where they multiply to form cancer-free red bone marrow. *Stem cells* produced by the bone marrow eventually develop into blood cells. (See Chapter 2 for more information on stem cells.)

### Types of Bone Marrow Transplants

An **allogenic bone marrow transplant** uses healthy bone marrow cells from a compatible donor, often a sibling. However, unless this is a perfect match, there is the danger that the recipient's body will reject the transplant. **Allogenic** (**al**-oh-**JEN**-ick) means originating within another.

In an **autologous bone marrow transplant**, the patient receives his own bone marrow cells, which have been harvested, cleansed, treated, and stored before the remaining bone marrow in the patient's body is destroyed. **Autologous** (aw-**TOL**-uh-guss) means originating within an individual.

*C.T. computerized tomography*

## Medical Devices

- An **orthotic** (or-**THOT**-ick) is a mechanical appliance, such as a leg brace or a splint, that is specially designed to control, correct, or compensate for impaired limb function.

- A **prosthesis** (pros-**THEE**-sis) is a substitute for a diseased or missing body part, such as a leg that has been amputated (plural, *prostheses*).

## Joints

- **Arthrodesis** (ar-throh-**DEE**-sis), also known as *surgical ankylosis*, is the surgical fusion (joining together) of two bones to stiffen a joint, such as an ankle, elbow, or shoulder (**arthr/o** means joint, and **-desis** means to bind, tie together). This procedure is performed to treat severe arthritis or a damaged joint. Compare with *arthrolysis*.

- **Arthrolysis** (ar-**THROL**-ih-sis) is the surgical loosening of an ankylosed joint (**arthr/o** means joint, and **-lysis** means loosening or setting free). Note: The suffix **-lysis** also means breaking down or destruction, and may indicate either a pathologic state or a therapeutic procedure. Compare with *arthrodesis*.

- **Arthroscopic surgery** (ar-throh-**SKOP**-ick) is a minimally invasive procedure for the treatment of the interior of a joint. For example, torn cartilage can be removed with the use of an arthroscope and instruments inserted through small incisions (Figure 3.23).

- **Chondroplasty** (**KON**-droh-**plas**-tee) is the surgical repair of damaged cartilage (**chondr/o** means cartilage, and **-plasty** means surgical repair).

- A **synovectomy** (sin-oh-**VECK**-toh-mee) is the surgical removal of a synovial membrane from a joint (**synov** means synovial membrane, and **-ectomy** means surgical removal). One use of this procedure, which can be performed endoscopically, is to repair joint damage caused by rheumatoid arthritis.

- **Viscosupplementations** (**vis**-ko **sup**-leh-men-**TAY**-shunz) are injections used to add a preparation of hyaluronic acid and related compounds to a joint, easing friction and making movement easier. This is often used to treat osteoarthritis, especially in the knees. *Synvisc* is one of the products used for this purpose.

## Joint Replacements

Based on its word parts, the term **arthroplasty** (**AR**-throh-**plas**-tee) means the surgical repair of a damaged joint (**arthr/o** means joint, and **-plasty** means surgical repair); however, this term has come to mean the surgical placement of an artificial joint. These procedures are named for the involved joint and the amount of the joint that is replaced (Figures 3.24 and 3.25).

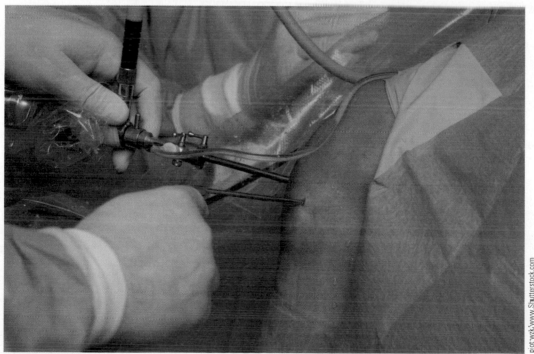

**FIGURE 3.23** During arthroscopic surgery, the physician is able to view the interior of the knee on a monitor.

- The joint replacement part is a prosthesis that is commonly referred to as an *implant*.

- A **total knee replacement** (TKR) means that all of the parts of the knee were replaced. This procedure is also known as a *total knee arthroplasty* (Figure 3.24).

- A **partial knee replacement** (PKR) describes a procedure in which only part of the knee is replaced.

- A **total hip replacement** (THR), also known as a *total hip arthroplasty*, is performed to restore a damaged hip to full function. During the surgery, a plastic lining is fitted into the acetabulum to restore a smooth surface. The head of the femur is removed and replaced with a metal ball attached to a metal shaft that is fitted into the femur (see Figure 3.25). These smooth surfaces restore the function of the hip joint.

- **Hip resurfacing** is an alternative to removing the head of the femur. Function is restored to the hip by placing a metal cap over the head of the femur to allow it to move smoothly over a metal lining in the acetabulum.

- **Revision surgery** is the replacement of a worn or failed implant.

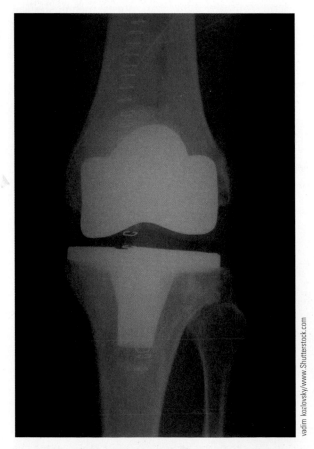

**FIGURE 3.24** Radiograph (x-ray) of a total knee replacement. On the film the metallic components appear brighter than the bone.

## Spinal Column

- A **percutaneous diskectomy** (**pcr**-kyou-**TAY**-nee-us dis-**KECK**-toh-mee) is performed to treat a herniated intervertebral disk. In this procedure, a thin tube is inserted through the skin of the back to suction out the ruptured disk or to vaporize it with a laser. *Percutaneous* means performed through the skin.

- **Percutaneous vertebroplasty** (**per**-kyou-**TAY**-nee-us **VER**-tee-broh-**plas**-tee) is performed to treat osteoporosis-related compression fractures (**vertebr/o** means vertebra, and **-plasty** means surgical repair). In this minimally invasive procedure, bone cement is injected to stabilize compression fractures within the spinal column.

- A **laminectomy** (**lam**-ih-**NECK**-toh-mee) is the surgical removal of a lamina or posterior portion of a vertebra (**lamin** means lamina, and **-ectomy** means surgical removal).

- **Spinal fusion** is a technique to immobilize part of the spine by joining together (fusing) two or more vertebrae. *Fusion* means to join together.

## Bones

- A **craniectomy** (**kray**-nee-**EK**-toh-mee) is the surgical removal of a portion of the skull (**crani** means skull, and **-ectomy** means surgical removal). This procedure is performed to treat craniostenosis or to relieve increased intracranial pressure due to swelling of the brain. The term *intracranial pressure* describes the amount of pressure inside the skull.

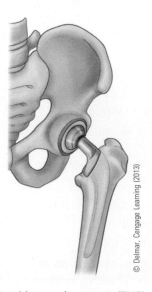

**FIGURE 3.25** Total hip replacement (THR).

- A **craniotomy** (**kray**-nee-**OT**-oh-mee) is a surgical incision or opening into the skull (**crani** means skull, and **-otomy** means a surgical incision). This procedure is performed to gain access to the brain to remove a tumor, to relieve intracranial pressure, or to obtain access for other surgical procedures.

- A **cranioplasty** (**KRAY**-nee-oh-**plas**-tee) is the surgical repair of the skull (**crani/o** means skull, and **-plasty** means surgical repair).

- **Osteoclasis** (**oss**-tee-**OCK**-lah-sis) is the surgical fracture of a bone to correct a deformity (**oste/o** means bone, and **-clasis** means to break).

- An **ostectomy** (oss-**TECK**-toh-mee) is the surgical removal of bone (**ost** means bone, and **-ectomy** means the surgical removal).

- **Osteoplasty** (**OSS**-tee-oh-**plas**-tee) is the surgical repair of a bone or bones (**oste/o** means bone, and **-plasty** means surgical repair).

- **Osteorrhaphy** (**oss**-tee-**OR**-ah-fee) is the surgical suturing, or wiring together, of bones (**oste/o** means bone, and **-rrhaphy** means surgical suturing).

- **Osteotomy** (**oss**-tee-**OT**-oh-mee) is the surgical cutting of a bone (**oste** means bone, and **-otomy** means a surgical incision). This may include removing part or all of a bone, or cutting into or through a bone.

- A **periosteotomy** (**pehr**-ee-**oss**-tee-**OT**-oh-mee) is an incision through the periosteum to the bone (**peri-** means surrounding, **oste** means bone, and **-otomy** means surgical incision).

## Treatment of Fractures

- **Closed reduction**, also known as *manipulation*, is the attempted realignment of the bone involved in a fracture or joint dislocation. The affected bone is returned to its normal anatomic alignment by manually applied force and then is usually immobilized to maintain the realigned position during healing.

- When a closed reduction is not practical, a surgical procedure known as an *open reduction* is required to realign the bone parts.

- **Immobilization**, also known as *stabilization*, is the act of holding, suturing, or fastening the bone in a fixed position with strapping or a cast.

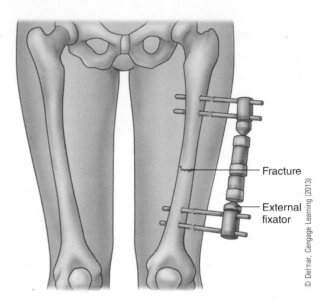

**FIGURE 3.26** *External fixation* of the femur stabilizes the bone and is removed after the bone has healed.

- **Traction** is a pulling force exerted on a limb in a distal direction in an effort to return the bone or joint to normal alignment.

### External and Internal Fixation

- **External fixation** is a fracture treatment procedure in which pins are placed through the soft tissues and bone so that an external appliance can be used to hold the pieces of bone firmly in place during healing. When healing is complete, the appliance is removed (Figure 3.26).

- **Internal fixation**, also known as *open reduction internal fixation* (ORIF), is a fracture treatment in which a plate or pins are placed directly into the bone to hold the broken pieces in place. This form of fixation is *not* usually removed after the fracture has healed (Figure 3.27).

## ABBREVIATIONS RELATED TO THE SKELETAL SYSTEM

Table 3.1 presents an overview of the abbreviations related to the terms introduced in this chapter. Note: To avoid errors or confusion, always be cautious when using abbreviations.

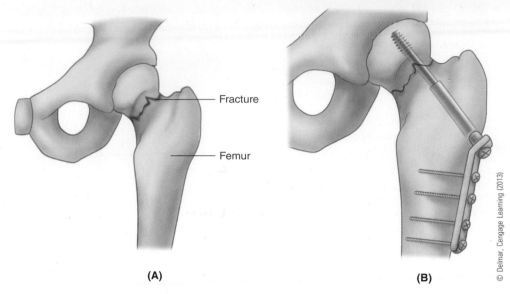

Fracture

Femur

© Delmar, Cengage Learning (2013)

(A)    (B)

**FIGURE 3.27** *Internal fixation* of fractured hip. (A) Fracture of the femoral neck. (B) *Internal fixation* pins are placed to stabilize the bone. These pins are not removed after the bone has healed.

## TABLE 3.1
## Abbreviations Related to the Skeletal System

| | |
|---|---|
| **bone density testing** = BDT | **BDT** = bone density testing |
| **closed reduction** = CR | **CR** = closed reduction |
| **fracture** = Fx | **Fx** = fracture |
| **osteoarthritis** = OA | **OA** = osteoarthritis |
| **osteoporosis** = OP | **OP** = osteoporosis |
| **partial knee replacement** = PKR | **PKR** = partial knee replacement |
| **polymyalgia rheumatica** = PMR | **PMR** = polymyalgia rheumatica |
| **rheumatoid arthritis** = RA | **RA** = rheumatoid arthritis |
| **total hip arthroplasty** = THA | **THA** = total hip arthroplasty |
| **total knee arthroplasty** = TKA | **TKA** = total knee arthroplasty |

**StudyWARE** **CONNECTION**

For more practice and to test your mastery of this material, go to the StudyWARE™ to play interactive games and complete the quiz for this chapter.

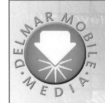

Downloadable audio is available for selected medical terms in this chapter to enhance your learning of medical terminology.

☐ **Workbook Practice**

Go to your workbook and complete the exercises for this chapter.

# LEARNING EXERCISES

## MATCHING WORD PARTS 1

Write the correct answer in the middle column.

| Definition | | Correct Answer | Possible Answers |
|---|---|---|---|
| 3.1. | hump | | ankyl/o |
| 3.2. | cartilage | | arthr/o |
| 3.3. | crooked, bent, stiff | | -um |
| 3.4. | joint | | kyph/o |
| 3.5. | singular noun ending | | chondr/i, chondr/o |

## MATCHING WORD PARTS 2

Write the correct answer in the middle column.

| Definition | | Correct Answer | Possible Answers |
|---|---|---|---|
| 3.6. | cranium, skull | | cost/o |
| 3.7. | rib | | crani/o |
| 3.8. | setting free, loosening | | -desis |
| 3.9. | spinal cord, bone marrow | | -lysis |
| 3.10. | to bind, tie together | | myel/o |

## MATCHING WORD PARTS 3

Write the correct answer in the middle column.

| Definition | | Correct Answer | Possible Answers |
|---|---|---|---|
| 3.11. | vertebrae | | oste/o |
| 3.12. | curved | | spondyl/o |

3.13.   swayback bent _____ **lord/o**

3.14.   synovial membrane _____ **synovi/o, synov/o**

3.15.   bone _____ **scoli/o**

## DEFINITIONS

Select the correct answer, and write it on the line provided.

3.16.   The shaft of a long bone is known as the _____.

   diaphysis          distal epiphysis          endosteum          proximal epiphysis

3.17.   Seven short _____ bones make up each ankle.

   carpal          metatarsal          phalanx          tarsal

3.18.   The upper portion of the sternum is the _____.

   clavicle          mandible          manubrium          xiphoid process

3.19.   A _____ is movable.

   cartilaginous joint          fibrous joint          suture joint          synovial joint

3.20.   The _____ bone is located just below the urinary bladder.

   ilium          ischium          pubis          sacrum

3.21.   The opening in a bone through which blood vessels, nerves, and ligaments pass

   is a _____.

   foramen          foramina          process          symphysis

3.22.   A/An _____ connects one bone to another bone.

   articular cartilage          ligament          synovial membrane          phalange

3.23.   The hip socket is known as the _____.

   acetabulum          malleolus          patella          trochanter

3.24.   The bones of the fingers and toes are known as the _____.

   carpals          metatarsals          tarsals          phalanges

3.25. A normal projection on the surface of a bone that serves as an attachment for muscles and tendons is

known as a/an _____.

    cruciate                exostosis                popliteal                process

## MATCHING STRUCTURES

Write the correct answer in the middle column.

| Definition | Correct Answer | Possible Answers |
|---|---|---|
| 3.26.  breast bone | _____ | clavicle |
| 3.27.  cheekbones | _____ | olecranon process |
| 3.28.  collar bone | _____ | sternum |
| 3.29.  kneecap | _____ | patella |
| 3.30.  point of the elbow | _____ | zygomatic |

## WHICH WORD?

Select the correct answer, and write it on the line provided.

3.31. The surgical procedure for loosening of an ankylosed joint is known as _____.

        arthrodesis               arthrolysis

3.32. The bone disorder of unknown cause that destroys normal bone structure and replaces it with fibrous

(scarlike) tissue is known as _____.

      fibrous dysplasia       Paget's disease

3.33. An _____ bone marrow transplant uses bone marrow from a donor.

         allogenic            autologous

3.34. A percutaneous _____ is performed to treat osteoporosis-related compression

fractures.

        diskectomy          vertebroplasty

3.35. The medical term for the form of arthritis that is commonly known as wear-and-tear arthritis

is _____.

        osteoarthritis      rheumatoid arthritis

## SPELLING COUNTS

Find the misspelled word in each sentence. Then write that word, spelled correctly, on the line provided.

3.36.   The medical term for the condition commonly known as low back pain is

lumbaego. ___lumbago___ ✓

3.37.   The surgical fracture of a bone to correct a deformity is known as osteclasis. ___Osteoclasis___ ✓

3.38.   Ankylosing spondilitis is a form of rheumatoid arthritis that primarily causes inflammation of the joints

between the vertebrae. ___Spondylitis___ ✓

3.39.   An osterrhaphy is the surgical suturing, or wiring together, of bones. ___Osteorhaphy___ ✓

3.40.   Crepetation is the grating sound heard when the ends of a broken bone move

together. ___Crepetation___ ✓

## ABBREVIATION IDENTIFICATION

Write the correct answer on the line provided.

3.41.   **BMT**        _____

3.42.   **CR**         _____

3.43.   **Fx**         _____

3.44.   **RA**         _____

3.45.   **TMJ**        _____

## TERM SELECTION

Select the correct answer, and write it on the line provided.

3.46.   The term meaning the death of bone tissue is _____.

osteitis deformans          osteomyelitis          osteonecrosis          osteoporosis

3.47.   An abnormal increase in the forward curvature of the lumbar spine is known

as _____.

kyphosis              lordosis              scoliosis              spondylosis

3.48.   The condition known as _____ is a congenital defect.

juvenile arthritis          osteoarthritis          rheumatoid arthritis          spina bifida

3.49.　A type of cancer that occurs in blood-making cells found in the red bone marrow is known as a/

　　　an _____.

　　　　　　chondroma　　　　　Ewing's sarcoma　　　　　myeloma　　　　　osteochondroma

3.50.　The bulging deposit that forms around the area of the break during the healing of a fractured bone is

　　　a _____.

　　　　　　callus　　　　　　　crepitation　　　　　　crepitus　　　　　　luxation

## SENTENCE COMPLETION

Write the correct term or terms on the lines provided.

3.51.　A/An _____ is performed to gain access to the brain or to relieve intracranial

　　　pressure.

3.52.　The partial displacement of a bone from its joint is known as _____.

3.53.　The procedure that stiffens a joint by joining two bones is _____. This is also

　　　known as surgical ankylosis.

3.54.　The surgical placement of an artificial joint is known as _____.

3.55.　A medical term for the condition commonly known as a bunion is _____.

## WORD SURGERY

Divide each term into its component word parts. Write these word parts, in sequence, on the lines provided. When necessary, use a slash (/) to indicate a combining vowel. (You may not need all of the lines provided.)

3.56.　**Hemarthrosis** is blood within a joint.

　　　_____　　　　_____　　　　_____　　　　_____

3.57.　An **osteochondroma** is a benign bony projection covered with cartilage.

　　　_____　　　　_____　　　　_____　　　　_____

3.58.　**Osteomalacia**, also known as adult rickets, is abnormal softening of bones in adults.

　　　_____　　　　_____　　　　_____　　　　_____

3.59.　**Periostitis** is an inflammation of the periosteum.

　　　_____　　　　_____　　　　_____　　　　_____

3.60.   **Spondylolisthesis** is the forward slipping movement of the body of one of the lower lumbar vertebrae on

the vertebra or sacrum below it.

_____        _____        _____        _____

## TRUE/FALSE

If the statement is true, write **True** on the line. If the statement is false, write **False** on the line.

3.61.   _____ Osteopenia is thinner-than-average bone density. This term is used to

describe the condition of someone who does not yet have osteoporosis, but is at risk for developing it.

3.62.   _____ Paget's disease is caused by a deficiency of calcium and vitamin D in early

childhood.

3.63.   _____ Costochondritis is an inflammation of the cartilage that connects a rib to the

sternum.

3.64.   _____ Dislocation is the partial displacement of a bone from its joint.

3.65.   _____ Arthroscopic surgery is a minimally invasive procedure for the treatment of

the interior of a joint.

## CLINICAL CONDITIONS

Write the correct answer on the line provided.

3.66.   When Bobby Kuhn fell out of a tree, the bone in his arm was bent and partially broken. Dr. Grafton

described this as a/an _____ fracture and told the family that this type of fracture

occurs primarily in children.

3.67.   Eduardo Sanchez was treated for an inflammation of the bone and bone marrow. The medical term for

this condition is _____.

3.68.   Beth Hubert's breast cancer spread to her bones. These new sites are referred to

as _____ _____ _____.

3.69.   Mrs. Morton suffers from dowager's hump. The medical term for this abnormal curvature of the spine

is _____.

3.70. Henry Turner wears a brace to compensate for the impaired function of his leg. The medical term for this orthopedic appliance is a/an _____.

3.71. As the result of a head injury in an auto accident, Sam Cheng required a/an _____ to relieve the rapidly increasing intracranial pressure.

3.72. Mrs. Gilmer has leukemia and requires a bone marrow transplant. Part of the treatment was the harvesting of her bone marrow so she could receive it later as a/an _____ bone marrow transplant.

3.73. Betty Greene has been running for several years; however, now her knees hurt. Dr. Morita diagnosed her condition as _____, which is an abnormal softening of the cartilage in these joints.

3.74. Patty Turner (age 7) has symptoms that include a skin rash, fever, slowed growth, fatigue, and swelling in the joints. She was diagnosed as having juvenile _____ arthritis.

3.75. Heather Lewis has a very sore shoulder. Dr. Plunkett diagnosed this as an inflammation of the bursa and said that Heather's condition is _____.

## WHICH IS THE CORRECT MEDICAL TERM?

Select the correct answer, and write it on the line provided

3.76. Rodney Horner is being treated for a _____ fracture in which the ends of the bones were crushed together.

        Colles'        comminuted        compound        spiral

3.77. Alex Jordon fell and injured her knee. Her doctor performed a/an _____ to surgically repair the damaged cartilage.

        arthroplasty        chondroma        chondroplasty        osteoplasty

3.78. Mrs. Palmer is at high risk for osteoporosis. To obtain a definitive evaluation of the status of her bone density, Mrs. Palmer's physician ordered a/an _____ test.

        dual x-ray absorptiometry        MRI        x-ray        ultrasonic bone density

3.79.　In an effort to return a fractured bone to normal alignment, Dr. Wong

ordered _____. This procedure exerts a pulling force on the distal end of the

affected limb.

|  |  |  |  |
|---|---|---|---|
| external fixation | immobilization | internal fixation | traction |

3.80.　Baby Juanita was treated for _____, which is a congenital deformity of the foot

involving the talus (ankle bones). Her family calls this condition clubfoot.

|  |  |  |  |
|---|---|---|---|
| osteomalacia | rickets | scoliosis | talipes |

## CHALLENGE WORD BUILDING

These terms are *not* found in this chapter; however, they are made up of the following familiar word parts. If you need help in creating the term, refer to your medical dictionary.

| poly- | arthr/o | -ectomy |
|---|---|---|
|  | chondr/o | -itis |
|  | cost/o | -malacia |
|  | crani/o | -otomy |
|  | oste/o | -pathy |
|  |  | -sclerosis |

3.81.　Abnormal hardening of bone is known as _____.

3.82.　The surgical removal of a rib or ribs is a/an _____.

3.83.　Any disease of cartilage is known as _____.

3.84.　A surgical incision into a joint is a/an _____.

3.85.　Inflammation of cartilage is known as _____.

3.86.　The surgical removal of a joint is a/an _____.

3.87.　Inflammation of more than one joint is known as _____.

3.88.　Any disease involving the bones and joints is known as _____.

3.89.　A surgical incision or division of a rib or ribs is a/an _____.

3.90.　Abnormal softening of the skull is known as _____.

## LABELING EXERCISES

Identify the numbered items on the accompanying figures.

3.91. _Cervical_ vertebrae

3.92. _Scapula_

3.93. _Humerus_

3.94. _Coccyx_

3.95. _Femur_

3.96. _Patella_

3.97. _Parietal_ bone

3.98. _Frontal_ bone

3.99. _Occipital_ bone

3.100. _Mandible_

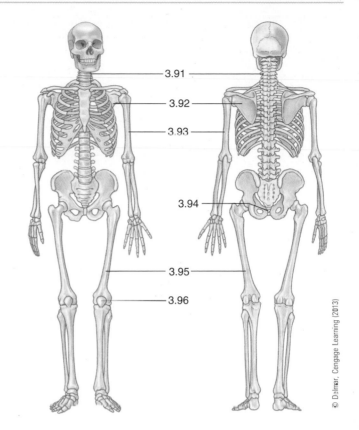

© Delmar, Cengage Learning (2013)

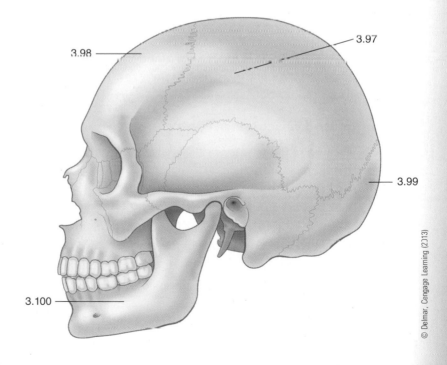

© Delmar, Cengage Learning (2013)

# THE HUMAN TOUCH
## Critical Thinking Exercise

The following story and questions are designed to stimulate critical thinking through class discussion or as a brief essay response. There are no right or wrong answers to these questions.

*Dr. Johnstone didn't like what he saw. The x-rays of Gladys Gwynn's hip showed a fracture of the femoral neck and severe osteoporosis of the hip. Mrs. Gwynn had been admitted to the orthopedic ward of Hamilton Hospital after a fall that morning at Sunny Meadows, an assisted-living facility. The accident had occurred when Sheri Smith, a new aide, lost her grip while helping Mrs. Gwynn in the shower.*

*A frail but alert and cheerful woman of 85, Mrs. Gwynn has osteoarthritis and osteoporosis that have forced her to rely on a walker. Although her finances were limited, she has been living at Sunny Meadows since her husband's death 4 years ago. Dr. Johnstone knew that she didn't have any close relatives, and he did not think that she had signed a Health Care Power of Attorney designating someone to help with medical decisions like this.*

*A total hip replacement would be the logical treatment for a younger patient because it could restore some of her lost mobility. However, for a frail patient like Mrs. Gwynn, internal fixation of the fracture might be the treatment of choice. This would repair the break, but not improve her mobility.*

*Dr. Johnstone needs to make a decision soon, but he knows that Mrs. Gwynn is groggy from pain medication. With one more look at the x-ray, Dr. Johnstone sighed and walked toward Mrs. Gwynn's room.*

## Suggested Discussion Topics

1. Because of the pain medication, Gladys Gwynn may not be able to speak for herself. Since she has no relatives to help, is it appropriate for Dr. Johnstone to make the decision about surgery for her? Under the circumstances, is it possible that when Gladys moved into Sunny Meadows they had her sign a Health Care Power of Attorney to someone at the facility?

2. Because the accident happened when Sheri Smith was helping Mrs. Gwynn, do you think Sheri should be held responsible for the accident? Given that Sheri is an employee of Sunny Meadows, should that facility be held responsible?

3. The recovery time for internal fixation surgery is shorter than that following a total hip replacement. The surgery is also less expensive and has a less strenuous recovery period; however, Mrs. Gwynn probably will not be able to walk again. Given the patient's condition, and the limited dollars available for health care, which procedure should be performed?

4. Would you have answered Question 3 differently if Mrs. Gwynn were your mother?

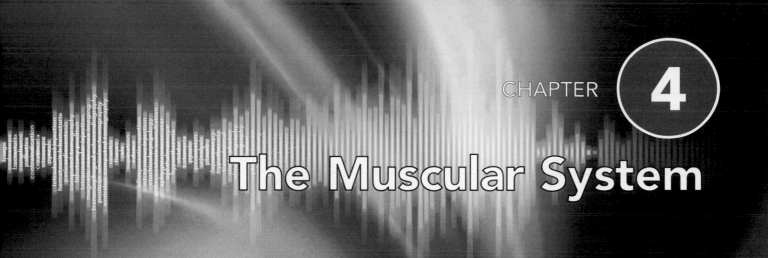

# The Muscular System

## Overview of
## STRUCTURES, COMBINING FORMS, AND FUNCTIONS OF THE MUSCULAR SYSTEM

| Major Structures | Related Combining Forms | Primary Functions |
| --- | --- | --- |
| Muscles | **muscul/o**, **my/o**, **myos/o** | Make body movement possible, hold body erect, move body fluids, and produce body heat. |
| Fascia | **fasci/o** | Cover, support, and separate muscles. |
| Tendons | **ten/o**, **tend/o**, **tendin/o** | Attach muscles to bones. |

## Vocabulary Related to **THE MUSCULAR SYSTEM**

This list contains essential word parts and medical terms for this chapter. These terms are pronounced in the StudyWARE™ and Audio CDs that are available for use with this text. These and the other important **primary terms** are shown in boldface throughout the chapter. *Secondary terms*, which appear in *orange* italics, clarify the meaning of primary terms.

### Word Parts

- [ ] **bi-** twice, double, two
- [ ] **-cele** hernia, tumor, swelling
- [ ] **dys-** bad, difficult, or painful
- [ ] **fasci/o** fascia, fibrous band
- [ ] **fibr/o** fibrous tissue, fiber
- [ ] **-ia** abnormal condition, disease, plural of **-ium**
- [ ] **-ic** pertaining to
- [ ] **kines/o, kinesi/o** movement
- [ ] **my/o** muscle
- [ ] **-plegia** paralysis, stroke
- [ ] **-rrhexis** rupture
- [ ] **tax/o** coordination, order
- [ ] **ten/o, tend/o, tendin/o** tendon, stretch out, extend, strain
- [ ] **ton/o** tone, stretching, tension
- [ ] **tri-** three

### Medical Terms

- [ ] **abduction** (ab-**DUCK**-shun)
- [ ] **adduction** (ah-**DUCK**-shun)
- [ ] **adhesion** (ad-**HEE**-zhun)
- [ ] **ataxia** (ah-**TACK**-see-ah)
- [ ] **atonic** (ah-**TON**-ick)
- [ ] **atrophy** (**AT**-roh-fee)
- [ ] **bradykinesia** (brad-ee-kih-**NEE**-zee-ah)
- [ ] **carpal tunnel syndrome** (**KAR**-pul)
- [ ] **chronic fatigue syndrome**
- [ ] **circumduction** (ser-kum-**DUCK**-shun)
- [ ] **contracture** (kon-**TRACK**-chur)
- [ ] **dorsiflexion** (dor-sih-**FLECK**-shun)
- [ ] **dyskinesia** (dis-kih-**NEE**-zee-ah)
- [ ] **dystonia** (dis-**TOH**-nee-ah)
- [ ] **electromyography** (ee-**leck**-troh-my-**OG**-rah-fee)
- [ ] **epicondylitis** (ep-ih-**kon**-dih-**LYE**-tis)
- [ ] **ergonomics** (er-goh-**NOM**-icks)
- [ ] **exercise physiologist** (**fiz**-ee-**OL**-oh-jist)

- [ ] **fasciitis** (fas-ee-**EYE**-tis)
- [ ] **fibromyalgia syndrome** (figh-broh-my-**AL**-jee-ah)
- [ ] **ganglion cyst** (**GANG**-glee-on **SIST**)
- [ ] **heel spur**
- [ ] **hemiparesis** (hem-ee-pah-**REE**-sis)
- [ ] **hemiplegia** (hem-ee-**PLEE**-jee-ah)
- [ ] **hernia** (**HER**-nee-ah)
- [ ] **hyperkinesia** (**high**-per-kye-**NEE**-zee-a)
- [ ] **hypotonia** (**high**-poh-**TOH**-nee-ah)
- [ ] **impingement syndrome** (im-**PINJ**-ment **SIN**-drohm)
- [ ] **insertion**
- [ ] **intermittent claudication** (klaw-dih-**KAY**-shun)
- [ ] **muscular dystrophy** (**DIS**-troh-fee)
- [ ] **myasthenia gravis** (my-as-**THEE**-nee-ah **GRAH**-vis)
- [ ] **myocele** (**MY**-oh-seel)
- [ ] **myoclonus** (my-oh-**KLOH**-nus)
- [ ] **myofascial release** (**my**-oh-**FASH**-ee-ahl)
- [ ] **myolysis** (my-**OL**-ih-sis)
- [ ] **myoparesis** (**my**-oh-**PAR**-eh-sis)
- [ ] **myorrhaphy** (my-**OR**-ah-fee)
- [ ] **neuromuscular** (new-roh-**MUS**-kyou-lar)
- [ ] **nocturnal myoclonus** (nock-**TER**-nal **my**-oh-**KLOH**-nus)
- [ ] **oblique** (oh-**BLEEK**)
- [ ] **paralysis** (pah-**RAL**-ih-sis)
- [ ] **paraplegia** (par-ah-**PLEE**-jee-ah)
- [ ] **physiatrist** (fiz-ee-**AT**-rist)
- [ ] **plantar fasciitis** (**PLAN**-tar fas-ee-**EYE**-tis)
- [ ] **polymyositis** (**pol**-ee-**my**-oh-**SIGH**-tis)
- [ ] **pronation** (proh-**NAY**-shun)
- [ ] **quadriplegia** (kwad-rih-**PLEE**-jee-ah)
- [ ] **range of motion testing**
- [ ] **sarcopenia** (sar-koh-**PEE**-nee-ah)
- [ ] **shin splint**
- [ ] **singultus** (sing-**GUL**-tus)
- [ ] **spasmodic torticollis** (spaz-**MOD**-ick tor-tih-**KOL**-is)
- [ ] **sphincter** (**SFINK**-ter)
- [ ] **sprain**
- [ ] **tenodesis** (ten-**ODD**-eh-sis)
- [ ] **tenosynovitis** (ten-oh-sin-oh-**VYE**-tis)
- [ ] **tenolysis** (ten-**OL**-ih-sis)
- [ ] **tenorrhaphy** (ten-**OR**-ah-fee)
- [ ] **transverse** (trans-**VERSE**)

## LEARNING GOALS

On completion of this chapter, you should be able to:

1. Describe the functions and structures of the muscular system, including muscle fibers, fascia, tendons, and the three types of muscle.

2. Recognize, define, pronounce, and spell the primary terms related to muscle movements, and explain how the muscles are named.

3. Recognize, define, pronounce, and spell the primary terms related to the pathology and the diagnostic and treatment procedures of the muscular system.

# ■ FUNCTIONS OF THE MUSCULAR SYSTEM

■ Muscles hold the body erect and make movement possible.

■ Muscle movement generates nearly 85% of the heat that keeps the body warm.

■ Muscles move food through the digestive system.

■ Muscle movements, such as walking, aid the flow of blood through veins as it returns to the heart.

■ Muscle action moves fluids through the ducts and tubes associated with other body systems.

# ■ STRUCTURES OF THE MUSCULAR SYSTEM

The muscular and skeletal systems are sometimes referred to jointly as the *musculoskeletal* system. Because of the interactions of these two systems, they provide the body with form, support, stability, and the ability to move.

The body has more than 600 muscles, which make up about 40–45% of the body's weight. Skeletal muscles are made up of fibers that are covered with fascia and are attached to bones by tendons.

## Muscle Fibers

**Muscle fibers** are the long, slender cells that make up muscles. Each muscle consists of a group of fibers that are bound together by connective tissue.

## Fascia

**Fascia** (**FASH**-ee-ah) is a band of connective tissue that envelops, separates, or binds together muscles or groups

of muscles (plural, *fasciae* or *fascias*). Fascia is flexible to allow muscle movements.

The term **myofascial** (**my**-oh-**FASH**-ee-ahl) means pertaining to muscle tissue and fascia (**my/o** means muscle, **fasci** means fascia, and **-al** means pertaining to).

## Tendons

■ A **tendon** is a narrow band of nonelastic, dense, fibrous connective tissue that attaches a muscle to a bone. Do not confuse tendons with *ligaments*, which are bands of fibrous tissue that form joints by connecting one bone to another bone (Figure 4.1). See Chapter 3 for more information on ligaments.

■ For example, the *patellar tendon* attaches muscles to the bottom of the patella (kneecap), and the *Achilles tendon* attaches the gastrocnemius muscle (the major muscle of the calf of the leg) to the heel bone (Figure 4.10).

■ An *aponeurosis* is a sheet-like fibrous connective tissue, which resembles a flattened tendon that serves as a fascia to bind muscles together or as a means of connecting muscle to bone (plural, *aponeuroses*). As an example, the abdominal aponeurosis can be seen in Figure 4.9.

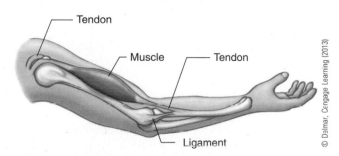

Tendon
Muscle — Tendon
Ligament

© Dalmar, Cengage Learning (2013)

**FIGURE 4.1** *Tendons* attach muscle to bone. *Ligaments* join bone to bone.

# ■ TYPES OF MUSCLE TISSUE

The three types of muscle tissue are *skeletal, smooth*, and *myocardial* (Figure 4.2). These muscle types are described according to their appearance and function.

## Skeletal Muscles

■ **Skeletal muscles** are attached to the bones of the skeleton and make body motions possible (Figure 4.2A).

**(A)** Skeletal muscle

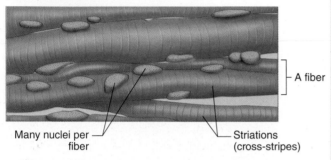

Many nuclei per fiber

Striations (cross-stripes)

A fiber

**(B)** Smooth muscle

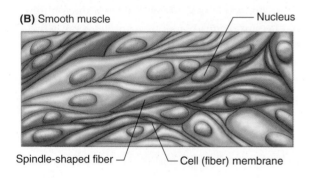

Nucleus

Spindle-shaped fiber

Cell (fiber) membrane

**(C)** Myocardial muscle

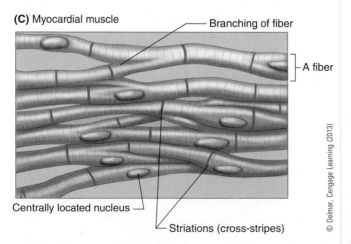

Branching of fiber

A fiber

Centrally located nucleus

Striations (cross-stripes)

© Delmar, Cengage Learning (2013)

**FIGURE 4.2** Types of muscle tissue. (A) Skeletal muscle. (B) Smooth muscle. (C) Myocardial muscle.

■ Skeletal muscles are also known as *voluntary muscles* because we have conscious (voluntary) control over these muscles.

■ Skeletal muscles are also known as *striated muscles* because under a microscope, the dark and light bands in the muscle fibers create a striped appearance. *Striated* means striped.

## Smooth Muscles

**Smooth muscles** are located in the walls of internal organs such as the digestive tract, blood vessels, and ducts leading from glands (Figure 4.2B). Their function is to move and control the flow of fluids through these structures.

■ Smooth muscles are also known as *involuntary muscles* because they are under the control of the autonomic nervous system and are *not* under voluntary control. The autonomic nervous system is discussed in Chapter 10.

■ Smooth muscles are also known as *unstriated muscles*. This is because they do *not* have the dark and light bands that produce the striped appearance seen in striated muscles.

■ Smooth muscles are also known as *visceral muscles* because they are found in hollow structures such as those of the digestive and urinary systems. *Visceral* means relating to the internal organs. These muscles are found in large internal organs, with the exception of the heart.

## Myocardial Muscle

**Myocardial muscles** (**my**-oh-**KAR**-dee-al), also known as *myocardium* or *cardiac muscle*, form the muscular walls of the heart (**my/o** means muscle, **cardi** means heart, and **-al** means pertaining to) (Figure 4.2C).

Myocardial muscle is like striated skeletal muscle in appearance, but is similar to smooth muscle in that its action is involuntary. It is the constant contraction and relaxation of the myocardial muscle that causes the heartbeat. This topic is discussed in Chapter 5.

**StudyWARE** **CONNECTION**

Watch the **Types of Muscle** animation in the StudyWARE™.

# MUSCLE CONTRACTION AND RELAXATION

A wide range of muscle movements are made possible by the combination of specialized muscle types, muscle innervation, and the organization of muscles into antagonistic muscle pairs.

## Muscle Innervation

**Muscle innervation** (**in**-err-**VAY**-shun) is the stimulation of a muscle by an impulse transmitted by a motor nerve. Motor nerves enable the brain to stimulate a muscle to contract. When the stimulation stops, the muscle relaxes. This information controls the body's voluntary muscular contractions. (Nerves are further described in Chapter 10.)

If the nerve impulse is disrupted due to an injury or disease, the muscle is unable to function properly. For example, it can be paralyzed or unable to contract properly. These conditions are described later in this chapter.

**Neuromuscular** (**new**-roh **MUS**-kyou-lar) means pertaining to the relationship between a nerve and muscle (**neur/o** means nerve, **muscul** means muscle, and **-ar** means pertaining to).

## Antagonistic Muscle Pairs

All muscles are arranged in antagonistic pairs. The term *antagonistic* refers to working in opposition to each other. Muscles within each pair are made up of specialized cells that can change length or shape by contracting and relaxing. When one muscle of the pair contracts, the opposite muscle of the pair relaxes. It is these contrasting motions that make contraction and relaxation possible.

■ **Contraction** is the tightening of a muscle. As the muscle contracts, it becomes shorter and thicker, causing the *belly* (center) of the muscle to enlarge.

■ **Relaxation** occurs when a muscle returns to its original form. As the muscle relaxes, it becomes longer and thinner, and the belly is no longer enlarged.

As an example, the triceps and biceps work as a pair to make movement of the arm possible (Figure 4.3).

# CONTRASTING MUSCLE MOTION

These muscle motions, which occur as pairs of opposites, are described in the following text and illustrated in Figures 4.4 through 4.8.

## Abduction and Adduction

**Abduction** (ab-**DUCK**-shun) is the movement of a limb (arm or leg) *away from* the midline of the body (**ab-** means away from, **duct** means to lead, and **-ion** means action). During abduction, the arm moves outward away from the side of the body. An *abductor* is a muscle that moves a body part away from the midline.

In contrast, **adduction** (ah-**DUCK**-shun) is the movement of a limb (arm or leg) *toward* the midline of the body (**ad-** means toward, **duct** means to lead, and **-ion** means action). During adduction, the arm moves inward toward the side of the body. An *adductor* is a muscle that moves a body part toward the midline (Figure 4.4).

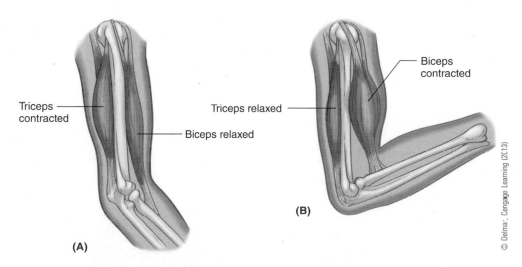

Triceps contracted

Biceps relaxed

Triceps relaxed

Biceps contracted

**(A)**

**(B)**

© Delmar, Cengage Learning (2C13)

**FIGURE 4.3** An antagonistic muscle pair of the upper arm. (A) During *extension*, the *triceps* is contracted and the *biceps* is *relaxed*. (B) During *flexion*, the *triceps* is relaxed and the *biceps* is contracted.

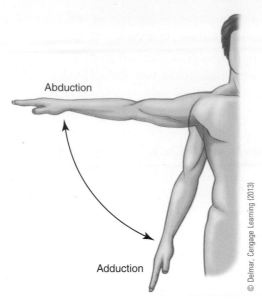

**FIGURE 4.4** *Abduction* moves the arm away from the body. *Adduction* moves the arm toward the body.

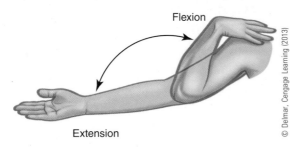

**FIGURE 4.5** *Extension* increases the angle of the elbow and moves the hand away from the body. *Flexion* decreases the angle of the elbow and moves the hand toward the body.

## Flexion and Extension

**Flexion** (**FLECK**-shun) means decreasing the angle between two bones by bending a limb at a joint (**flex** means to bend, and **-ion** means action). During flexion, the knee or elbow is bent. A *flexor muscle* bends a limb at a joint.

In contrast, **extension** means increasing the angle between two bones or the straightening out of a limb (**ex-** means away from, **tens** means to stretch out, and **-ion** means action). During extension, the knee or elbow is straightened. An *extensor muscle* straightens a limb at a joint (Figure 4.5).

- **Hyperextension** is the extreme or overextension of a limb or body part beyond its normal limit. For example, movement of the head far backward or far forward beyond the normal range of motion causes hyperextension of the muscles of the neck.

## Elevation and Depression

**Elevation** is the act of raising or lifting a body part. For example, the elevation of the *levator anguli oris* muscles of the face raises the corners of the mouth into a smile. A *levator* is a muscle that raises a body part.

In contrast, **depression** is the act of lowering a body part. The *depressor anguli oris*, for example, lowers the corner of the mouth into a frown. A *depressor* muscle lowers a body part. See Figure 4.9 for illustrations of some of the muscles of the face.

## Rotation and Circumduction

**Rotation** is a circular movement around an axis such as the shoulder joint. An *axis* is an imaginary line that runs lengthwise through the center of the body, and rotation turns a bone on its own axis.

In contrast, **circumduction** (**ser**-kum-**DUCK**-shun) is the circular movement at the far end of a limb. An example of circumduction is the swinging motion of the far end of the arm (Figure 4.6).

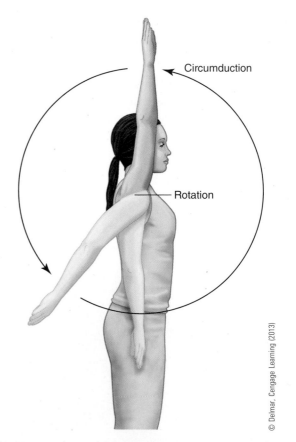

**FIGURE 4.6** *Rotation* is a circular movement around an axis such as the shoulder joint. *Circumduction* is the circular movement at the far end of a limb.

- A *rotator muscle* turns a body part on its axis. For example, the head of the **humerus** (**HYUM**-er-us), which is the bone of the upper arm, rotates within the shoulder joint.

- The *rotator cuff* is the group of muscles and their tendons that hold the head of the humerus securely in place as it rotates within the shoulder joint (Figure 4.13).

## Supination and Pronation

**Supination** (**soo**-pih-**NAY**-shun) is the act of rotating the arm or the leg so that the palm of the hand or sole of the foot is turned forward or upward. An easy way to remember this is to think of carrying a bowl of soup.

In contrast, **pronation** (proh-**NAY**-shun) is the act of rotating the arm or leg so that the palm of the hand or sole of the foot is turned downward or backward (Figure 4.7).

## Dorsiflexion and Plantar Flexion

**Dorsiflexion** (**dor**-sih-**FLECK**-shun) is the movement that bends the foot *upward* at the ankle. Pointing the toes and foot upward decreases the angle between the top of the foot and the front of the leg (Figure 4.8).

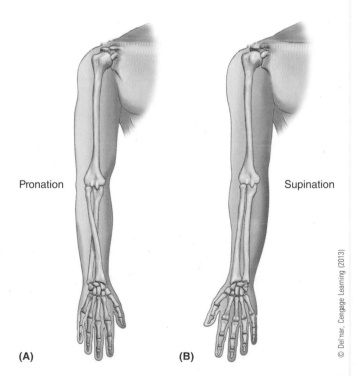

**FIGURE 4.7** (A) *Pronation* is turning the arm so the palm of the hand is turned downward. (B) *Supination* is turning the arm so that the palm of the hand is turned upward.

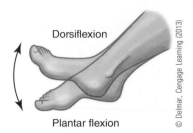

**FIGURE 4.8** *Dorsiflexion* bends the foot upward at the ankle. *Plantar flexion* bends the foot downward at the ankle.

In contrast, **plantar flexion** (**PLAN**-tar **FLECK**-shun) is the movement that bends the foot *downward* at the ankle. *Plantar* means pertaining to the sole of the foot. Pointing the toes and foot downward increases the angle between the top of the foot and the front of the leg (Figure 4.8).

## ■ HOW MUSCLES ARE NAMED

As you study this section, refer to Figures 4.9 through 4.12.

In Figures 4.9 and 4.10, many of the *superficial* muscles are labeled. These muscles are so called because they are located near the surface, just under the skin.

### Muscles Named for Their Origin and Insertion

The movements of skeletal muscles are made possible by two points of attachment. These are known as the origin and insertion, and some muscles are also named for these points.

- The **origin** is where the muscle begins, and it is located nearest the midline of the body or on a less movable part of the skeleton. The origin is the less movable attachment.

- The **insertion** is where the muscle ends by attaching to a bone or tendon. In contrast to the origin, the insertion is the more movable attachment, and it is the farthest point from the midline of the body.

- The *sternocleidomastoid muscle*, for example, helps bend the neck and rotate the head (Figures 4.9 and 4.11). This muscle is named for its two points of origin, which are **stern/o** meaning breastbone and **cleid/o** meaning collar bone. The **mastoid** muscle inserts at one point of insertion into the mastoid process. (This is part of the temporal bone that is located just behind the ear).

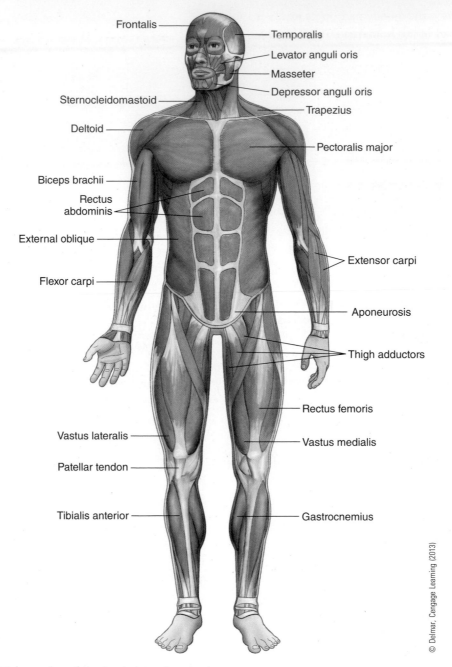

Frontalis — — Temporalis

— Levator anguli oris

— Masseter

— Depressor anguli oris

Sternocleidomastoid — — Trapezius

Deltoid — — Pectoralis major

Biceps brachii —

Rectus abdominis —

External oblique — — Extensor carpi

Flexor carpi — — Aponeurosis

— Thigh adductors

— Rectus femoris

Vastus lateralis — — Vastus medialis

Patellar tendon —

Tibialis anterior — — Gastrocnemius

© Delmar, Cengage Learning (2013)

**FIGURE 4.9** Superficial muscles of the body (anterior view).

## Muscles Named for Their Action

Some muscles are named for their action, such as flexion or extension.

- For example, the *flexor carpi muscles* and the *extensor carpi muscles* are the pair of muscles that make flexion (bending) and extension (straightening) of the wrist possible (Figure 4.9). *Carpi* means wrist or wrist bones.

## Muscles Named for Their Location

Some muscles are named for their location on the body or the organ they are near.

- The **pectoralis major** (**peck**-toh-**RAY**-lis), for example, is a thick, fan-shaped muscle situated on the anterior chest wall (Figure 4.9). *Pectoral* means relating to the chest.

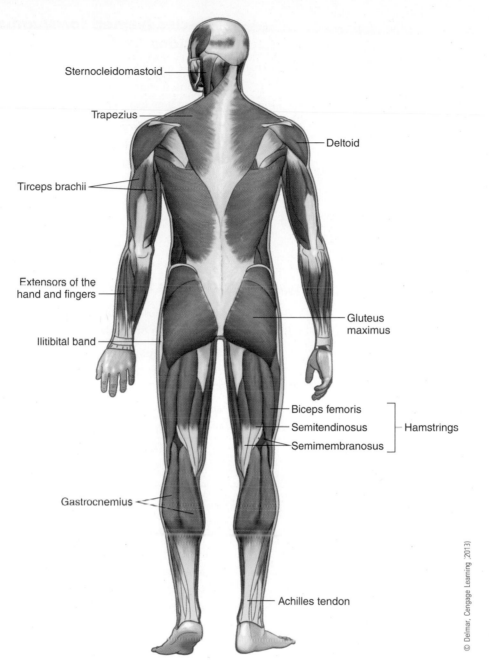

**FIGURE 4.10**  Superficial muscles of the body (posterior view).

■ **Lateralis** means toward the side. For example: the **vastus lateralis** (lat-er-**AY**-lis) is a muscle toward the outer side of the leg.

■ **Medialis** means toward the midline. The **vastus medialis** (mee-dee-**AY**-lis) is a muscle toward the midline of the leg. These muscles are part of the quadriceps that flex and extend the leg at the knee. (These muscles can be located on Figure 4.9.)

## Muscles Named for Fiber Direction

Some muscles are named for the direction in which their fibers run (Figure 4.12).

■ **Oblique** (oh-**BLEEK**) means slanted or at an angle. As an example, the *external oblique* and *internal oblique* muscles have a slanted alignment.

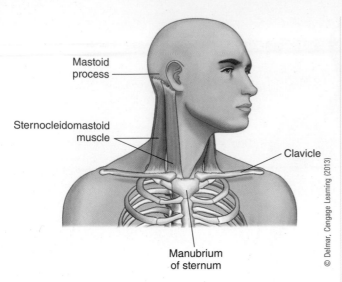

**FIGURE 4.11** The *sternocleidomastoid muscle* is named for its *origins* and *insertion*.

## Muscles Named for Number of Divisions

Muscles may be named according to the number of divisions forming them. See the muscles of the arm in Figure 4.3 as examples of this.

■ The **biceps brachii** (**BYE**-seps **BRAY**-kee-eye), also known as the *biceps*, is formed from two divisions (**bi-** means two, and **-ceps** means head).

■ The **triceps brachii** (**TRY**-seps **BRAY**-kee-eye), also known as the *triceps*, is formed from three divisions (**tri-** means three, and **-ceps** means head).

■ These muscles flex and extend the upper arm.

## Muscles Named for Their Size or Shape

Some muscles are named because they are broad or narrow, or large or small.

■ The **gluteus maximus** (**GLOO**-tee-us **MAX**-ih-mus) is the largest muscle of the buttock (Figure 4.10). *Maximus* means great or large.

■ Other muscles are named because they are shaped like a familiar object. For example, the **deltoid muscle** (**DEL**-toyd), located on the shoulder, is shaped like an inverted triangle, which is the Greek letter *delta*.

■ **Rectus** (**RECK**-tus) means in straight alignment with the vertical axis of the body. As an example, the *rectus abdominis* and *rectus femorus* (below, under "Select Muscles and Their Functions") have straight alignment.

■ A **sphincter** (**SFINK**-ter) is a ring-like muscle that tightly constricts the opening of a passageway. A sphincter is named for the passage involved. As an example, the *anal sphincter* closes the anus.

■ **Transverse** (trans-**VERSE**) means in a crosswise direction. An example is the *transverse abdominis* muscle in the abdomen, which has a crosswise alignment.

## Muscles Named for Strange Reasons

Some muscles, such as the hamstrings, have seemingly strange names. The reason this group of muscles is so named is because these are the muscles by which a butcher hangs a slaughtered pig.

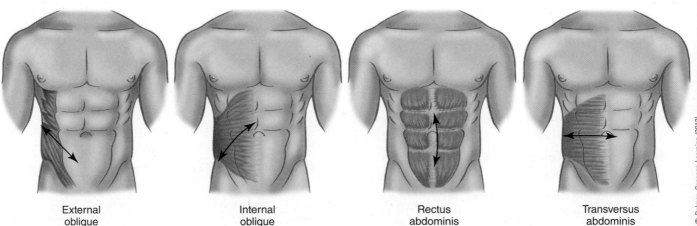

| External oblique | Internal oblique | Rectus abdominis | Transversus abdominis |

**FIGURE 4.12** Many of the muscles of the trunk are named for their direction.

- The **hamstring group**, located at the back of the upper leg, consists of three separate muscles: the *biceps femoris*, *semitendinosus*, and *semimembranosus* muscles. The primary functions of the hamstrings are knee flexion and hip extension (Figure 4.10).

# ■ SELECT MUSCLES AND THEIR FUNCTIONS

Each of the body's 600 muscles has a specific role. Here are just a few listed with their function.

## Muscles of the Head

- The **frontalis** (fron-**TAY**-lis), or *occipitofrontalis*, muscle is in the forehead. It raises and lowers the eyebrows.
- The **temporalis** (tem-poh-**RAY**-lis) muscle moves the lower jaw up and back to close the mouth.
- The **masseter** (mah-**SEE**-ter) muscle, which is one of the strongest in the body, moves the lower jaw up to close the mouth when chewing.

## Muscles of the Trunk

- In the male, the **pectoralis major** makes up the bulk of the chest muscles. In the female, this muscle lies under the breast.
- The **external oblique** and **internal oblique muscles** are found in the abdomen. The external oblique muscles flex and rotate the vertebral column. They also flex the torso and compress the abdomen. The internal oblique muscles flex the spine, support the abdominal contents, help breathe, and rotate the spine.
- The **rectus abdominis** (ab-**DOM**-ih-nus) helps flex the trunk, assists in breathing, and supports the spine.
- The **transverse abdominis** is located on the side of the abdomen. This *core* muscle is engaged when a person laughs or coughs.

## Muscles of the Shoulders and Arms

- The **deltoid** forms the muscular cap of the shoulder (Figures 4.9 and 4.10).
- The **trapezius** (trah-**PEE**-zee-us) muscle moves the head and shoulder blade.
- The **biceps brachii**, located in the anterior upper arm, flexes the elbow.
- The **triceps brachii**, located in the posterior upper arm, extends the elbow.

## Muscles of the Legs

- The **rectus femoris** (**FEM**-or-iss) extends the leg at the knee.
- The **quadriceps femoris** is made up of four muscles, including the vastus lateralis and vastus medialis, which flex and extend the leg at the knee.
- The **hamstring group** is involved in knee flexion and hip extension.
- The **gastrocnemius** (gas-trok-**NEE**-mee-uhs) is the calf muscle that flexes the knee and bends the foot downward. The name comes from the Latin for "stomach of the leg," because of the way this muscle bulges out.

# ■ MEDICAL SPECIALTIES RELATED TO THE MUSCULAR SYSTEM

- An **exercise physiologist** (fiz-ee-**OL**-oh-jist) is a specialist who works under the supervision of a physician to develop, implement, and coordinate exercise programs, and administer medical tests to promote physical fitness.
- A **neurologist** (new-**ROL**-oh-jist) is a physician who specializes in treating the causes of paralysis and similar muscular disorders in which there is a loss of function.
- A **physiatrist** (fiz-ee-**AT**-rist) is a physician who specializes in physical medicine and rehabilitation with the focus on restoring function. *Rehabilitation* is restoration, following disease, illness, or injury, of the ability to function in a normal or near-normal manner.
- A **sports medicine physician** specializes in treating sports-related injuries of the bones, joints, and muscles.

# ■ PATHOLOGY OF THE MUSCULAR SYSTEM

## Fibers, Fascia, and Tendons

- **Fasciitis** (fas-ee-**EYE**-tis), which is also spelled *fascitis*, is inflammation of a fascia (**fasci** means fascia, and **-itis** means inflammation).
- **Fibromyalgia syndrome** (figh-broh-my-**AL**-jee-ah) is a debilitating chronic condition characterized by fatigue; diffuse or specific muscle, joint, or bone pain;

and a wide range of other symptoms (**fibr/o** means fibrous tissue, **my** means muscle, and **-algia** means pain). *Debilitating* means a condition causing weakness. Contrast fibromyalgia syndrome with *chronic fatigue syndrome*.

- **Tenosynovitis** (**ten**-oh-**sin**-oh-**VYE**-tis) is an inflammation of the sheath surrounding a tendon. (**ten/o** means tendon, **synov** means synovial membrane, and **-itis** means inflammation).

- **Tendinitis** (**ten**-dih-**NIGH**-tis), sometimes spelled *tendonitis*, is an inflammation of the tendons caused by excessive or unusual use of the joint (**tendin** means tendon, and **-itis** means inflammation). The terms *tenonitis* and *tenontitis* also mean tendinitis.

## Chronic Fatigue Syndrome

**Chronic fatigue syndrome** (CFS) is a disorder of unknown cause that affects many body systems. It is discussed in this chapter because many of the symptoms are similar to those of the fibromyalgia syndrome.

- CFS is a debilitating and complex disorder characterized by profound fatigue that is not improved by bed rest and may be made worse by physical or mental activity.

## Muscle Disorders

- An **adhesion** (ad-**HEE**-zhun) is a band of fibrous tissue that holds structures together abnormally. Adhesions can form in muscles or in internal organs, as the result of an injury or surgery. The term *frozen shoulder* refers to adhesions forming in the capsule of connective tissue in the shoulder, tightening around the shoulder joint.

- **Atrophy** (**AT**-roh-fee) means weakness or wearing away of body tissues and structures. Atrophy of a muscle or muscles can be caused by pathology or by disuse of the muscle over a long period of time.

- **Myalgia** (my-**AL**-jee-ah) is tenderness or pain in the muscles (**my** means muscle, and **-algia** means pain).

- A **myocele** (**MY**-oh-seel) is the herniation (protrusion) of muscle substance through a tear in the fascia surrounding it (**my/o** means muscle, and **-cele** means a hernia). A **hernia** (**HER**-nee-ah) is the protrusion of a part of a structure through the tissues normally containing it.

- **Myolysis** (my-**OL**-ih-sis) is the degeneration of muscle tissue (**my/o** means muscle, and **-lysis** means destruction or breaking down in disease).

*Degeneration* means deterioration or breaking down. *Deterioration* means the process of becoming worse.

- **Myorrhexis** (my-oh-**RECK**-sis) is the rupture or tearing of a muscle (**my/o** means muscle, and **-rrhexis** means rupture).

- **Polymyositis** (pol-ee-**my**-oh-**SIGH**-tis) is a muscle disease characterized by the simultaneous inflammation and weakening of voluntary muscles in many parts of the body (**poly-** means many, **myos** means muscle, and **-itis** means inflammation). The affected muscles are typically those closest to the trunk or torso, and the resulting weakness can be severe.

- **Sarcopenia** (sar-koh-**PEE**-nee-ah) is the loss of muscle mass, strength, and function that come with aging (**sarc/o** means flesh, and **-penia** means deficiency). A weight or resistance training program can significantly improve muscle mass and slow, but not stop, this process.

## Muscle Tone

**Muscle tone** is the state of balanced muscle tension (contraction and relaxation) that makes normal posture, coordination, and movement possible.

- **Atonic** (ah-**TON**-ick) means lacking normal muscle tone or strength (**a-** means without, **ton** means tone, and **-ic** means pertaining to).

- **Dystonia** (dis-**TOH**-nee-ah) is a condition of abnormal muscle tone that causes the impairment of voluntary muscle movement (**dys-** means bad, **ton** means tone, and **-ia** means condition).

- **Hypotonia** (high-poh-**TOH**-nee-ah) is a condition in which there is diminished tone of the skeletal muscles (**hypo-** means deficient, **ton** means tone, and **-ia** means condition).

## Muscle Movement

- **Ataxia** (ah-**TACK**-see-ah) is the lack of muscle coordination during voluntary movement (**a-** means without, **tax** means coordination, and **-ia** means condition). These movements, which are often shaky and unsteady, are most frequently caused by abnormal activity in the cerebellum (see Chapter 10).

- A **contracture** (kon-**TRACK**-chur) is the permanent tightening of fascia, muscles, tendons, ligaments, or skin that occurs when normally elastic connective tissues are replaced with nonelastic fibrous tissues. The most common causes of contractures are scarring or the lack of use due to immobilization or inactivity.

- **Intermittent claudication** (klaw-dih-**KAY**-shun) is pain in the leg muscles that occurs during exercise and is relieved by rest. *Intermittent* means coming and going at intervals, and *claudication* means limping. This condition, which is due to poor circulation, is associated with peripheral vascular disease (see Chapter 5).

- A **spasm** is a sudden, involuntary contraction of one or more muscles. Also known as a *charley horse*, especially when occurring in the leg.

- A **cramp** is a painful localized muscle spasm often named for its cause, such as menstrual cramps or writer's cramp.

- **Spasmodic torticollis** (spaz-**MOD**-ick **tor**-tih-**KOL**-is), also known as *wryneck*, is a stiff neck due to spasmodic contraction of the neck muscles that pull the head toward the affected side. *Spasmodic* means relating to a spasm, and *torticollis* means a contraction, or shortening, of the muscles of the neck.

## Muscle Function

- **Bradykinesia** (brad-ee-kih-**NEE**-zee-ah) is extreme slowness in movement (**brady-** means slow, **kines** means movement, and **-ia** means condition). This is one of the symptoms of Parkinson's disease, which is discussed in Chapter 10.

- **Dyskinesia** (dis-kih-**NEE**-zee-ah) is the distortion or impairment of voluntary movement such as a tic or spasm (**dys-** means bad, **kines** means movement, and **-ia** means condition). A *tic* is a spasmodic muscular contraction that often involves parts of the face. Although these movements appear purposeful, they are not under voluntary control.

- **Hyperkinesia** (high-per-kye-**NEE**-zee-ah), also known as *hyperactivity*, is abnormally increased muscle function or activity (**hyper-** means excessive, **kines** means movement, and **-ia** means condition).

## Myoclonus

**Myoclonus** (my-oh-**KLOH**-nus) is the sudden, involuntary jerking of a muscle or group of muscles (**my/o** means muscle, **clon** mean violent action, and **-us** is a singular noun ending).

- **Nocturnal myoclonus** (nock-**TER**-nal my-oh-**KLOH**-nus) is jerking of the limbs that can occur normally as a person is falling asleep. *Nocturnal* means pertaining to night.

- **Singultus** (sing-**GUL**-tus), also known as *hiccups*, is myoclonus of the diaphragm that causes the characteristic hiccup sound with each spasm.

## Myasthenia Gravis

**Myasthenia gravis (MG)** (**my**-as-**THEE**-nee-ah **GRAH**-vis) is a chronic autoimmune disease that affects the neuromuscular junction (where the neuron activates muscle to contract) and produces serious weakness of voluntary muscles. Muscles that control eye movement, facial expression, chewing, talking, and swallowing are often affected by this condition. *Myasthenia* means muscle weakness (**my** means muscle, and **-asthenia** means weakness or lack of strength). *Gravis* comes from the Latin word meaning grave or serious.

## Muscular Dystrophy

The condition commonly known as **muscular dystrophy** (**DIS**-troh-fee) is properly referred to in the plural, which is *muscular dystrophies*. This general term describes a group of more than 30 genetic diseases that are characterized by progressive weakness and degeneration of the skeletal muscles that control movement, without affecting the nervous system. There is no specific treatment to stop or reverse any form of muscular dystrophy. Two of the most common forms are:

- *Duchenne muscular dystrophy* (DMD) is the most common form of muscular dystrophy in children. This condition affects primarily boys with onset between the ages of 3 and 5 years. The disorder progresses rapidly so that most of these boys are unable to walk by age 12 and later need a respirator to breathe.

- *Becker muscular dystrophy* (BMD) is very similar to, but less severe than, Duchenne muscular dystrophy.

## Repetitive Stress Disorders

**Repetitive stress disorders**, also known as *repetitive motion disorders*, are a variety of muscular conditions that result from repeated motions performed in the course of normal work, daily activities, or recreation such as sports. The symptoms caused by these frequently repeated motions involve muscles, tendons, nerves, and joints.

- **Compartment syndrome** involves the compression of nerves and blood vessels due to swelling within the enclosed space created by the fascia that separates groups of muscles. This syndrome can be caused by trauma, tight bandages or casts, or by repetitive activities such as running.

- **Overuse injuries** are minor tissue injuries that have not been given time to heal. These injuries can be caused by spending hours at the computer keyboard or by lengthy sports training sessions.

- **Overuse tendinitis** (ten-dih-**NIGH**-tis), also known as *overuse tendinosis*, is an inflammation of tendons caused by excessive or unusual use of a joint (**tendin-** means tendon, and **-itis** means inflammation).

- **Stress fractures**, which are also overuse injuries, are discussed in Chapter 3.

## Myofascial Pain Syndrome

**Myofascial pain syndrome** (**my**-oh-**FASH**-ee-ahl) is a chronic pain disorder that affects muscles and fascia throughout the body. This condition, which is caused by the development of trigger points, produces local and referred muscle pain. *Trigger points* are tender areas that most commonly develop where the fascia comes into contact with a muscle. *Referred pain* describes pain that originates in one area of the body, but is felt in another.

## Rotator Cuff Injuries

- **Impingement syndrome** (im-**PINJ**-ment) occurs when inflamed and swollen tendons are caught in the narrow space between the bones within the shoulder joint. A common sign of impingement syndrome is discomfort when raising your arm above your head.

- **Rotator cuff tendinitis** (ten-dih-**NIGH**-tis) is an inflammation of the tendons of the rotator cuff (Figure 4.13). This condition is often named for the cause, such as *tennis shoulder* or *pitcher's shoulder*.

- A **ruptured rotator cuff** develops when rotator cuff tendinitis is left untreated or if the overuse continues. This occurs as the irritated tendon weakens and tears (Figure 4.13).

## Carpal Tunnel Syndrome

**Carpal tunnel syndrome** symptoms occur when the tendons that pass through the carpal tunnel are chronically overused and become inflamed and swollen. The carpal tunnel is a narrow, bony passage under the carpal ligament that is located one-fourth of an inch below the inner surface of the wrist. The median nerve and the tendons that bend the fingers pass through this tunnel (Figure 4.14). *Carpal* means pertaining to the wrist.

- This swelling of carpal tunnel syndrome creates pressure on the median nerve as it passes through the tunnel.

- **Carpal tunnel release** is the surgical enlargement of the carpal tunnel or cutting of the carpal ligament to relieve the pressure on tendons and nerves.

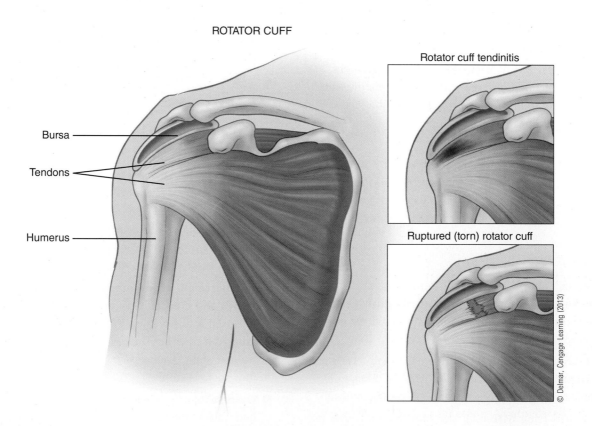

ROTATOR CUFF

Rotator cuff tendinitis

Ruptured (torn) rotator cuff

Bursa

Tendons

Humerus

© Delmar, Cengage Learning (2013)

**FIGURE 4.13** Diagrammatic views of the *rotator cuff* in health (left) and with injuries (right).

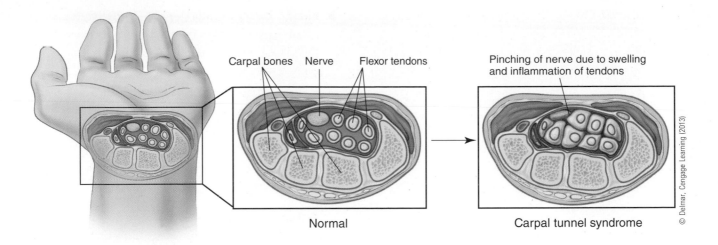

Carpal bones   Nerve   Flexor tendons

Pinching of nerve due to swelling
and inflammation of tendons

Normal

Carpal tunnel syndrome

© Delmar, Cengage Learning (2013)

**FIGURE 4.14** When the tendons that pass through the carpal tunnel become inflamed and swollen, they pinch the nerve and cause *carpal tunnel syndrome*.

## Ganglion Cyst

A **ganglion cyst** (**GANG**-glee-on **SIST**) is a harmless fluid-filled swelling that occurs most commonly on the outer surface of the wrist. This condition, which can be caused by repeated minor injuries, is usually painless and does not require treatment. (Do not confuse this use of the term *ganglion* here with the nerve ganglions described in Chapter 10.)

## Epicondylitis

**Epicondylitis** (**ep**-ih-**kon**-dih-**LYE**-tis) is inflammation of the tissues surrounding the elbow (**epi-** means on, **condyl** means condyle, and **-itis** means inflammation). *Condyle* refers to the round prominence at the end of a bone.

- *Lateral epicondylitis*, also known as *tennis elbow*, is characterized by pain on the outer side of the forearm.

- *Medial epicondylitis*, also known as *golfer's elbow*, is characterized by pain on the palm-side of the forearm.

## Ankle and Foot Problems

- A **heel spur** is a calcium deposit in the plantar fascia near its attachment to the calcaneus (heel) bone that can be one of the causes of *plantar fasciitis*.

- **Plantar fasciitis** (**PLAN**-tar **fas**-ee-**EYE**-tis) is an inflammation of the plantar fascia on the sole of the foot. This condition causes foot or heel pain when walking or running (Figure 4.15).

## Sports Injuries

The following injuries are frequently associated with sports overuse; however, some may also be caused by other forms of trauma.

- A **sprain** is an injury to a joint, such as an ankle, knee, or wrist, which usually occurs when a ligament is wrenched or torn (Figure 4.16).

- A **strain** is an injury to the body of the muscle or to the attachment of a tendon. Strains usually are associated with overuse injuries that involve a stretched or torn muscle or tendon attachment.

- A **shin splint** is a painful condition caused by the *tibialis anterior* muscle tearing away from the tibia (shin bone). Shin splints can develop in the anterolateral (front and

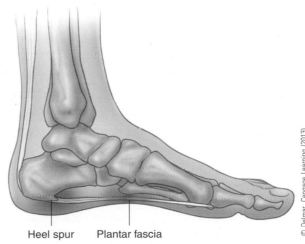

Heel spur   Plantar fascia

© Delmar, Cengage Learning (2013)

**FIGURE 4.15** A *heel spur* and *plantar fasciitis*.

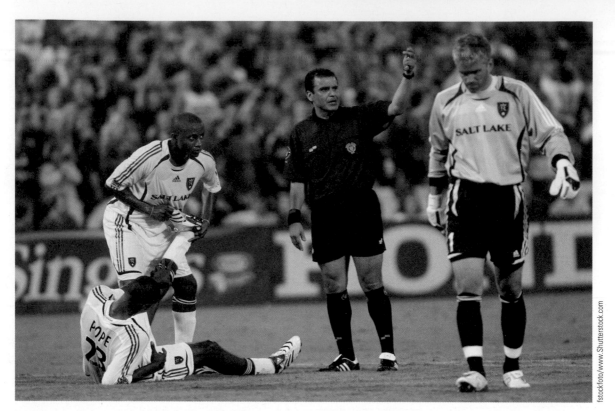

**FIGURE 4.16** A *sprained ankle* involving one or more wrenched or torn ligaments is a common sports injury.

side) muscles or in the posteromedial (back and middle) muscles of the lower leg (Figures 4.10 and 4.11). This type of injury is usually caused by repeated stress to the lower leg, such as running on hard surfaces.

■ A **hamstring injury** can be a strain or tear on any of the three hamstring muscles that straighten the hip and bend the knee. When these muscles contract too quickly, an injury can occur that is characterized by sudden and severe pain in the back of the thigh.

■ **Achilles tendinitis** (**ten**-dih-**NIGH**-tis) is a painful inflammation of the Achilles tendon caused by excessive stress being placed on that tendon.

■ **Iliotibial band syndrome** (ITBS) (**ill**-ee-oh-**TIB**-ee-al) is an overuse injury. The iliotibial band runs from the hip bone, diagonally across the leg to the tibia. ITBS is caused by this band rubbing against bone, often in the area of the knee.

## Spinal Cord Injuries

As described in Chapter 3, the spinal cord is surrounded and protected by the bony vertebrae. This protection is essential because the spinal cord is soft, with the consistency of toothpaste.

■ The type of paralysis caused by a **spinal cord injury** (SCI) is determined by the level of the vertebra closest to the injury. The higher on the spinal cord the injury occurs, the greater the area of the body that may be affected.

■ An injury occurs when a vertebra is broken and a piece of the broken bone is pressing into the spinal cord. The cord can also be injured if the vertebrae are pushed or pulled out of alignment.

■ When the spinal cord is injured, the ability of the brain to communicate with the body below the level of the injury may be reduced or lost altogether. When that happens, the affected parts of the body will not function normally.

■ An *incomplete injury* means that the person has some function below the level of the injury, even though that function isn't normal.

■ A *complete injury* means that there is complete loss of sensation and muscle control below the level of the injury; however, a complete injury does not mean that there is no hope of any improvement.

## Types of Paralysis

**Paralysis** (pah-**RAL**-ih-sis) is the loss of sensation and voluntary muscle movements in a muscle through disease or injury to its nerve supply. Damage can be either temporary or permanent (plural, *paralyses*).

■ **Myoparesis** (**my**-oh-**PAR**-eh-sis) is a weakness or slight muscular paralysis (**my/o** means muscle, and **-paresis** means partial or incomplete paralysis).

■ **Hemiparesis** (**hem**-ee-pah-**REE**-sis) is slight paralysis or weakness affecting one side of the body (**hemi-** means half, and **-paresis** means partial or incomplete paralysis). Contrast hemiparesis with *hemiplegia*.

■ **Hemiplegia** (**hem**-ee-**PLEE**-jee-ah) is total paralysis affecting only one side of the body (**hemi-** means half, and **-plegia** means paralysis). This form of paralysis is usually associated with a stroke or brain damage. Damage to one side of the brain causes paralysis on the opposite side of the body. An individual affected with hemiplegia is known as a *hemiplegic*. Contrast with *hemiparesis*.

■ **Paraplegia** (**par**-ah-**PLEE**-jee-ah) is the paralysis of both legs and the lower part of the body. An individual affected with paraplegia is known as a *paraplegic*.

■ **Quadriplegia** (**kwad** rih **PLEE**-jee-ah) is paralysis of all four extremities (**quadr/i** means four, and **-plegia** means paralysis). An individual affected with quadriplegia is known as a *quadriplegic*.

■ **Cardioplegia** (**kar**-dee-oh-**PLEE**-jee-ah) is paralysis of heart muscle (**cardi/o** means heart, and **-plegia** means paralysis). Although this can be caused by a direct blow or trauma, it is more commonly induced intentionally to perform complicated surgery.

**StudyWARE CONNECTION**

Watch the **Spinal Cord Injuries** animation in the StudyWARE™.

# ■ DIAGNOSTIC PROCEDURES OF THE MUSCULAR SYSTEM

■ **Deep tendon reflexes** (DTR) are tested with a reflex hammer that is used to strike a tendon (Figure 4.17). A *reflex* is an involuntary response to a stimulus. No response or an abnormal response can indicate a disruption of the nerve supply to the involved muscles. Reflexes also are lost in deep coma or because of medication such as heavy sedation.

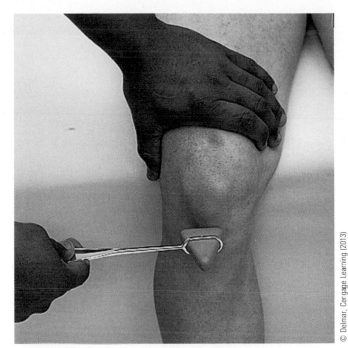

(A)

© Delmar, Cengage Learning (2013)

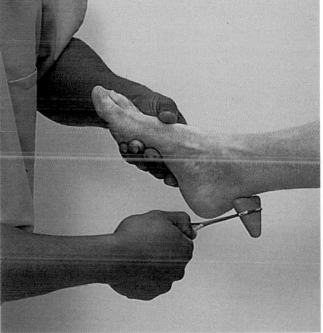

(B)

© Delmar, Cengage Learning (2013)

**FIGURE 4.17** Assessment of *deep tendon reflexes.* (A) Testing the *patellar reflex.* (B) Testing the *Achilles tendon reflex.*

■ **Range-of-motion testing** (ROM) is a diagnostic procedure to evaluate joint mobility and muscle strength (Figure 4.18). Range-of-motion exercises are used to increase strength, flexibility, and mobility.

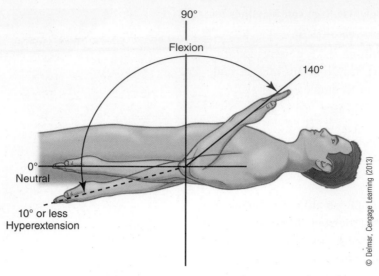

**FIGURE 4.18** *Range-of-motion testing* is used to evaluate joint mobility. The results are expressed in degrees.

■ **Electromyography** (EMG) (ee-**leck**-troh-my-**OG**-rah-fee) is a diagnostic test that measures the electrical activity within muscle fibers in response to nerve stimulation (**electr/o** means electricity, **my/o** means muscle, and **-graphy** means the process of producing a picture or record). The resulting record is called an *electromyogram*. Electromyography is most frequently used when people have symptoms of weakness, and examination shows impaired muscle strength.

■ A **muscle biopsy** involves removal of a plug of tissue for examination. A biopsy needle is commonly used to obtain this specimen, which is later used for examination.

## ■ TREATMENT PROCEDURES OF THE MUSCULAR SYSTEM

### Medications

■ An **antispasmodic**, also known as an *anticholinergic*, is administered to suppress smooth muscle contractions of the stomach, intestine, or bladder. For example, *atropine* is an antispasmodic that can be administered preoperatively to relax smooth muscles during surgery.

■ A **skeletal muscle relaxant** is administered to relax certain muscles and to relieve the stiffness, pain, and discomfort caused by strains, sprains, or other muscle injuries. These medications act on the central nervous system and may have a negative interaction with alcohol and some antidepressants (see Chapter 10).

■ A **neuromuscular blocker**, also known as a *neuromuscular blocking agent*, is a drug that causes temporary paralysis by blocking the transmission of nerve stimuli to the muscles. These drugs are used as an adjunct to anesthesia during surgery to cause skeletal muscles to relax. As used here, *adjunct* means in addition to.

### Ergonomics

**Ergonomics** (er-goh-**NOM**-icks) is the study of the human factors that affect the design and operation of tools and the work environment. This term is usually applied to the design of equipment and workspaces, with the goal of reducing injuries, strain, and stress.

### Treatment Techniques

■ **Myofascial release** (**my**-oh-**FASH**-ee-ahl) is a specialized soft-tissue manipulation technique used to ease the pain of conditions such as fibromyalgia syndrome, myofascial pain syndrome, movement restrictions, temporomandibular joint disorders (TMJ), and carpal tunnel syndrome.

■ **Occupational therapy** (OT) consists of activities to promote recovery and rehabilitation to assist patients in performing the **activities of daily living** (ADL), which include grooming, eating, and dressing.

■ **Physical therapy** (PT) is treatment to prevent disability or restore function through the use of exercise, heat, massage, or other techniques.

■ **Therapeutic ultrasound** uses high-frequency sound waves to treat muscle injuries by generating heat deep within muscle tissue. This heat eases pain, reduces muscle spasms, and accelerates healing by increasing the flow of blood into the target tissues.

■ **Transcutaneous electrical nerve stimulation** (TENS) uses a device that delivers electrical impulses through the skin, which cause changes in muscles. This is discussed further in Chapter 15.

## *Rice*

The most common first aid treatment of muscular injuries is known by the acronym ***RICE***. These letters stand for *Rest, Ice, Compression,* and *Elevation.* Rest and ice are recommended for the first few days after the injury to ease pain. Compression, such as wrapping with a stretch bandage, and elevation help minimize swelling.

After the first few days, as the pain decreases, using heat, accompanied by stretching and light exercises, helps bring blood to the injured area to speed healing.

## Fascia

■ A **fasciotomy** (**fash**-ee-**OT**-oh-mee) is a surgical incision through the fascia to relieve tension or pressure (**fasci** means fascia, and **-otomy** means a surgical incision). Without this procedure, which is commonly used to treat compartment syndrome, the pressure causes a loss of circulation that damages the affected tissues.

■ **Fascioplasty** (**FASH**-ee-oh **plas**-tee) is the surgical repair of a fascia (**fasci/o** means fascia, and **-plasty** means surgical repair).

## Tendons

■ **Tenodesis** (ten-**ODD**-eh-sis) is the surgical suturing of the end of a tendon to a bone (**ten/o** means tendon, and **-desis** means to bind or tie together). *Tenodesis* is the opposite of *tenolysis.*

■ **Tenolysis** (ten-**OL**-ih-sis), also known as *tendolysis,* is the release of a tendon from adhesions (**ten/o** means tendon, and **-lysis** means to set free). *Tenolysis* is the opposite of *tenodesis.*

■ **Tenorrhaphy** (ten-**OR**-ah-fee) is the surgical suturing together of the divided ends of a tendon (**ten/o** means tendon, and **-rrhaphy** means surgical suturing).

## Muscles

■ **Myorrhaphy** (my-**OR**-ah-fee) is the surgical suturing a muscle (**my/o** means muscle, and **-rrhaphy** means surgical suturing).

■ A **myotomy** (my-**OT**-oh-mee) is a surgical incision into a muscle (**my** means muscle, and **-otomy** means surgical incision).

## ■ ABBREVIATIONS RELATED TO THE MUSCULAR SYSTEM

Table 4.1 presents an overview of the abbreviations related to the terms introduced in this chapter. Note: To avoid errors or confusion, always be cautious when using abbreviations.

**TABLE 4.1**
**Abbreviations Related to the Muscular System**

| | |
|---|---|
| **activities of daily living** = ADL | **ADL** = activities of daily living |
| **carpal tunnel syndrome** = CTS | **CTS** = carpal tunnel syndrome |
| **electromyography** = EMG | **EMG** = electromyography |
| **fibromyalgia syndrome** = FMS | **FMS** = fibromyalgia syndrome |
| **hemiplegia** = hemi | **hemi** = hemiplegia |
| **intermittent claudication** = IC | **IC** = intermittent claudication |
| **muscular dystrophy** = MD | **MD** = muscular dystrophy |
| **myasthenia gravis** = MG | **MG** = myasthenia gravis |
| **occupational therapy** = OT | **OT** = occupational therapist |
| **polymyositis** = PM | **PM** = polymyositis |
| **quadriplegia, quadriplegic** = quad | **quad** = quadriplegia, quadriplegic |
| **repetitive stress disorder** = RSD | **RSD** = repetitive stress disorder |

CFS — a

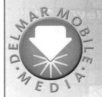

**StudyWARE CONNECTION**

For more practice and to test your mastery of this material, go to the StudyWARE™ to play interactive games and complete the quiz for this chapter.

*Downloadable audio is available for selected medical terms in this chapter to enhance your learning of medical terminology.*

☐ **Workbook Practice**

Go to your workbook and complete the exercises for this chapter.

# LEARNING EXERCISES

## MATCHING WORD PARTS 1

Write the correct answer in the middle column.

| Definition | Correct Answer | Possible Answers |
|---|---|---|
| 4.1. abnormal condition | _____ | -cele |
| 4.2. fascia | _____ | fasci/o |
| 4.3. fibrous tissue | _____ | fibr/o |
| 4.4. hernia, swelling | _____ | -ia |
| 4.5. movement | _____ | kines/o, kinesi/o |

## MATCHING WORD PARTS 2

Write the correct answer in the middle column.

| Definition | Correct Answer | Possible Answers |
|---|---|---|
| 4.6. coordination | _____ | my/o |
| 4.7. muscle | _____ | -rrhexis |
| 4.8. rupture | _____ | tax/o |
| 4.9. tendon | _____ | tend/o |
| 4.10. tone | _____ | ton/o |

## MATCHING MUSCLE DIRECTIONS AND POSITIONS

Write the correct answer in the middle column.

| Definition | Correct Answer | Possible Answers |
|---|---|---|
| 4.11. crosswise | _____ | lateralis |
| 4.12. ringlike | _____ | oblique |

| | | |
|---|---|---|
| 4.13. | slanted at an angle | _____ | rectus |
| 4.14. | straight | _____ | sphincter |
| 4.15. | toward the side | _____ | transverse |

## DEFINITIONS

Select the correct answer, and write it on the line provided.

4.16. The _____ muscles are under voluntary control.

       involuntary        nonstriated        skeletal        visceral

4.17. A/An _____ is a calcium deposit in the plantar fascia near its attachment to the

calcaneus bone.

       heel spur        impingement syndrome        overuse injury        shin splint

4.18. Turning the hand so the palm is upward is called _____.

       extension        flexion        pronation        supination

4.19. One of the symptoms of Parkinson's disease is _____, which is extreme slowness of

movement.

       bradykinesia        dyskinesia        hypotonia        hyperactivity

4.20. A/An _____ is a physician who specializes in physical medicine and rehabilitation

with the focus on restoring function.

       exercise physiologist        physiatrist        physiologist        rheumatologist

4.21. The term _____ means pertaining to muscle tissue and fascia.

       aponeurosis        fibrous sheath        myocardium        myofascial

4.22. A/An _____ is a narrow band of nonelastic, fibrous connective tissue that attaches

a muscle to a bone.

       aponeurosis        fascia        ligament        tendon

4.23. A band of fibers that holds structures together abnormally is a/an _____. These

bands can form as the result of an injury or surgery.

       adhesion        aponeurosis        atrophy        contracture

4.24. The paralysis of both legs and the lower part of the body is known as _____.

      hemiparesis           hemiplegia           paraplegia           quadriplegia

4.25. The surgical suturing of the end of a tendon to a bone is known as _____.

      tenodesis           tenorrhaphy           tendinosis           tenolysis

## MATCHING STRUCTURES

Write the correct answer in the middle column.

| Definition | Correct Answer | Possible Answers |
|---|---|---|
| 4.26. heart muscle | _____ | gluteus maximus |
| 4.27. buttock muscle | _____ | myocardial |
| 4.28. fibrous connective tissue | _____ | sphincter |
| 4.29. muscular cap of shoulder | _____ | tendon |
| 4.30. ring-like muscle | _____ | deltoid |

## WHICH WORD?

Select the correct answer, and write it on the line provided.

4.31. An injury to the body of the muscle or the attachment of a tendon is known as a/

an _____. These are usually associated with overuse injuries that involve a

wrenched or torn muscle or tendon attachment.

      sprain           strain

4.32. A _____ is a drug that causes temporary paralysis by blocking the transmission of

nerve stimuli to the muscles.

      neuromuscular blocker           skeletal muscle relaxant

4.33. The condition of abnormal muscle tone that causes the impairment of voluntary muscle movement is

known as _____.

      ataxia           dystonia

4.34. Inflamed and swollen tendons caught in the narrow space between the bones within the shoulder joint

cause the condition known as _____.

impingement syndrome          intermittent claudication

4.35. The _____ forms the muscular cap of the shoulder.

triceps brachii          deltoid

## SPELLING COUNTS

Find the misspelled word in each sentence. Then write that word, spelled correctly, on the line provided.

4.36. An antispasmydic is administered to suppress smooth muscle contractions of the stomach, intestine, or

bladder. _____

4.37. The medical term for hiccups is singulutas. _____

4.38. Myasthenia gravus is a chronic autoimmune disease that affects the neuromuscular junction and

produces serious weakness of voluntary muscles. _____

4.39. A ganglian cyst is a harmless fluid-filled swelling that occurs most commonly on the outer surface of the

wrist. _____

4.40. Pronetion is the movement that turns the palm of the hand downward or

backward. _____

## ABBREVIATION IDENTIFICATION

Write the correct answer on the line provided.

4.41. **CTS**          _____

4.42. **DTR**          _____

4.43. **ROM**          _____

4.44. **RSD**          _____

4.45. **SCI**          _____

## TERM SELECTION

Select the correct answer, and write it on the line provided.

4.46. The term _____ means the rupture or tearing of a muscle.

myocele          myorrhaphy          myorrhexis          myotomy

4.47.  The term meaning the degeneration of muscle tissue is _____.

       myoclonus              myolysis              myocele              myoparesis

4.48.  The term _____ means abnormally increased muscle function or activity.

       hyperkinesia           hypertonia            dyskinesia           hypotonia

4.49.  A/An _____ injury can be a strain or tear on any of the three muscles that

       straighten the hip and bend the knee.

       Achilles tendon        hamstring             myofascial           shin splint

4.50.  The specialized soft-tissue manipulation technique used to ease the pain of conditions such as fibromy-

       algia syndrome, movement restrictions, and temporomandibular joint disorders is known

       as _____.

       myofascial release     occupational therapy        RICE        therapeutic ultrasound

## SENTENCE COMPLETION

Write the correct term or terms on the lines provided.

4.51.  An inflammation of the tissues surrounding the elbow is known as _____.

4.52.  The movement during which the knees or elbows are bent to decrease the angle of the joints is known

       as _____.

4.53.  Pain in the leg muscles that occurs during exercise and is relieved by rest is known

       as _____. This condition is due to poor circulation and is associated with periph-

       eral vascular disease.

4.54.  A weakness or slight muscular paralysis is known as _____.

4.55.  A stiff neck due to spasmodic contraction of the neck muscles that pull the head toward the affected side

       is known as _____ or wryneck.

## WORD SURGERY

Divide each term into its component word parts. Write these word parts, in sequence, on the lines provided.
When necessary, use a slash (/) to indicate a combining vowel. (You may not need all of the lines provided.)

4.56.  **Electromyography** is a diagnostic test that measures the electrical activity within muscle fibers.

       _____    _____    _____    _____

4.57.    **Hyperkinesia** means abnormally increased muscle function or activity.

_____    _____    _____    _____

4.58.    **Myoclonus** is the sudden, involuntary jerking of a muscle or group of muscles.

_____    _____    _____    _____

4.59.    **Polymyositis** is a muscle disease characterized by the simultaneous inflammation and weakening of voluntary muscles in many parts of the body.

_____    _____    _____    _____

4.60.    **Sarcopenia** is the loss of muscle mass, strength, and function that comes with aging.

_____    _____    _____    _____

## TRUE/FALSE

If the statement is true, write **True** on the line. If the statement is false, write **False** on the line.

4.61.    _____ Overuse tendinitis is inflammation of tendons caused by excessive or unusual use of a joint.

4.62.    _____ Hemiplegia is the total paralysis of the lower half of the body.

4.63.    _____ A spasm is a sudden, involuntary contraction of one or more muscles.

4.64.    _____ Ataxia is the distortion of voluntary movement such as in a tic or spasm.

4.65.    _____ Striated muscles are located in the walls of internal organs such as the digestive tract, blood vessels, and ducts leading from glands.

## CLINICAL CONDITIONS

Write the correct answer on the line provided.

4.66.    George Quinton developed a swelling on the outer surface of his wrist. His doctor diagnosed this as being a/an _____ and explained that this was a harmless fluid-filled swelling.

4.67.    Raul Valladares has a protrusion of a muscle substance through a tear in the fascia surrounding it. This condition is known as a/an _____ .

4.68.    Louisa Ferraro experienced _____ of her leg muscles due to the disuse of these muscles over a long period of time.

4.69. Jasmine Franklin has _____. This is a condition in which there is diminished tone of the skeletal muscles.

4.70. Carolyn Goodwin complained of profound fatigue that is not improved by bed rest and was made worse by physical or mental activity. After ruling out other causes, her physician diagnosed her condition as being _____ syndrome.

4.71. Chuan Lee, who is a runner, required treatment for _____

_____. This condition is a painful inflammation of the Achilles tendon caused by excessive stress being placed on that tendon.

4.72. For the first several days after his fall, Bob Hill suffered severe muscle pain. This condition is known as _____.

4.73. Jorge Guendulay could not play for his team because of a/an _____. This is a painful condition caused by the muscle tearing away from the tibia.

4.74. Due to a spinal cord injury, Marissa Giannati suffers from _____, which is paralysis of all four limbs.

4.75. Duncan McDougle has slight paralysis on one side of his body. This condition, which was caused by a stroke, is known as _____.

## WHICH IS THE CORRECT MEDICAL TERM?

Select the correct answer, and write it on the line provided.

4.76. The term *muscular* _____ describes a group of genetic diseases characterized by progressive weakness and degeneration of the skeletal muscles.

      atonic             ataxia             dystonia             dystrophy

4.77. The surgical enlargement of the carpal tunnel or cutting of the carpal ligament to relieve nerve pressure is called _____.

    carpal tunnel syndrome     compartment     carpal tunnel release     myofascial pain
                             syndrome                               syndrome

4.78. During _____, the arm moves inward and toward the side of the body.

      abduction             adduction             circumduction             rotation

4.79.    A surgical incision into a muscle is known as _____.

myoccle            myorrhaphy            myotomy            fascioplasty

4.80.    The term _____ means bending the foot upward at the ankle.

abduction        dorsiflexion            elevation            plantar flexion

## CHALLENGE WORD BUILDING

These terms are *not* found in this chapter; however, they are made up of the following familiar word parts. If you need help in creating the term, refer to your medical dictionary.

| poly- | card/o | -desis |
|---|---|---|
| | fasci/o | -ectomy |
| | herni/o | -itis |
| | my/o | -necrosis |
| | sphincter/o | -otomy |
| -algia | -pathy |
| | | -rrhaphy |

4.81.    Any abnormal condition of skeletal muscles is known as _____.

4.82.    Pain in several muscle groups is known as _____.

4.83.    The death of individual muscle fibers is known as _____.

4.84.    Surgical suturing of torn fascia is known as _____.

4.85.    Based on word parts, the removal of multiple muscles is known as _____.

4.86.    The surgical attachment of a fascia to another fascia or to a tendon is known

as _____.

4.87.    Inflammation of the muscle of the heart is known as _____.

4.88.    The surgical removal of fascia is a/an _____.

4.89.    The surgical suturing of a defect in a muscular wall, such as the repair of a hernia, is a/

an _____.

4.90.    An incision into a sphincter muscle is a/an _____.

## LABELING EXERCISES

Identify the movements in the accompanying figures by writing the correct term on the line provided.

4.91. _____

4.92. _____

4.93. _____

4.94. _____

4.95. _____

4.96. _____

4.97. _____

4.98. _____

4.99. _____

4.100. _____

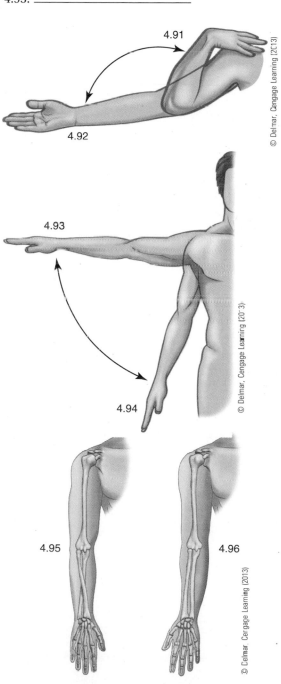

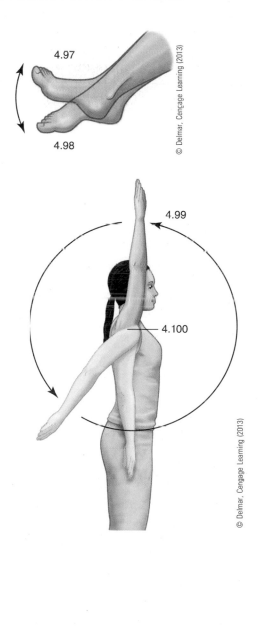

# THE HUMAN TOUCH

# Critical Thinking Exercise

The following story and questions are designed to stimulate critical thinking through class discussion or as a brief essay response. There are no right or wrong answers to these questions.

*"Leg muscles save back muscles ... Mandatory OSHA meeting Tuesday at noon. Bring lunch," states the company memo. Sandor Padilla, a 28-year-old cargo loader, sighs, "Third meeting this year, and it's not even June yet!" He has only two minutes to reach the tarmac. "Oh well, cargo waits for no man," he thinks as he jogs off to work.*

*Sandor enjoys his job. It keeps him fit, but lets his mind follow more creative avenues. Today, his thoughts stray to his daughter Reina's fifth birthday party, just two weeks away. "A pony or a clown? Hot dogs or tacos?" he muses. Single parenting has its moments. As he is busy thinking of other things, the heavy crate slips, driving him into a squatting position that injures his thigh muscles. His cry of pain brings Janet Wilson, his supervisor, running to help.*

*The first aid station ices his leg to reduce swelling and pain. After the supervisor completes the incident report, Sandor is taken to the emergency room. Dr. Basra, the orthopedic specialist on call, diagnoses myorrhexis of the left rectus femoris. A myorrhaphy is required to treat this injury. After several days in the hospital, Sandor is sent home with a Vicodin prescription for pain and orders for physical therapy sessions three times a week. He is not expected to return to work for at least 90 days.*

*AirFreight Systems receives the first report of injury and compares it with the supervisor's incident report. Ruling: Safety Violation. No Liability. Return to work in 30 days or dismissal.*

## Suggested Discussion Topics

1. On what basis do you think AirFreight determined that this was a safety violation?
2. Use lay terms to explain Sandor's injury and the treatment that was required.
3. Sandor knows how to handle heavy loads safely; however, the crate may have slipped because he was busy thinking about his daughter's birthday party and not about his work. Could the responsibility for this accident be considered negligence on Sandor's part? Do you think Sandor should be held responsible or is blameless in this situation?
4. It was determined that AirFreight was not responsible for the accident. Therefore, do you think the company should take away Sandor's job if he does not return in 30 calendar days?

# The Cardiovascular System

## Overview of
## STRUCTURES, COMBINING FORMS, AND FUNCTIONS OF THE CARDIOVASCULAR SYSTEM

| Major Structures | Related Combining Forms | Primary Functions |
| --- | --- | --- |
| Heart | **card/o, cardi/o** | Receives blood from the veins and pumps blood into the arteries. |
| Blood Vessels | **angl/o, vas/o** | Transport blood to and from all areas of the body. |
| Arteries | **arteri/o** | Transport blood away from the heart to all parts of the body. |
| Capillaries | **capill/o** | Permit the exchange of nutrients and waste products between the blood and the cells. |
| Veins | **phleb/o, ven/o** | Return blood from all body parts to the heart. |
| Blood | **hem/o, hemat/o** | Brings oxygen and nutrients to the cells and carries away waste. |

# Vocabulary Related to **THE CARDIOVASCULAR SYSTEM**

This list contains essential word parts and medical terms for this chapter. These terms are pronounced in the StudyWARE™ and Audio CDs that are available for use with this text. These and the other important **primary terms** are shown in boldface throughout the chapter. *Secondary terms*, which appear in *orange* italics, clarify the meaning of primary terms.

## Word Parts

- ☐ **angi/o** blood or lymph vessel
- ☐ **aort/o** aorta
- ☐ **arteri/o** artery
- ☐ **ather/o** plaque, fatty substance
- ☐ **brady-** slow
- ☐ **cardi/o** heart
- ☐ **-crasia** a mixture or blending
- ☐ **-emia** blood, blood condition
- ☐ **erythr/o** red
- ☐ **hem/o, hemat/o** blood, relating to the blood
- ☐ **leuk/o** white
- ☐ **phleb/o** vein
- ☐ **tachy-** fast, rapid
- ☐ **thromb/o** clot
- ☐ **ven/o** vein

## Medical Terms

- ☐ **ACE inhibitor**
- ☐ **anemia** (ah-**NEE**-mee-ah)
- ☐ **aneurysm** (**AN**-you-rizm)
- ☐ **angina** (an-**JIH**-nuh)
- ☐ **angioplasty** (**AN**-jee-oh-**plas**-tee)
- ☐ **anticoagulant** (**an**-tih-koh-**AG**-you-lant)
- ☐ **aplastic anemia** (ay-**PLAS**-tick ah-**NEE**-mee-ah)
- ☐ **arrhythmia** (ah-**RITH**-mee-ah)
- ☐ **atherectomy** (**ath**-er-**ECK**-toh-mee)
- ☐ **atheroma** (**ath**-er-**OH**-mah)
- ☐ **atherosclerosis** (**ath**-er-oh-skleh-**ROH**-sis)
- ☐ **atrial fibrillation** (**AY**-tree-al fih-brih-**LAY**-shun)
- ☐ **automated external defibrillator** (dee-**fih**-brih-**LAY**-ter)
- ☐ **beta-blocker**
- ☐ **blood dyscrasia** (dis-**KRAY**-zee-ah)
- ☐ **bradycardia** (**brad**-ee-**KAR**-dee-ah)
- ☐ **cardiac arrest**
- ☐ **cardiac catheterization** (**KAR**-dee-ack **kath**-eh-ter-eye-**ZAY**-shun)
- ☐ **cardiomyopathy** (**kar**-dee-oh-my-**OP**-pah-thee)
- ☐ **carotid endarterectomy** (kah-**ROT**-id **end**-ar-ter-**ECK**-toh-mee)
- ☐ **cholesterol** (koh-**LES**-ter-ol)

- ☐ **chronic venous insufficiency**
- ☐ **coronary thrombosis** (**KOR**-uh-**nerr**-ee throm-**BOH**-sis)
- ☐ **defibrillation** (dee-**fih**-brih-**LAY**-shun)
- ☐ **diuretic** (**dye**-you-**RET**-ick)
- ☐ **electrocardiogram** (ee-**leck**-troh-**KAR**-dee-oh-gram)
- ☐ **embolism** (**EM**-boh-lizm)
- ☐ **embolus** (**EM**-boh-lus)
- ☐ **endocarditis** (**en**-doh-kar-**DYE**-tis)
- ☐ **erythrocytes** (eh-**RITH**-roh-sights)
- ☐ **hemoglobin** (**hee**-moh-**GLOH**-bin)
- ☐ **hemolytic anemia** (**hee**-moh-**LIT**-ick ah-**NEE**-mee-ah)
- ☐ **hemostasis** (**hee**-moh-**STAY**-sis)
- ☐ **ischemic heart disease** (iss-**KEE**-mick)
- ☐ **leukemia** (loo-**KEE**-mee-ah)
- ☐ **leukocytes** (**LOO**-koh-sites)
- ☐ **leukopenia** (**loo**-koh-**PEE**-nee-ah)
- ☐ **megaloblastic anemia** (**MEG**-ah-loh-**blas**-tick ah-**NEE**-mee-ah)
- ☐ **myelodysplastic syndrome** (**my**-eh-loh-dis-**PLAS**-tick **SIN**-drohm)
- ☐ **myocardial infarction** (**my**-oh-**KAR**-dee-al in-**FARK**-shun)
- ☐ **orthostatic hypotension** (**or**-thoh-**STAT**-ick **high**-poh-**TEN**-shun)
- ☐ **pericardium** (**pehr**-ih-**KAR**-dee-um)
- ☐ **pernicious anemia** (per-**NISH**-us ah-**NEE**-mee-ah)
- ☐ **phlebitis** (**fleh**-**BYE**-tis)
- ☐ **Raynaud's disease** (ray-**NOHZ**)
- ☐ **septicemia** (**sep**-tih-**SEE**-mee-ah)
- ☐ **sickle cell anemia**
- ☐ **tachycardia** (**tack**-ee-**KAR**-dee-ah)
- ☐ **temporal arteritis** (**TEM**-poh-**ral ar**-teh-**RYE**-tis)
- ☐ **thallium stress test** (**THAL**-ee-um)
- ☐ **thrombocytopenia** (**throm**-boh-**sigh**-toh-**PEE**-nee-ah)
- ☐ **thrombolytic** (**throm**-boh-**LIT**-ick)
- ☐ **thrombosis** (throm-**BOH**-sis)
- ☐ **thrombotic occlusion** (throm-**BOT**-ick ah-**KLOO**-zhun)
- ☐ **thrombus** (**THROM**-bus)
- ☐ **transfusion reaction**
- ☐ **valvulitis** (**val**-view-**LYE**-tis)
- ☐ **varicose veins** (**VAR**-ih-kohs **VAYNS**)
- ☐ **ventricular fibrillation** (ven-**TRICK**-you-lar fih-brih-**LAY**-shun)
- ☐ **ventricular tachycardia** (ven-**TRICK**-you-lar **tack**-ee-**KAR**-dee-ah)

# ■ FUNCTIONS OF THE CARDIOVASCULAR SYSTEM

The cardiovascular system consists of the heart, blood vessels, and blood. **Cardiovascular** (kar-dee-oh-VAS-kyou-lar) means pertaining to the heart and blood vessels (**cardi/o** means heart, **vascul** means blood vessels, and **-ar** means pertaining to).

These structures work together to efficiently pump blood to all body tissues.

■ Blood is a fluid tissue that transports oxygen and nutrients to the body tissues.

■ Blood returns some waste products from these tissues to the kidneys and carries carbon dioxide back to the lungs.

■ Blood cells also play important roles in the immune system (see Chapter 6), and in the endocrine system (see Chapter 13).

# ■ STRUCTURES OF THE CARDIOVASCULAR SYSTEM

The major structures of the cardiovascular system are the heart, blood vessels, and blood.

## The Heart

The **heart** is a hollow, muscular organ located in the thoracic cavity, between the lungs (Figure 5.1). It is a very effective pump that furnishes the power to maintain the blood flow needed throughout the entire body (Figures 5.2 and 5.3). The *apex* is the lower tip of the heart.

## The Pericardium

The **pericardium** (pehr-ih-KAR-dee-um), also known as the *pericardial sac*, is the double-walled membranous sac that encloses the heart (**peri-** means surrounding, **cardi** means heart, and **-um** is a singular noun ending). *Membranous* means pertaining to membrane, which is a thin layer of pliable tissue that covers or encloses a body part.

■ The *parietal pericardium* is a fibrous sac that surrounds and protects the heart.

■ *Pericardial fluid* is found between these two layers, where it acts as a lubricant to prevent friction as the heart beats.

■ The *visceral pericardium* is the inner layer of the pericardium that also forms the outer layer of the heart. When referred to as the outer layer of the heart, it is known as the *epicardium* (Figure 5.4).

## The Walls of the Heart

The walls of the heart are made up of these three layers: the epicardium, myocardium, and endocardium (Figure 5.4).

■ The **epicardium** (ep-ih-KAR-dee-um) is the external layer of the heart and the inner layer of the pericardium (**epi-** means upon, **cardi** means heart, and **-um** is a singular noun ending).

■ The **myocardium** (my-oh-KAR-dee-um) is the middle and thickest of the heart's three layers (**my/o** means muscle, **cardi** means heart, and **-um** is a singular noun ending). Also known as *myocardial muscle*, this consists of specialized cardiac muscle tissue that is capable of the constant contraction and relaxation of this muscle that creates the pumping movement that is necessary to maintain the flow of blood throughout the body. Myocardial muscle is discussed in Chapter 4.

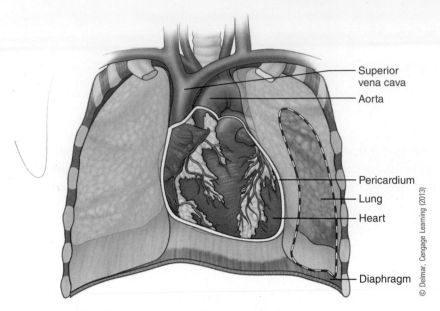

**FIGURE 5.1** The heart is located in the thoracic cavity between the lungs.

- Superior vena cava
- Aorta
- Pericardium
- Lung
- Heart
- Diaphragm

© Delmar, Cengage Learning (2013)

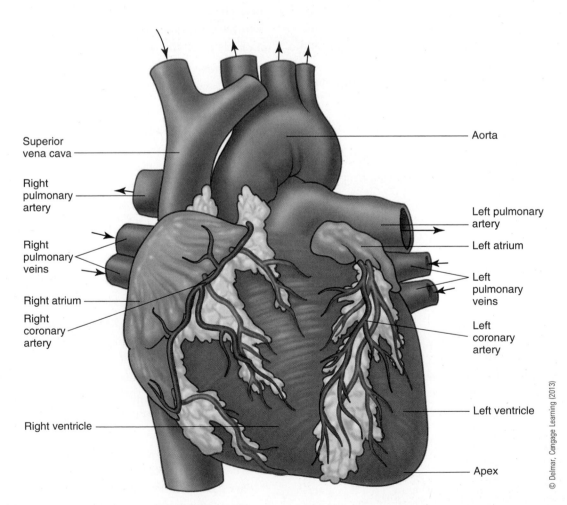

- Superior vena cava
- Right pulmonary artery
- Right pulmonary veins
- Right atrium
- Right coronary artery
- Right ventricle
- Aorta
- Left pulmonary artery
- Left atrium
- Left pulmonary veins
- Left coronary artery
- Left ventricle
- Apex

© Delmar, Cengage Learning (2013)

**FIGURE 5.2** Anterior external view of the heart.

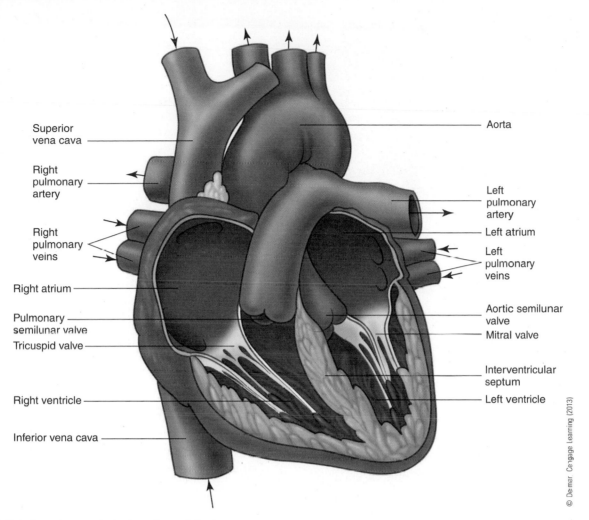

**FIGURE 5.3** Anterior cross-section view of the heart.

■ The **endocardium** (**en**-doh-**KAR**-dee-um), which consists of epithelial tissue, is the inner lining of the heart (**endo-** means within, **cardi** means heart, and **-um** is a singular noun ending). This is the surface that comes into direct contact with the blood as it is being pumped through the heart.

## Blood Supply to the Myocardium

The myocardium, which beats constantly, must have a continuous supply of oxygen and nutrients plus prompt waste removal to survive. If for any reason this blood supply is disrupted, the myocardium of the affected area dies.

The **coronary arteries** (**KOR**-uh-**nerr**-ee), which supply oxygen-rich blood to the myocardium, are shown in red in Figure 5.6. The veins, which are shown in blue, remove waste products from the myocardium.

## The Chambers of the Heart

The heart is divided into four chambers, each of which has a specialized function (Figure 5.3):

■ The **atria** (**AY**-tree-ah) are the two upper chambers of the heart, and these chambers are divided by *interatrial septum*. (A *septum* is a wall that separates two chambers.)

■ The atria are the receiving chambers, and all blood enters the heart through these chambers. The singular form of *atria* is *atrium*.

■ The **ventricles** (**VEN**-trih-kuhls) are the two lower chambers of the heart, and these chambers are divided by the *interventricular septum*.

■ The walls of the ventricles are thicker than those of the atria because the ventricles must pump blood throughout the entire body.

■ The term *ventricle* is also defined as a normal hollow chamber of the brain (see Chapter 10).

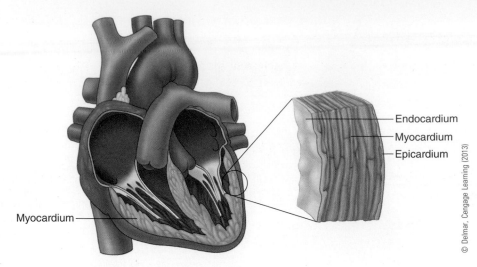

Endocardium
Myocardium
Epicardium

© Delmar, Cengage Learning (2013)

Myocardium

**FIGURE 5.4** A simplified view of the tissues of the heart walls.

## The Valves of the Heart

The flow of blood through the heart is controlled by four valves as described in this section. If any of these valves is not working correctly, blood cannot flow properly through the heart and cannot be pumped effectively to all parts of the body (Figures 5.3 and 5.5).

■ The **tricuspid valve** (try-**KUS**-pid) controls the opening between the right atrium and the right ventricle. The term *tricuspid* means having three cusps (points), and this describes the shape of this valve.

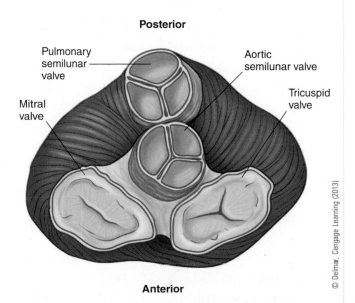

**Posterior**

Pulmonary semilunar valve

Aortic semilunar valve

Mitral valve

Tricuspid valve

**Anterior**

© Delmar, Cengage Learning (2013)

**FIGURE 5.5** The valves of the heart viewed from above with the atria removed.

■ The **pulmonary semilunar valve** (**PULL**-mah-**nair**-ee sem-ee-**LOO**-nar) is located between the right ventricle and the pulmonary artery. *Pulmonary* means pertaining to the lungs, and *semilunar* means half-moon. This valve is shaped like a half-moon.

■ The **mitral valve** (**MY**-tral) is located between the left atrium and left ventricle. *Mitral* means shaped like a bishop's miter (hat). This valve is also known as the *bicuspid valve* because *bicuspid* means having two cusps (points), which describes the shape of this valve.

■ The **aortic semilunar valve** (ay-**OR**-tick sem-ee-**LOO**-nar) is located between the left ventricle and the aorta. *Aortic* means pertaining to the aorta. *Semilunar* means half-moon, which describes the shape of this valve.

■ The flow of blood through the heart is summarized in Table 5.1. The red arrows indicate oxygenated blood, and blue arrows indicate deoxygenated blood. *Oxygenated* means oxygen rich, or containing an adequate supply of oxygen. *Deoxygenated* means oxygen poor, or not yet containing an adequate supply of oxygen.

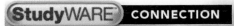

**StudyWARE** **CONNECTION**

Watch the **Blood Flow Through the Heart** animation in the StudyWARE™.

## TABLE 5.1
### Blood Flow Through the Heart

| | |
|---|---|
| ↓ | The **right atrium** (RA) receives oxygen-poor blood from all tissues, except the lungs, through the superior and inferior venae cavae. Blood flows out of the RA through the tricuspid valve into the right ventricle. |
| ↓ | The **right ventricle** (RV) pumps the oxygen-poor blood through the pulmonary semilunar valve and into the pulmonary artery, which carries it to the lungs. |
| ↓ | The **left atrium** (LA) receives oxygen-rich blood from the lungs through the four pulmonary veins. The blood flows out of the LA, through the mitral valve, and into the left ventricle. |
| ↓ | The **left ventricle** (LV) receives oxygen-rich blood from the left atrium. Blood flows out of the LV through the aortic semilunar valve and into the aorta, which carries it to all parts of the body, except the lungs. |
| ↓ | Oxygen-poor blood is returned by the venae cavae to the right atrium, and the cycle continues. |

## Systemic and Pulmonary Circulation

Blood is pumped through the systemic and pulmonary circulation systems. Together the blood in these systems brings oxygen to the cells and removes waste products from the cells (Figure 5.6).

**Pulmonary circulation** is the flow of blood only between the heart and lungs.

- The **pulmonary arteries** carry deoxygenated blood out of the right ventricle and into the lungs. This is the only place in the body where deoxygenated blood is carried by arteries instead of veins.

- In the lungs, carbon dioxide from the body is exchanged for oxygen from the inhaled air.

- The **pulmonary veins** carry the oxygenated blood from the lungs into the left atrium of the heart. This is the only place in the body where veins carry oxygenated blood.

**Systemic circulation** includes the flow of blood to all parts of the body *except* the lungs.

- Oxygenated blood flows out of the left ventricle and into arterial circulation.

- The veins carry deoxygenated blood into the right atrium.

- From here, the blood flows into the pulmonary circulation before being pumped out of the heart into the arteries again.

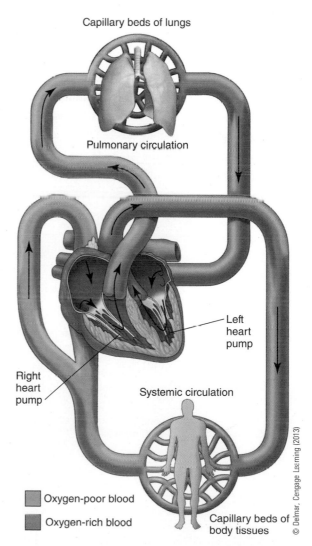

FIGURE 5.6 Systemic and pulmonary blood circulation.

Capillary beds of lungs

Pulmonary circulation

Left heart pump

Right heart pump

Systemic circulation

Oxygen-poor blood

Oxygen-rich blood

Capillary beds of body tissues

© Delmar, Cengage Learning (2013)

## The Heartbeat

The **heartbeat** is the ability to pump blood effectively throughout the body; the contraction and relaxation (beating) of the heart must occur in exactly the correct sequence.

- The rate and regularity of the heartbeat is determined by *electrical impulses* from nerves that stimulate the myocardium of the chambers of the heart. (The specialized myocardial muscles that make this pumping action possible are described in Chapter 4.)

- Also known as the *conduction system*, these electrical impulses are controlled by the sinoatrial (SA) node, atrioventricular (AV) node, and the bundle of His (Figure 5.7).

### The Sinoatrial Node

- The **sinoatrial node** (**sigh**-noh-**AY**-tree-ahl), which is often referred to as the *SA node*, is located in the posterior wall of the right atrium near the entrance of the superior vena cava (Figure 5.7).

- The SA node establishes the basic rhythm and rate of the heartbeat. For this reason, it is known as the *natural pacemaker* of the heart.

- Electrical impulses from the SA node start each wave of muscle contraction in the heart.

- The impulse in the right atrium spreads over the muscles of both atria, causing them to contract simultaneously. This contraction forces blood into the ventricles.

### The Atrioventricular Node

- The impulses from the SA node also travel to the **atrioventricular node** (**ay**-tree-oh-ven-**TRICK**-you-lar), which is also known as the *AV node*.

- The AV node is located on the floor of the right atrium near the interatrial septum (Figure 5.7). From here, it transmits the electrical impulses onward to the bundle of His.

### The Bundle of His

- The **bundle of His** (**HISS**) is a group of fibers located within the interventricular septum. These fibers carry an electrical impulse to ensure the sequence of the heart contractions (Figure 5.7). These electrical impulses travel onward to the right and left ventricles and the Purkinje fibers.

- **Purkinje fibers** (per-**KIN**-jee) are specialized conductive fibers located within the walls of the ventricles. These fibers relay the electrical impulses to the cells of the ventricles, and it is this stimulation that causes the ventricles to contract. This contraction

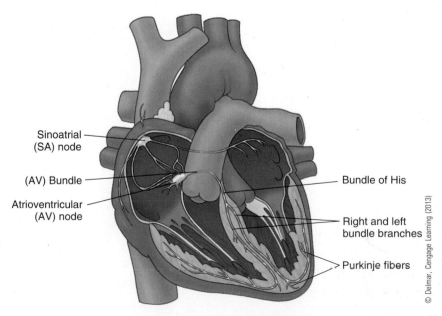

Sinoatrial (SA) node

(AV) Bundle

Atrioventricular (AV) node

Bundle of His

Right and left bundle branches

Purkinje fibers

© Delmar, Cengage Learning (2013)

**FIGURE 5.7** An electrical impulse from the SA node travels to the AV node and causes the ventricle to contract.

of the ventricles forces blood out of the heart and into the aorta and pulmonary arteries (Figure 5.7).

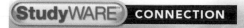

**CONNECTION**

Watch the **Electrical Stimulation of the Heart** animation in the StudyWARE™.

## Electrical Waves

The activities of the electrical conduction system of the heart can be visualized as wave movements on a monitor or an electrocardiogram. The term *sinus rhythm* refers to the normal beating of the heart (Figures 5.8 and 5.16A).

- The *P wave* is due to the stimulation (contraction) of the atria.

- The *QRS complex* shows the stimulation (contraction) of the ventricles. The atria relax as the ventricles contract.

- The *T wave* is the recovery (relaxation) of the ventricles.

## ■ THE BLOOD VESSELS

There are three types of blood vessels: arteries, capillaries, and veins. These vessels form the arterial and venous circulatory systems (Figures 5.9 and 5.10).

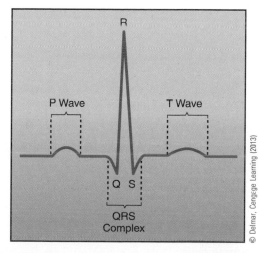

**FIGURE 5.8** The waves of contraction and relaxation of the heart can be visualized on a monitor or as an electrocardiogram (EKG or ECG).

## Arteries

- The **arteries** are large blood vessels that carry blood away from the heart to all regions of the body.

- The walls of the arteries are composed of three layers. This structure makes the arteries muscular and elastic so they can expand and contract with the pumping beat of the heart. The term *endarterial* means within an artery or pertaining to the inner portion of an artery.

- *Arterial blood* is bright red in color because it is oxygen rich. The pumping action of the heart causes blood to spurt out when an artery is cut.

- The **aorta** (ay-**OR**-tah) is the largest blood vessel in the body. It begins from the left ventricle of the heart and forms the main trunk of the arterial system (Figures 5.2 and 5.9).

- The **carotid arteries** (kah-**ROT**-id) are the major arteries that carry blood upward to the head.

- The *common carotid artery* is located on each side of the neck.

- It divides into the *internal carotid artery*, which brings oxygen-rich blood to the brain.

- The *external carotid artery* brings blood to the face.

- Any disruption in this blood flow can result in a stroke or other brain damage.

- The **arterioles** (ar-**TEE**-ree-ohlz) are the smaller, thinner branches of arteries that deliver blood to the capillaries. As it enters one end of the capillary bed, it is here that the rate of flow of arterial blood slows.

## Capillaries

**Capillaries** (**KAP**-uh-**ler**-eez), which are only one epithelial cell in thickness, are the smallest blood vessels in the body. The capillaries form networks of expanded vascular beds that have the important role of delivering oxygen and nutrients to the cells of the tissues (Figure 5.11).

- The capillaries further slow the flow of blood to allow plasma to flow into the tissues. It is here that the exchange of oxygen, nutrients, and waste materials occur within the surrounding cells.

- After leaving the cells, 90% of this fluid, which is now oxygen poor and contains some waste products, enter the opposite end of the capillary bed through the venules.

- The 10% of this fluid that is left behind in the tissues becomes lymph. This is explained in Chapter 6.

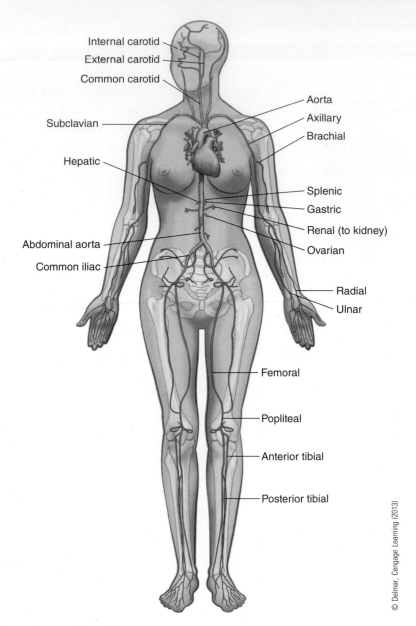

Internal carotid
External carotid
Common carotid
Subclavian
Hepatic
Abdominal aorta
Common iliac

Aorta
Axillary
Brachial
Splenic
Gastric
Renal (to kidney)
Ovarian
Radial
Ulnar
Femoral
Popliteal
Anterior tibial
Posterior tibial

© Delmar, Cengage Learning (2013)

**FIGURE 5.9** Anterior view of arterial circulation.

## Veins

**Veins** form a low-pressure collecting system to return oxygen-poor blood to the heart (Figures 5.10 through 5.12).

■ **Venules** (**VEN**-youls) are the smallest veins that join to form the larger veins.

■ The walls of the veins are thinner and less elastic than those of the arteries.

■ The venous blood continues its flow at an increased speed as it continues its return journey to the heart. *Venous* means relating to, or contained in, the veins.

■ Veins have valves that enable blood to flow only toward the heart and to prevent it from flowing away from the heart (Figure 5.12).

■ *Superficial veins* are located near the body surface.

■ *Deep veins* are located within the tissues and away from the body surface.

### The Venae Cavae

■ The **venae cavae** (**VEE**-nee **KAY**-vee) are the two largest veins in the body. These are the veins that return blood into the heart (singular, *vena cava*).

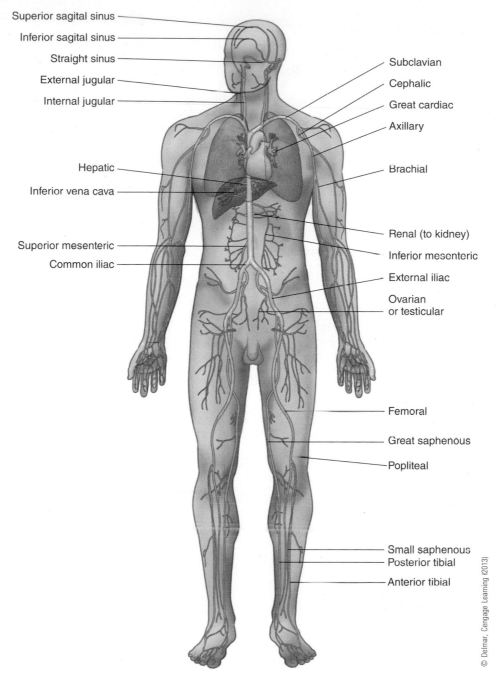

**FIGURE 5.10** Anterior view of venous circulation.

- The *superior vena cava* transports blood from the upper portion of the body to the heart (Figures 5.2 and 5.3).

- The *inferior vena cava* transports blood from the lower portion of the body to the heart (Figure 5.3).

## Pulse and Blood Pressure

- The **pulse** is the rhythmic pressure against the walls of an artery caused by the contraction of the heart. The *pulse rate* is discussed in Chapter 15.

- **Blood pressure** is the measurement of the amount of systolic and diastolic pressure exerted against the walls of the arteries. How to record blood pressure is discussed in Chapter 15. See Table 5.3 for blood pressure classifications.

- **Systolic pressure** (sis-**TOL**-ick), which occurs when the ventricles contract, is the highest pressure against the walls of an artery. The term *systole* means contraction of the heart, and *systolic* means pertaining to this contraction phase.

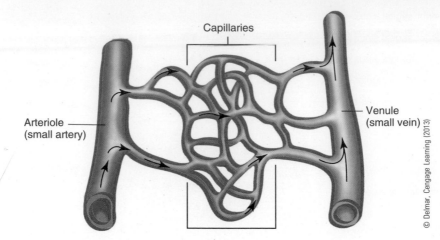

Capillaries

Arteriole
(small artery)

Venule
(small vein)

© Delmar, Cengage Learning (2013)

**FIGURE 5.11** Oxygen-rich arterial blood is delivered by arterioles to the capillaries. After the oxygen has been extracted, the oxygen-poor blood is returned to circulation as venous blood.

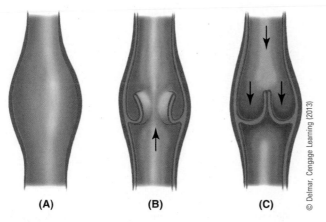

(A)                (B)                (C)

© Delmar, Cengage Learning (2013)

**FIGURE 5.12** Veins contain valves to prevent the backward flow of blood. (A) External view of the vein shows wider area of valve. (B) Internal view with the valve open as blood flows through it toward the heart. (C) Internal view with the valve closed to prevent the backflow of blood.

- **Diastolic pressure** (dye-ah-**STOL**-ick), which occurs when the ventricles are relaxed, is the lowest pressure against the walls of an artery. The term *diastole* means relaxation of the heart, and *diastolic* means pertaining to this relaxation phase.

# BLOOD

Blood is the fluid tissue in the body. It is composed of 55% liquid plasma and 45% formed elements. As you study these elements, refer to Figure 5.13.

## Plasma

**Plasma** (**PLAZ**-mah) is a straw-colored fluid that contains nutrients, hormones, and waste products. Plasma is 91%

water. The remaining 9% consists mainly of proteins, including the clotting proteins.

- **Serum** (**SEER**-um) is plasma fluid after the blood cells and the clotting proteins have been removed.

- **Fibrinogen** (figh-**BRIN**-oh-jen) and **prothrombin** (proh-**THROM**-bin) are the clotting proteins found in plasma. They have an important role in clot formation to control bleeding.

## Formed Elements of the Blood

The formed elements of blood include erythrocytes, leukocytes, and thrombocytes.

### Erythrocytes

**Erythrocytes** (eh-**RITH**-roh-sights), also known as *red blood cells* (RBC), are mature red blood cells produced by the red bone marrow (**erythr/o** means red, and **-cytes** means cells). The primary role of these cells is to transport oxygen to the tissues.

This oxygen is transported by **hemoglobin** (**hee**-moh-**GLOH**-bin), which is the oxygen-carrying blood protein pigment of the erythrocytes (**hem/o** means blood, and **-globin** means protein).

### Leukocytes

**Leukocytes** (**LOO**-koh-sites), also known as *white blood cells* (WBC), are the blood cells involved in defending the body against infective organisms and foreign substances (**leuk/o** means white, and **-cytes** means cells). The following are the major groups of leukocytes:

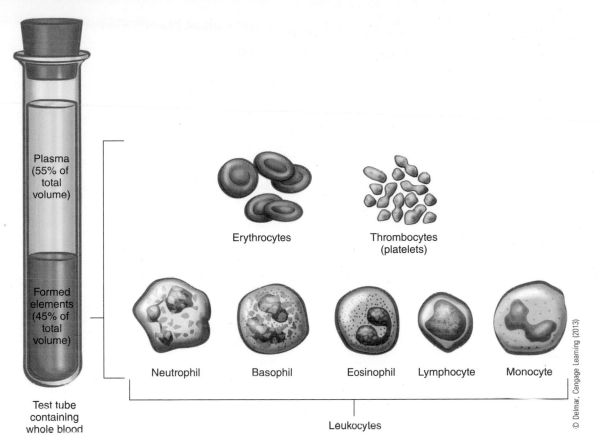

Plasma
(55% of
total
volume)

Formed
elements
(45% of
total
volume)

Test tube
containing
whole blood

Erythrocytes

Thrombocytes
(platelets)

Neutrophil    Basophil    Eosinophil    Lymphocyte    Monocyte

Leukocytes

© Delmar, Cengage Learning (2013)

**FIGURE 5.13** The major fluid and formed components of blood. The formed elements include erythrocytes, thrombocytes, and leukocytes.

- **Neutrophils** (**NEW**-troh-fills), which are formed in red bone marrow, are the most common type of WBC. Through phagocytosis, neutrophils play a major role in the immune system's defense against pathogens, including bacteria, viruses, and fungi. *Phagocytosis* is the process of destroying pathogens by surrounding and swallowing them. (Neutrophils are discussed further in Chapter 6.)

- **Basophils** (**BAY**-soh-fills), which are also formed in red bone marrow, are the least common type of WBC. Basophils are responsible for causing the symptoms of allergies.

- **Eosinophils** (**ee**-oh-**SIN**-oh-fills) are formed in red bone marrow and then migrate to tissues throughout the body. Here these cells destroy parasitic organisms and play a major role in allergic reactions.

- **Lymphocytes** (**LIM**-foh-sights) are formed in red bone marrow, in lymph nodes, and in the spleen. Lymphocytes identify foreign substances and germs (bacteria or viruses) in the body and produce antibodies that specifically target them. (Lymphocytes are discussed further in Chapter 6.)

- **Monocytes** (**MON**-oh-sights) are formed in red bone marrow, lymph nodes, and the spleen. Through phagocytosis, monocytes provide immunological defenses against many infectious organisms.

## Thrombocytes

**Thrombocytes** (**THROM**-boh-sights), which are also known as *platelets*, are the smallest formed elements of the blood. They play an important role in the clotting of blood (**thromb/o** means clot, and -**cytes** means cells).

- When a blood vessel is damaged, the thrombocytes are activated and become sticky.

- This action causes the thrombocytes to clump together to form a clot to stop the bleeding.

## Blood Types

**Blood types** are classified according to the presence or absence of certain antigens. (An *antigen* is any substance that the body regards as being foreign.)

The four major blood types are **A**, **AB**, **B**, and **O**. The A, AB, and B groups are based on the presence of the A or

B antigens or both on the red blood cells. In contrast, in type O blood both the A and B antigens are absent.

## The Rh Factor

The **Rh factor** defines the presence or absence of the Rh antigen on red blood cells. The Rh factor was so named because this antigen was first found in rhesus monkeys.

- About 85% of Americans have the Rh antigen, and these individuals are described as being *Rh positive* (Rh+).

- The remaining 15% of Americans *do not have* the Rh antigen, and these individuals are described as being *Rh negative* (Rh–).

- The Rh factor is an important consideration in cross-matching blood for transfusions (see Chapter 15).

- The Rh factor can cause difficulties when an Rh-positive infant is born to an Rh-negative mother (see Chapter 14).

## Blood Gases

**Blood gases** are gases that are normally dissolved in the liquid portion of blood. The major blood gases are *oxygen* ($O_2$), *carbon dioxide* ($CO_2$), and *nitrogen* ($N_2$).

## ■ MEDICAL SPECIALTIES RELATED TO THE CARDIOVASCULAR SYSTEM

- A **cardiologist** (**kar**-dee-**OL**-oh-jist) is a physician who specializes in diagnosing and treating abnormalities, diseases, and disorders of the heart (**cardi** means heart, and **-ologist** means specialist).

- A **hematologist** (**hee**-mah-**TOL**-oh-jist) is a physician who specializes in diagnosing and treating abnormalities, diseases, and disorders of the blood and blood-forming tissues (**hemat** means blood, and **-ologist** means specialist).

- A **vascular surgeon** is a physician who specializes in the diagnosis, medical management, and surgical treatment of disorders of the blood vessels.

## ■ PATHOLOGY OF THE CARDIOVASCULAR SYSTEM

Disorders of the heart can be congenital (present from or before birth) or can develop at any time throughout life.

## Congenital Heart Defects

**Congenital heart defects** are structural abnormalities caused by the failure of the heart to develop normally before birth. *Congenital* means present at birth. Some congenital heart defects are apparent at birth, whereas others may not be detected until later in life.

## Coronary Artery Disease (CAD)

**Coronary artery disease** (CAD) is atherosclerosis of the coronary arteries that reduces the blood supply to the heart muscle. This creates an insufficient supply of oxygen that can cause angina (pain), a myocardial infarction (heart attack), or death. *End-stage coronary artery disease* is characterized by unrelenting angina pain and a severely limited lifestyle.

## Atherosclerosis

**Atherosclerosis** (ath-er-**oh**-skleh-**ROH**-sis) is hardening and narrowing of the arteries caused by a buildup of cholesterol plaque on the interior walls of the arteries (**ather/o** means plaque or fatty substance, and **-sclerosis** means abnormal hardening) (Figures 5.14 and 5.15).

- This type of **plaque** (**PLACK**), which is found within the lumen of an artery, is a fatty deposit that is similar to the buildup of rust inside a pipe. (This substance is not the same as *dental plaque*, which is discussed in Chapter 8.) The *lumen* is the opening within these vessels through which the blood flows.

- The plaque can protrude outward into the lumen from the wall of the blood vessel or protrude inward into the wall of the vessel.

- An **atheroma** (ath-er-**OH**-mah), which is a characteristic of atherosclerosis, is a deposit of plaque on or within the arterial wall (**ather** means plaque, and **-oma** means tumor).

## Ischemic Heart Disease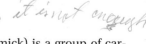

**Ischemic heart disease** (iss-**KEE**-mick) is a group of cardiac disabilities resulting from an insufficient supply of oxygenated blood to the heart. These diseases are usually associated with coronary artery disease. *Ischemic* means pertaining to the disruption of the blood supply. (See also *ischemic stroke* in Chapter 10.)

- **Ischemia** (iss-**KEE**-mee-ah) is a condition in which there is an insufficient supply of oxygen in the tissues due to a restricted blood flow to a part of the body

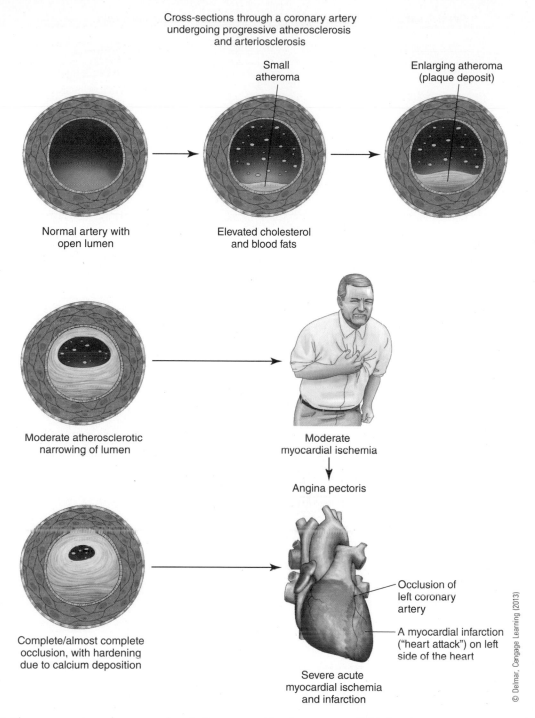

Cross-sections through a coronary artery undergoing progressive atherosclerosis and arteriosclerosis

Small atheroma

Enlarging atheroma (plaque deposit)

Normal artery with open lumen

Elevated cholesterol and blood fats

Moderate atherosclerotic narrowing of lumen

Moderate myocardial ischemia

Angina pectoris

Complete/almost complete occlusion, with hardening due to calcium deposition

Occlusion of left coronary artery

A myocardial infarction ("heart attack") on left side of the heart

Severe acute myocardial ischemia and infarction

© Delmar, Cengage Learning (2013)

**FIGURE 5.14** The progression of coronary heart disease resulting in a myocardial infarction.

(**isch** means to hold back, and **-emia** means blood). For example, *cardiac ischemia* is the lack of blood flow and oxygen to the heart muscle.

## Angina

**Angina** (an-**JIH**-nuh), also known as *angina pectoris*, is a condition in which severe episodes of chest pain occur due to an inadequate blood flow to the myocardium.

These episodes are due to ischemia of the heart muscle and often progressively worsen as the blood flow continues to be compromised, until a myocardial infarction occurs.

- *Stable angina* occurs during exertion (exercise) and resolves with rest.

- *Unstable angina* may occur either during exertion or rest, and is a precursor to a myocardial infarction.

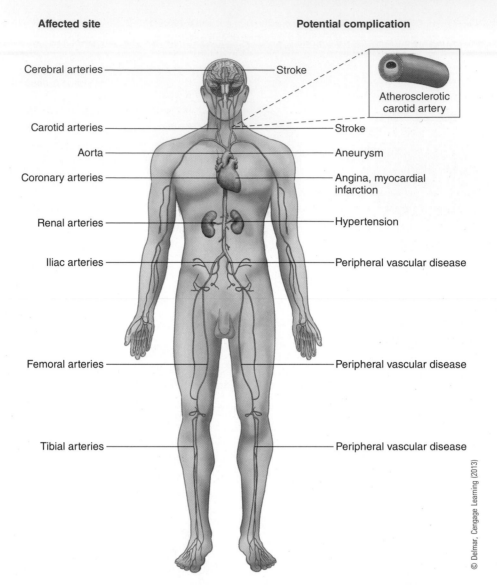

Affected site                                Potential complication

Cerebral arteries —————————————— Stroke

Atherosclerotic carotid artery

Carotid arteries ——————————————— Stroke

Aorta ————————————————————— Aneurysm

Coronary arteries ————————————— Angina, myocardial infarction

Renal arteries ———————————————— Hypertension

Iliac arteries ————————————————— Peripheral vascular disease

Femoral arteries —————————————— Peripheral vascular disease

Tibial arteries ———————————————— Peripheral vascular disease

© Delmar, Cengage Learning (2013)

**FIGURE 5.15** The sites affected by atherosclerosis (left column) and the potential complications of this condition (right column).

## Myocardial Infarction

A **myocardial infarction** (**my**-oh-**KAR**-dee-al in-**FARK**-shun), commonly known as a *heart attack*, is the occlusion (blockage) of one or more coronary arteries caused by plaque buildup. As used here, *occlusion* means total blockage.

■ The term *infarction* means a sudden insufficiency of blood.

■ An *infarct* is a localized area of dead tissue caused by a lack of blood.

■ This damage to the myocardium impairs the heart's ability to pump blood throughout the body (Figure 5.14).

■ The most frequently recognized symptoms of a myocardial infarction include pain or pressure in the middle of the chest that may spread to the back, jaw, or left arm. Many individuals having a heart attack have mild symptoms or none at all.

■ Women are more likely to have atypical symptoms, including weakness and fatigue.

## Heart Failure

**Heart failure**, which is also referred to as *congestive heart failure (CHF)*, occurs most commonly in the elderly. In this chronic condition the heart is unable to pump out all of the blood that it receives. The decreased pumping action causes the congestion. The term *congestion* describes a fluid buildup.

- *Left-sided heart failure* causes an accumulation of fluid in the lungs also known as *pulmonary edema*. This occurs because the left side of the heart is unable to efficiently pump oxygen-rich blood from the lungs to the rest of the body (see Chapter 7). The increase in pressure in the veins of the lungs results in localized fluid accumulation.

- *Right-sided heart failure* causes fluid buildup throughout the rest of the body. This occurs because the right side of the heart is unable to efficiently pump blood throughout the rest of the body. Due to the pressure of gravity, this edema, or swelling, is first noticeable in the feet and legs. As this swelling worsens, it can also affect the liver, gastrointestinal tract, or the arms.

- **Cardiomegaly** (**kar**-dee-oh-**MEG**-ah-lee) is the abnormal enlargement of the heart that is frequently associated with heart failure as the heart enlarges in an effort to compensate for its decreased pumping ability (**cardi/o** means heart, and **-megaly** means enlargement).

## Carditis

**Carditis** (kar-**DYE**-tis) is an inflammation of the heart (**card** means heart, and **-itis** means inflammation). Note the spelling of *carditis*: In this term, the word root (combining form) **card/o** is used to avoid having a double *i* when it is joined with the suffix **-itis**.

- **Endocarditis** (**en**-doh-kar-**DYE**-tis) is an inflammation of the inner lining of the heart (**endo-** means within, **card** means heart, and **-itis** means inflammation).

- **Bacterial endocarditis** is an inflammation of the lining or valves of the heart caused by the presence of bacteria in the bloodstream. One cause of this condition is bleeding during dental surgery because it allows bacteria from the mouth to enter the bloodstream.

- **Pericarditis** (**pehr**-ih-kar-**DYE**-tis) is an inflammation of the pericardium (**peri-** means surrounding, **card** means heart, and **-itis** means inflammation). This inflammation causes an accumulation of fluid within the pericardial sac, and this excess fluid restricts the beating of the heart, thereby reducing the ability of the heart to pump blood throughout the body.

- **Myocarditis** (**my**-oh-kar-**DYE**-tis) is an uncommon condition that is an inflammation of the myocardium (heart muscle) that develops as a complication of a viral infection (**my/o** means muscle, **card** means heart, and **-itis** means inflammation).

## Diseases of the Myocardium

- **Cardiomyopathy** (**kar**-dee-oh-my-**OP**-pah-thee) is the term used to describe all diseases of the heart muscle (**cardi/o** means heart, **my/o** means muscle, and **-pathy** means disease).

- *Dilated cardiomyopathy* is a disease of the heart muscle that causes the heart to become enlarged and to pump less strongly. The progression of this condition is usually slow and only presents with symptoms when quite advanced. *Dilated* means the expansion of a hollow structure.

## Heart Valves

- A **heart murmur** is an abnormal blowing or clicking sound heard when listening to the heart or a neighboring large blood vessels. Heart murmurs are most often caused by defective heart valves, but do not usually require surgery unless they affect the patient's quality of life.

- **Valvulitis** (**val**-view-**LYE**-tis) is an inflammation of a heart valve (**valvul** means valve, and **-itis** means inflammation).

- **Valvular prolapse** (**VAL**-voo-lar proh-**LAPS**) is the abnormal protrusion of a heart valve that results in the inability of the valve to close completely (**valvul** means valve, and **-ar** means pertaining to). *Prolapse* means the falling or dropping down of an organ or internal part. This condition is named for the affected valve, such as a *mitral valve prolapse*.

- **Valvular stenosis** (steh-**NOH**-sis) is a condition in which there is narrowing, stiffening, thickening, or blockage of one or more valves of the heart. *Stenosis* is the abnormal narrowing of an opening. These conditions are named for the affected valve, such as *aortic valve stenosis*.

## Cardiac Arrest and Arrhythmia

An **arrhythmia** (ah-**RITH**-mee-ah) is the loss of the normal rhythm of the heartbeat. This can be a minor, temporary episode, or it can be a fatal event. The severity of this episode depends on how much the heart's ability to pump blood is compromised. Rather than being an abnormality in the heart muscle, arrhythmias are usually caused by an abnormality in the electrical conduction system of the heart.

■ **Asystole** (ay-**SIS**-toh-lee), known as a *flat line* (**a-** means without, and **systole** means contraction), is the complete lack of electrical activity in the heart. The resulting lack of heart contractions, with no blood pumping from the heart and no blood flow through the body, is one of the conditions required for a medical practitioner to certify death.

■ **Cardiac arrest** is an event in which the heart abruptly stops beating or develops an arrhythmia that prevents it from pumping blood effectively.

■ **Sudden cardiac death** results when treatment of cardiac arrest is not provided within a few minutes.

■ **Bradycardia** (**brad**-ee-**KAR**-dee-ah) is an abnormally slow resting heart rate (**brady-** means slow, **card** means heart, and **-ia** means abnormal condition). The term *bradycardia* is usually applied to a *heartbeat rate* of less than 60 beats per minute. This condition is the opposite of *tachycardia*.

■ **Tachycardia** (**tack**-ee-**KAR**-dee-ah) is an abnormally rapid resting heart rate (**tachy-** means rapid, **card** means heart, and **-ia** means abnormal condition). The term *tachycardia* is usually applied to a heartbeat rate of greater than 100 beats per minute. This condition is the opposite of *bradycardia*.

■ **Palpitation** (**pal**-pih-**TAY**-shun) is a pounding or racing heartbeat with or without irregularity in rhythm. This condition is associated with certain heart disorders; however, it can also occur during a panic attack (see Chapter 10).

## Atrial and Ventricular Fibrillations

The term **fibrillation** (**fih**-brih-**LAY**-shun) describes a rapid and uncontrolled heartbeat. The addition of the term *atrial* or *ventricular* identifies which heart chambers are affected.

■ **Atrial fibrillation** (**AY**-tree-al **fih**-brih-**LAY**-shun), also known as *A-fib*, occurs when the normal rhythmic contractions of the atria are replaced by rapid, irregular twitching of the muscular heart wall. This causes an irregular and quivering action of the atria (Figure 5.16B).

Some of the increased electrical impulses reach the ventricles, and this makes them contract more rapidly and less efficiently than normal, causing an irregular rate of 80–180 beats per minute or more.

■ **Paroxysmal supraventricular tachycardia** (**par**-ock-**SIZ**-mal **soo**-prah-ven-**TRICK**-you-lar **tack**-ee-**KAR**-dee-ah), also known as *PSVT*, is an episode that begins and ends abruptly during which there are very rapid and regular heartbeats that originate in the atrium or in the AV node (Figure 5.16C). *Paroxysmal* means pertaining to sudden occurrence. Compare *PSVT* with *ventricular tachycardia*.

■ **Ventricular fibrillation** (ven-**TRICK**-you-lar **fih**-brih-**LAY**-shun), also known as *V-fib*, consists of rapid, irregular, and useless contractions of the ventricles. Instead of pumping strongly, the heart muscle quivers ineffectively. This condition is the cause of many sudden cardiac deaths (Figure 5.16D).

■ **Ventricular tachycardia** (ven-**TRICK**-you-lar **tack**-ee-**KAR**-dee-ah), also known as *V-tach*, is a very rapid heartbeat that begins within the ventricles. This condition is potentially fatal because the heart is beating so rapidly that it is unable to adequately pump blood through the body. For some patients, this condition can be controlled with an automated implantable cardioverter-defibrillator. Compare *V-tach* with *paroxysmal supraventricular tachycardia*.

## Blood Vessel Abnormalities

■ **Vasculitis** (**vas**-kyou-**LYE**-tis) is the inflammation of a blood vessel (**vascul** means blood vessels, and **-itis** means inflammation). There are many types of vasculitis, including phlebitis (under "Veins") and *angiitis* or *arteritis* (inflammation of the arteries).

■ **Polyarteritis** (**pol**-ee-**ar**-teh-**RYE**-tis) is a form of vasculitis involving several medium and small arteries at the same time (**poly-** means many, **arter** means artery, and **-itis** mean inflammation). Polyarteritis is a rare but serious blood vessel disease that occurs when certain immune cells attack the affected arteries.

■ **Temporal arteritis** (**TEM**-poh-**ral ar**-teh-**RYE**-tis), also known as *giant cell arteritis*, is a form of vasculitis that can cause headaches, visual impairment, jaw pain, and other symptoms. It is diagnosed when a biopsy shows the presence of abnormally large cells. Temporal arteritis can cause unilateral or bilateral blindness, and more rarely, a stroke.

■ **Angiostenosis** (**AN**-jee-oh-steh-**NOH**-sis) is the abnormal narrowing of a blood vessel (**angi/o** means vessel, and **-stenosis** means abnormal narrowing).

■ A **hemangioma** (hee-**man**-jee-**OH**-mah) is a benign tumor made up of newly formed blood vessels (**hem** means blood, **angi** means blood or lymph vessel, and **-oma** means tumor) (see birthmarks in Chapter 12).

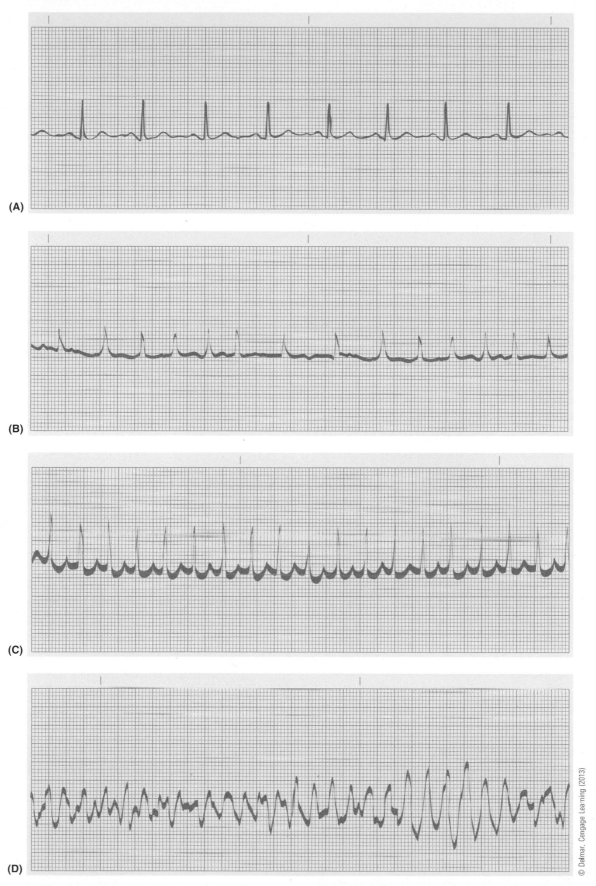

**FIGURE 5.16** Electrocardiograms showing disruptions of heart rhythms. (A) Normal sinus rhythm. (B) Atrial fibrillation. (C) Paroxysmal supraventricular tachycardia. (D) Ventricular fibrillation.

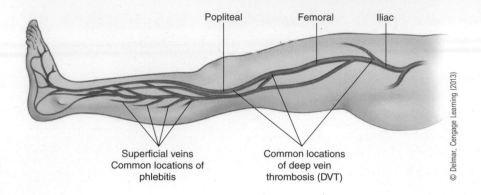

Popliteal   Femoral   Iliac

Superficial veins
Common locations of
phlebitis

Common locations
of deep vein
thrombosis (DVT)

© Delmar, Cengage Learning (2013)

**FIGURE 5.17** Common sites for the development of phlebitis and deep vein thrombosis.

■ **Hypoperfusion** (**high**-poh-per-**FYOU**-zhun) is a deficiency of blood passing through an organ or body part. *Perfusion* is the flow of blood through the vessels of an organ.

## Arteries

■ An **aneurysm** (**AN**-you-rizm) is a localized weak spot or balloon-like enlargement of the wall of an artery. The rupture of an aneurysm can be fatal because of the rapid loss of blood. Aneurysms are named for the artery involved such as *aortic aneurysm*, *abdominal aortic aneurysm*, and *popliteal aneurysm*.

■ **Arteriosclerosis** (ar-**tee**-ree-oh-skleh-**ROH**-sis), also known as *hardening of the arteries*, is any of a group of diseases characterized by thickening and the loss of elasticity of arterial walls (**arteri/o** means artery, and **-sclerosis** mean abnormal hardening).

■ **Arteriostenosis** (ar-**tee**-ree-oh-steh-**NOH**-sis) is the abnormal narrowing of an artery or arteries (**arteri/o** means artery, and **-stenosis** means abnormal narrowing).

## Veins

■ **Chronic venous insufficiency**, also known as *venous insufficiency*, is a condition in which venous circulation is inadequate due to partial vein blockage or to the leakage of venous valves. This condition primarily affects the feet and ankles, and the leakage of venous blood into the tissues causes discoloration of the skin.

■ **Phlebitis** (fleh-**BYE**-tis) is the inflammation of a vein (**phleb** means vein, and **-itis** means inflammation). It

is also known as *thrombophlebitis*, because the walls of the vein are often infiltrated and a clot (thrombus) formed. This condition usually occurs in a superficial vein (Figure 5.17).

■ **Varicose veins** (**VAR**-ih-kohs **VAYNS**) are abnormally swollen veins that usually occur in the superficial veins of the legs. This condition occurs when the valves in these veins do not function properly, so blood pools in the veins, causing them to enlarge.

## Thromboses and Embolisms

Thromboses and embolisms are serious conditions that can result in the blockage of a blood vessel.

### Thrombosis

A **thrombosis** (throm-**BOH**-sis) is the abnormal condition of having a thrombus (**thromb** means clot, and **-osis** means abnormal condition or disease) (Figure 5.18). The plural form is *thromboses*.

A **thrombus** (**THROM**-bus) is a blood clot attached to the interior wall of an artery or vein (**thromb** means clot, and **-us** is a singular noun ending) (plural, *thrombi*).

■ A **thrombotic occlusion** (throm-**BOT**-ick ah-**KLOO**-zhun) is the blocking of an artery by a thrombus. *Thrombotic* means caused by a thrombus. As used here, *occlusion* means blockage.

■ A **coronary thrombosis** (**KOR**-uh-**nerr**-ee throm-**BOH**-sis) is damage to the heart muscle caused by a thrombus blocking a coronary artery (**coron** means crown, and **-ary** means pertaining to, and **thromb** means clot, and **-osis** means abnormal condition).

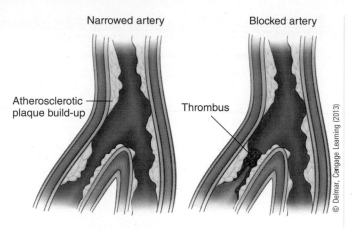

**FIGURE 5.18** A thrombus is a blood clot attached to the interior wall of an artery or vein.

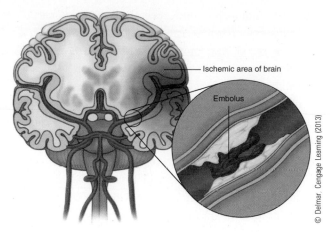

**FIGURE 5.19** An embolus is a foreign object circulating in the blood.

■ A **deep vein thrombosis** (DVT), also known as a *deep venous thrombosis*, is the condition of having a thrombus attached to the interior wall of a deep vein. Sometimes such a blockage forms in the legs of a bedridden patient or in someone who has remained seated too long in an airplane or car. The danger is that the thrombus (clot) will break loose and travel to a lung where it can be fatal by causing a blockage (Figure 5.17).

## Embolism

An **embolism** (EM-boh-lizm) is the sudden blockage of a blood vessel by an embolus (**embol** means something inserted, and **-ism** means condition). The embolism is often named for the causative factor, such as an *air embolism* or a *fat embolism* (Figure 5.19), or its location, such as *pulmonary embolism*.

■ An **embolus** (EM-boh-lus) is a foreign object, such as a blood clot, a quantity of air or gas, or a bit of tissue or tumor that is circulating in the blood (**embol** means something inserted, and **-us** is a singular noun ending) (plural, *emboli*).

## Peripheral Vascular Diseases

**Peripheral vascular diseases** are disorders of blood vessels that are located outside of the heart and brain. These conditions usually involve narrowing of the vessels that carry blood to the legs, arms, stomach, or kidneys.

■ **Peripheral arterial occlusive disease** (per-IH-feh-**ral** ar-TEE-ree-al oh-KLOO-siv), also known as *peripheral artery disease*, is an example of a peripheral vascular disease that is caused by atherosclerosis. This condition is a common and serious problem affecting

more than 20% of all patients over 70 years of age. Impaired circulation to the extremities and vital organs can cause changes in the skin color and temperature. It is also involved with *intermittent claudication*, which is discussed in Chapter 4.

■ **Raynaud's disease** (ray-NOHZ) is a peripheral arterial occlusive disease in which intermittent attacks are triggered by cold or stress. The symptoms, which are due to constricted circulation, include pallor (paleness), cyanosis (blue color), and redness of the fingers and toes.

## Blood Disorders

■ **Blood dyscrasia** (dis-KRAY-zee-ah) is any pathologic condition of the cellular elements of the blood (**dys-** means bad, and **-crasia** means a mixture or blending).

■ **Hemochromatosis** (hee-moh-kroh-mah-TOH-sis), also known as *iron overload disease*, is a genetic disorder in which the intestines absorb too much iron (**hem/o** means blood, **chromat** means color, and **-osis** means abnormal condition or disease). The excess iron that is absorbed enters the bloodstream and accumulates in organs where it causes damage.

■ **Leukopenia** (loo-koh-PEE-nee-ah) is a decrease in the number of disease-fighting white blood cells circulating in the blood (**leuk/o** means white, and **-penia** means deficiency). This condition, which is also known as a *low white blood cell count*, places the patient at an increased of risk of developing or having difficulty fighting infections.

■ **Polycythemia** (pol-ee-sy-THEE-mee-ah) is an abnormal increase in the number of red cells in the blood due to excess production of these cells by the bone marrow.

- **Septicemia** (**sep**-tih-**SEE**-mee-ah) is often associated with severe infections caused by the presence of bacteria in the blood. Also known as **bacteremia** (**bacter** means bacteria, and -**emia** means a blood condition), this condition can begin with a sudden onset of symptoms that include a spiking fever, chills, rapid breathing, and rapid heart rate. Septicemia can lead to *sepsis*, which is a systemic bacterial infection in the bloodstream.

- **Thrombocytopenia** (**throm**-boh-**sigh**-toh-**PEE**-nee-ah) is a condition in which there is an abnormally small number of platelets circulating in the blood (**thromb/o** means clot, **cyt/o** means cell, and -**penia** means deficiency). Because these cells help the blood to clot, this condition is sometimes associated with abnormal bleeding.

- **Thrombocytosis** (**throm**-boh-sigh-**TOH**-sis) is an abnormal increase in the number of platelets in the circulating blood (**thromb/o** means clot, **cyt** means cell, and -**osis** means abnormal condition).

- A **hemorrhage** (**HEM**-or-idj) is the loss of a large amount of blood in a short time (**hem/o** means blood, and -**rrhage** means bleeding). This term also means *to bleed*.

- A **transfusion reaction** is a serious and potentially fatal complication of a blood transfusion in which a severe immune response occurs because the patient's blood and the donated blood do not match.

## Cholesterol

- **Cholesterol** (koh-**LES**-ter-ol) is a fatty substance that travels through the blood and is found in all parts of the body. It aids in the production of cell membranes, some hormones, and vitamin D. Some cholesterol comes from dietary sources, and some is created by the liver. Excessively high levels of certain types of cholesterol can lead to heart disease (Table 5.2).

- **Hyperlipidemia** (**high**-per-**lip**-ih-**DEE**-mee-ah) is the general term used to describe elevated levels of cholesterol and other fatty substances in the blood (**hyper-** means excessive, **lipid** means fat, and -**emia** means blood condition).

## TABLE 5.2
### Interpreting Cholesterol Levels

| | |
|---|---|
| **Total cholesterol** is measured in terms of milligrams (mg) per deciliter (dL) of blood. A *milligram* is equal to one-thousandth of a gram. A *deciliter* is equal to one-tenth of a liter | *Desirable levels* are below 200 mg/dL. *Borderline high levels* are 200–239 mg/dL. *High levels* are 240 mg/dL and above. |
| **Low-density lipoprotein cholesterol** (LDL) is referred to as *bad cholesterol* because excess quantities of LDL contribute to plaque buildup in the arteries. | *Optimal levels* are below 100 mg/dL. *Near optimal* levels are 100–129 mg/dL. *Borderline high* levels are 130–159 mg/dL. *High levels* are 160–189 mg/dL. *Very high levels* are 190 mg/dL and above. |
| **High-density lipoprotein cholesterol** (HDL) is referred to as *good cholesterol* because it carries unneeded cholesterol back to the liver for processing and does not contribute to plaque buildup. | *Bad levels* are below 40 mg/dL. *Better levels* are between 40 and 59 mg/dL. *Best levels* are 60 mg/dL and above. |
| **Triglycerides** (try-**GLIS**-er-eyeds) are combinations of *fatty acids* attached to glycerol that are also found normally in the blood in limited quantities. | *Desirable levels* are below 150 mg/dL. *Borderline high levels* are 150–199 mg/dL. *High levels* are 200–499 mg/dL. *Very high levels* are 500 mg/dL and above. |

*Source:* National Heart, Lung, and Blood Institute, 2010.

### Leukemia

- **Myelodysplastic syndrome** (**my**-eh-loh-dis-**PLAS**-tick) is a group of bone marrow disorders that are characterized by the insufficient production of one or more types of blood cells due to dysfunction of the bone marrow.

- **Leukemia** (loo-**KEE**-mee-ah) is a type of cancer characterized by a progressive increase in the number of abnormal leukocytes (white blood cells) found in blood-forming tissues, other organs, and in the circulating blood (**leuk** means white, and **-emia** means blood condition).

### Anemias

**Anemia** (ah-**NEE**-mee-ah) is a lower-than-normal number of erythrocytes (red blood cells) in the blood (**an-** means without or less than, and **-emia** means blood condition). The severity of this condition is usually measured by a decrease in the amount of hemoglobin in the blood. When inadequate hemoglobin is present, all parts of the body receive less oxygen and have less energy than is needed to function properly.

- **Aplastic anemia** (ay-**PLAS**-tick ah-**NEE**-mee-ah) is characterized by an absence of *all* formed blood elements caused by the failure of blood cell production in the bone marrow (**a-** means without, **plast** means growth, and **-ic** means pertaining to). Anemia, a low red blood cell count, leads to fatigue and weakness. Leukopenia, a low white blood cell count, causes an increased risk of infection. Thrombocytopenia, a low platelet count, results in bleeding especially from mucous membranes and skin.

- **Hemolytic anemia** (**hee**-moh-**LIT**-ick ah-**NEE**-mee-ah) is characterized by an inadequate number of circulating red blood cells due to the premature destruction of red blood cells by the spleen (**hem/o** means relating to blood, and **-lytic** means to destroy). *Hemolytic* means pertaining to breaking down of red blood cells.

- **Iron-deficiency anemia** is the most common form of anemia. Iron, an essential component of hemoglobin, is normally obtained through food intake and by recycling iron from old red blood cells. Without sufficient iron to help create hemoglobin, blood cannot carry oxygen effectively.

- **Megaloblastic anemia** (**MEG**-ah-loh-**blas**-tick ah-**NEE**-mee-ah) is a blood disorder characterized by anemia in which the red blood cells are larger than normal (**mega-** means large, **blast** means immature, and **-tic** means pertaining to). This condition usually results from a deficiency of folic acid or of vitamin $B_{12}$.

- **Pernicious anemia** (per-**NISH**-us ah-**NEE**-mee-ah) is caused by a lack of the protein *intrinsic factor* (IF) that helps the body absorb vitamin $B_{12}$ from the gastrointestinal tract. Vitamin $B_{12}$ is necessary for the formation of red blood cells.

- **Sickle cell anemia** is a genetic disorder that causes abnormal hemoglobin, resulting in some red blood cells assuming an abnormal sickle shape. This sickle shape interferes with normal blood flow, resulting in damage to most of the body systems. The genetic transmission of sickle cell anemia is discussed in Chapter 2.

- **Thalassemia** (thal-ah-**SEE**-mee-ah) is an inherited blood disorder that causes mild or severe anemia due to reduced hemoglobin and fewer red blood cells than normal. *Cooley's anemia* is the name that is sometimes used to refer to any type of thalassemia that requires treatment with regular blood transfusions.

## Hypertension

**Hypertension** (HTN), commonly known as *high blood pressure*, is the elevation of arterial blood pressure to a level that is likely to cause damage to the cardiovascular system. Hypertension is the opposite of *hypotension*.

- *Essential hypertension*, also known as *primary hypertension* or *idiopathic hypertension*, is consistently elevated blood pressure of unknown cause. *Idiopathic* means a disease of unknown cause. The classifications of blood pressure for adults with this condition are summarized in Table 5.3.

- *Secondary hypertension* is caused by a different medical problem, such as a kidney disorder or a tumor on the adrenal glands. When the other problem is cured, the secondary hypertension is usually resolved.

- *Malignant hypertension* is characterized by very high blood pressure. This condition, which can be fatal, is usually accompanied by damage to the organs, the brain, and optic nerves, or failure of the heart and kidneys.

## Hypotension

**Hypotension** (**high**-poh-**TEN**-shun) is lower-than-normal arterial blood pressure. Symptoms can include dizziness, light-headedness, or fainting. *Hypotension* is the opposite of *hypertension*.

**TABLE 5.3**
**Blood Pressure Classifications for Adults**

| Category | Systolic (mm Hg) Top Number | Diastolic (mm Hg) Bottom Number |
|---|---|---|
| Normal blood pressure | less than 120 | less than 80 |
| Pre-hypertension | between 120 and 139 | between 80 and 89 |
| Stage 1 Hypertension | between 140 and 159 | between 90 and 99 |
| Stage 2 Hypertension | 160 or higher | 100 or higher |

■ **Orthostatic hypotension** (or-thoh-**STAT**-ick **high**-poh-**TEN**-shun), also known as *postural hypotension*, is low blood pressure that occurs upon standing up. *Orthostatic* means relating to an upright or standing position.

## ■ DIAGNOSTIC PROCEDURES OF THE CARDIOVASCULAR SYSTEM

■ **Blood tests** and **ultrasonic diagnostic procedures** are discussed in Chapter 15.

■ **Angiography** (an-jee-**OG**-rah-fee) is a radiographic (x-ray) study of the blood vessels after the injection of a contrast medium (**angi/o** means blood vessel, and **-graphy** means the process of recording). The resulting film is an *angiogram* (Figure 5.20).

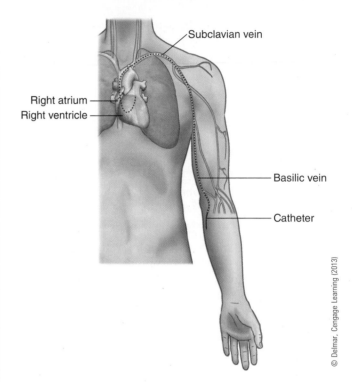

Subclavian vein
Right atrium
Right ventricle
Basilic vein
Catheter

© Delmar, Cengage Learning (2013)

**FIGURE 5.21** In *cardiac catheterization* is a catheter is passed into a vein or artery and then guided into the heart.

■ **Cardiac catheterization** (**KAR**-dee-ack kath-eh-ter-eye-**ZAY**-shun) is a diagnostic procedure in which a catheter is passed into a vein or artery and then guided into the heart (Figure 5.21). When the catheter is in place, a contrast medium is introduced to produce an angiogram to determine how well the heart is working. This procedure is also used during treatment. See the section on clearing blocked arteries later in this chapter.

■ **Digital subtraction angiography** (DSA) combines angiography with computerized components to clarify the view of the area of interest by removing the soft tissue and bones from the images.

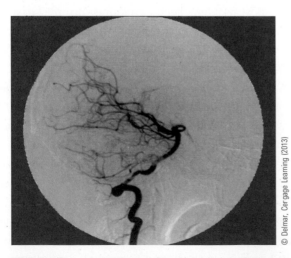

© Delmar, Cengage Learning (2013)

**FIGURE 5.20** In angiography, the blood vessels (in black) are made visible through the use of a contrast medium.

- **Duplex ultrasound** is a diagnostic procedure to image the structures of the blood vessels and the flow of blood through these vessels. This is a combination of *diagnostic ultrasound* to show the structure of the blood vessels and *Doppler ultrasound* to show the movement of the red blood cells through these vessels. Diagnostic and Doppler ultrasounds are discussed in Chapter 15.

- **Phlebography** (fleh-**BOG**-rah-fee), also known as *venography*, is a radiographic test that provides an image of the leg veins after a contrast dye is injected into a vein in the patient's foot (**phleb/o** means vein, and **-graphy** means the process of recording). The resulting film is a *phlebogram*. This is a very accurate test for detecting deep vein thrombosis.

## Electrocardiography

**Electrocardiography** (ee-**leck**-troh-kar-dee-**OG**-rah-fee) is the noninvasive process of recording the electrical

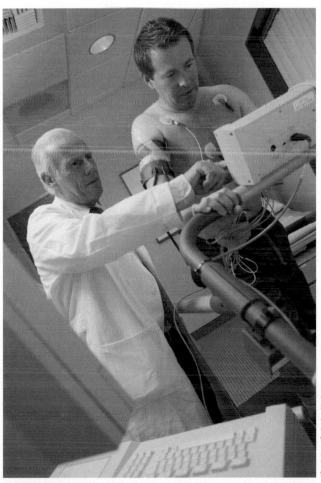

**FIGURE 5.22** In *electrocardiography*, the electrical activity of the myocardium is captured and externally recorded by electrodes placed on the skin.

activity of the myocardium (**electr/o** means electric, **cardi/o** means heart, and **graphy** means the process of recording a picture or record) (Figure 5.22). A *noninvasive* procedure does not require the insertion of an instrument or device through the skin or a body opening for diagnosis or treatment.

- An **electrocardiogram** (ee-**leck**-troh-**KAR**-dee-oh-gram) (EKG or ECG) is a record of the electrical activity of the myocardium (**electr/o** means electric, **cardi/o** means heart, and **-gram** means picture or record) (Figure 5.16).

- A **Holter monitor** is a portable electrocardiograph that is worn by an ambulatory patient to continuously monitor the heart rates and rhythms over a 24- or 48-hour period.

- A **stress test** is performed to assess cardiovascular health and function during and after stress. This involves monitoring with an electrocardiogram while the patient exercises on a treadmill, or is injected with a chemical to increase the patient's heart rate if he or she is unable to use a treadmill. The test can also be performed in conjunction with an echocardiogram (see Chapter 15).

- A **thallium stress test** (**THAL**-ee-um) is performed to evaluate how well blood flows through the coronary arteries of the heart muscle during exercise by injecting a small amount of thallium into the bloodstream. If it is not taken up equally by all heart muscle cells, it shows a decrease in blood flow to part of the heart.

## ▉ TREATMENT PROCEDURES OF THE CARDIOVASCULAR SYSTEM

### Medications

Many heart conditions are controlled with medications; however, successful treatment depends on patient compliance. *Compliance* is the accuracy and consistency with which the patient follows the physician's instructions.

### Antihypertensives

An **antihypertensive** (**an**-tih-**high**-per-**TEN**-siv) is a medication administered to lower blood pressure. Some of these drugs are also used to treat other heart conditions.

- An **ACE inhibitor** (*angiotensin-converting enzyme*) blocks the action of the enzyme that causes the blood vessels to contract, resulting in hypertension.

When this enzyme is blocked, the blood vessels are able to dilate (enlarge), and this reduces the blood pressure. These medications are used primarily to treat hypertension and heart failure. *Angiotensin II receptor blockers (ARBs)* have a similar action and effect.

■ A **beta-blocker** reduces the workload of the heart by slowing the rate of the heartbeat. They are commonly prescribed to lower blood pressure, relieve angina, or to treat heart failure.

■ **Calcium channel blocker agents** cause the heart and blood vessels to relax by decreasing the movement of calcium into the cells of these structures. This relaxation reduces the workload of the heart by increasing the supply of blood and oxygen. Some calcium channel blocking agents are used to treat hypertension or to relieve and control angina.

■ A **diuretic** (**dye**-you-**RET**-ick) is administered to stimulate the kidneys to increase the secretion of urine to rid the body of excess sodium and water. These medications are administered to treat hypertension and heart failure by reducing the amount of fluid circulating in the blood.

## Additional Medications

■ An **antiarrhythmic** (**an**-tih-ah-**RITH**-mick) is a medication administered to control irregularities of the heartbeat.

■ An **anticoagulant** (**an**-tih-koh-**AG**-you-lant) slows coagulation and prevents new clots from forming. *Coagulation* is the process of clotting blood (see Coumadin).

■ **Aspirin** taken in a very small daily dose, such as 81 mg, which is commonly known as *baby aspirin*, may be recommended to reduce the risk of a heart attack or stroke by reducing the ability of the blood to clot.

■ **Cholesterol-lowering drugs**, such as *statins*, are used to combat hyperlipidemia by reducing the undesirable cholesterol levels in the blood.

■ **Coumadin**, which is a brand name for *warfarin*, is an anticoagulant administered to prevent blood clots from forming or growing larger. This medication is often prescribed for patients with clotting difficulties, certain types of heartbeat irregularities, or after a heart attack or heart valve replacement surgery.

■ **Digitalis** (**dij**-ih-**TAL**-is), also known as *digoxin*, strengthens the contraction of the heart muscle, slows the heart rate, and helps eliminate fluid from body

tissues. It is often used to treat heart failure or certain types of arrhythmias.

■ A **thrombolytic** (**throm**-boh-**LIT**-ick), also known as a *clot-busting drug*, dissolves or causes a thrombus to break up (**thromb/o** means clot, and **-lytic** means to destroy).

■ **Tissue plasminogen activator** (TPA) (plaz-**MIN**-oh-jen) is a thrombolytic that is administered to some patients having a heart attack or stroke. If administered within a few hours after symptoms begin, this medication can dissolve the damaging blood clots.

■ A **vasoconstrictor** (**vas**-oh-kon-**STRICK**-tor) causes blood vessels to narrow. Examples of these medications include antihistamines and decongestants. A vasoconstrictor is the opposite of a *vasodilator*.

■ A **vasodilator** (**vas**-oh-dye-**LAYT**-or) causes blood vessels to expand. A vasodilator is the opposite of a *vasoconstrictor*.

■ **Nitroglycerin** (**nye**-troh-**GLIH**-sih-rin) is a vasodilator that is prescribed to prevent or relieve the pain of angina by dilating the blood vessels to the heart. This increases the blood flow and oxygen supply to the heart. Nitroglycerin can be administered sublingually (under the tongue), transdermally (through the skin), or orally as a spray.

## Clearing Blocked Arteries

■ **Angioplasty** (**AN**-jee-oh-**plas**-tee) is the technique of mechanically widening a narrowed or obstructed blood vessel (**angi/o** means blood vessel, and **-plasty** means surgical repair). The narrowing is typically caused by atherosclerosis.

■ **Percutaneous transluminal coronary angioplasty** (PTCA) is also known as a *balloon angioplasty*. This is a procedure in which a small balloon on the end of a catheter is used to open a partially blocked coronary artery by flattening the plaque deposit and stretching the lumen (Figure 5.23).

■ **Laser angioplasty** (**AN**-jee-oh-**plas**-tee) involves a laser on the end of a catheter, which uses beams of light to remove the plaque deposit. It can be used separately or in conjunction with PTCA.

■ A **stent** is a wire-mesh tube that is commonly placed after the artery has been opened. This provides support to the arterial wall, keeps the plaque from expanding again, and prevents restenosis (Figure 5.24).

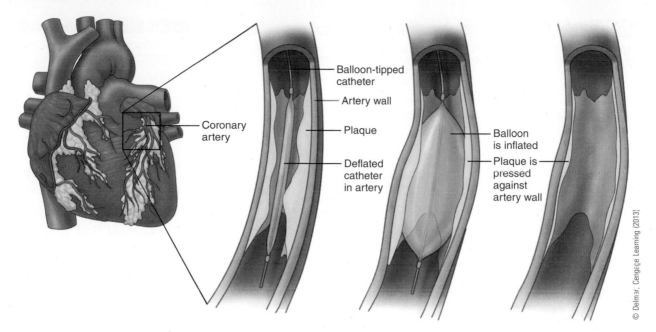

**FIGURE 5.23** *Balloon angioplasty* is performed to reopen a blocked coronary artery.

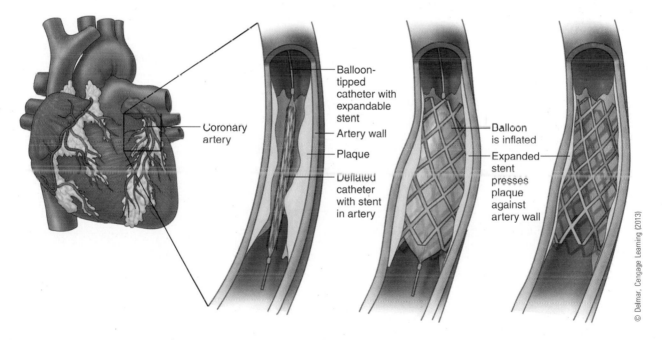

**FIGURE 5.24** A *stent* is put in place to prevent *restenosis* of a treated artery.

- **Restenosis** describes the condition when an artery that has been opened by angioplasty closes again (**re-** means again, and **-stenosis** means narrowing).

- An **atherectomy** (**ath**-er-**ECK**-toh-mee) is the surgical removal of plaque buildup from the interior of an artery (**ather** means plaque, and **-ectomy** means surgical removal). A stent may be put in place after the atherectomy to prevent the artery from becoming blocked again.

- A **carotid endarterectomy** (kah-**ROT**-id **end**-ar-ter-**ECK**-toh-mee) is the surgical removal of the lining of a portion of a clogged carotid artery leading to the brain. This procedure is performed to reduce the risk of a stroke caused by a disruption of the blood flow to the brain. Strokes are discussed in Chapter 10.

## Coronary Artery Bypass Graft

**Coronary artery bypass graft** (CABG) is also known as *bypass surgery* (Figure 5.25). In this operation, which requires opening the chest, a piece of vein from the leg or chest is implanted on the heart to replace a blocked coronary artery and to improve the flow of blood to the heart.

■ A **minimally invasive coronary artery bypass**, also known as a *keyhole bypass* or a *buttonhole bypass*, is an alternative technique for some bypass patients. This procedure is performed with the aid of a fiberoptic camera through small openings between the ribs.

## Treatment of Cardiac Arrhythmias

■ **Defibrillation** (dee-**fih**-brih-**LAY**-shun), also known as *cardioversion*, is the use of electrical shock to restore the heart's normal rhythm. This shock is provided by a device known as a *defibrillator* (Figure 5.26).

■ An **automated external defibrillator** (AED) is designed for use by nonprofessionals in emergency situations when defibrillation is required. This piece of equipment automatically samples the electrical rhythms of the heart and if necessary, externally shocks the heart to restore a normal cardiac rhythm.

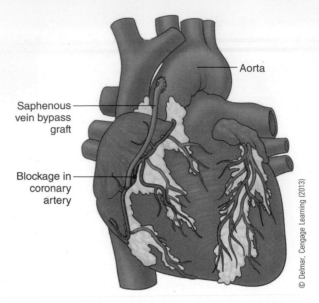

Aorta

Saphenous vein bypass graft

Blockage in coronary artery

© Delmar, Cengage Learning (2013)

**FIGURE 5.25** *Coronary artery bypass surgery* is performed to allow the flow of blood by placing vein grafts to bypass blocked arteries.

■ An **artificial pacemaker** is used primarily as treatment for bradycardia or atrial fibrillation. This electronic device can be attached externally or implanted under the skin with connections leading into the heart to regulate the heartbeat.

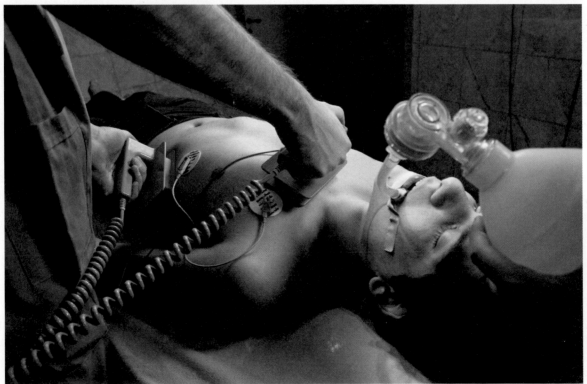

iStockphoto/Niko Guido

**FIGURE 5.26** *Defibrillation* uses electrical shock to attempt to restore the heart to its usual rhythm.

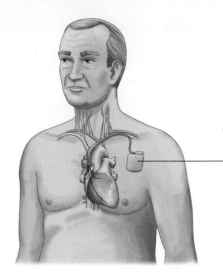

Automated implantable cardioverter-defibrillator

© Delmar, Cengage Learning (2013)

**FIGURE 5.27** An *automated implantable cardioverter-defibrillator* constantly regulates the heartbeat and if necessary, acts as an automatic defibrillator.

- An **automated implantable cardioverter-defibrillator** (**KAR**-dee-oh-**ver**-ter dee-**fib**-rih-**LAY**-ter) (AICD) is a double-action pacemaker. (1) It constantly regulates the heartbeat to ensure that the heart does not beat too slowly. (2) If a dangerous disruption of the heart's rhythm occurs, it acts as an automatic defibrillator (Figure 5.27).

- **Valvoplasty** (**VAL**-voh-**plas**-tee), also known as *valvuloplasty*, is the surgical repair or replacement of a heart valve (**valv/o** means valve, and -**plasty** means surgical repair).

- **Cardiopulmonary resuscitation**, commonly known as *CPR*, is an emergency procedure for life support consisting of artificial respiration and manual external cardiac compression. *Cardiopulmonary* means pertaining to the heart and lungs.

- *Compression-only resuscitation* can be effective in keeping a patient suffering from cardiac arrest alive until professional responders arrive, although artificial respiration is still recommended for children, drowning victims, and drug overdoses.

## Blood Vessels, Blood, and Bleeding

- An **aneurysmectomy** (**an**-you-riz-**MECK**-toh-mee) is the surgical removal of an aneurysm (**aneurysm** means aneurysm, and -**ectomy** means surgical removal).

- An **aneurysmorrhaphy** (**an**-you-riz-**MOR**-ah-fee), also known as *aneurysmoplasty*, is the surgical suturing of an aneurysm (**aneurysm/o** means aneurysm, and -**rrhaphy** means surgical suturing).

- An **arteriectomy** (**ar**-teh-ree-**ECK**-toh-mee) is the surgical removal of part of an artery (**arteri** means artery, and -**ectomy** means surgical removal).

- **Hemostasis** (**hee**-moh-**STAY**-sis) means to stop or control bleeding (**hem/o** means blood, and -**stasis** means stopping or controlling). This could be accomplished by the formation of a blood clot by the body or through the external application of pressure to block the flow of blood.

- **Plasmapheresis** (**plaz**-mah-feh-**REE**-sis), also known as *plasma exchange*, is the removal of whole blood from the body and separation of the blood's cellular elements. The red blood cells and platelets are suspended in saline or a plasma substitute and returned to the circulatory system. For blood donors, this makes more frequent donations possible. Patients with certain autoimmune disorders receive their own red blood cells and platelets back cleansed of antibodies.

## ABBREVIATIONS RELATED TO THE CARDIOVASCULAR SYSTEM

Table 5.4 presents an overview of the abbreviations related to the terms introduced in this chapter. Note: To avoid errors or confusion, always be cautious when using abbreviations.

## TABLE 5.4
## Abbreviations Related to the Cardiovascular System

| | |
|---|---|
| atrial fibrillation = A-fib | **A-fib** = atrial fibrillation |
| automated external defibrillator = AED | **AED** = automated external defibrillator |
| automated implantable cardioverter-defibrillator = AICD | **AICD** = automated implantable cardioverter-defibrillator |
| cardiac catheterization = card cath, CC | **card cath, CC** = cardiac catheterization |
| chronic venous insufficiency = CVI | **CVI** = chronic venous insufficiency |
| coronary artery bypass graft = CABG | **CABG** = coronary artery bypass graft |
| coronary artery disease = CAD | **CAD** = coronary artery disease |
| electrocardiogram = EKG, ECG | **EKG, ECG** = electrocardiogram |
| hypertension = HTN | **HTN** = hypertension |
| myocardial infarction = MI | **MI** = myocardial infarction |
| peripheral artery disease = PAD | **PAD** = peripheral artery disease |
| peripheral vascular disease = PVD | **PVD** = peripheral vascular disease |
| thallium stress test = TST | **TST** = thallium stress test |
| tissue plasminogen activator = tPA | **tPA** = tissue plasminogen activator |
| ventricular fibrillation = V-fib | **V-fib** = ventricular fibrillation |

### StudyWARE CONNECTION

For more practice and to test your mastery of this material, go to the StudyWARE™ to play interactive games and complete the quiz for this chapter.

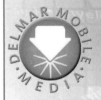

Downloadable audio is available for selected medical terms in this chapter to enhance your learning of medical terminology.

### ☐ Workbook Practice

Go to your workbook and complete the exercises for this chapter.

# LEARNING EXERCISES

## MATCHING WORD PARTS 1

Write the correct answer in the middle column.

| Definition | Correct Answer | Possible Answers |
|---|---|---|
| 5.1. aorta | _____ | **angi/o** |
| 5.2. artery | _____ | **aort/o** |
| 5.3. plaque, fatty substance | _____ | **arteri/o** |
| 5.4. relating to blood or lymph vessels | _____ | **ather/o** |
| 5.5. slow | _____ | **brady-** |

## MATCHING WORD PARTS 2

Write the correct answer in the middle column.

| Definition | Correct Answer | Possible Answers |
|---|---|---|
| 5.6. blood or blood condition | _____ | **cardi/o** |
| 5.7. heart | _____ | **-crasia** |
| 5.8. mixture or blending | _____ | **ven/o** |
| 5.9. red | _____ | **-emia** |
| 5.10. vein | _____ | **erythr/o** |

## MATCHING WORD PARTS 3

Write the correct answer in the middle column.

| Definition | Correct Answer | Possible Answers |
|---|---|---|
| 5.11.    white | _____ | **hem/o** |
| 5.12.    vein | _____ | **leuk/o** |
| 5.13.    fast, rapid | _____ | **phleb/o** |
| 5.14.    clot | _____ | **tachy-** |
| 5.15.    blood, relating to blood | _____ | **thromb/o** |

## DEFINITIONS

Select the correct answer, and write it on the line provided.

5.16.    The term meaning white blood cells is _____.

      erythrocytes       leukocytes       platelets       thrombocytes

5.17.    Commonly known as the natural pacemaker, the medical name of the structure is

the _____.

      atrioventricular node      bundle of His      Purkinje fiber      sinoatrial node

5.18.    The myocardium receives its blood supply from the _____ arteries.

      aorta      coronary arteries      inferior vena cava      superior vena cava

5.19.    The _____ are formed in red bone marrow and then migrate to tissues throughout

the body. These blood cells destroy parasitic organisms and play a major role in allergic reactions.

      basophils      eosinophils      erythrocytes      monocytes

5.20.    The bicuspid valve is also known as the _____ valve.

      aortic      mitral      pulmonary      tricuspid

5.21.    The _____ pumps blood into the pulmonary artery, which carries it to the lungs.

      left atrium      left ventricle      right atrium      right ventricle

5.22.  The _____ are the smallest formed elements in the blood, and they play an impor-

tant role in blood clotting.

erythrocytes              leukocytes              monocytes              thrombocytes

5.23.  A foreign object, such as a bit of tissue or air, circulating in the blood is known as a/

an _____.

embolism              embolus              thrombosis              thrombus

5.24.  The _____ carries blood to all parts of the body except the lungs.

left atrium        left ventricle        right atrium        right ventricle

5.25.  The _____ are the most common type of white blood cell.

erythrocytes              leukocytes              neutrophils              thrombocytes

## MATCHING STRUCTURES

Write the correct answer in the middle column.

| Definition | Correct Answer | Possible Answers |
|---|---|---|
| 5.26.  a hollow, muscular organ | _____ | endocardium |
| 5.27.  cardiac muscle | _____ | epicardium |
| 5.28.  external layer of the heart | _____ | heart |
| 5.29.  inner lining of the heart | _____ | myocardium |
| 5.30.  sac enclosing the heart | _____ | pericardium |

## WHICH WORD?

Select the correct answer, and write it on the line provided.

5.31.  High-density _____ is also known as good cholesterol.

lipoprotein cholesterol        total cholesterol

5.32.  An abnormally slow resting heart rate is described as _____.

bradycardia              tachycardia

5.33. In _____ fibrillation, instead of pumping strongly, the heart muscle quivers

ineffectively.

       atrial                ventricular

5.34. The highest pressure against the blood vessels is _____ pressure, and it occurs

when the ventricles contract.

       diastolic             systolic

5.35. The diagnostic procedure that images the structures of the blood vessels and the flow of blood through

these vessels is known as _____.

      digital angiography      duplex ultrasound

## SPELLING COUNTS

Find the misspelled word in each sentence. Then write that word, spelled correctly, on the line provided.

5.36. The autopsy indicated that the cause of death was a ruptured aneuryism. _____

5.37. A deficiency of blood passing through an organ or body part is known as

hypoprefusion. _____

5.38. An arrhythemia is an abnormal heart rhythm in which the heartbeat is faster or slower than

normal. _____

5.39. Reynaud's disease is a condition with symptoms that include of intermittent attacks of pallor, cyanosis,

and redness of the fingers and toes. _____

5.40. An automated implantable cardioverter-defibrilator is a double-action

pacemaker. _____

## ABBREVIATION IDENTIFICATION

In the space provided, write the words that each abbreviation stands for.

5.41. **CAD** _____

5.42. **EKG, ECG** _____

5.43. **A-fib** _____

5.44. **MI** _____

5.45. **VF** _____

## TERM SELECTION

Select the correct answer, and write it on the line provided.

5.46.    The systemic condition often associated with severe infections caused by the presence of bacteria in the

blood is known as _____.

dyscrasia             endocarditis             pericarditis             septicemia

5.47.    A/An _____ reduces the workload of the heart by slowing the rate of the heartbeat.

ACE inhibitor             beta-blocker             calcium blocker             statin inhibitor

5.48.    The blood disorder characterized by anemia in which the red blood cells are larger than normal is known

as _____ anemia.

aplastic             hemolytic             megaloblastic             pernicious

5.49.    A/An _____ is administered to lower high blood pressure.

antiarrhythmic             antihypertensive             aspirin             diuretic

5.50.    A bacterial infection of the lining or valves of the heart is known as bacterial _____.

endocarditis             myocarditis             pericarditis             valvulitis

## SENTENCE COMPLETION

Write the correct term or terms on the lines provided.

5.51.    Plasma with the clotting proteins removed is known as _____.

5.52.    Having an abnormally small number of platelets in the circulating blood is known

as _____.

5.53.    The surgical removal of the lining of a portion of a clogged carotid artery leading to the brain is known as

a/an _____.

5.54.    The abnormal protrusion of a heart valve that results in the inability of the valve to close completely is

known as a/an _____ _____.

5.55.    The medication _____ is prescribed to prevent or relieve the pain of angina by

dilating the blood vessels to the heart.

## WORD SURGERY

Divide each term into its component word parts. Write these word parts, in sequence, on the lines provided. When necessary, use a slash (/) to indicate a combining vowel. (You may not need all of the lines provided.)

5.56.   **Aneurysmorrhaphy** means the surgical suturing a ruptured aneurysm.

_____   _____   _____   _____

5.57.   **Aplastic** anemia is characterized by an absence of *all* formed blood elements.

_____   _____   _____   _____

5.58.   **Electrocardiography** is the process of recording the electrical activity of the myocardium.

_____   _____   _____   _____

5.59.   **Polyarteritis** is a form of vasculitis involving several medium and small arteries at the same time.

_____   _____   _____   _____

5.60.   **Valvoplasty** is the surgical repair or replacement of a heart valve.

_____   _____   _____   _____

## TRUE/FALSE

If the statement is true, write **True** on the line. If the statement is false, write **False** on the line.

5.61.   _____ A thrombus is a clot or piece of tissue circulating in the blood.

5.62.   _____ Hemochromatosis is also known as iron overload disease.

5.63.   _____ Plasmapheresis is the removal of whole blood from the body, separation of

its cellular elements, and reinfusion of these cellular elements suspended in saline or a plasma substitute.

5.64.   _____ A vasoconstrictor is a drug that enlarges the blood vessels.

5.65.   _____ Peripheral vascular disease is a disorder of the blood vessels located outside

the heart and brain.

## CLINICAL CONDITIONS

Write the correct answer on the line provided.

5.66.   Alberta Fleetwood has a/an _____. This condition is a benign tumor made up of

newly formed blood vessels.

5.67.   After his surgery, Ramon Martinez developed a deep vein _____ in his leg.

5.68. During her pregnancy, Polly Olson suffered from abnormally swollen veins in her legs. The medical term for this condition is _____ veins.

5.69. Thomas Wilkerson suffers from episodes of severe chest pain due to inadequate blood flow to the myocardium. This is a condition is known as _____.

5.70. When Mr. Klein stands up too quickly, his blood pressure drops. His physician describes this as postural or _____.

5.71. Juanita Gomez was diagnosed as having _____. This bone marrow disorder is characterized by the insufficient production of one or more types of blood cells.

5.72. Dr. Lawson read her patient's _____. This diagnostic record is also known as an ECG or EKG.

5.73. Jason Turner suffered from cardiac arrest. The paramedics arrived promptly and saved his life by using _____ (CPR).

5.74. Darlene Nolan was diagnosed as having a deep vein thrombosis. Her doctor immediately prescribed a/an _____ to cause the thrombus to dissolve.

5.75. Hamilton Edwards Sr. suffers from _____ (IHD). This is a group of cardiac disabilities resulting from an insufficient supply of oxygenated blood to the heart.

## WHICH IS THE CORRECT MEDICAL TERM?

Select the correct answer, and write it on the line provided.

5.76. A/An _____, which is a characteristic of atherosclerosis, is a deposit of plaque on or within the arterial wall.

    vasculitis    angiostenosis    arteriosclerosis    atheroma

5.77. The term _____ means to stop or control bleeding.

    hemochromatosis    hemostasis    plasmapheresis    transfusion reaction

5.78. Inflammation of a vein is known as _____.

    arteriostenosis    endocarditis    phlebitis    carditis

5.79.    Blood _____ is any pathologic condition of the cellular elements of the blood.

>           anemia            dyscrasia         hemochromatosis        septicemia

5.80.    The surgical removal of an aneurysm is a/an _____.

>           aneurysmectomy        aneurysmoplasty      aneurysmorrhaphy      aneurysmotomy

## CHALLENGE WORD BUILDING

These terms are *not* found in this chapter; however, they are made up of the following familiar word parts. If you need help in creating the term, refer to your medical dictionary.

| | | |
|---|---|---|
| **peri-** | **angi/o** | **-itis** |
| | **arter/o** | **-necrosis** |
| | **cardi/o** | **-rrhaphy** |
| | **phleb/o** | **-rrhexis** |
| | **-ectomy** | **-stenosis** |

5.81.    Inflammation of an artery or arteries is known as _____.

5.82.    The surgical removal of a portion of a blood vessel is a/an _____.

5.83.    The abnormal narrowing of the lumen of a vein is known as _____.

5.84.    The surgical removal of a portion of the tissue surrounding the heart is a/an _____.

5.85.    To surgically suture the wall of the heart is a/an _____.

5.86.    Rupture of a vein is known as _____.

5.87.    The suture repair of any vessel, especially a blood vessel, is a/an _____.

5.88.    Rupture of the heart is known as _____.

5.89.    To suture the tissue surrounding the heart is a/an _____.

5.90.    The tissue death of the walls of the blood vessels is known as _____.

## LABELING EXERCISES

Identify the numbered items in the accompanying figures.

5.91.  superior _____

5.92.  right _____

5.93.  right _____

5.94.  left pulmonary _____

5.95.  left pulmonary _____

5.96.  pulmonary _____ valve

5.97.  _____ valve

5.98.  _____

5.99.  _____ semilunar valve

5.100. _____ valve

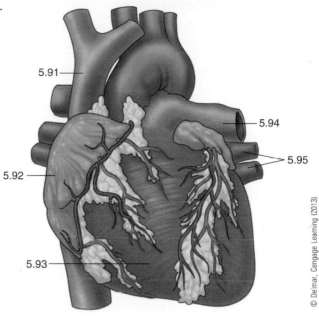

© Delmar, Cengage Learning (2013)

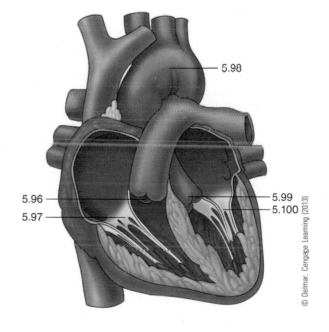

© Delmar, Cengage Learning (2013)

# THE HUMAN TOUCH
## Critical Thinking Exercise

The following story and questions are designed to stimulate critical thinking through class discussion or as a brief essay response. There are no right or wrong answers to these questions.

*Randi Marchant, a 42-year-old waitress, was vacuuming the family room when she felt that painful squeezing in her chest again. Third time today, but this one really hurt. She sat down to catch her breath and stubbed out the cigarette she had left smoldering in the half-filled ashtray by the couch. Randi's husband, Jimmy, and stepdaughter Melonie had pestered her until she finally had taken time off work to see her doctor. Dr. Harris found that her blood pressure was 158/88—probably owing to the noon rush stress at work, she rationalized. At least her cholesterol test was only 30 points above average this time. It had been slowly coming down, even though she cheated on her diet.*

*Another wave of pain tightened its icy fingers around her heart, and the pain moved up into both sides of her jaw. Randi thought, "Probably just a little heartburn. Since the pain doesn't radiate down my left arm, it couldn't be my heart, could it?"*

*"Don't think about the pain," she told herself. "Think of something else. Melonie's prom dress needs altering." Randi fell to the floor, clutching her chest, just as Melonie walked in. She saw her stepmother slumped on the floor and screamed, "Oh my God! Help, somebody, help!"*

## Suggested Discussion Topics

1. What information in the story indicates that Randi might be a candidate for heart disease?
2. Discuss why Randi thought this was not a heart attack.
3. What can Melonie do immediately to try to save Randi's life?
4. Assuming that Randi is suffering a myocardial infarction, discuss why it is important that she receive appropriate treatment quickly.

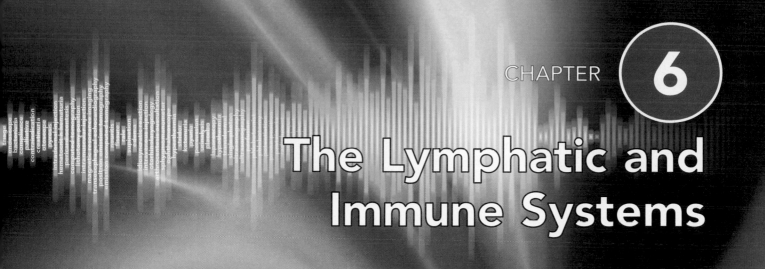

# The Lymphatic and Immune Systems

## Overview of
## STRUCTURES, COMBINING FORMS, AND FUNCTIONS OF THE LYMPHATIC AND IMMUNE SYSTEMS

| Major Structures | Related Combining Forms | Primary Functions |
|---|---|---|
| Lymph | **lymph/o** | The fluid that removes cellular waste products, pathogens, and dead blood cells from the tissues. |
| Lymphatic Vessels and Ducts | **lymphangi/o** | The capillaries, vessels, and ducts that return lymph from the tissues to the venous bloodstream. |
| Lymph Nodes | **lymphaden/o** | Bean-shaped structures of the lymphatic system where pathogens and other harmful substances are filtered from the lymph by specialized cells of the immune system. |
| Tonsils and Adenoids | **tonsill/o, adenoid/o** | Lymphoid structures of the lymphatic system that protect the entry to the respiratory system. |
| Spleen | **splen/o** (Note: this combining form is spelled with only one e.) | A sac-like mass of lymphoid tissue with protective roles in both the immune and lymphatic systems. |
| Bone Marrow | **myel/o** | Produces lymphocytes, which are specialized leukocytes (white blood cells). **Myel/o** also means spinal cord (see Chapter 10). |
| Lymphocytes | **lymphocyt/o** | Specialized leukocytes that play important roles in the immune reactions. |
| Thymus | **thym/o** | A gland located in the upper chest with specialized roles in both the lymphatic and immune systems. |

## Vocabulary Related to THE LYMPHATIC AND IMMUNE SYSTEMS

This list contains essential word parts and medical terms for this chapter. These terms are pronounced in the StudyWARE™ and Audio CDs that are available for use with this text. These and the other important **primary terms** are shown in boldface throughout the chapter. *Secondary terms*, which appear in *orange* italics, clarify the meaning of primary terms.

### Word Parts

- ☐ **anti-** against
- ☐ **carcin/o** cancerous
- ☐ **immun/o** immune, protection, safe
- ☐ **lymph/o** lymph, lymphatic tissue
- ☐ **lymphaden/o** lymph node or gland
- ☐ **lymphangi/o** lymph vessel
- ☐ **neo-, ne/o** new, strange
- ☐ **-oma** tumor, neoplasm
- ☐ **onc/o** tumor
- ☐ **phag/o** eat, swallow
- ☐ **-plasm** formative material of cells
- ☐ **sarc/o** flesh, connective tissue
- ☐ **splen/o** spleen
- ☐ **-tic** pertaining to
- ☐ **tox/o** poison, poisonous

### Medical Terms

- ☐ **acquired immunodeficiency syndrome** (**im**-you-noh-deh-**FISH**-en-see)
- ☐ **allergen** (**AL**-er-jen)
- ☐ **anaphylaxis** (**an**-ah-fih-**LACK**-sis)
- ☐ **antibiotics**
- ☐ **antibody** (**AN**-tih-**bod**-ee)
- ☐ **antifungal** (**an**-tih-**FUNG**-gul)
- ☐ **antigen** (**AN**-tih-jen)
- ☐ **antigen-antibody reaction**
- ☐ **autoimmune disorder** (aw-toh-ih-**MYOUN**)
- ☐ **bacilli** (bah-**SILL**-eye)
- ☐ **bacteria** (back-**TEER**-ree-ah)
- ☐ **candidiasis** (kan-dih-**DYE**-ah-sis)
- ☐ **carcinoma** (**kar**-sih-**NOH**-mah)
- ☐ **carcinoma in situ** (**kar**-sih-**NOH**-mah in **SIGH**-too)
- ☐ **complement system** (**KOM**-pleh-ment)
- ☐ **cytokines** (**SIGH**-toh-kyens)
- ☐ **cytomegalovirus** (sigh-toh-**meg**-ah-loh-**VYE**-rus)
- ☐ **cytotoxic drug** (sigh-toh-**TOK**-sick)
- ☐ **ductal carcinoma in situ** (**DUCK**-tal **kar**-sih-**NOH**-mah in **SIGH**-too)
- ☐ **hemolytic** (**hee**-moh-**LIT**-ick)

- ☐ **herpes zoster** (**HER**-peez **ZOS**-ter)
- ☐ **Hodgkin's lymphoma** (**HODJ**-kinz lim-**FOH**-mah)
- ☐ **human immunodeficiency virus** (**im**-you-noh-deh-**FISH**-en-see)
- ☐ **immunodeficiency disorder** (**im**-you-noh-deh-**FISH**-en-see)
- ☐ **immunoglobulins** (**im**-you-noh-**GLOB**-you-lins)
- ☐ **immunosuppressant** (**im**-you-noh-soo-**PRES**-ant)
- ☐ **immunotherapy** (ih-**myou**-noh-**THER**-ah-pee)
- ☐ **infectious mononucleosis** (**mon**-oh-**new**-klee-**OH**-sis)
- ☐ **infiltrating ductal carcinoma** (in-**FILL**-trate-ing **DUK**-tal kar-sih-**NOH**-mah)
- ☐ **interferons** (**in**-ter-**FEAR**-onz)
- ☐ **lymphadenitis** (lim-**fad**-eh-**NIGH**-tis)
- ☐ **lymphadenopathy** (lim-**fad**-eh-**NOP**-ah-thee)
- ☐ **lymphangioma** (lim-**fan**-jee-**OH**-mah)
- ☐ **lymphedema** (**lim**-feh-**DEE**-mah)
- ☐ **lymphocytes** (**LIM**-foh-sights)
- ☐ **lymphoma** (lim-**FOH**-mah)
- ☐ **lymphoscintigraphy** (**lim**-foh-sin-**TIH**-grah-fee)
- ☐ **macrophage** (**MACK**-roh-fayj)
- ☐ **malaria** (mah-**LAY**-ree-ah)
- ☐ **mammography** (mam-**OG**-rah-fee)
- ☐ **metastasis** (meh-**TAS**-tah-sis)
- ☐ **metastasize** (meh-**TAS**-tah-sighz)
- ☐ **myoma** (my-**OH**-mah)
- ☐ **myosarcoma** (my-oh-sahr-**KOH**-mah)
- ☐ **non-Hodgkin's lymphoma** (non-**HODJ**-kinz lim-**FOH**-mah)
- ☐ **opportunistic infection** (op-ur-too-**NIHS**-tick)
- ☐ **osteosarcoma** (**oss**-tee-oh-sar-**KOH**-mah)
- ☐ **parasite** (**PAR**-ah-sight)
- ☐ **rabies** (**RAY**-beez)
- ☐ **rickettsia** (rih-**KET**-see-ah)
- ☐ **rubella** (roo-**BELL**-ah)
- ☐ **sarcoma** (sar-**KOH**-mah)
- ☐ **spirochetes** (**SPY**-roh-keets)
- ☐ **splenomegaly** (splee-noh-**MEG**-ah-lee)
- ☐ **staphylococci** (staf-ih-loh-**KOCK**-sigh)
- ☐ **streptococci** (strep-toh-**KOCK**-sigh)
- ☐ **systemic reaction**
- ☐ **teletherapy** (tel-eh-**THER**-ah-pee)
- ☐ **toxoplasmosis** (tock-soh-plaz-**MOH**-sis)
- ☐ **varicella** (var-ih-**SEL**-ah)

## LEARNING GOALS

On completion of this chapter, you should be able to:

1. Describe the major functions and structures of the lymphatic and immune systems.

2. Identify the medical specialists who treat disorders of the lymphatic and immune systems.

3. Recognize, define, spell, and pronounce the primary terms related to the structures,

functions, pathology, and the diagnostic and treatment procedures of the lymphatic and immune systems.

4. Recognize, define, spell, and pronounce the primary terms related to oncology.

# FUNCTIONS OF THE LYMPHATIC SYSTEM

The three main functions of the lymphatic system are to:

1. Absorb fats and fat-soluble vitamins through the lacteals of the small intestine.

2. Remove waste products from the tissues, and cooperate with the immune system in destroying invading pathogens.

3. Return filtered lymph to the veins at the base of the neck.

## Absorption of Fats and Fat-Soluble Vitamins

Food is digested in the small intestine, which is lined with small fingerlike projections known as *villi*. Each *villus* (singular) contains lacteals and blood vessels.

■ **Lacteals** (**LACK**-tee-ahlz) are specialized structures of the lymphatic system that absorb those fats that cannot be transported by the bloodstream. These dietary fats are transformed in the cells of the lacteals. The lymphatic vessels then return them to the venous circulation so they can be used throughout the body as nutrients.

■ The blood vessels absorb the nutrients, fats, and fat-soluble vitamins from the digested food directly into the bloodstream for use throughout the body. This is discussed further in Chapter 8.

## Interstitial Fluid and Lymph Creation

**Interstitial fluid** (**in**-ter-**STISH**-al), which is also known as *intercellular* or *tissue fluid*, is plasma from arterial

blood that flows out of the arterioles and into the capillaries, and then flows into the spaces between the cells of the tissues.

■ This fluid delivers nutrients, oxygen, and hormones to the cells.

■ When interstitial fluid leaves the cells, it brings with it waste products and protein molecules that were created within the cells. About 90% of this fluid returns to the bloodstream.

**Lymph** (**limf**) is made up of the remaining 10% of the returning interstitial fluid. Lymph is a clear, watery fluid containing electrolytes and proteins. It plays essential roles in the lymphatic system as it works in close cooperation with the immune system

■ Lymph collects the protein molecules created within the cells as it leaves. Lymph also removes dead cells, debris, and pathogens (including cancer cells) that were still left in the intercellular spaces.

■ The lymph enters very small capillaries within the tissues and then flows into progressively larger vessels and ducts as it travels in a one-way trip upward toward the neck.

■ At this stage, the lymph begins to play an active role in cooperation with the immune system to protect the body against invading microorganisms and diseases. These functions are described in the discussion of the immune system.

# STRUCTURES OF THE LYMPHATIC SYSTEM

Many of the structures of the lymphatic system cooperate and also perform roles in other body systems.

## Lymphatic Circulation

The **lymphatic circulatory system** and blood circulatory system work closely together, and because of these similarities the lymphatic circulatory system is often referred to as the *secondary circulatory system*. However, it is also very important to understand the differences in these two systems. While studying this section, compare Figure 6.1 with Figures 5.9 and 5.10 in Chapter 5.

- Blood circulates throughout the entire body in a loop, pumped by the heart. The bloodstream flows in an open system in which it leaves and reenters the blood vessels through the capillaries

- Since the lymphatic system does not have a pump-like organ, it must depend on the pumping motion of muscles to move the fluid upward.

- Lymph flows in only one direction. From its point of origin, lymph can move only upward until it returns to the circulatory system at the base of the neck. Once lymph enters a lymphatic capillary, it must continue this upward flow.

- Blood is filtered by the kidneys, and waste products are excreted by the urinary system. Lymph is filtered by lymph nodes, which are located along lymphatic vessels. These nodes contain specialized cells of the immune system.

- The color of blood makes the arteries and veins readily visible. Since lymph is a clear fluid, the lymphatic vessels are not readily visible.

## Lymphatic Capillaries

**Lymphatic capillaries** are microscopic, blind-ended tubes located near the surface of the body with capillary walls that are only one cell in thickness. These cells separate briefly to allow the lymph to enter the capillary. Then the action of the cells as they close forces the lymph to flow upward and forward (Figure 6.2).

## Lymphatic Vessels and Ducts

Lymph flows from the lymphatic capillaries into the progressively larger **lymphatic vessels**, which are located deeper within the tissues. Like veins, lymphatic vessels have valves to prevent the backward flow of lymph.

The larger lymphatic vessels eventually join together to form two ducts. Each duct drains a specific part of the body and returns the lymph to the venous circulation (Figure 6.1).

- The **right lymphatic duct** collects lymph from the right side of the head and neck, the upper right quadrant of the body, and the right arm. The right lymphatic duct empties into the right subclavian vein. The *subclavian* vein is the proximal part of the main vein of the arm.

- The **thoracic duct**, which is the largest lymphatic vessel in the body, collects lymph from the left side of the head and neck, the upper left quadrant of the trunk, the left arm, the entire lower portion of the trunk, and both legs. The thoracic duct empties into the left subclavian vein.

## Lymph Nodes

Each small, bean-shaped **lymph node** contains specialized lymphocytes that are capable of destroying pathogens. Unfiltered lymph flows into the nodes, and here the lymphocytes destroy harmful substances such as bacteria, viruses, and malignant cells. Additional structures within the node filter the lymph to remove other impurities. After these processes are complete, the lymph leaves the node and continues its journey to become part of the venous circulation again.

There are between 400 and 700 lymph nodes located along the larger lymphatic vessels, and approximately half of these nodes are in the abdomen. Most of the other nodes are positioned on the branches of the larger lymphatic vessels throughout the body. The exceptions are the three major groups of lymph nodes that are named for their locations (Figure 6.1).

- **Cervical lymph nodes** (**SER**-vih-kal) are located along the sides of the neck (**cervic** means neck, and **-al** means pertaining to).

- **Axillary lymph nodes** (**AK**-sih-**lar**-ee) are located under the arms in the area known as the armpits (**axill** means armpit, and **-ary** means pertaining to).

- **Inguinal lymph nodes** (**ING**-gwih-nal) are located in the inguinal (groin) area of the lower abdomen (**inguin** means groin, and **-al** means pertaining to).

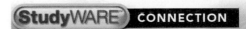

Watch the **Lymph Nodes** animation in the StudyWARE™.

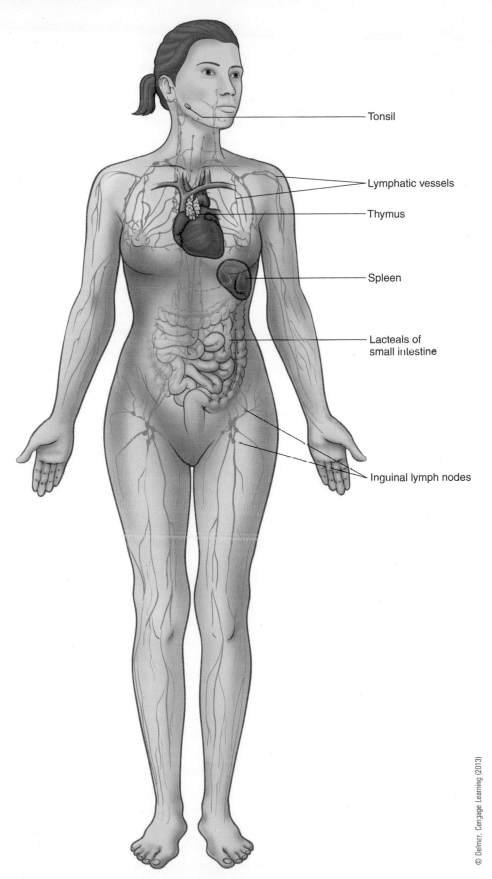

Tonsil

Lymphatic vessels

Thymus

Spleen

Lacteals of
small intestine

Inguinal lymph nodes

**FIGURE 6.1** The vessels and organs of the lymphatic system; only inguinal lymph nodes are labeled.

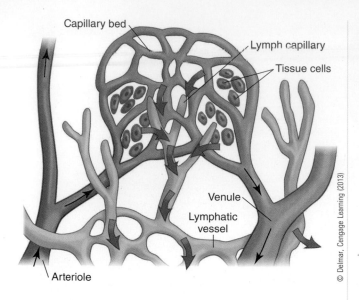

Labels: Capillary bed, Lymph capillary, Tissue cells, Venule, Lymphatic vessel, Arteriole

© Delmar, Cengage Learning (2013)

**FIGURE 6.2** *Lymph capillaries* begin as blind-ended tubes. Lymph enters between the cells of the capillary wall and flows into progressively larger lymphatic vessels.

## Lymphocytes

**Lymphocytes** (**LIM**-foh-sights), also known as *lymphoid cells*, are leukocytes that are formed in bone marrow as stem cells (**lymph/o** means lymph, and **-cytes** means cells). There are three types of lymphocytes: natural killer cells, B cells, and T cells.

■ Lymphocytes undergo further maturation and differentiation in lymphoid tissues throughout the body. These changes enable these lymphocytes to act as specialized antibodies that are capable of attacking specific antigens. *Maturation* means the process of becoming mature. *Differentiation* means to be modified to perform a specific function.

■ **Natural killer cells** (NK cells) play an important role in the killing of cancer cells and cells infected by viruses.

## B Cells

■ **B cells**, also known as *B lymphocytes*, are specialized lymphocytes that produce antibodies. Each lymphocyte makes a specific antibody that is capable of destroying a specific antigen.

■ B cells are most effective against viruses and bacteria that are circulating in the blood. When a B cell is confronted with the antigen that it is coded to destroy, that B cell is transformed into a plasma cell.

■ **Plasma cells** develop from B cells and secrete a large volume of antibodies coded to destroy specific antigens.

## T Cells

■ **T cells**, also known as *T lymphocytes*, belong to a group of leukocytes known as lymphocytes. These cells, which get the 'T' in their name from their origin in the thymus, play a central role in cell-mediated immunity.

■ **Cytokines** (**SIGH**-toh-kyens) are a group of proteins such as interferons and interleukins released primarily by the T cells. These cells act as intracellular signals to begin the immune response.

■ **Interferons** (**in**-ter-**FEAR**-onz) (IFNs) are produced in response to the presence of antigens, particularly viruses or tumor cells. Interferons activate the immune system, fight viruses by slowing or stopping their multiplication, and signal other cells to increase their defenses.

■ **Interleukins** (**in**-ter-**LOO**-kinz) play multiple roles in the immune system, including directing B and T cells to divide and proliferate.

# ■ ADDITIONAL STRUCTURES OF THE LYMPHATIC SYSTEM

The remaining structures of this body system are made up of lymphoid tissue. The term *lymphoid* means pertaining to the lymphatic system or resembling lymph or lymphatic tissue. Although these structures consist of lymphoid tissue, their primary roles are in conjunction with the immune system (Figure 6.3).

## The Tonsils

The **tonsils** (**TON**-sils) are three masses of lymphoid tissue that form a protective ring around the back of the nose and upper throat (Figure 6.4). The tonsils play an important role in the immune system by preventing pathogens from entering the respiratory system when breathing through the nose and mouth.

■ The **adenoids** (**AD**-eh-noids), also known as the *nasopharyngeal tonsils*, are located in the nasopharynx, which is the upper part of the pharynx and is described in Chapter 7.

■ The **palatine tonsils** (**PAL**-ah-tine) are located on the left and right sides of the throat in the area that is visible at the back of the mouth. *Palatine* describes the hard and soft palates that form the roof of the mouth.

■ The **lingual tonsils** (**LING**-gwal) are located at the base of the tongue; however, they are not readily visible. *Lingual* means pertaining to the tongue.

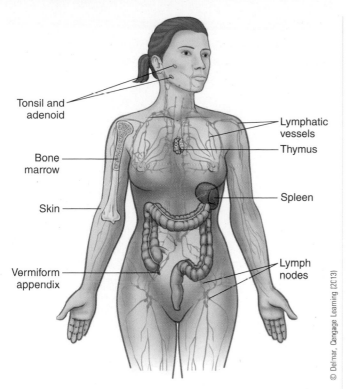

**FIGURE 6.3** Structures consisting of lymphoid tissues play many important roles in the immune system.

## The Thymus Gland

The **thymus** (**THIGH**-mus), which is a mass of lymphoid tissue located above the heart, reaches its greatest size at puberty and becomes smaller with age.

- As part of the endocrine system, the thymus secretes a hormone that stimulates the maturation of lymphocytes into T cells (see Chapter 13).

- These T cells, which are essential to the immune system, leave the thymus through the bloodstream and the lymphatic system.

## The Vermiform Appendix

The **vermiform appendix**, commonly referred to as the *appendix*, hangs from the lower portion of the cecum, which is the first section of the large intestine. Although its purpose was unknown for many years, recent research indicates that the appendix may play an important role in the immune system.

## The Spleen

The **spleen** is a sac-like mass of lymphoid tissue located in the left upper quadrant of the abdomen, just inferior to

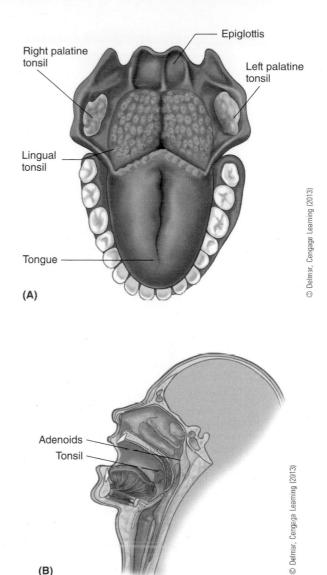

**(A)**

**(B)**

**FIGURE 6.4** The *tonsils* form a protective ring around the entrance to the respiratory system.

(below) the diaphragm and posterior to (behind) the stomach (Figure 6.5).

- The spleen filters microorganisms and other foreign material from the blood.

- The spleen forms *lymphocytes* and *monocytes*, which are specialized leukocytes (white blood cells) with roles to play in the immune system.

- The spleen has the **hemolytic** (**hee**-moh-**LIT**-ick) function of destroying worn-out erythrocytes (red blood cells) and releasing their hemoglobin for reuse (**hem/o** means blood, and **-lytic** means to destroy).

- The spleen also stores extra erythrocytes (red blood cells) and maintains the appropriate balance between these cells and the plasma of the blood.

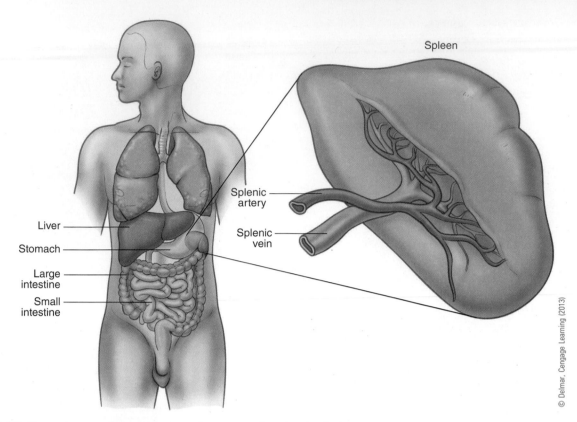

Spleen

Splenic artery

Splenic vein

Liver

Stomach

Large intestine

Small intestine

© Delmar, Cengage Learning (2013)

**FIGURE 6.5** The spleen performs important functions related to both the immune and cardiovascular systems.

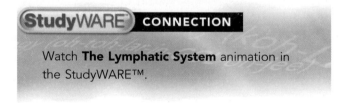

**StudyWARE CONNECTION**

Watch **The Lymphatic System** animation in the StudyWARE™.

# ■ FUNCTIONS AND STRUCTURES OF THE IMMUNE SYSTEM

The primary function of the immune system is to maintain good health and to protect the body from harmful substances such as:

- *Pathogens*, which are disease-producing microorganisms.

- *Allergens*, which are substances that produce allergic reactions.

- *Toxins*, which are poisonous or harmful substances.

- *Malignant cells*, which are potentially life-threatening cancer cells.

The immune system first attempts to prevent the entry of these harmful substances into the body. If harmful substances do gain entry into the body, the immune system immediately begins working to destroy them.

- The immune system uses a complex system of chemical signaling between specialized cells to identify, attack, and remember antigens.

- This is accomplished by coordinating a highly specific response based on the type of antigen and differentiating it from the body's own tissues to avoid attacking itself.

- After encountering an antigen once, the immune system's "memory" of the invader enables the body to mount a more efficient future defense against that antigen.

## The Immune System's First Line of Defense

Unlike other body systems, the immune system is not contained within a single set of organs or vessels. Instead, its functions use structures from several other body systems. The first line of defense includes:

- **Intact skin** that wraps the body in a physical barrier to prevent invading organisms from entering the body. *Intact* means that there are no cuts, scrapes, open sores, or breaks in the skin. The skin is also covered with an *acid mantle* that makes it an inhospitable environment for most bacteria.

- The **respiratory system** traps breathed-in foreign matter with nose hairs and the moist mucous membrane lining of the respiratory system. The tonsils form a protective ring around the entrance to the throat. If foreign matter gets past these barriers, coughing and sneezing help expel it from the respiratory system.

- The **digestive system** uses the acids and enzymes produced by the stomach to destroy invaders that are swallowed or consumed with food.

- The structures of the **lymphatic system** and specialized leukocytes (white blood cells) work together in specific ways to attack and destroy pathogens that have succeeded in entering the body.

## The Antigen-Antibody Reaction

An **antigen-antibody reaction**, also known as the *immune reaction*, involves binding antigens to antibodies. This reaction labels a potentially dangerous antigen so it can be recognized and destroyed by other cells of the immune system.

- An **antigen** (**AN**-tih-jen) is any substance that the body regards as being foreign. This includes viruses, bacteria, toxins, and transplanted tissues. The immune system immediately responds to the presence of any antigen. (Figure 6.6).

- **Tolerance** refers to an acquired unresponsiveness to a specific antigen. The term is also used to describe a decline in the effective response to a drug, usually due to repeated use.

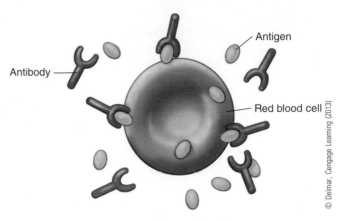

**FIGURE 6.6** Antibodies bind together foreign antigens to neutralize them and to flag them for destruction by the microphages.

© Delmar, Cengage Learning (2013)

- An **antibody** (**AN**-tih-**bod**-ee) is a disease-fighting protein created by the immune system in response to the presence of a specific antigen (the prefix **anti**- means against). The terms *antibody* and *immunoglobulin* are often used interchangeably.

## Immunoglobulins

- **Immunoglobulins** (**im**-you-noh-**GLOB**-you-lins) bind with specific antigens in the antigen-antibody response. The five primary types of immunoglobulins, which are secreted by plasma cells, are also known as antibodies (Table 6.1).

## TABLE 6.1
### Immunoglobulins and Their Roles

*Immunoglobulin G* (IgG) is the most abundant class of antibodies, and they are found in blood serum and lymph. These antibodies are active against bacteria, fungi, viruses, and foreign particles.

*Immunoglobulin A* (IgA) is the class of antibodies produced predominantly against ingested antigens. These antibodies are found in body secretions such as saliva, sweat, or tears, and function to prevent the attachment of viruses and bacteria to the epithelial surfaces that line most organs.

*Immunoglobulin M* (IgM) is the class of antibodies that are found in circulating body fluids. These are the first antibodies to appear in response to an initial exposure to an antigen.

*Immunoglobulin D* (IgD) is the class of antibodies found only on the surface of B cells. These antibodies are important in B cell activation.

*Immunoglobulin E* (IgE) is the class of antibodies produced in the lungs, skin, and mucous membranes. These antibodies are responsible for allergic reactions.

Note: Synthetic immunoglobulins, which are used as medications, are discussed later in this chapter.

## Phagocytes

**Phagocytes** (**FAG**-oh-sights) are specialized leukocytes that act as part of the antigen-antibody reaction by destroying substances such as cell debris, dust, pollen, and pathogens by the process of phagocytosis (**phag/o** means to eat or swallow, and **-cyte** means cell). *Phagocytosis* is the process of destroying pathogens by surrounding and swallowing them. Phagocytes include monocytes, macrophages, dendritic cells, and mast cells. Mast cells are discussed in Chapter 12.

- **Monocytes** are leukocytes that provide immunological defenses against many infectious organisms. Macrophages derive from monocytes after they leave the bloodstream and enter into the tissue. Monocytes replenish macrophages and dendritic cells.

- A **macrophage** (**MACK**-roh-fayj) is a type of leukocyte that surrounds and kills invading cells (**macro-** means large, and **-phage** means a cell that eats). Macrophages also remove dead cells and stimulate the action of other immune cells.

- **Dendritic cells** (den-**DRIT**-ic) are specialized leukocytes that patrol the body searching for antigens that produce infections. When such a cell is found, the dendritic cell grabs it, swallows, and alerts B and T cells to act against this specific antigen.

## The Complement System

**The complement system** (**KOM**-pleh-ment) is a group of proteins that normally circulate in the blood in an inactive form. When needed, these cells complement the ability of antibodies to ward off pathogens by combining with them to dissolve and remove pathogenic bacteria and other foreign cells. *Complement* means to complete or make whole.

## Immunity

**Immunity** is the state of being resistant to a specific disease. This resistance can be present naturally or it can be acquired.

- **Natural immunity**, which is also known as *passive immunity*, is resistance to a disease present without the administration of an antigen or exposure to a disease. Natural immunity is either present at birth or it is passed from the mother to her child through breast milk.

- **Acquired immunity** is obtained by having had a contagious disease. Being *vaccinated* against a contagious disease provides protection against that disease, such

as measles or polio, without having been exposed to the risk of actually having the disease.

- A *vaccine* is a preparation containing an antigen, consisting of whole or partial disease-causing organisms, which have been killed or weakened. For some diseases, such as tetanus (discussed in Chapter 10), a periodic booster shot is required to maintain the effectiveness of the immunity.

- *Vaccination* provides protection against the disease; however, for some conditions a periodic booster is required to maintain the effectiveness of the immunization.

# ■ MEDICAL SPECIALTIES RELATED TO THE LYMPHATIC AND IMMUNE SYSTEMS

- The lymphatic and immune systems work in close cooperation to protect and maintain the health of the body. Some functions and structures of these systems are performed by specialized structures or shared structures. Some medical specialists treat disorders that affect both of these body systems.

- An **allergist** (**AL**-er-jist) specializes in diagnosing and treating conditions of altered immunologic reactivity, such as allergic reactions.

- An **immunologist** (**im**-you-**NOL**-oh-jist) specializes in diagnosing and treating disorders of the immune system (**immun** means protected, and **-ologist** means specialist).

- A **lymphologist** (lim-**FOL**-oh-jist) is a physician who specializes in diagnosing and treating disorders of the lymphatic system (**lymph** means lymphatic system, and **-ologist** means specialist).

- An **oncologist** (ong-**KOL**-oh-jist) is a physician specializing in the diagnosing and treatment of malignant disorders such as tumors and cancer (**onc** mean tumor, and **-ologist** means specialist).

# ■ PATHOLOGY AND DIAGNOSTIC PROCEDURES OF THE LYMPHATIC SYSTEM

- **Lymphadenitis** (lim-**fad**-eh-**NIGH**-tis), commonly known as *swollen glands*, is an inflammation of the lymph nodes (**lymphaden** means lymph node, and

-**itis** means inflammation). The terms *lymph nodes* and *lymph glands* are sometimes used interchangeably. Swelling of the lymph nodes is frequently an indication of an infection.

- **Lymphadenopathy** (lim-**fad**-eh-**NOP**-ah-thee) is any disease process affecting a lymph node or nodes (**lymphaden/o** means lymph node, and -**pathy** means disease).

- A **lymphangioma** (lim-**fan** jee-**OH**-mah) is a benign tumor formed by an abnormal collection of lymphatic vessels due to a congenital malformation of the lymphatic system (**lymph** means lymph, **angi** means lymph vessel, and -**oma** means tumor).

- **Splenomegaly** (**splee**-noh-**MEG**-ah lee) is an abnormal enlargement of the spleen (**splen/o** means spleen, and -**megaly** means enlargement). This condition can be due to bleeding caused by an injury, an infectious disease such as mononucleosis, or abnormal functioning of the immune system.

- **Splenorrhagia** (**splee**-noh-**RAY**-jee-ah) is bleeding from the spleen (**splen/o** means spleen, and -**rrhagia** means bleeding).

- **Tonsillitis** and **tonsillectomy** are discussed in Chapter 1.

- **Lymphoscintigraphy** (lim-foh-sin-**TIH**-grah-fee) is a diagnostic test that is performed to detect damage or malformations of the lymphatic vessels. A radioactive substance is injected into lymph ducts, and a scanner or probe is used to follow the movement of the substance on a computer screen. This technique is used to find a sentinel node.

## Lymphedema

**Lymphedema** (**lim**-feh-**DEE**-mah) is swelling of the tissues due to an abnormal accumulation of lymph fluid within the tissues (**lymph** means lymph, and -**edema** means swelling). This is not the type of swelling that occurs due to an injury such as a sprained ankle. It is caused by damage to the lymphatic system that prevents lymph from draining properly. Because lymph is rich in protein, which is an environment that pathogens thrive in, lymphedema is often associated with infections.

- **Primary lymphedema** is a hereditary condition of the lymphatic system that develops with swelling beginning in the feet and progressing into the ankles and in an upward direction along the legs. The disorder occurs most frequently in females when the symptoms begin to appear during puberty.

- **Secondary lymphedema** is caused by damage to lymphatic vessels that is most frequently due to cancer treatment, surgery, trauma, or burns.

- Primary and secondary lymphedema are most commonly treated with compression and exercise to control the swelling and to minimize the infections. Although this treatment helps, at this time it is not possible to cure lymphedema.

- **Bioimpedance spectroscopy** (**BYE**-oh-im-**pee**-dens) is a noninvasive method of diagnosing lymphedema. It measures the resistance to an electrical current passed through the affected limb, with abnormally low results showing a buildup of lymph. If this condition can be diagnosed with this technique at an early stage, there is hope that it will not develop any further.

## PATHOLOGY AND DIAGNOSTIC PROCEDURES OF THE IMMUNE SYSTEM

The effectiveness of the immune system depends upon the individual's:

- *General health.* If the immune system is compromised by poor health, it cannot be fully effective.

- *Age.* Older individuals usually have more acquired immunity; however, their immune system tends to respond less quickly or effectively to new challenges.

- *Age.* Babies and very young children do not yet have as much acquired immunity, and their bodies sometimes have difficulty resisting challenges to the immune system.

- *Heredity.* Genes and genetic disorders affect the individual's general health and the functioning of his or her immune system.

## Allergic Reactions

- An **allergic reaction** occurs when the body's immune system reacts to a harmless allergen such as pollen, food, or animal dander as if it were a dangerous invader.

- An **allergy**, also known as *hypersensitivity*, is an overreaction by the body to a particular antigen. For *allergic rhinitis*, an allergic reaction to airborne allergens, see Chapter 7.

- An **allergen** (**AL**-er-jen) is a substance that produces an allergic reaction in an individual.

■ A **localized allergic response**, also known as a *cellular response*, includes redness, itching, and burning where the skin has come into contact with an allergen. For example, contact with poison ivy can cause a localized allergic response in the form of an itchy rash (see Chapter 12). Although the body reacts mildly the first time it is exposed to the allergen, sensitivity is established, and future contacts can cause much more severe symptoms.

■ A **systemic reaction**, which is also described as **anaphylaxis** (**an**-ah-fih-**LACK**-sis) or as *anaphylactic shock*, is a severe response to an allergen. As shown in Figure 6.7, the symptoms of this response develop quickly. Without prompt medical aid, the patient can die within a few minutes.

■ A *scratch test* is a diagnostic test to identify commonly troublesome allergens such as tree pollen and ragweed. Swelling and itching indicate an allergic reaction (Figure 6.8).

■ **Antihistamines** are medications administered to relieve or prevent the symptoms of hay fever, which is a common allergy to wind-borne pollens, and other types of allergies. Antihistamines work by preventing the effects of *histamine*, which is a substance produced by the body that causes the itching, sneezing, runny nose, and watery eyes of an allergic reaction.

## Autoimmune Disorders

An **autoimmune disorder** (**aw**-toh-ih-**MYOUN**), also known as an *autoimmune disease*, is any of a large group of diseases characterized by a condition in which the immune system produces antibodies against its own tissues, mistaking healthy cells, tissues, or organs for antigens.

■ This abnormal functioning of the immune system appears to be genetically transmitted and predominantly occurs in women during the childbearing years.

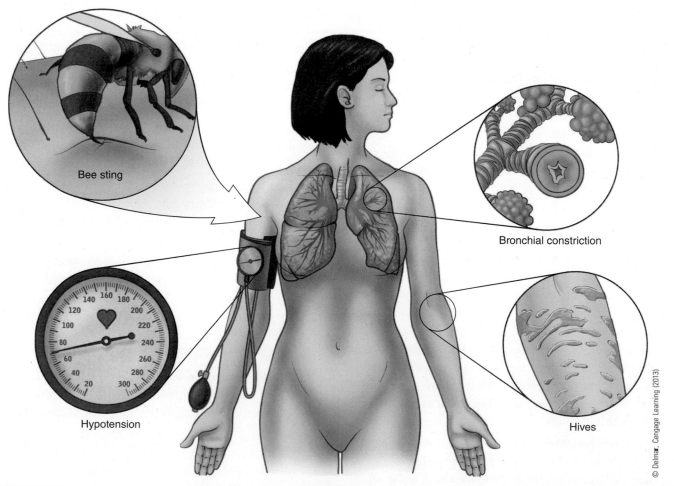

Bee sting

Bronchial constriction

Hypotension

Hives

© Delmar, Cengage Learning (2013)

**FIGURE 6.7** A severe anaphylactic allergic reaction involves several body systems and requires prompt treatment. Shown here are the many systems that may respond to a bee sting.

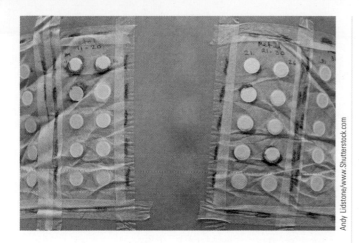

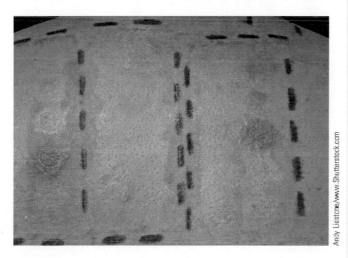

**FIGURE 6.8** In scratch tests, allergens are placed on the skin, the skin is scratched, and the allergen is labeled. Reactions usually begin to occur within 20 minutes.

■ It is estimated that 3% of Americans have an autoimmune disorder, with women affected 2.7 times more often than men. Autoimmune disorders affect most body systems. For examples, see Table 6.2.

## Immunodeficiency Disorders

An **immunodeficiency disorder** (**im**-you-noh-deh-**FISH**-en-see) occurs when the immune response is compromised. *Compromised* means weakened or not functioning properly.

### HIV: Human Immunodeficiency Virus

The **human immunodeficiency virus** (**im**-you-noh-deh-**FISH**-en-see), commonly known as *HIV*, is a bloodborne infection in which the virus damages or kills the T cells of the immune system, causing it to progressively fail, thus leaving the body at risk of developing many life-threatening opportunistic infections (Figure 6.9). Medical intervention including reverse transcriptase (RT), protease, and fusion inhibitors can now prolong the patient's life, especially if administered starting in the early stages of HIV.

■ An **opportunistic infection** (**op**-ur-too-**NIHS**-tick) is caused by a pathogen that does not normally produce an illness in healthy humans. However, when the host is debilitated, these pathogens are able to cause an infection. *Debilitated* means weakened by another condition.

■ **Acquired immunodeficiency syndrome**, commonly known as *AIDS*, is the most advanced and fatal stage of an HIV infection.

## TABLE 6.2
### Examples of Autoimmune Disorders and the Affected Body Systems

| Body System | Autoimmune Disorder |
| --- | --- |
| Skeletal System | *Rheumatoid arthritis* affects joints and connective tissue. |
| Muscular System | *Myasthenia gravis* affects nerve and muscle synapses. |
| Cardiovascular System | *Pernicious anemia* affects the red blood cells. |
| Digestive System | *Crohn's disease* affects the intestines, ileum, or the colon. |
| Nervous System | *Multiple sclerosis* affects the brain and spinal cord. |
| Integumentary System | *Scleroderma* affects the skin and connective tissues. |
| Endocrine System | *Graves' disease* affects the thyroid gland. |

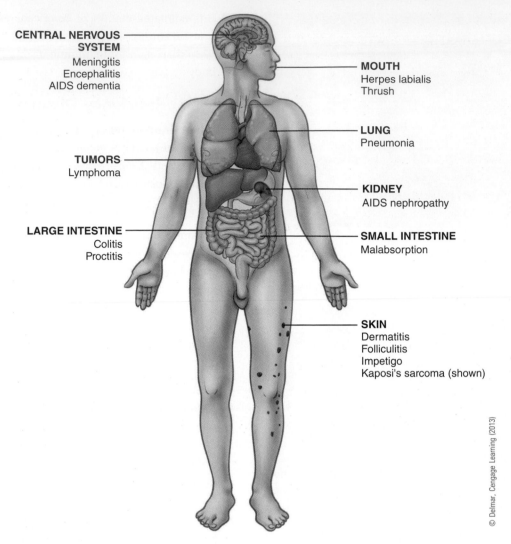

CENTRAL NERVOUS
SYSTEM
Meningitis
Encephalitis
AIDS dementia

MOUTH
Herpes labialis
Thrush

LUNG
Pneumonia

TUMORS
Lymphoma

KIDNEY
AIDS nephropathy

LARGE INTESTINE
Colitis
Proctitis

SMALL INTESTINE
Malabsorption

SKIN
Dermatitis
Folliculitis
Impetigo
Kaposi's sarcoma (shown)

© Delmar, Cengage Learning (2013)

**FIGURE 6.9** Pathologies associated with Acquired immunodeficiency syndrome (AIDS). (Each condition is discussed in the appropriate body system chapter.)

- **Kaposi's sarcoma** (**KAP**-oh-seez sar-**KOH**-mah) is an example of an opportunistic infection that is frequently associated with HIV. This cancer causes patches of abnormal tissue to grow under the skin; in the lining of the mouth, nose, and throat; or in other organs.

- **ELISA**, which is the acronym for *enzyme-linked immunosorbent assay*, is a blood test used to screen for the presence of HIV antibodies.

- A **Western blot test** is a blood test that produces more accurate results than the ELISA test. The Western blot test is performed to confirm the diagnosis when the results of the ELISA test are positive. This is necessary because the ELISA test sometimes produces a *false positive* result in which the test erroneously indicates the presence of HIV.

# TREATMENT OF THE IMMUNE SYSTEM

A variety of treatment procedures are used to correct or control the symptoms of disorders of the immune system.

## Immunotherapy

**Immunotherapy** (ih-**myou**-noh-**THER**-ah-pee), also called *biological therapy*, is a disease treatment that involves either stimulating or repressing the immune response (**immun/o** means immune, and **-therapy** means treatment).

- In the treatment of cancers, immunotherapy is used to stimulate the immune response to fight the malignancy. *Stimulate* means to cause greater activity.

- In the treatment of allergies, immunotherapy is used to repress the body's sensitivity to a particular allergen. *Repress* means to decrease or stop a normal response. This treatment is also known as *allergy desensitization*.

## Antibody Therapy

- **Synthetic immunoglobulins**, also known as *immune serum*, are used as a postexposure preventive measure against certain viruses, including rabies and some types of hepatitis. *Postexposure* means that the patient has been exposed to the virus, for example, by being bitten by an animal with rabies. The goal of this treatment is to prevent the disease from developing by providing temporary immunity.

- **Synthetic interferon** is used in the treatment of multiple sclerosis, hepatitis C, and some cancers.

- **Monoclonal antibodies** are any of a class of antibodies produced in the laboratory by identical offspring of a clone of specific cells. These artificially produced antibodies are used to enhance the patient's immune response to certain malignancies, including some non-Hodgkin's lymphoma, melanoma, breast cancer, and colon cancer. *Monoclonal* means pertains to a single clone of cells. As used here, a *clone* is an exact replica of a group of bacteria.

## Immunosuppression

**Immunosuppression** (im-you-noh-sup-**PRESH**-un) is treatment to repress or interfere with the ability of the immune system to respond to stimulation by antigens.

- An **immunosuppressant** (im-you-noh-soo-**PRES**-ant) is a substance that prevents or reduces the body's normal immune response. This medication is administered to prevent the rejection of donor tissue and to depress autoimmune disorders.

- A **corticosteroid drug** (kor-tih-koh-**STEHR**-oid) is a hormone-like preparation administered primarily as an anti-inflammatory and as an immunosuppressant. The natural production of corticosteroids by the endocrine system is discussed in Chapter 13.

- A **cytotoxic drug** (sigh-toh-**TOK**-sick) is a medication that kills or damages cells (**cyt/o** means cell, **tox** means poison, and **-ic** means pertaining to). These drugs are used as

immunosuppressants or as antineoplastics. *Antineoplastics* are discussed under "Chemotherapy" later in this chapter.

## PATHOGENIC ORGANISMS

A **pathogen** (**PATH**-oh-jen) is a microorganism that causes a disease in humans. A *microorganism* is a living organism that is so small it can be seen only with the aid of a microscope. *Pathogenic* means capable of producing disease (Figure 6.10).

### Bacteria

**Bacteria** (back-**TEER**-ree-ah) are one-celled microscopic organisms (singular, *bacterium*). Most bacteria are not harmful to humans. The following bacteria are pathogenic:

- **Bacilli** (bah-**SILL**-eye) are rod-shaped spore-forming bacteria (**bacilli** means rod shaped). (The singular is *bacillus*.)

- **Anthrax** (**AN**-thraks) is a contagious disease that can be transmitted through livestock infected with *bacillus anthracis*. Spores grown in laboratories have been used in biological warfare.

- A **rickettsia** (rih-**KET**-see-ah) is a small bacterium that lives in lice, fleas, ticks, and mites (plural, *rickettsiae*). *Rocky Mountain spotted fever* is caused by a rickettsia that is transmitted to humans by the bite of an infected tick.

- **Spirochetes** (**SPY**-roh-keets) are long, slender spiral-shaped bacteria that have flexible walls and are capable of movement.

- **Lyme disease** (**LIME**) is caused by a spirochete belonging to the genus *Borrelia*. Lyme disease, which can affect the joints, heart, and central nervous system, is transmitted by the bite of an infected deer tick. Syphilis is also caused by spirochetes (see Chapter 14).

- **Staphylococci** (staf-ih-loh-**KOCK**-sigh) are a group of about 30 species of bacteria that form irregular groups or clusters resembling grapes (**staphyl/o** means clusters or bunches of grapes, and **-cocci** means spherical bacteria). (The singular is *staphylococcus*.) Most staphylococci are harmless and reside normally on the skin and mucous membranes of humans and other organisms; however, others are capable of producing very serious infections.

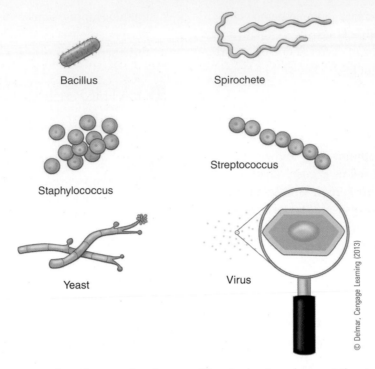

**FIGURE 6.10** Shown here are examples of types of pathogens. The single virus shown at the right is magnified to illustrate details of its structure.

- **Staphylococcus aureus** (**staf**-ih-loh-**KOCK**-us OR-ee-us), also known as *staph aureus*, is a form of staphylococci that often infects wounds and causes serious problems such as toxic shock syndrome or food poisoning.

- **Streptococci** (**strep**-toh-**KOCK**-sigh) are bacteria that form a chain (**strept/o** means twisted chain, and -**cocci** means spherical bacteria). (The singular is *streptococcus.*) Many streptococcal species are harmless; however, other members of this group are responsible for serious illnesses such as strep throat, meningitis (see Chapter 10), endocarditis (see Chapter 5), and necrotizing fasciitis (see Chapter 12).

## Septic Shock

**Septic shock** is a serious condition that occurs when an overwhelming bacterial infection affects the body. Toxins that are released by pathogens can produce direct tissue damage, resulting in low blood pressure.

This damage causes vital organs (the brain, heart, kidneys, and liver) not to function properly or to fail completely. Septic shock occurs most frequently in the very old and the very young. It also occurs in those with underlying or debilitating illnesses.

## Antibiotic-Resistant Bacteria

**Antibiotic-resistant bacteria** occur when antibiotics fail to kill all of the bacteria they target. When this occurs, the surviving bacteria become resistant to this particular drug. As more and more bacteria become resistant to first-line antibiotics, the consequences are severe because the illness lasts longer, and the risks of complications and death increase.

Originally these infections were nosocomial (hospital acquired), but now these antibiotic-resistant bacteria are increasingly common in the general population.

**Methicillin-resistant** *Staphylococcus aureus*, commonly known as *MRSA*, is one of several types of bacteria that are now resistant to most antibiotics.

- The first symptom of MRSA looks like small, red bumps with a black top. These bumps soon become abscesses that require immediate care.

- MRSA infections are serious, difficult to treat, can be fatal, and often occur repeatedly as breaks in the skin allow the bacteria entry. These infections are becoming increasingly present in the general population.

## Fungus and Yeast Infections

A **fungus** (**FUNG**-gus) is a simple parasitic organism (plural, *fungi*). Some of these fungi are harmless to humans; others are pathogenic. **Tinea pedis**, commonly known as *athlete's foot*, is a fungal infection that develops between the toes (see Chapter 12).

Yeast is a type of fungus. An example is **candidiasis** (**kan**-dih-**DYE**-ah-sis), is also known as a *yeast infection*. These infections occur on the skin or mucous membranes in warm, moist areas such as the vagina or mouth and are caused by the pathogenic yeast *Candida albicans*. *Oral thrush* is a yeast infection that occurs in the mouth, whereas *vaginal candidiasis* occurs in the vagina (see Chapter 14).

## Parasites

A **parasite** (**PAR**-ah-sight) is a plant or animal that lives on or within another living organism at the expense of that organism.

- **Malaria** (mah-**LAY**-ree-ah) is caused by a parasite that lives in certain mosquitoes and is transferred to humans by the bite of an infected mosquito. Symptoms develop from 7 days to 4 weeks after being infected and include fever, shaking chills, headache, muscle aches, and tiredness.

- **Toxoplasmosis** (**tock**-soh-plaz-**MOH**-sis) is another example of a parasite that is most commonly transmitted from pets to humans by contact with contaminated animal feces. A pregnant woman should avoid such contact because it can transmit diseases in the developing child such as *microcephalus* (an abnormally small head and underdeveloped brain) or *hydrocephalus* (excess cerebrospinal fluid accumulates in the ventricles of the brain).

- **West Nile virus** is also spread to humans by the bite of an infected mosquito. A mild form of this condition has flu-like symptoms. A more severe variety spreads to the spinal cord and brain. West Nile virus is a member of the *Flavivirus* genus, which also includes the viruses that cause dengue fever.

- **Lyme disease** is transmitted to humans by the bite of an infected blacklegged tick. The tick becomes infected by having bitten a deer infected with the bacterium *Borrelia burgdorferi*. The symptoms of Lyme disease include fever, headache, fatigue, and a characteristic skin rash known as *erythema migrans*. If untreated, Lyme disease can spread to the joints, heart, and nervous system.

## Viral Infections

**Viruses** (**VYE**-rus-ez) are very small infectious agents that live only by invading other cells. After invading the cell, the virus reproduces and then breaks the wall of the infected cell to release the newly formed viruses. These viruses spread to other cells and repeat the process.

- **Influenza** (**in**-floo-**EN**-zah), commonly known as the *flu*, is a highly contagious viral respiratory infection that usually occurs in seasonal epidemics. Flu symptoms include fever, sore throat, muscle aches, cough, runny nose, and fatigue. Complications can include pneumonia. A vaccine is available annually to protect against the most common strains of influenza.

- **Measles** are an acute, highly contagious infection that is transmitted by respiratory droplets of the *rubeola virus*. Symptoms include a red, itchy rash over the entire body, a high fever, runny nose, and coughing. Serious complications of measles can include *photophobia*, which is a serious sensitivity to light.

- **Mumps** is an acute viral infection that is characterized by the swelling of the parotid glands, which are the salivary glands located just in front of the ears. In adults, mumps can also cause painful swelling of the ovaries or testicles.

- **Rubella** (roo-**BELL**-ah), also known as *German measles* or *3-day measles*, is a viral infection characterized by a low-grade fever, swollen glands, inflamed eyes, and a fine, pink rash. Although not usually severe or long lasting, rubella is serious in a woman during early pregnancy because it can cause defects in a developing fetus.

- The **measles, mumps, and rubella vaccination** (MMR) immunization can prevent these three viral conditions and should be administered in early childhood.

- **Rabies** (**RAY**-beez) is an acute viral infection that is transmitted to humans through the bite or saliva of an infected animal. An infected animal is said to be *rabid*. If risk is suspected, it is necessary to undergo testing immediately so that postexposure treatment can be started as quickly as possible. Without testing and treatment, the signs and symptoms of rabies usually occur 30 to 90 days after the bite, and once symptoms have developed, rabies is almost always fatal.

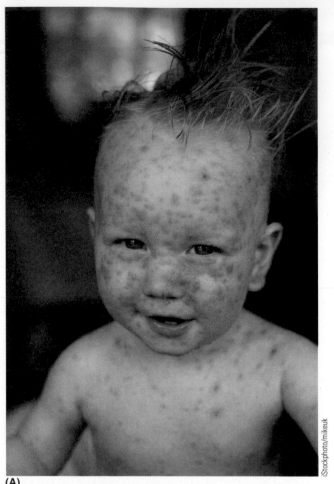

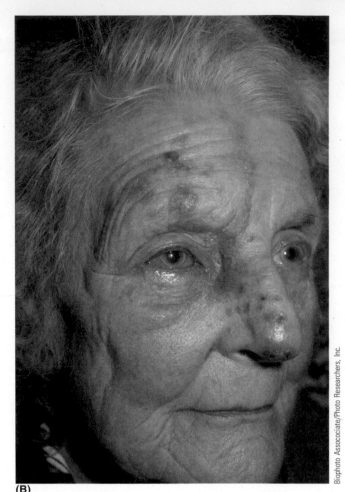

**(A)**

**(B)**

**FIGURE 6.11** Varicella, or chickenpox (A), is caused by the varicella zoster virus, which can remain dormant until later in life when it erupts as herpes zoster, or shingles (B).

## Herpesviruses

The group of herpesviruses, which includes *varicella zoster*, *Epstein-Barr*, *cytomegalovirus*, and *herpes simplex*, causes a variety of diseases in humans.

- **Cytomegalovirus** (**sigh**-toh-**meg**-ah-loh-**VYE**-rus) (CMV) is found in most body fluids (**cyt/o** means cell, **megal/o** means large, **vir** means virus, and **-us** is a singular noun ending). It is most often present as a *silent infection* in which the individual has no signs or symptoms of the infection, although it can potentially cause a serious illness when the individual has a weakened immune system, or when it is transmitted from the mother to her unborn child. This transmission can cause serious congenital disabilities to the child.

- **Varicella** (var-ih-**SEL**-ah), also known as *chickenpox*, is caused by the herpes virus *Varicella zoster* and is highly contagious. This condition is characterized by a fever and a rash consisting of hundreds of itchy, fluid-filled blisters that burst and form crusts.

- **Herpes zoster** (**HER**-peez **ZOS**-ter), which is also known as *shingles*, is an acute viral infection characterized by painful skin eruptions that follow the underlying route of an inflamed nerve. This inflammation occurs when the dormant varicella (chickenpox) virus is reactivated later in life. A vaccine is available to prevent shingles; however, this treatment can be effective only if it is administered promptly.

■ **Infectious mononucleosis** (**mon**-oh-**new**-klee-**OH**-sis), also known as *mono*, is caused by the Epstein-Barr virus (EBV). This condition is characterized by fever, a sore throat, and enlarged lymph nodes. Swelling of the spleen or liver involvement can also develop.

## Medications to Control Infections

■ **Antibiotics** are medications capable of inhibiting growth or killing pathogenic bacterial microorganisms (**anti-** means against, **bio** means life, and **-tic** means pertaining to). *Inhibit* means to slow the growth or development. Antibiotics are effective against most bacterial infections; however, they are not effective against viral infections.

■ A **bactericide** (back-**TEER**-ih-sighd) is a substance that causes the death of bacteria (**bacteri** means bacteria, and **-cide** means causing death). This group of antibiotics includes penicillins and cephalosporins.

■ A *bacteriostatic* agent slows or stops the growth of bacteria (**bacteri** means bacteria, and **-static** means causing control). This group of antibiotics includes tetracycline, sulfonamide, and erythromycin.

■ An **antifungal** (**an**-tih-**FUNG**-gul) is an agent that destroys or inhibits the growth of fungi (**anti-** means against, **fung** means fungus, and **-al** means pertaining to). Lotrimin is an example of a topical antifungal that is applied to treat or prevent athlete's foot. This type of medication is also known as an *antimycotic*.

■ An **antiviral drug** (**an**-tih-**VYE**-ral), such as acyclovir, is used to treat viral infections or to provide temporary immunity (**anti-** means against, **vir** means virus, and **-al** means pertaining to).

## ■ ONCOLOGY

**Oncology** (ong-**KOL**-oh-jee) is the study of the prevention, causes, and treatment of tumors and cancer (**onc** means tumor, and **-ology** means study of). Most cancers are named for the part of the body where the cancer originated. Cancer can attack all body systems and is the second leading cause of death in the United States after heart conditions.

## Tumors

A **tumor**, which is also known as a **neoplasm** (**neo-** means new or strange, and **-plasm** means formation), is an abnormal growth of body tissue. Within this mass, the multiplication of cells is uncontrolled, abnormal, rapid, and progressive.

A *benign tumor* is not a form of cancer, and it is not life-threatening. For example, a **myoma** (my-**OH**-mah) is a benign tumor made up of muscle tissue (**my** means muscle, and **-oma** means tumor). Although this type of tumor is not life threatening, it can cause damage as the tumor grows and places pressure on adjacent structures.

A *malignant tumor* is a form of cancer. It is capable of spreading to distant body sites, including to other body systems, and it is potentially life threatening. For example, a **myosarcoma** (my-oh-sahr-**KOH**-mah) is a malignant tumor derived from muscle tissue (**my/o** means muscle, **sarc** means flesh, and **-oma** means tumor).

■ **Angiogenesis** (an-jee-oh-**JEN**-eh-sis) is the process through which a tumor supports its growth by creating its own blood supply (**angi/o** means vessel, and **-genesis** means reproduction). Angiogenesis is the opposite of *antiangiogenesis*.

■ **Antiangiogenesis** (an-tih-an-jee-oh-**JEN**-eh-sis) is a form of treatment that disrupts the blood supply to the tumor (**anti-** means against, **angi/o** means vessel, and **-genesis** means reproduction). Antiangiogenesis is the opposite of *angiogenesis*.

## Cancer

**Cancer** is a class of diseases characterized by the uncontrolled division of cells and the ability of these cells to invade other tissues, either by invasion through direct growth into adjacent tissue or by spreading into distant sites by metastasizing.

■ To **metastasize** (meh-**TAS**-tah-sighz) is the process by which cancer spreads from one place to another. The cancer moves from the primary site and metastasizes (spreads) to a secondary site.

■ A **metastasis** (meh-**TAS**-tah-sis) is the new cancer site that results from the spreading process (**meta-** means beyond, and **-stasis** means stopping). The metastasis can be in the same body system or within another body system at a distance from the primary site (plural, *metastases*).

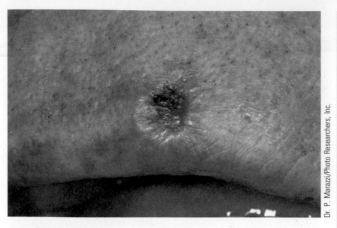

Dr. P. Marazzi/Photo Researchers, Inc.

**FIGURE 6.12** Basal cell carcinoma of the lip. This type of malignant tumor occurs in the basal cell layer of the epidermis.

## Carcinomas

A **carcinoma** (**kar**-sih-**NOH**-mah) is a malignant tumor that occurs in epithelial tissue (**carcin** means cancer, and **-oma** means tumor) (Figure 6.12). Epithelial tissue forms the protective covering for all of the internal and external surfaces of the body.

■ Carcinomas tend to infiltrate and produce metastases (new cancer sites) that can affect any organ or part of the body. (*Infiltrate* means to gain access to.)

■ A **carcinoma in situ** (**kar**-sih-**NOH**-mah in **SIGH**-too) is a malignant tumor in its original position that has not yet disturbed or invaded the surrounding tissues. *In situ* means in the place where the cancer first occurred.

■ For example, an **adenocarcinoma** (**ad**-eh-noh-**kar**-sih-**NOH**-mah) is any one of a large group of carcinomas derived from glandular tissue (**aden/o** means gland, **carcin** means cancer, and **-oma** means tumor).

## Sarcomas

A **sarcoma** (sar-**KOH**-mah) is a malignant tumor that arises from connective tissues, including hard, soft, and liquid connective tissues (**sarc** means flesh, and **-oma** means tumor) (plural, *sarcomas* or *sarcomata*).

■ *Hard-tissue sarcomas* arise from bone or cartilage (see Chapter 3). For example, an **osteosarcoma** (**oss**-tee-oh-sar-**KOH**-mah) is a hard-tissue sarcoma that usually involves the upper shaft of the long bones, pelvis, or knee (**oste/o** means bone, **sarc** means flesh, and **-oma** means tumor).

■ *Soft-tissue sarcomas* are cancers of the muscle, fat, fibrous tissue, blood and lymphatic vessels, or other supporting tissue, including the synovial tissues that line the cavities of joints. For example, a **synovial sarcoma** (sih-**NOH**-vee-al sar-**KOH**-mah) is a tumor of the tissues surrounding a synovial joint such as the knees or elbows.

■ *Liquid-tissue sarcomas* arise from blood and lymph. For example, **leukemia** (loo-**KEE**-mee-ah) is a cancer of the white blood-forming cells in the bone marrow (**leuk/o** means white, and **-emia** means pertaining to blood). See Chapter 5 for more about leukemia.

## Staging Tumors

**Staging** is the process of classifying tumors by how far the disease has progressed, the potential for its responding to therapy, and the patient's prognosis. Specific staging systems are used for different types of cancer (Figure 6.13).

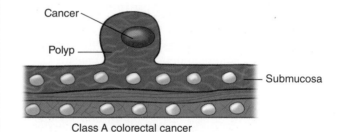

Class A colorectal cancer

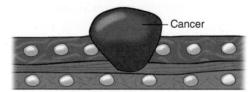

Class B colorectal cancer

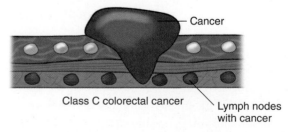

Class C colorectal cancer

© Delmar, Cengage Learning (2013)

**FIGURE 6.13** Stages of colorectal cancer. *Class A:* The cancerous tumor has formed within a polyp inside the colon, but has not yet invaded the surrounding tissue. *Class B:* The cancer has invaded the underlying tissue. *Class C:* The cancer has spread to the underlying tissues and nearby lymph nodes.

## Lymphomas

**Lymphoma** (lim-**FOH**-mah) is a general term applied to malignancies affecting lymphoid tissues (**lymph** means lymph, and **-oma** means tumor). This includes lymph nodes, the spleen, liver, and bone marrow. The two most common types of lymphomas are Hodgkin's lymphoma and non-Hodgkin's lymphoma.

- **Hodgkin's lymphoma** (**HODJ**-kinz lim-**FOH**-mah), also known as *Hodgkin's disease*, is distinguished from other lymphomas by the presence of large, cancerous lymphocytes known as *Reed-Sternberg cells*.

- **Non-Hodgkin's lymphoma** is the term used to describe all other lymphomas *other than* Hodgkin's lymphoma. There are many different types of non-Hodgkin's lymphoma, some aggressive (fast growing) and some indolent (slow growing).

## Breast Cancer

**Breast cancer** is a carcinoma that develops from the cells of the breast and can spread to adjacent lymph nodes and other body sites (Figure 6.14). There are several types of breast cancer named for their location or amount of spreading.

- **Ductal carcinoma in situ** is breast cancer at its earliest stage before the cancer has broken through the wall of the milk duct. At this stage, the cure rate is nearly 100%.

- **Infiltrating ductal carcinoma** (in-**FILL**-trate-ing **DUK**-tal kar-sih-**NOH**-mah), also known as *invasive ductal carcinoma*, starts in the milk duct, breaks through the wall of that duct, and invades the fatty breast tissue. This form of cancer accounts for the majority of all

breast cancers. *Infiltrating* and *invasive* are terms used to describe cancer that has spread beyond the layer of tissue in which it developed and is now growing into surrounding, healthy tissues.

- **Infiltrating lobular carcinoma**, also known as *invasive lobular carcinoma*, is cancer that starts in the milk glands (lobules), breaks through the wall of the gland, and invades the fatty tissue of the breast. Once this cancer reaches the lymph nodes, it can rapidly spread to distant parts of the body.

- **Inflammatory breast cancer** (IBC) is a rare but aggressive form of breast cancer. IBC grows rapidly, and the symptoms include pain, rapid increase in the breast size, redness or a rash on the breast, and swelling of nearby lymph nodes. Most breast cancers are detected by mammography, ultrasound, or self-examination. In contrast, IBC can be detected only by magnetic resonance imaging (MRI).

- *Male breast cancer* can occur in the small amount of breast tissue that is normally present in men. The types of cancers are similar to those occurring in women.

### Stages of Breast Cancer

Breast cancer is described as one of the following stages that depend to the size of the cancer, the lymph node involvement, and the presence of metastases (spreading).

| | |
|---|---|
| Stage 0: | Cancer cells are found only in one location, such as ductal carcinoma in situ. |
| Stage I: | Cancer cells have moved beyond the duct but have not yet reached the lymph nodes. |
| Stage II: | Cancer has increased in size, and/or has reached the axillary (armpit) lymph nodes. |
| Stage III: | Cancer has spread to the cervical (neck) lymph nodes and/or the tissues surrounding the breast, such as the chest wall or skin. |
| Stage IV: | Cancer has spread to other organs, most commonly the brain, lungs, liver, or bones. This is also known as invasive cancer. |

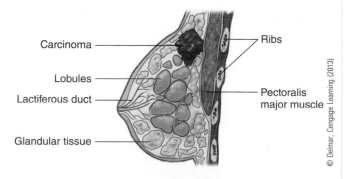

Carcinoma
Lobules
Lactiferous duct
Glandular tissue
Ribs
Pectoralis major muscle

© Delmar, Cengage Learning (2013)

**FIGURE 6.14** Most breast cancers are initially detected as a lump. When this lump is malignant, it is a form of carcinoma.

### Detection of Breast Cancer

Early detection of breast cancer is important and uses the following techniques.

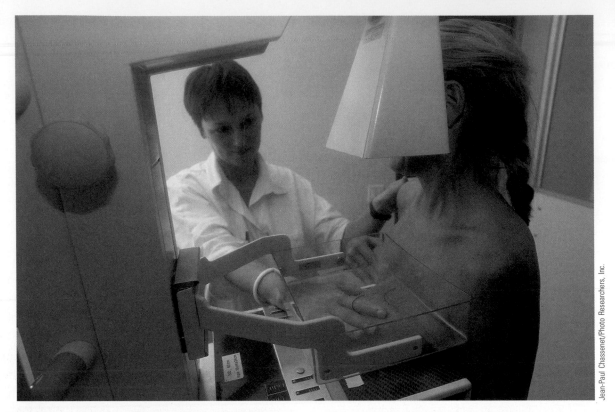

**FIGURE 6.15** In mammography, the breast is gently flattened and radiographed from various angles.

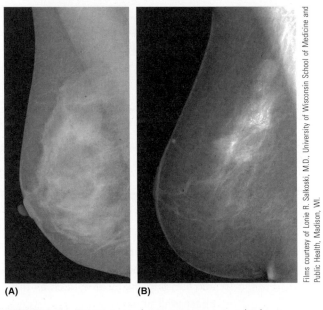

(A)          (B)

**FIGURE 6.16** (A) A normal mammogram in which no abnormal mass is visible. (B) A mammogram in which breast cancer is visible.

■ **Breast self-examination** is a self-care procedure for the early detection of breast cancer. The focus of self-examination is checking for a new lump or for changes in an existing lump, shape of the nipple, or the skin covering the breast.

■ **Professional palpation of the breast** is performed to feel the texture, size, and consistency of the breast. Palpation is explained in Chapter 15.

■ **Mammography** (mam-**OG**-rah-fee) is a radiographic examination of the breasts to detect the presence of tumors or precancerous cells (**mamm/o** means breast, and **-graphy** means the process of producing a picture or record) (Figure 6.15). The resulting record is a *mammogram* (Figure 6.16).

■ **Ultrasound** is used as an initial follow-up test when an abnormality is found by mammography. (Ultrasound is discussed in Chapter 15.)

■ A **needle breast biopsy** is a technique in which an x-ray-guided needle is used to remove small samples of tissue from the breast. It is less painful and disfiguring than a surgical biopsy.

■ A **surgical biopsy** (**BYE**-op-see) is the removal of a small piece of tissue for examination to confirm a diagnosis (**bi-** means pertaining to life, and **-opsy** means view of). After a diagnosis has been established, treatment is then planned based on the stage of the cancer.

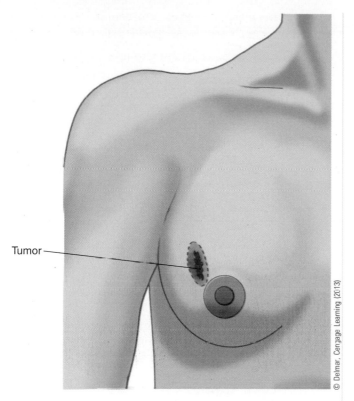

**FIGURE 6.17** A lumpectomy is the removal of the cancerous tissue plus a margin of healthy tissue.

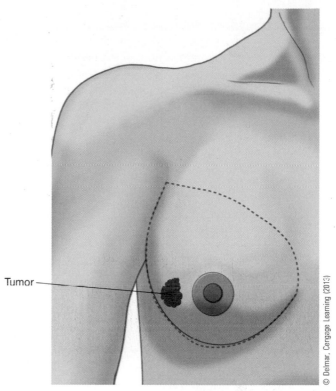

**FIGURE 6.18** A modified radical mastectomy is the removal of the entire breast and the adjacent lymph nodes.

- A *sentinel node biopsy* is a biopsy of the first lymph node to come into contact with cancer cells as they leave the organ of origination and start spreading into the rest of the body. After the sentinel lymph node has been identified, only this and the other affected nodes are removed for biopsy.

- **Lymph node dissection** is a surgical procedure in which all of the lymph nodes in a major group are removed to determine or slow the spread of cancer in this area. For example, an *axillary lymph node dissection (ALND)* is sometimes performed as part of the surgical treatment of the breast.

## Surgical Treatment of Breast Cancer

- A **lumpectomy** is the surgical removal of only the cancerous tissue with the surrounding margin of normal tissue (Figure 6.17). The remainder of the tissue of the affected breast is not removed.

- A **mastectomy** (mas-**TECK**-toh-mee) is the surgical removal of the entire breast and nipple (**mast** means breast, and **-ectomy** means surgical removal). Although simply described as a mastectomy, this procedure often includes the removal of axillary lymph nodes under the adjacent arm.

- A **radical mastectomy** is the surgical removal of an entire breast and many of the surrounding tissues.

- A **modified radical mastectomy** is the surgical removal of the entire breast and all of the axillary lymph nodes under the adjacent arm (Figure 6.18).

## Breast Reconstruction

As an alternative to wearing an external prosthesis, which simulates the shape of the breast within a bra, many women who have undergone a mastectomy elect to have breast reconstruction.

- *Immediate breast reconstruction* begins during the same surgery as the mastectomy when an "expander" is placed to replace the tissue that was removed.

- *Delayed breast reconstruction* may be necessary if the surgery is to be followed by radiation treatment. Several different techniques are used to restore the size and shape of the missing breast.

## ■ CANCER TREATMENTS

The most common forms of treatment for all types of cancer are surgery, chemotherapy, and radiation therapy.

## Surgery

Most commonly, cancer surgery involves removing the malignancy plus a margin of normal surrounding tissue. It may also involve the removal of one or more nearby lymph nodes to detect whether the cancer has started to spread.

Other types of cancer surgery include:

- Laser surgery, which uses targeted beams of light to destroy cancer cells

- Cryosurgery, in which cancerous cells are frozen and destroyed using a substance such as liquid nitrogen

## Chemotherapy

**Chemotherapy** is the use of chemical agents and drugs in combinations selected to destroy malignant cells and tissues.

- **Chemoprevention** (**kee**-moh-pree-**VEN**-shun) is the use of natural or synthetic substances such as drugs or vitamins to reduce the risk of developing cancer, or to reduce the chance that cancer will recur. Chemoprevention may also be used to reduce the size or slow the development of an existing tumor.

- An **antineoplastic** (**an**-tih-nee-oh-**PLAS**-tick) is a medication that blocks the development, growth, or proliferation of malignant cells (**anti-** means against, **ne/o** means new, **plast** means growth or formation, and **-ic** means pertaining to). *Proliferation* means to increase rapidly.

- **Cytotoxic drugs**, which are also used for both immunosuppression and chemotherapy, are discussed earlier in this chapter.

## Radiation Therapy

With the goal of destroying only the cancerous tissues while sparing healthy tissues, **radiation therapy** is used in the treatment of some cancers (Figure 6.19).

- **Brachytherapy** (**brack**-ee-**THER**-ah-pee) is the use of radioactive materials in contact with or implanted into the tissues to be treated (**brachy-** means short, and **-therapy** means treatment).

- **Teletherapy** (**tel**-eh-**THER**-ah-pee) is radiation therapy administered at a distance from the body (**tele-** means distant, and **-therapy** means treatment). With the assistance of three-dimensional computer imaging, it is possible to aim doses more precisely.

## Additional Cancer Treatment Therapies

- **Targeted therapy** is a developing form of anti-cancer drug therapy that uses drugs or other substances to identify and attack specific cancer cells without

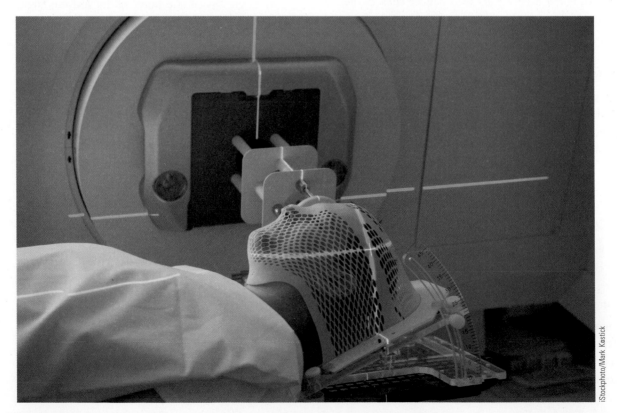

**FIGURE 6.19** Radiation therapy destroys cancerous cells while sparing healthy tissues.

iStockphoto/Mark Kostick

harming normal cells. A monoclonal antibody is a type of targeted therapy.

- After the primary cancer treatments have been completed to decrease the chance that a cancer will recur, sometimes **adjuvant therapy** (**AD**-jeh-vant) is used. The term *adjuvant* refers to an agent intended to increase the effectiveness of a drug; however, adjuvant treatments for cancer can also include chemotherapy, hormone therapy, radiation, immunotherapy, or targeted therapy.

- **Clinical trials** involve testing new and promising cancer treatments that have not yet received Food and Drug Administration (FDA) approval on patients who agree to be part of the research.

## ABBREVIATIONS RELATED TO THE LYMPHATIC AND IMMUNE SYSTEMS

Table 6.3 presents an overview of the abbreviations related to the terms introduced in this chapter. Note: To avoid errors or confusion, always be cautious when using abbreviations.

**StudyWARE    CONNECTION**

For more practice and to test your mastery of this material, go to the StudyWARE™ to play interactive games and complete the quiz for this chapter.

☐ **Workbook Practice**

Go to your workbook and complete the exercises for this chapter.

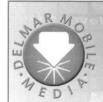

*Downloadable audio is available for selected medical terms in this chapter to enhance your learning of medical terminology.*

### TABLE 6.3
### Abbreviations Related to the Lymphatic and Immune Systems

| | |
|---|---|
| antibody = A, Ab | **A, Ab** = antibody |
| antigen = AG, Ag | **AG, Ag** = antigen |
| carcinoma = CA, Ca | **CA, Ca** = carcinoma |
| carcinoma in situ = CIS | **CIS** = carcinoma in situ |
| ductal carcinoma in situ = DCIS | **DCIS** = ductal carcinoma in situ |
| herpes zoster = HZ | **HZ** = herpes zoster |
| Hodgkin's lymphoma = HL | **HL** = Hodgkin's lymphoma |
| immunoglobulin = IG | **IG** = immunoglobulin |
| lymphedema – LE | **LE** = lymphedema |
| measles, mumps, and rubella vaccination = MMR | **MMR** = measles, mumps, and rubella vaccination |
| metastasis = MET | **MET** = metastasis |
| metastasize = met | **met** = metastasize |
| non-Hodgkin's lymphoma = NHL | **NHL** = non-Hodgkin's lymphoma |
| varicella = VSZ | **VSZ** = varicella |

## MATCHING WORD PARTS 1

Write the correct answer in the middle column.

| Definition | Correct Answer | Possible Answers |
|---|---|---|
| 6.1. against | _____ | anti- |
| 6.2. eat, swallow | _____ | lymphaden/o |
| 6.3. lymph node | _____ | lymphangi/o |
| 6.4. lymph vessel | _____ | phag/o |
| 6.5. poison | _____ | tox/o |

## MATCHING WORD PARTS 2

Write the correct answer in the middle column.

| Definition | Correct Answer | Possible Answers |
|---|---|---|
| 6.6. flesh | _____ | immun/o |
| 6.7. formative material of cells | _____ | onc/o |
| 6.8. protection, safe | _____ | -plasm |
| 6.9. spleen | _____ | sarc/o |
| 6.10. tumor | _____ | splen/o |

## MATCHING TYPES OF PATHOGENS

Write the correct answer in the middle column.

| Definition | Correct Answer | Possible Answers |
|---|---|---|
| 6.11. bacteria capable of movement | _____ | parasites |
| 6.12. chain-forming bacteria | _____ | spirochetes |

6.13.   cluster-forming bacteria        _____        staphylococci

6.14.   live only by invading cells        _____        streptococci

6.15.   live within other organisms        _____        viruses

## DEFINITIONS

Select the correct answer, and write it on the line provided.

6.16.   The _____ has/have a hemolytic function.

    appendix             lymph nodes             spleen             tonsils

6.17.   Inflammation of the lymph nodes is known as _____.

    angiogenesis         lymphadenitis         lymphedema         lymphoma

6.18.   The medical term for the condition commonly known as shingles is _____.

    cytomegalovirus         herpes zoster         rubella         varicella

6.19.   Proteins who activate the immune system, fight viruses by slowing or stopping their multiplication, and

    signal other cells to increase their defenses are known as _____.

    T cells         immunoglobulins         interferons         synthetic immunoglobulins

6.20.   The _____ plays specialized roles in both the lymphatic and immune systems.

    bone marrow             liver             spleen             thymus

6.21.   The protective ring of lymphoid tissue around the back of the nose and upper throat is formed by

    the _____.

    lacteals             lymph nodes             tonsils             villi

6.22.   Secondary _____ can be caused by cancer treatments, burns, or injuries.

    lymphadenitis         lymphangioma         lymphadenopathy         lymphedema

6.23.   Fats that cannot be transported by the bloodstream are absorbed by the _____ that

    are located in the villi that line the small intestine.

    lacteals             lymph nodes             B cells             spleen

6.24.   The parasite _____ is most commonly transmitted from pets to humans by contact

    with contaminated animal feces.

    herpes zoster         malaria         rabies         toxoplasmosis

6.25. A/An _____ is a type of leukocyte that surrounds and kills invading cells. This type of cell also removes dead cells and stimulates the action of other immune cells.

B lymphocyte          macrophage          platelet          T lymphocyte

## MATCHING STRUCTURES

Write the correct answer in the middle column.

| Definition | Correct Answer | Possible Answers |
| --- | --- | --- |
| 6.26. filter harmful substances from lymph | _____ | complement system cells |
| 6.27. lymphoid tissue hanging from the lower portion of the cecum | _____ | intact skin |
| 6.28. combine with antibodies to dissolve foreign cells | _____ | lymph nodes |
| 6.29. stores extra erythrocytes | _____ | spleen |
| 6.30. wraps the body in a physical barrier | _____ | vermiform appendix |

## WHICH WORD?

Select the correct answer, and write it on the line provided.

6.31. The _____ act as intracellular signals to begin the immune response.

cytokines          macrophages

6.32. A _____ drug is a medication that kills or damages cells.

corticosteroid          cytotoxic

6.33. The _____ develop from B cells and secrete large bodies of antibodies coded to destroy specific antigens.

Reed-Sternberg cells          plasma cells

6.34. The antibody therapy known as _____ is used to treat multiple sclerosis, hepatitis C, and some cancers.

monoclonal antibodies          synthetic interferon

6.35.   Infectious mononucleosis is caused by a _____.

        spirochete              virus

## SPELLING COUNTS

Find the misspelled word in each sentence. Then write that word, spelled correctly, on the line provided.

6.36.   A sarkoma is a malignant tumor that arises from connective tissue. _____

6.37.   The adanoids, which are also known as the nasopharyngeal tonsils, are located in the

        nasopharynx. _____

6.38.   Lymphiscintigraphy is a diagnostic test that is performed to detect damage or malformations of the lym-

        phatic vessels. _____

6.39.   Antiobiotics are commonly used to combat bacterial infections. _____

6.40.   Varichella is commonly known as chickenpox. _____

## ABBREVIATION IDENTIFICATION

In the space provided, write the words that each abbreviation stands for.

6.41.   **CIS**          _____

6.42.   **DCIS**         _____

6.43.   **LE**           _____

6.44.   **MMR**          _____

6.45.   **Ag**           _____

## TERM SELECTION

Select the correct answer, and write it on the line provided.

6.46.   _____ is the process through which a tumor supports its growth by creating its

        own blood supply.

                metastasis          angiogenesis          neoplasm          malignant tumor

6.47.   An opportunistic infection that is frequently associated with HIV is _____.

            Hodgkin's disease      Kaposi's sarcoma      myasthenia gravis      tinea pedis

6.48.   Malaria is caused by a _____ that is transferred to humans by the bite of an

infected mosquito.

parasite              rickettsiae             spirochete              virus

6.49.   Bacilli, which are rod-shaped, spore-forming bacteria, cause _____.

Lyme disease          measles                 rubella                 anthrax

6.50.   Swelling of the parotid glands is a symptom of _____.

measles               mumps                   shingles                rubella

## SENTENCE COMPLETION

Write the correct term on the line provided.

6.51.   A severe systemic reaction to an allergen causing serious symptoms that develop very quickly is known

as _____.

6.52.   In _____, radioactive materials are implanted into the tissues to be treated.

6.53.   When testing for HIV, a/an _____ test produces more accurate results than the

ELISA test.

6.54.   A/An _____ is a benign tumor formed by an abnormal collection of lymphatic

vessels.

6.55.   After primary cancer treatments have been completed, _____ therapy is used to

decrease the chances that the cancer will recur.

## WORD SURGERY

Divide each term into its component word parts. Write these word parts, in sequence, on the lines provided.
When necessary, use a slash (/) to indicate a combining vowel. (You may not need all of the lines provided.)

6.56.   An **antineoplastic** is a medication that blocks the development, growth, or proliferation of malignant

cells.

_____          _____          _____          _____

6.57.   **Metastasis** is the new cancer site that results from the spreading process.

_____          _____          _____          _____

6.58.   **Osteosarcoma** is a hard-tissue sarcoma that usually involves the upper shaft of the long bones, pelvis, or

knee.

_____        _____        _____        _____

6.59.   **Cytomegalovirus** is a member of the *herpesvirus* family that causes a variety of diseases.

_____        _____        _____        _____

6.60.   **Antiangiogenesis** is a form of cancer treatment that disrupts the blood supply to the tumor.

_____        _____        _____        _____

## TRUE/FALSE

If the statement is true, write **True** on the line. If the statement is false, write **False** on the line.

6.61.   _____ Inflammatory breast cancer is the most aggressive and least common form of breast cancer.

6.62.   _____ Lymph carries nutrients and oxygen to the cells.

6.63.   _____ A myosarcoma is a benign tumor derived from muscle tissue.

6.64.   _____ Reed-Sternberg cells are present in Hodgkin's lymphoma.

6.65.   _____ Septic shock is caused by a viral infection.

## CLINICAL CONDITIONS

Write the correct answer on the line provided.

6.66.   Dr. Wei diagnosed her patient as having an enlarged spleen due to damage caused by his injuries. The

medical term for this condition is _____.

6.67.   At the beginning of the treatment of Juanita Phillips' breast cancer, a/an _____

breast biopsy was performed using an x-ray-guided needle.

6.68.   Mr. Grossman described his serious illness as being caused by a "superbug infection." His doctor

describes these bacteria as being _____.

6.69.   Dorothy Peterson was diagnosed with breast cancer. She and her doctor agreed upon treating this surgi-

cally with a/an _____. This is a procedure in which the cancerous tissue with a

margin of normal tissue are removed.

6.70.   Every day since his kidney transplant, Mr. Lanning must take a/an _____ to

prevent rejection of the donor organ.

6.71.  Rosita Sanchez is 2 months pregnant, and she and her doctor are worried because her rash was diagnosed as _____. They are concerned because this condition can produce defects in Rosita's developing child.

6.72.  Tarana Inglis took _____ to relieve the symptoms of her allergies.

6.73.  The _____ virus is spread to humans through the bite of an infected mosquito. The more severe variety spreads to the spinal cord and brain.

6.74.  John Fogelman was diagnosed with having a/an _____. This is a malignant tumor that arises from connective tissues, including hard, soft, and liquid tissues.

6.75.  Jane Doe is infected with HIV. One of her medications is acyclovir, which is a/an _____ drug.

## WHICH IS THE CORRECT MEDICAL TERM?

Select the correct answer, and write it on the line provided.

6.76.  The _____ are specialized lymphocytes that produce antibodies. Each lymphocyte makes a specific antibody that is capable of destroying a specific antigen.

|  B cells | bacilli | immunoglobulins | T cells |
|---|---|---|---|

6.77.  Any of a large group of diseases characterized by a condition in which the immune system produces antibodies against its own tissues is known as a/an _____ disorder.

| autoimmune | allergy | rubella | immunodeficiency |
|---|---|---|---|

6.78.  The _____ lymph nodes are located in the groin.

| axillary | cervical | inguinal | subcutaneous |
|---|---|---|---|

6.79.  A/An _____ is any one of a large group of carcinomas derived from glandular tissue.

| adenocarcinoma | lymphoma | myosarcoma | myoma |
|---|---|---|---|

6.80.  A/An _____ drug is used either as an immunosuppressant or as an antineoplastic.

| corticosteroid | cytotoxic | immunoglobulin | monoclonal |
|---|---|---|---|

## CHALLENGE WORD BUILDING

These terms are *not* found in this chapter; however, they are made up of the following familiar word parts. If you need help in creating the term, refer to your medical dictionary.

| | |
|---|---|
| **adenoid/o** | **-ectomy** |
| **lymphaden/o** | **-itis** |
| **lymphang/o** | **-ology** |
| **immun/o** | **-oma** |
| **splen/o** | **-rrhaphy** |
| **tonsill/o** | |
| **thym/o** | |

6.81.  The study of the immune system is known as _____.

6.82.  Surgical removal of the spleen is a/an _____.

6.83.  Inflammation of the thymus is known as _____.

6.84.  Inflammation of the lymph vessels is known as _____.

6.85.  The term meaning to suture the spleen is _____.

6.86.  The surgical removal of the adenoids is a/an _____.

6.87.  The surgical removal of a lymph node is a/an _____.

6.88.  A tumor originating in the thymus is known as _____.

6.89.  Inflammation of the tonsils is known as _____.

6.90.  Inflammation of the spleen is known as _____.

## LABELING EXERCISES

Identify the numbered items on the accompanying figures on the next page.

6.91.  tonsils and _____

6.92.  Lymphocytes are formed in bone _____

6.93.  large intestine and _____

6.94.  _____

6.95. _____

6.96. _____ lymph nodes

6.97. Right _____ empties into the right subclavian vein.

6.98. _____ duct

6.99. _____ lymph nodes

6.100. _____ lymph nodes

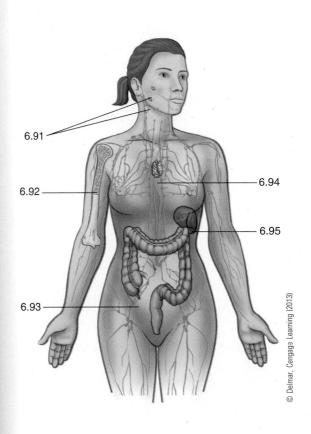

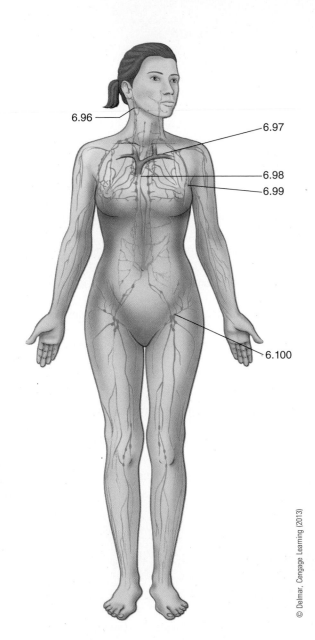

© Delmar, Cengage Learning (2013)

© Delmar, Cengage Learning (2013)

# THE HUMAN TOUCH
## Critical Thinking Exercise

The following story and questions are designed to stimulate critical thinking through class discussion or as a brief essay response. There are no right or wrong answers to these questions.

*Hernani Fermin, a 35-year-old married father, was diagnosed HIV positive 2 years ago. He is a sales representative for a nationally recognized pharmaceutical company, and his hectic travel schedule was beginning to take a toll on his health. A few weeks ago, his doctor suggested he rethink his career goals. "You know, stress and this disease don't mix," Dr. Wettstein reminded him, "Why don't you look for something closer to home?"*

*That evening over lasagna, his wife, Emily, suggested teaching. Hernani had enjoyed sharing the challenging concepts of math and science with seventh graders during the 6 years he had taught in a rural school upstate. It was only the financial demands of Kim and Kili's birth 7 years ago that had tempted him into the better-paying field of pharmaceuticals.*

*Hernani sent out resumes for the next 5 weeks. Finally, one was well received by South Hills Middle School. They had an opening in their math department, plus a need for someone to coach after-school athletics, and they wanted to meet with him. He hadn't interviewed since the twins were born. He thought about the questions normally asked—would there be some questions about his health? Being HIV positive shouldn't have any bearing on his ability to teach, but parents might be concerned about having him coach. And it might disqualify him for the school's health insurance policy. Hernani believed in honesty, but what would happen if he revealed his HIV status?*

## Suggested Discussion Topics

1. Do you think Hernani should reveal his HIV status to South Hills Middle School? If so, why? If not, why not?

2. Do you think South Hills Middle School would hire Hernani for a coaching job if they knew he was HIV positive? Why or why not? Would the possibility of a team or coaching injury, and the bloodborne transmission of HIV, affect their decision?

3. If South Hills Middle School decided that Hernani was not suitable for a coaching job, would they still consider him for the teaching position?

4. How would you feel if your child were in a class Hernani was teaching or on one of the teams he was coaching? Why?

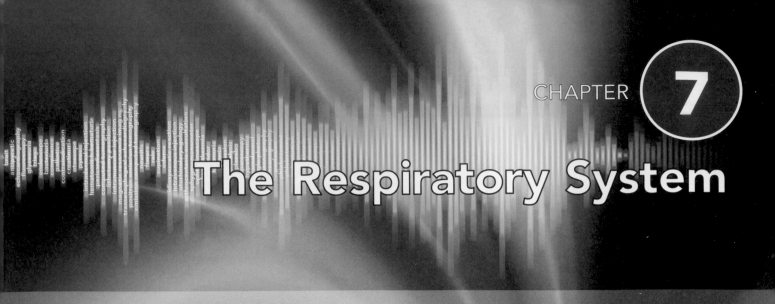

## CHAPTER 7

# The Respiratory System

## Overview of
## STRUCTURES, COMBINING FORMS, AND FUNCTIONS OF THE RESPIRATORY SYSTEM

| Major Structures | Related Combining Forms | Primary Functions |
| --- | --- | --- |
| Nose | **nas/o** | Exchanges air during inhaling and exhaling; warms, moisturizes, and filters inhaled air. |
| Sinuses | **sinus/o** | Produce mucus for the nasal cavities, make bones of the skull lighter, aid in sound production. |
| Pharynx | **pharyng/o** | Transports air back and forth between the nose and the trachea. |
| Larynx | **laryng/o** | Makes speech possible. |
| Epiglottis | **epiglott/o** | Closes off the trachea during swallowing. |
| Trachea | **trache/o** | Transports air back and forth between the pharynx and the bronchi. |
| Bronchi | **bronch/o, bronchi/o** | Transports air from the trachea into the lungs. |
| Alveoli | **alveol/o** | Air sacs that exchange gases with the pulmonary capillary blood. |
| Lungs | **pneum/o, pneumon/o, pulmon/o** | Bring oxygen into the body, and remove carbon dioxide and some water waste from the body. |

## Vocabulary Related to **THE RESPIRATORY SYSTEM**

This list contains essential word parts and medical terms for this chapter. These terms are pronounced in the StudyWARE™ and Audio CDs that are available for use with this text. These and the other important **primary terms** are shown in boldface throughout the chapter. *Secondary terms*, which appear in *orange* italics, clarify the meaning of primary terms.

## Word Parts

- ☐ **bronch/o, bronchi/o** bronchial tube, bronchus
- ☐ **laryng/o** larynx, throat
- ☐ **nas/o** nose
- ☐ **ox/i, ox/o, ox/y** oxygen
- ☐ **pharyng/o** throat, pharynx
- ☐ **phon/o** sound, voice
- ☐ **pleur/o** pleura, side of the body
- ☐ **-pnea** breathing
- ☐ **pneum/o, pneumon/o, pneu-** lung, air
- ☐ **pulm/o, pulmon/o** lung
- ☐ **sinus/o** sinus
- ☐ **somn/o** sleep
- ☐ **spir/o** to breathe
- ☐ **thorac/o, thorax** chest, pleural cavity
- ☐ **trache/o, trachea** windpipe

## Medical Terms

- ☐ **alveoli** (al-**VEE**-oh-lye)
- ☐ **anoxia** (ah-**NOCK**-see-ah)
- ☐ **antitussive** (an-tih-**TUSS**-iv)
- ☐ **aphonia** (ah-**FOH**-nee-ah)
- ☐ **asbestosis** (ass-beh-**STOH**-sis)
- ☐ **asphyxia** (ass-**FICK**-see-ah)
- ☐ **asthma** (**AZ**-mah)
- ☐ **atelectasis** (at-ee-**LEK**-tah-sis)
- ☐ **bradypnea** (brad-ihp-**NEE**-ah)
- ☐ **bronchodilator** (brong-koh-dye-**LAY**-tor)
- ☐ **bronchorrhea** (brong-koh-**REE**-ah)
- ☐ **bronchoscopy** (brong-**KOS**-koh-pee)
- ☐ **bronchospasm** (brong-koh-spazm)
- ☐ **Cheyne-Stokes respiration** (**CHAYN-STOHKS**)
- ☐ **croup** (**KROOP**)
- ☐ **cyanosis** (sigh-ah-**NOH**-sis)
- ☐ **cystic fibrosis** (**SIS**-tick figh-**BROH**-sis)

- ☐ **diphtheria** (dif-**THEE**-ree-ah)
- ☐ **dysphonia** (dis-**FOH**-nee-ah)
- ☐ **dyspnea** (**DISP**-nee-ah)
- ☐ **emphysema** (em-fih-**SEE**-mah)
- ☐ **empyema** (em-pye-**EE**-mah)
- ☐ **endotracheal intubation** (en-doh-**TRAY**-kee-al **in**-too-**BAY**-shun)
- ☐ **epistaxis** (ep-ih-**STACK**-sis)
- ☐ **hemoptysis** (hee-**MOP**-tih-sis)
- ☐ **hemothorax** (hee-moh-**THOH**-racks)
- ☐ **hypercapnia** (high-per-**KAP**-nee-ah)
- ☐ **hyperpnea** (high-perp-**NEE**-ah)
- ☐ **hypopnea** (high-poh-**NEE**-ah)
- ☐ **hypoxemia** (high-pock-**SEE**-mee-ah)
- ☐ **hypoxia** (high-**POCK**-see-ah)
- ☐ **laryngectomy** (lar-in-**JECK**-toh-mee)
- ☐ **laryngitis** (lar-in-**JIGH**-tis)
- ☐ **laryngoscopy** (lar-ing-**GOS**-koh-pee)
- ☐ **laryngospasm** (lah-**RING**-goh-spazm)
- ☐ **mediastinum** (mee-dee-as-**TYE** num)
- ☐ **nebulizer** (**NEB**-you-lye-zer)
- ☐ **otolaryngologist** (oh-toh-lar-in-**GOL**-oh-jist)
- ☐ **pertussis** (per-**TUS**-is)
- ☐ **pharyngitis** (fah-rin-**JIGH**-tis)
- ☐ **phlegm** (**FLEM**)
- ☐ **pleurisy** (**PLOOR**-ih-see)
- ☐ **pleurodynia** (ploor-oh-**DIN**-ee-ah)
- ☐ **pneumoconiosis** (new-moh-koh-nee-**OH**-sis)
- ☐ **pneumonectomy** (new-moh-**NECK**-toh-mee)
- ☐ **pneumonia** (new-**MOH**-nee-ah)
- ☐ **pneumothorax** (new-moh-**THOR**-racks)
- ☐ **polysomnography** (pol-ee-som-**NOG**-rah-fee)
- ☐ **pulmonologist** (pull-mah-**NOL**-oh-jist)
- ☐ **pulse oximeter** (ock-**SIM**-eh-ter)
- ☐ **pyothorax** (pye-oh-**THOH**-racks)
- ☐ **sinusitis** (sigh-nuh-**SIGH**-tis)
- ☐ **sleep apnea** (**AP**-nee-ah)
- ☐ **spirometer** (spih-**ROM**-eh-ter)
- ☐ **tachypnea** (tack-ihp-**NEE**-ah)
- ☐ **thoracentesis** (thoh-rah-sen-**TEE**-sis)
- ☐ **thoracotomy** (thoh-rah-**KOT**-toh-mee)
- ☐ **tracheostomy** (tray-kee-**OS**-toh-mee)
- ☐ **tracheotomy** (tray-kee-**OT**-oh-mee)
- ☐ **tuberculosis** (too-ber-kew-**LOH**-sis)

## LEARNING GOALS

On completion of this chapter, you should be able to:

1. Describe the major functions of the respiratory system.

2. Name and describe the structures of the respiratory system.

3. Recognize, define, spell, and pronounce the primary terms related to the pathology and the diagnostic and treatment procedures of the respiratory system.

## ◼ FUNCTIONS OF THE RESPIRATORY SYSTEM

The functions of the respiratory system are to:

◼ Deliver air to the lungs.

◼ Convey oxygen from the inhaled air to the blood for delivery to the body cells.

◼ Expel the waste products (carbon dioxide and a small amount of water) returned to the lungs by the blood through exhalation.

◼ Produce the airflow through the larynx that makes speech possible.

## ◼ STRUCTURES OF THE RESPIRATORY SYSTEM

The **respiratory system** supplies the blood with oxygen for transportation to the cells in all parts of the body (Figure 7.1). Oxygen is vital to the survival and function of these cells. The respiratory system also removes carbon dioxide and some water waste from the body. For descriptive purposes, the respiratory system is divided into upper and lower respiratory tracts (Figures 7.1 and 7.2).

◼ The **upper respiratory tract** consists of the nose (nostrils), mouth, pharynx, epiglottis, larynx, and trachea. (Figure 7.2)

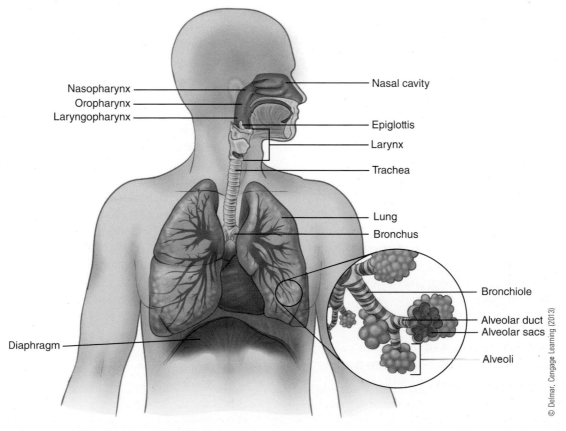

Nasopharynx
Oropharynx
Laryngopharynx
Nasal cavity
Epiglottis
Larynx
Trachea
Lung
Bronchus
Bronchiole
Alveolar duct
Alveolar sacs
Alveoli
Diaphragm

© Delmar, Cengage Learning (2013)

**FIGURE 7.1** Structures of the respiratory system.

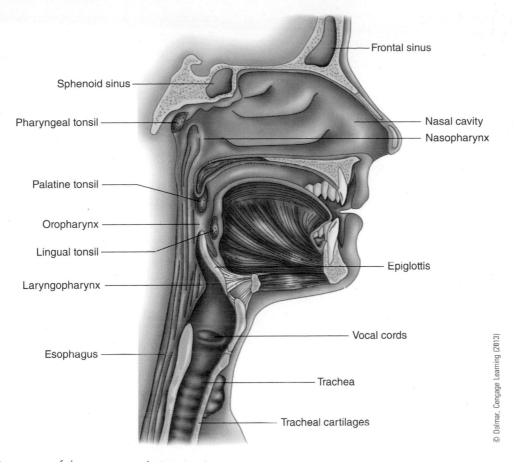

Frontal sinus

Sphenoid sinus

Pharyngeal tonsil

Nasal cavity

Nasopharynx

Palatine tonsil

Oropharynx

Lingual tonsil

Epiglottis

Laryngopharynx

Esophagus

Vocal cords

Trachea

Tracheal cartilages

© Delmar, Cengage Learning (2013)

**FIGURE 7.2** Structures of the upper respiratory tract.

- The **lower respiratory tract** consists of the bronchial tree and lungs. These structures are located within and protected by the **thoracic cavity** (thoh-**RAS**-ick), or **thorax**, also known as the *rib cage*.

- The upper respiratory tract and the bronchial tree of the lower respiratory tract are sometimes referred to as the *airway*.

## The Nose

Air enters the body through the **nose** and passes through the *nasal cavity*, which is the interior portion of the nose.

- The *nostrils* are the external openings of the nose.

- The **nasal septum** (**NAY**-zal **SEP**-tum) is a wall of cartilage that divides the nose into two equal sections. A *septum* is a wall that separates two chambers.

- **Cilia** (**SIL**-ee-ah), the thin hairs located just inside the nostrils, filter incoming air to remove debris. The *nostrils* are the external openings of the nose.

- **Mucous membranes** (**MYOU**-kus) line the nose. These specialized tissues also line the digestive, reproductive, and urinary systems as well as other parts of the respiratory system.

- **Mucus** (**MYOU**-kus) is a slippery secretion produced by the mucous membranes that protects and lubricates these tissues. In the nose, mucus helps moisten, warm, and filter the air as it enters. Notice that mucous and mucus have different spellings; however, they share the same pronunciation. Mucous is the name of the tissue (which comes first, both anatomically and alphabetically); mucus is the secretion that flows from the tissue.

- The **olfactory receptors** (ol-**FACK**-toh-ree) are nerve endings that act as the receptors for the sense of smell. They are also important to the sense of taste. These receptors are located in the mucous membrane in the upper part of the nasal cavity.

## The Tonsils

The **tonsils** and **adenoids** are part of the lymphatic system described in Chapter 6. They help protect the body from infection coming through the nose or the mouth. The tonsils, also called the *palatine tonsils*, are located at the back of the mouth. The adenoids, also called the *nasopharyngeal tonsils*, are higher up, behind the nose and the roof of the mouth.

## The Paranasal Sinuses

The **paranasal sinuses**, which are air-filled cavities lined with mucous membrane, are located in the bones of the skull (**para-** means near, **nas** means nose, and **-al** means pertaining to). A *sinus* can be a sac or cavity in any organ or tissue; however, the term *sinus* most commonly refers to the paranasal sinuses.

The functions of these sinuses are (1) to make the bones of the skull lighter, (2) to help produce sound by giving resonance to the voice, and (3) to produce mucus to provide lubrication for the tissues of the nasal cavity. The sinuses are connected to the nasal cavity via short ducts. The four pairs of paranasal sinuses are located on either side of the nose and are named for the bones in which they are located.

■ The **frontal sinuses** are located in the frontal bone just above the eyebrows. An infection here can cause severe pain in this area.

■ The **sphenoid sinuses**, which are located in the sphenoid bone behind the eye and under the pituitary gland, are close to the optic nerves, and an infection here can damage vision.

■ The **maxillary sinuses**, which are the largest of the paranasal sinuses, are located in the maxillary bones under the eyes. An infection in these sinuses can cause pain in the posterior maxillary teeth.

■ The **ethmoid sinuses**, which are located in the ethmoid bones between the nose and the eyes, are irregularly shaped air cells that are separated from the orbital (eye) cavity by only a thin layer of bone.

## The Pharynx

The **pharynx** (**FAR**-inks), which is commonly known as the *throat*, receives the air after it passes through the nose or mouth, as well as food. (Its role in the digestive system is discussed in Chapter 8.)

The pharynx is made up of three divisions (Figure 7.2):

■ The **nasopharynx** (**nay**-zoh-**FAR**-inks), which is the first division, is posterior to the nasal cavity and continues downward to behind the mouth (**nas/o** means nose, and **-pharynx** means throat). This portion of the pharynx is used only by the respiratory system for the transport of air and opens into the oropharynx.

■ The **oropharynx** (**oh**-roh-**FAR**-inks), which is the second division, is the portion that is visible when looking into the mouth (**or/o** means mouth, and **-pharynx** means throat). The oropharynx is shared by the respiratory and digestive systems and transports air, food, and fluids downward to the laryngopharynx.

■ The **laryngopharynx** (lah-**ring**-goh-**FAR**-inks), which is the third division, is also shared by both the respiratory and digestive systems (**laryng/o** means larynx, and **-pharynx** means throat). Air, food, and fluids continue downward to the openings of the esophagus and trachea where air enters the trachea and food and fluids flow into the esophagus. See the later section "Protective Swallowing Mechanisms."

## Larynx

The **larynx** (**LAR**-inks), also known as the *voice box*, is a triangular chamber located between the pharynx and the trachea (Figure 7.3).

■ The larynx is protected and supported by a series of nine separate cartilages. The *thyroid cartilage* is the largest, and when enlarged it projects from the front of the throat and is commonly known as the *Adam's apple*.

■ The larynx contains the *vocal cords*. During breathing, the cords are separated to let air pass. During speech, they close together, and sound is produced as air is expelled from the lungs, causing the cords to vibrate against each other.

## Protective Swallowing Mechanisms

The respiratory and digestive systems share part of the pharynx. During swallowing, there is the risk of a blocked airway or aspiration pneumonia caused by food or water going into the trachea and entering the lungs, instead of

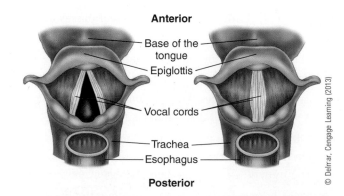

**FIGURE 7.3** View of the larynx and vocal cords from above. Shown on the left, the vocal cords are open during breathing. On the right, the vocal cords vibrate together during speech.

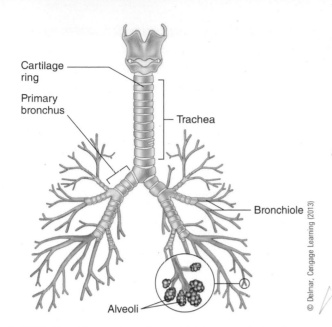

© Delmar, Cengage Learning (2013)

Cartilage ring
Primary bronchus
Trachea
Bronchiole
Alveoli

**FIGURE 7.4** The trachea, bronchial tree, and alveoli.

going into the esophagus. Two protective mechanisms act automatically during swallowing to ensure that *only* air goes into the lungs:

- The soft palate, which is the muscular posterior portion of the roof of the mouth, moves up and backward during swallowing to close off the nasopharynx. This prevents food or liquid from going up into the nose. Structures of the mouth are discussed further in Chapter 8.

- At the same time, the **epiglottis** (**ep**-ih-**GLOT**-is), which is a lid-like structure located at the base of the tongue, swings downward and closes off the laryngopharynx so that food does not enter the trachea and the lungs.

## The Trachea

- The role of the **trachea** (**TRAY**-kee-ah) is to transport air to and from the lungs. This tube, which is commonly known as the *windpipe*, is located directly in front of the esophagus.

- The trachea is held open by a series of flexible C-shaped cartilage rings that make it possible for the trachea to compress so that food can pass down the esophagus (Figure 7.4).

**Study**WARE  **CONNECTION**

Watch the **Respiratory Safeguards** animation in the StudyWARE™.

## The Bronchi

The **bronchi** (**BRONG**-kee) are two large tubes, also known as *primary bronchi*, which branch out from the trachea and convey air into the two lungs (singular, *bronchus*, pronounced **BRONG**-kus). Because of the similarity of these structures to an inverted tree, this is referred to as the *bronchial tree* (Figures 7.1 and 7.4).

- Within the lung, each primary bronchus divides and subdivides into increasingly smaller **bronchioles** (**BRONG**-kee-ohlz), which are the smallest branches of the bronchi.

## The Alveoli

**Alveoli** (al-**VEE**-oh-lye), also known as *air sacs*, are the very small grapelike clusters found at the end of each bronchiole (singular, *alveolus*, pronounced al-**VEE**-oh-lus). The alveoli are where the exchange of oxygen and carbon dioxide takes place. Each lung contains millions of alveoli (Figures 7.1 and 7.4).

- During respiration, the alveoli are filled with air from the bronchioles.

- A network of microscopic pulmonary capillaries surrounds the alveoli. **Pulmonary** (**PULL**-mah-**nair**-ee) means relating to or affecting the lungs.

- The exchange of oxygen and carbon dioxide between the air inside the alveoli and the blood in the pulmonary capillaries occurs through the thin, elastic walls of the alveoli.

- The alveoli produce a detergent-like substance, known as a *surfactant*, which reduces the surface tension of the fluid in the lungs. This makes the alveoli more stable so they do not collapse when an individual exhales. Premature babies often lack adequate surfactant.

## The Lungs

The **lungs**, which are the essential organs of respiration, are divided into lobes (Figure 7.5). A *lobe* is a subdivision or part of an organ.

- The **right lung** is larger and has three lobes: the upper, middle, and lower (or superior, middle, and inferior).

- The **left lung** has only two lobes, the upper and lower, due to space restrictions because the heart is located on that side of the body.

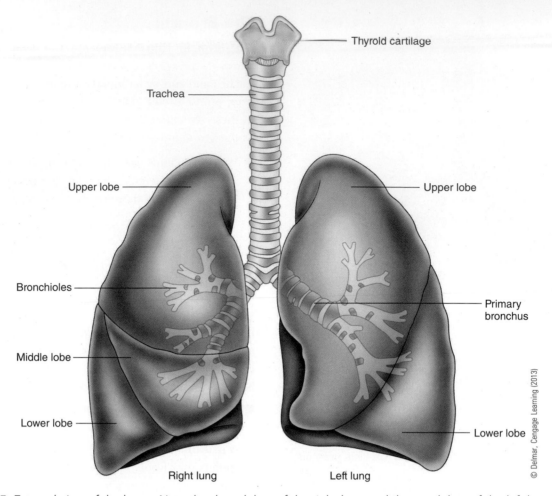

Thyroid cartilage

Trachea

Upper lobe

Upper lobe

Bronchioles

Primary bronchus

Middle lobe

Lower lobe

Lower lobe

Right lung

Left lung

© Delmar, Cengage Learning (2013)

**FIGURE 7.5** External view of the lungs. Note the three lobes of the right lung and the two lobes of the left lung.

## The Mediastinum

The **mediastinum** (**mee**-dee-as-**TYE**-num) is the middle section of the chest cavity and is located between the lungs. This cavity contains connective tissue and organs, including the heart and its veins and arteries, the esophagus, trachea, bronchi, the thymus gland, and lymph nodes (Figure 7.6).

## The Pleura

The **pleura** (**PLOOR**-ah) is a thin, moist, and slippery membrane that covers the outer surface of the lungs and lines the inner surface of the thoracic cavity (Figure 7.6).

■ The **parietal pleura** (pah-**RYE**-eh-tal) is the outer layer of the pleura. It lines the walls of the thoracic cavity, covers the diaphragm, and forms the sac containing each lung. The parietal pleura is attached to the chest wall. *Parietal* means relating to the walls of a cavity.

■ The **visceral pleura** (**VIS**-er-al), which is the inner layer of pleura that covers each lung, is attached directly to the lungs. *Visceral* means relating to the internal organs.

■ The **pleural cavity**, also known as the *pleural space*, is the thin fluid-filled space between the parietal and visceral pleural membranes. The fluid acts as a lubricant, allowing the membranes to slide easily over each other during respiration.

## The Diaphragm

The **diaphragm** (**DYE**-ah-fram), also known as the *thoracic diaphragm*, is a dome-shaped sheet of muscle that separates the thoracic cavity from the abdomen. It is the contraction and relaxation of this muscle that makes breathing possible.

■ The **phrenic nerves** (**FREN**-ick) stimulate the diaphragm and cause it to contract (Figure 7.7).

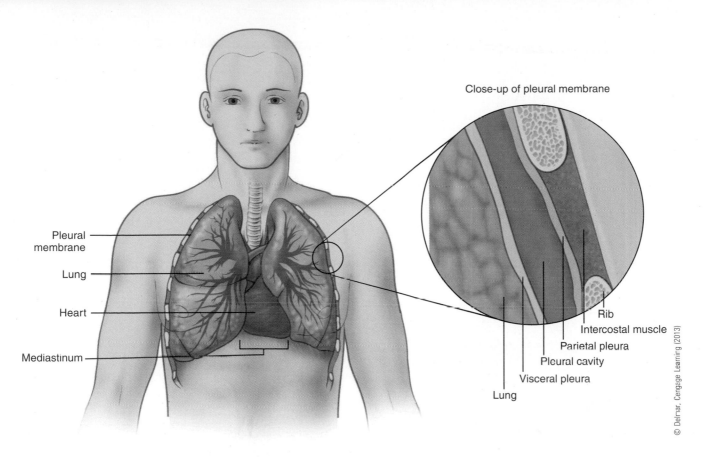

Close-up of pleural membrane

Pleural membrane

Lung

Heart

Mediastinum

Rib
Intercostal muscle
Parietal pleura
Pleural cavity
Visceral pleura
Lung

© Delmar, Cengage Learning (2013)

**FIGURE 7.6** The pleura allows the lungs to move smoothly within the chest.

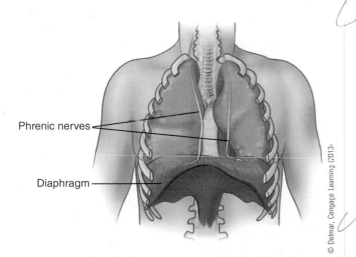

Phrenic nerves

Diaphragm

© Delmar, Cengage Learning (2013)

**FIGURE 7.7** The diaphragm is controlled by the phrenic nerves.

■ Note: the word *diaphragm* refers to a dividing structure, so the term is also used to describe a contraceptive device that separates the vagina from the cervix.

## ■ RESPIRATION

**Respiration**, or breathing, is the exchange of oxygen for carbon dioxide that is essential to life. A single respiration, or *breath*, consists of one inhalation and one exhalation (Figure 7.8). *Ventilation* is another word for moving air in and out of the lungs.

## Inhalation and Exhalation

**Inhalation** (**in**-hah-**LAY**-shun) is the act of taking in air as the diaphragm contracts and pulls downward (Figure 7.8 left). This action causes the thoracic cavity to expand. This produces a vacuum within the thoracic cavity that draws air into the lungs.

**Exhalation** (**ecks**-hah-**LAY**-shun) is the act of breathing out. As the diaphragm relaxes, it moves upward, causing the thoracic cavity to become narrower. This action forces air out of the lungs (Figure 7.8 right).

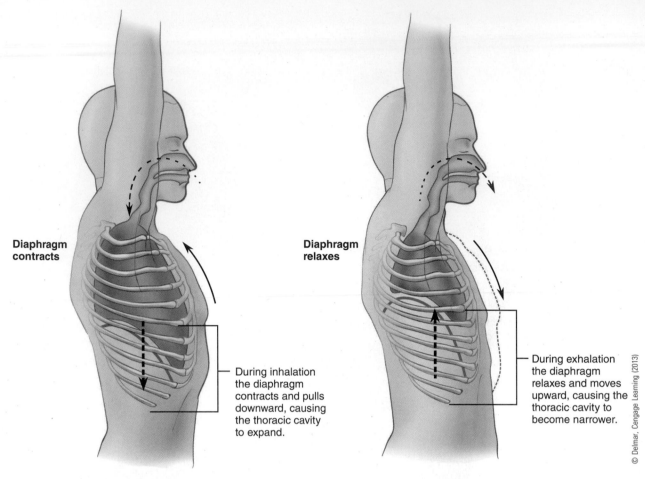

**Diaphragm contracts**

During inhalation the diaphragm contracts and pulls downward, causing the thoracic cavity to expand.

**Diaphragm relaxes**

During exhalation the diaphragm relaxes and moves upward, causing the thoracic cavity to become narrower.

© Delmar, Cengage Learning (2013)

**FIGURE 7.8** Movements of the diaphragm and thoracic cavity produce inhalation (left) and exhalation (right).

## External Respiration

**External respiration** is the act of bringing air in and out of the lungs from the outside environment and in the process, exchanging oxygen for carbon dioxide (Figure 7.9).

■ As air is *inhaled* into the alveoli, oxygen immediately passes into the surrounding capillaries and is carried by the erythrocytes (red blood cells) to all body cells.

■ At the same time, the waste product carbon dioxide that has passed into the bloodstream is transported into the air spaces of the lungs to be *exhaled*.

## Internal Respiration

**Internal respiration**, which is also known as *cellular respiration*, is the exchange of gases within the cells of the blood and tissues (Figure 7.9).

■ In this process, oxygen passes from the bloodstream into the cells.

■ The cells give off the waste product carbon dioxide, and this passes into the bloodstream.

■ The bloodstream transports the carbon dioxide to the lungs, where it is expelled during exhalation.

## ■ MEDICAL SPECIALTIES RELATED TO THE RESPIRATORY SYSTEM

■ An **otolaryngologist** (**oh**-toh-**lar**-in-**GOL**-oh-jist), also known as an **ENT** (ear, nose, throat), is a physician with specialized training in the diagnosis and treatment of diseases and disorders of the head and neck (**ot/o** means ear, **laryng/o** means larynx, and **-ologist** means specialist).

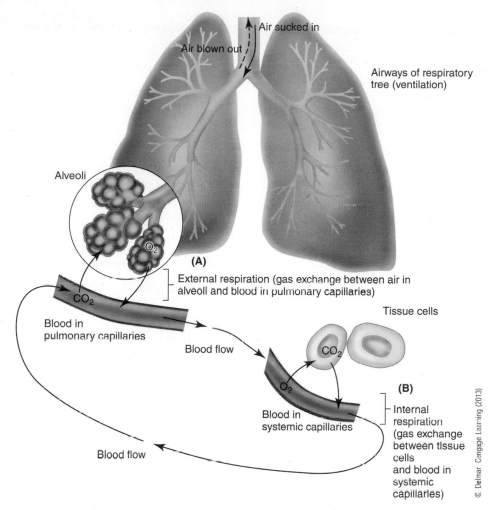

**FIGURE 7.9** External and internal respiration compared. (A) External respiration occurs in the lungs. (B) Internal respiration occurs at the cellular level within the blood and tissues.

- A **pulmonologist** (**pull**-mah-**NOL**-oh-jist) is a physician who specializes in diagnosing and treating diseases and disorders of the respiratory system (**pulmon** means lung, and **-ologist** means specialist).

- A **thoracic surgeon** performs operations on the organs inside the thorax, or chest, including the heart, lungs, and esophagus.

# ◼ PATHOLOGY OF THE RESPIRATORY SYSTEM

## Chronic Obstructive Pulmonary Disease

**Chronic obstructive pulmonary disease** (COPD) is a group of lung diseases in which the bronchial airflow is obstructed, making it hard to breathe. Chronic obstructive pulmonary disease, which is most often caused by long-term smoking, is generally permanent and progressive. Most people with COPD suffer from two related conditions: chronic bronchitis and emphysema.

## Chronic Bronchitis

**Chronic bronchitis** (brong-**KYE**-tis) is a disease in which the airways have become inflamed due to recurrent exposure to an inhaled irritant, usually cigarette smoke (**bronch** means bronchus, and **-itis** means inflammation). An increase in the number and size of mucus-producing cells results in excessive mucus production and a thickening of the walls of the air passages. This causes chronic coughing, difficulty getting air in and out of the lungs, and sometimes also bacterial lung infections.

## *Emphysema*

**Emphysema** (**em**-fih-SEE-mah) is the progressive, long-term loss of lung function, usually due to smoking. Emphysema is characterized by (1) a decrease in the total number of alveoli, (2) the enlargement of the remaining alveoli, and (3) the progressive destruction of the walls of these remaining alveoli.

As the alveoli are destroyed, breathing becomes increasingly rapid, shallow, and difficult. In an effort to compensate for the loss of capacity, the lungs chronically overinflate and the rib cage stays partially expanded all the time, resulting in a slightly rounded shape called a *barrel chest* (Figure 7.10).

## Asthma

**Asthma** (**AZ**-mah) is a chronic inflammatory disease of the bronchial tubes, often triggered by an allergic reaction. Asthma is characterized by episodes of severe breathing difficulty, coughing, and wheezing. These episodes are known as *asthmatic attacks*.

*Wheezing* is a breathing sound caused by a partially obstructed airway. The frequency and severity of asthmatic attacks is influenced by a variety of factors, including allergens, environmental agents, exercise, and infection.

- Figure 7.11A shows the exterior of the airway before an attack. Figure 7.11B shows the factors within and surrounding the airway that cause breathing difficulty during an attack.

- **Airway inflammation** is the swelling and clogging of the bronchial tubes with mucus. This usually occurs after the airway has been exposed to inhaled allergens.

- A **bronchospasm** (**brong**-koh-spazm) is a contraction of the smooth muscle in the walls of the bronchi and bronchioles, tightening and squeezing the airway shut (**bronch/o** means bronchi, and **-spasm** means involuntary contraction).

- *Exercise-induced asthma* is the narrowing of the airways that develops after 5 to 15 minutes of physical exertion. This also can be due to cold weather or allergies.

- A person who suffers from asthma is known as an *asthmatic*.

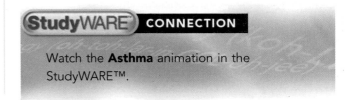

**StudyWARE CONNECTION**

Watch the **Asthma** animation in the StudyWARE™.

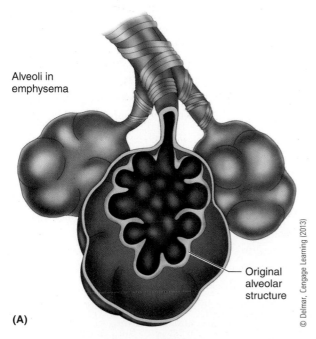

Alveoli in emphysema

Original alveolar structure

**(A)**

© Delmar, Cengage Learning (2013)

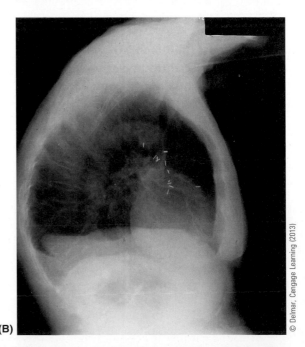

**(B)**

© Delmar, Cengage Learning (2013)

**FIGURE 7.10** Emphysema. (A) Changes in the alveoli as the disease progresses. (B) Lateral x-ray showing lung enlargement and abnormal barrel chest in emphysema. (Note: the short white lines shown in the x-ray are surgical clips.)

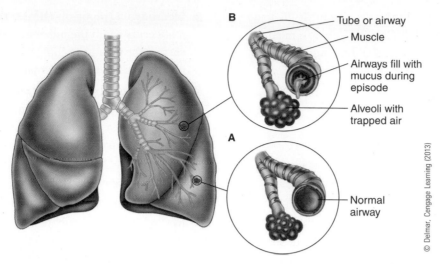

B
— Tube or airway
— Muscle
— Airways fill with mucus during episode
— Alveoli with trapped air

A
— Normal airway

© Delmar, Cengage Learning (2013)

**FIGURE 7.11** Changes in the airways during an asthma episode. (A) Before the episode, the muscles are relaxed and the airways are open. (B) During the episode, the muscles tighten and the airways fill with mucus.

## UPPER RESPIRATORY DISEASES

- **Upper respiratory infections** (URI) and *acute nasopharyngitis* are among the terms used to describe the *common cold*. An upper respiratory infection can be caused by any one of 200 different viruses, the most common of which is the *human rhinovirus*.

- **Allergic rhinitis** (rye-**NIGH**-tis), commonly referred to as an *allergy*, is an allergic reaction to airborne allergens that causes an increased flow of mucus (**rhin** means nose, and **-itis** means inflammation). Allergies are discussed in Chapter 6.

- **Croup** (**KROOP**) is an acute respiratory infection in children and infants characterized by obstruction of the larynx, hoarseness, and swelling around the vocal cords resulting in a barking cough and stridor. *Stridor* is a harsh, high-pitched sound caused by a blockage present when breathing in.

- **Diphtheria** (dif-**THEE**-ree-ah) is an acute bacterial infection of the throat and upper respiratory tract. The diphtheria bacteria produce toxins that can damage the heart muscle and peripheral nerves. Through immunization the disease is now largely prevented.

- **Epistaxis** (**ep**-ih-**STACK**-sis), also known as a *nose-bleed*, is bleeding from the nose that may be caused by dry air, an injury, medication to prevent blood clotting, or high blood pressure.

- **Influenza** (in-flew-**EN**-zah), also known as the *flu*, is an acute, highly contagious viral infection character-ized by respiratory inflammation, fever, chills, and muscle pain. Influenza is spread by respiratory dro-plets and occurs most commonly in epidemics during the colder months. There are many strains of the influenza virus. Some strains can be prevented by annual immunization.

- **Pertussis** (per-**TUS**-is), also known as *whooping cough*, is a contagious bacterial infection of the upper respiratory tract that is characterized by recurrent bouts of a paroxysmal cough, followed by breathless-ness and a noisy inspiration. *Paroxysmal* means sud-den or spasmlike. Childhood immunization against diphtheria, pertussis, and tetanus are given together (DPT); however, the incidence of pertussis is on the rise.

- **Rhinorrhea** (rye-noh-**REE**-ah), also known as a *runny nose*, is the watery flow of mucus from the nose (**rhin/o** means nose, and **-rrhea** means abnormal discharge).

- **Sinusitis** (**sigh**-nuh-**SIGH**-tis) is an inflammation of the sinuses (**sinus** means sinus, and **-itis** means inflammation).

### Pharynx and Larynx

- **Pharyngitis** (fah-rin-**JIGH**-tis), also known as a *sore throat*, is an inflammation of the pharynx (**pharyng** means pharynx, and **-itis** means inflammation). It is often a symptom of a cold, flu, or sinus infection.

- A **laryngospasm** (lah-**RING**-goh-spazm) is the sudden spasmodic closure of the larynx (**laryng/o** means larynx, and **spasm** means a sudden involuntary contraction). It is sometimes associated with gastroesophageal reflux disease (GERD), which is discussed in Chapter 8.

## Voice Disorders

- **Aphonia** (ah-**FOH**-nee-ah) is the loss of the ability of the larynx to produce normal speech sounds (**a-** means without, **phon** means sound or voice, and **-ia** means abnormal condition).

- **Dysphonia** (dis-**FOH**-nee-ah) is difficulty in speaking, which may include any impairment in vocal quality, including hoarseness, weakness, or the cracking of a boy's voice during puberty (**dys-** means bad, **phon** means sound or voice, and **-ia** means abnormal condition).

- **Laryngitis** (lar-in-**JIGH**-tis) is an inflammation of the larynx (**laryng** means larynx, and **-itis** means inflammation). This term is also commonly used to describe voice loss that is caused by this inflammation.

## Trachea and Bronchi

- **Tracheorrhagia** (tray-kee-oh-**RAY**-jee-ah) is bleeding from the mucous membranes of the trachea (**trache/o** means trachea, and **-rrhagia** means bleeding).

- **Bronchiectasis** (brong-kee-**ECK**-tah-sis) is the permanent dilation of the bronchi, caused by chronic infection and inflammation (**bronch/i** means bronchus, and **-ectasis** means stretching or enlargement).

- **Bronchorrhea** (brong-koh-**REE**-ah) is an excessive discharge of mucus from the bronchi (**bronch/o** means bronchus, and **-rrhea** means abnormal flow). This is often caused by chronic bronchitis or asthma.

## Pleural Cavity

- **Pleurisy** (**PLOOR**-ih-see), also known as *pleuritis*, is an inflammation of the pleura, the membranes that cover the lungs and line the pleural cavity. Pleurisy, which causes pleurodynia, may result from trauma, tuberculosis, connective tissue disease, or an infection (**pleur** means pleura, and **-isy** is a noun ending).

- **Pleurodynia** (ploor-oh-**DIN**-ee-ah) is a sharp pain that occurs when the inflamed membranes rub against each other with each inhalation (**pleur/o** means pleura, and **-dynia** means pain).

- **Pleural effusion** (eh-**FEW**-zhun) is the excess accumulation of fluid in the pleural space. This produces a feeling of breathlessness because it prevents the lung from fully expanding. *Effusion* is the escape of fluid from blood or lymphatic vessels into the tissues or into a body cavity (Figure 7.12).

- **Pyothorax** (pye-oh-**THOH**-racks), also known as *empyema of the pleural cavity*, is the presence of pus in the pleural cavity between the layers of the pleural membrane (**py/o** means pus, and **-thorax** means chest).

- **Empyema** (em-pye-**EE**-mah) refers to a collection of pus in a body cavity.

- **Hemothorax** (hee-moh-**THOH**-racks) is a collection of blood in the pleural cavity (**hem/o** means blood, and **-thorax** means chest). This condition often results from chest trauma, such as a stab wound, or it can be caused by disease or surgery.

- A **pneumothorax** (new-moh-**THOR**-racks) is the accumulation of air in the pleural space resulting in a pressure imbalance that causes the lung to fully or partially collapse (**pneum/o** means lung or air, and **-thorax** means chest). This can have an external cause, such as a stab wound through the chest wall, or can occur when there is a lung-disease-related rupture in the pleura that allows air to leak into the pleural space (Figure 7.13).

## Lungs

- **Acute respiratory distress syndrome** (ARDS) is a lung condition usually caused by trauma, pneumonia, smoke or fumes, inhaled vomit, or sepsis. *Sepsis* is a systemic

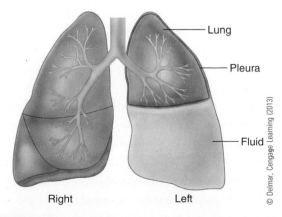

© Delmar, Cengage Learning (2013)

**FIGURE 7.12** In pleural effusion, excess fluid in the pleural cavity prevents the lung from fully expanding.

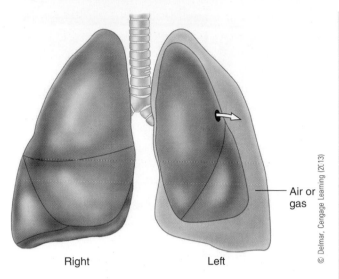

**FIGURE 7.13** Pneumothorax is an accumulation of air or gas in the pleural space that causes the lung to collapse. In the left lung, a perforation in the pleura allowed air to escape into the pleural space.

bacterial infection in the bloodstream. ARDS is a life-threatening condition in which inflammation in the lungs and fluid in the alveoli lead to low levels of oxygen in the blood.

■ **Atelectasis** (**at**-ee-**LEK**-tah-sis), or *collapsed lung*, is the incomplete expansion of part or all of a lung due to a blockage of the air passages or pneumothorax (**atel** means incomplete, and **-ectasis** means stretching or enlargement).

■ **Pulmonary edema** (eh-**DEE**-mah) is an accumulation of fluid in lung tissues, especially the alveoli. *Edema* means swelling. Pulmonary edema is often a symptom of heart failure and is discussed in Chapter 5.

■ **Pulmonary embolism** (**EM**-boh-lizm) is the sudden blockage of a pulmonary artery by foreign matter or by an embolus that has formed in the leg or pelvic region.

■ **Pneumorrhagia** (**new**-moh-**RAY**-jee-ah) is bleeding from the lungs (**pneum/o** means lungs, and **-rrhagia** means bleeding).

## Tuberculosis

**Tuberculosis** (too-**ber**-kew-**LOH**-sis) (TB), which is an infectious disease caused by *Mycobacterium tuberculosis*, usually attacks the lungs; however, it can also affect other parts of the body. Pleurisy and coughing up blood (hemoptysis) can be symptoms of TB in the lungs.

■ TB occurs most commonly in individuals whose immune systems are weakened by another condition such as AIDS. A healthy individual can carry latent TB

without showing symptoms of the disease. *Latent* means present but not active.

■ *Multidrug-resistant tuberculosis* is a dangerous form of tuberculosis because the germs have become resistant to the effect of the primary TB drugs.

## Pneumonia Named for the Affected Lung Tissue

**Pneumonia** (new-**MOH**-nee-ah) is a serious inflammation of the lungs in which the alveoli and air passages fill with pus and other fluids (**pneumon** means lung, and **-ia** means abnormal condition). Pneumonia is most commonly caused by an infection and often follows a cold, flu, chronic illness, or other condition that weakens the immune system and its ability to stave off infection.

There are two types of bacterial pneumonia named for the parts of the lungs affected (Figure 7.14). These are:

■ **Bronchopneumonia** (**brong**-koh-new-**MOH**-nee-ah) is a localized form of pneumonia that often affects the bronchioles (**bronch/o** means bronchial tubes, **pneumon** means lung, and **-ia** means abnormal condition). Bronchopneumonia often leads to lobar pneumonia.

■ **Lobar pneumonia** affects larger areas of the lungs, often including one or more sections, or lobes, of a lung. *Double pneumonia* is lobar pneumonia involving both lungs and is usually a form of bacterial pneumonia.

## Pneumonia Named for the Causative Agent

As many as 30 causes of pneumonia have been identified; however, the most common causative agents are air pollution, bacteria, fungi, viruses, and inhaled liquid or chemicals.

■ **Aspiration pneumonia** (**ass**-pih-**RAY**-shun) can occur when a foreign substance, such as vomit, is inhaled into the lungs. As used here, *aspiration* means inhaling or drawing a foreign substance into the upper respiratory tract.

■ **Bacterial pneumonia** is most commonly caused by *Streptococcus pneumoniae*. *Pneumococcal pneumonia* is the only form of pneumonia that can be prevented through vaccination.

■ **Community-acquired pneumonia** is a type of pneumonia that results from contagious infection outside of a hospital or clinic.

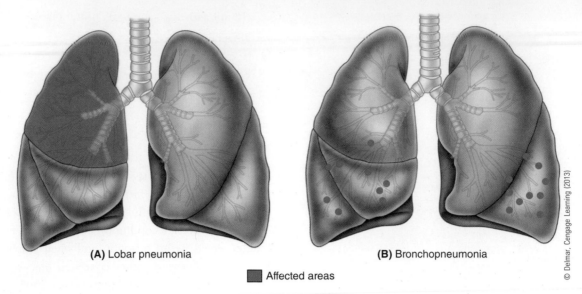

**(A)** Lobar pneumonia        **(B)** Bronchopneumonia

☐ Affected areas

© Delmar, Cengage Learning (2013)

**FIGURE 7.14** Types of pneumonia are usually named for the area of the lung that is involved, or for the causative agent. (A) Lobar pneumonia affects larger areas of the lungs. (B) Bronchopneumonia affects the bronchioles and surrounding alveoli.

- **Hospital-acquired pneumonia**, or *nosocomial pneumonia*, is a type of pneumonia contracted during a stay in the hospital when a patient's defenses are impaired. Patients on a respirator are particularly at risk. *Nosocomial* means hospital-acquired.

- **Walking pneumonia**, also known as *mycoplasma pneumonia*, is a milder but longer-lasting form of the disease caused by the bacteria *Mycoplasma pneumoniae*. It gets its name from the fact that the patient is often not bedridden.

- **Pneumocystis pneumonia** (**new**-moh-**SIS**-tis new-**MOH**-nee-ah) is an opportunistic infection caused by the yeast-like fungus *Pneumocystis carinii*. Opportunistic infections are discussed in Chapter 6.

- **Viral pneumonia**, which can be caused by several different types of viruses, accounts for approximately a third of all pneumonias.

### Interstitial Lung Disease

**Interstitial lung disease** (**in**-ter-**STISH**-al) refers to a group of almost 200 disorders that cause inflammation and scarring of the alveoli and their supporting structures. *Interstitial* means relating to spaces within or around a tissue or an organ. In these lung conditions the tissue around the alveoli becomes scarred or stiff, leading to a reduction of oxygen being transferred to the blood.

- **Pulmonary fibrosis** (figh-**BROH**-sis), or *interstitial fibrosis*, is the progressive formation of scar tissue in the lung, resulting in decreased lung capacity and

increased difficulty in breathing (**fibros** means fibrous connective tissue, and **-is** is the noun ending). *Fibrosis* is a condition in which normal tissue is replaced by fibrotic (hardened) tissue.

Many connective tissue diseases such as rheumatoid arthritis, scleroderma, and lupus can cause pulmonary fibrosis, as can environmental toxins such as asbestos and silica. Pulmonary fibrosis can also occur without a known cause.

### Environmental and Occupational Interstitial Lung Diseases

- **Pneumoconiosis** (**new**-moh-**koh**-nee-**OH**-sis) is any fibrosis of the lung tissues caused by dust in the lungs after prolonged environmental or occupational contact (**pneum/o** means lung, **coni** means dust, and **-osis** means abnormal condition or disease).

- **Anthracosis** (**an**-thrah-**KOH**-sis), also known as *coal miner's pneumoconiosis* or *black lung disease*, is caused by coal dust in the lungs (**anthrac** means coal dust, and **-osis** means abnormal condition or disease).

- **Asbestosis** (**ass**-beh-**STOH**-sis) is caused by asbestos particles in the lungs and usually occurs after working with asbestos (**asbest** means asbestos, and **-osis** means abnormal condition or disease).

- **Silicosis** (**sill**-ih-**KOH**-sis) is caused by inhaling silica dust in the lungs and usually occurs after working in occupations including foundry work, quarrying, ceramics, glasswork, and sandblasting (**silic** means glass, and **-osis** means abnormal condition or disease).

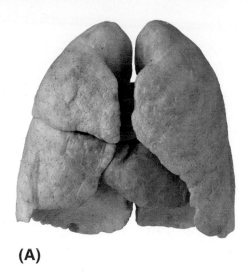 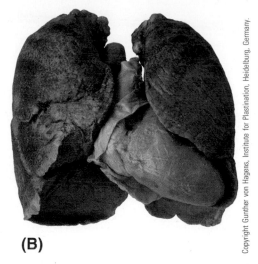

(A)   (B)

**FIGURE 7.15** Photographs of actual lung and heart specimens. (A) Healthy lungs of a nonsmoker. (B) Damaged lungs of a smoker.

## Cystic Fibrosis

**Cystic fibrosis** (**SIS**-tick figh-**BROH**-sis) is a life-threatening genetic disorder in which the lungs and pancreas are clogged with large quantities of abnormally thick mucus. This results in damage to the lungs, poor growth, and nutritional deficiencies. Treatments for cystic fibrosis include:

- *Pancreatic enzymes* to aid the digestive system
- *Antibiotics* to prevent and treat lung infections
- *Bronchodilators* to keep airways open
- *Chest percussion*, which is a therapeutic technique to remove excess mucus from the lungs. This is often performed with the patient positioned at an angle to allow gravity to help drain the secretions. Percussion is described in Chapter 15.

## Lung Cancer

**Lung cancer**, which is the leading cause of cancer death in the United States, is a condition in which cancer cells form in the tissues of the lung. Important risk factors for lung cancer are smoking and inhaling secondhand smoke (Figure 7.15).

## Breathing Disorders

The general term *breathing disorders* describes abnormal changes in the rate or depth of breathing. Specific terms describe in greater detail the changes that are occurring (Figure 7.16).

- **Eupnea** (youp-**NEE**-ah) is easy or normal breathing (**eu-** means good, and **-pnea** means breathing). This is the baseline for judging some breathing disorders (Figure 7.16A). Eupnea is the opposite of *apnea*.
- **Apnea** (**AP**-nee-ah) is the temporary absence of spontaneous respiration (**a-** means without, and **-pnea** means breathing) (Figure 7.16D). It is a common respiratory problem in premature infants. Apnea is the opposite of *eupnea*.
- **Bradypnea** (brad-ihp-**NEE**-ah) is an abnormally slow rate of respiration, usually of less than 10 breaths per minute (**brady-** means slow, and **-pnea** means breathing) (Figure 7.16C). Bradypnea is the opposite of *tachypnea*.
- **Cheyne-Stokes respiration** (**CHAYN-STOHKS**) is an irregular pattern of breathing characterized by alternating rapid or shallow respiration followed by slower respiration or apnea (Figure 7.16E). This pattern sometimes occurs in comatose patients or those nearing death.
- **Tachypnea** (tack-ihp-**NEE**-ah) is an abnormally rapid rate of respiration usually of more than 20 breaths per minute (**tachy-** means rapid, and **-pnea** means breathing) (Figure 7.16B). Tachypnea is the opposite of *bradypnea*.
- **Dyspnea** (**DISP**-nee-ah), also known as *shortness of breath (SOB)*, is difficult or labored breathing (**dys-** means painful, and **-pnea** means breathing). Shortness of breath is frequently one of the first symptoms of heart failure. It can also be caused by strenuous physical exertion or can be due to lung damage that produces dyspnea even at rest.

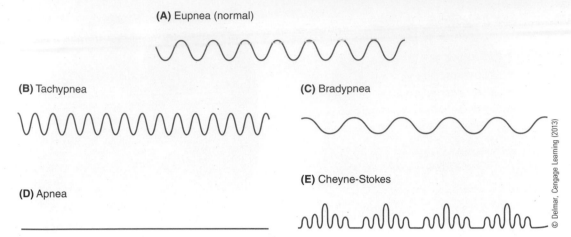

**FIGURE 7.16** Respiratory patterns. (A) Eupnea is normal breathing. (B) Tachypnea is abnormally rapid breathing. (C) Bradypnea is abnormally slow breathing. (D) Apnea is the absence of breathing. (E) Cheyne-Stokes is an alternating series of abnormal patterns.

■ **Hyperpnea** (**high**-perp-**NEE**-ah), which is commonly associated with exertion, is breathing that is deeper and more rapid than is normal at rest (**hyper-** means excessive, and **-pnea** means breathing). Hyperpnea may also occur at high altitude, or be caused by anemia or sepsis. Hyperpnea is the opposite of *hypopnea.*

■ **Hypopnea** (**high**-poh-**NEE**-ah) is shallow or slow respiration (**hypo-** means decreased, and **-pnea** means breathing). Hypopnea is the opposite of *hyperpnea.*

■ **Hyperventilation** (**high**-per-**ven**-tih-**LAY**-shun) is an abnormally rapid rate of deep respiration that is usually associated with anxiety (**hyper-** means excessive, and **-ventilation** means breathing). This decreases the level of carbon dioxide in the blood, causing dizziness and tingling in the fingers and toes.

## Sleep-Related Breathing Disorders

Sleep related breathing disorders are characterized by disruptions of normal breathing patterns that only occur during sleep and are associated with higher risks of cardiovascular disease and strokes.

■ **Sleep apnea** is a potentially serious disorder in which breathing repeatedly stops and starts during sleep for long-enough periods to cause a measurable decrease in blood oxygen levels. *Obstructive sleep apnea* is caused by the muscles at the back of the throat relaxing and narrowing the airways.

■ *Snoring*, which can be a symptom of sleep apnea, is noisy breathing caused by vibration of the soft palate.

## Coughing

■ **Expectoration** (eck-**SPEK**-toh-**rate**) is the act of coughing up and spitting out saliva, mucus, or other body fluid (**expector/o** means to cough up, and **-ation** means state or action).

■ **Hemoptysis** (hee-**MOP**-tih-sis) is the expectoration of blood or blood-stained sputum derived from the lungs or bronchial tubes as the result of a pulmonary or bronchial hemorrhage (**hem/o** means blood, and **-ptysis** means spitting).

## Lack of Oxygen

■ **Airway obstruction**, commonly known as *choking*, occurs when food or a foreign object partially or completely blocks the airway and prevents air from entering or leaving the lungs. This can be a life-threatening emergency requiring immediate action through the performance of the *abdominal thrust maneuver.* This is also known as the *Heimlich maneuver.*

■ **Anoxia** (ah-**NOCK**-see-ah) is the absence of oxygen from the body's tissues and organs even though there is an adequate flow of blood (**an-** means without, **ox** means oxygen, and **-ia** means abnormal condition). If anoxia continues for more than 4 to 6 minutes, irreversible brain damage can occur.

■ **Hypoxia** (high-**POCK**-see-ah) is the condition of having deficient oxygen levels in the body's tissues and organs; however, it is less severe than anoxia (**hyp-** means deficient, **ox** means oxygen, and **-ia** means abnormal condition). This condition can be caused by a variety of factors, including head trauma, carbon monoxide poisoning, suffocation, and high altitudes. Compare with *hypoxemia*.

■ *Altitude hypoxia*, also known as *altitude sickness*, is a condition that can be brought on by the decreased oxygen in the air at higher altitudes, usually above 8,000 feet.

■ **Asphyxia** (ass-**FICK**-see-ah) is the loss of consciousness that occurs when the body cannot get the oxygen it needs to function. Asphyxia can be caused by choking, suffocation, drowning, or inhaling gases such as carbon monoxide.

■ *Asphyxiation* is a state of asphyxia or suffocation. In this life-threatening condition, oxygen levels in the blood drop quickly, carbon dioxide levels rise, and unless the patient's breathing is restored within a few minutes, death or serious brain damage follows.

■ **Cyanosis** (sigh-ah-**NOH**-sis) is a bluish discoloration of the skin and mucous membranes caused by a lack of adequate oxygen in the blood (**cyan** means blue, and **-osis** means abnormal condition or disease).

■ **Hypercapnia** (high-per-**KAP**-nee-ah) is the abnormal buildup of carbon dioxide in the blood (**hyper-** means excessive, **capn** means carbon dioxide, and **-ia** means abnormal condition).

■ **Hypoxemia** (high-pock-**SEE**-mee-ah) is the condition of having low oxygen levels in the blood, usually due to respiratory disorders or heart conditions (**hyp-** means deficient, **ox** means oxygen, and **-emia** means blood). Compare with *hypoxia*.

■ **Respiratory failure** (RF), also known as *respiratory acidosis*, is a condition in which the level of oxygen in the blood becomes dangerously low (hypoxemia) or the level of carbon dioxide becomes dangerously high (hypercapnia). It is a medical emergency that can result from a chronic condition or develop suddenly.

■ **Smoke inhalation** is damage to the lungs in which particles from a fire coat the alveoli and prevent the normal exchange of gases.

## Sudden Infant Death Syndrome

**Sudden infant death syndrome** (SIDS) is the sudden and unexplainable death of an apparently healthy sleeping infant between the ages of 2 months and 6 months. Although the cause of SIDS is still unknown, it is suspected to be a heart problem or interruption in breathing.

The recommendation that infants sleep on their back or side instead of facedown has reduced the incidence of SIDS.

# ■ DIAGNOSTIC PROCEDURES OF THE RESPIRATORY SYSTEM

■ The *respiratory rate*, which is an important vital sign, is discussed in Chapter 15. It is a count of the number of breaths (one inhalation and one exhalation) per minute.

■ *Respiratory sounds* such as *rale*, *rhonchi*, and *stridor* provide information about the condition of the lungs and pleura. These are described in Chapter 15.

■ **Bronchoscopy** (brong-**KOS**-koh pee) is the visual examination of the bronchi using a bronchoscope (**bronch/o** means bronchus, and **-scopy** means direct visual examination). A *bronchoscope* is a flexible, fiber-optic device that is passed through the nose or mouth and down the airways. It can also be used for operative procedures, such as tissue repair or the removal of a foreign object.

■ A **chest x-ray** (CXR), also known as *chest imaging*, is a valuable tool for diagnosing pneumonia, lung cancer, pneumothorax, pleural effusion, tuberculosis, and emphysema (Figure 7.10B).

■ **Laryngoscopy** (lar-ing-**GOS**-koh-pee) is the visual examination of the larynx and vocal cords using a flexible or rigid laryngoscope inserted through the mouth (**laryng/o** means larynx, and **-scopy** means a direct visual examination). *Indirect laryngoscopy* is a simpler version of this test in which the larynx is viewed by shining a light on an angled mirror held at the back of the soft palate.

■ A **peak flow meter** is an inexpensive handheld device used to let patients with asthma measure air flowing out of the lungs, revealing any narrowing of the airways in advance of an asthma attack (Figure 7.17).

■ **Polysomnography** (pol-ee-som-**NOG**-rah-fee), also known as a *sleep study*, measures physiological activity during sleep and is often performed to detect nocturnal defects in breathing associated with sleep apnea (**poly-** means many, **somn/o** means sleep, and **-graphy** means the process of recording).

■ **Pulmonary function tests** (PFTs) are a group of tests that measure volume and flow of air by using a spirometer. These tests are measured against a norm for the individual's age, height, and sex.

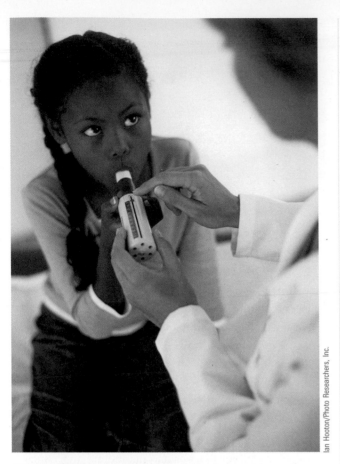

Ian Hooton/Photo Researchers, Inc.

**FIGURE 7.17** A peak flow meter is often used to measure how quickly a patient with asthma can expel air.

- A **spirometer** (spih-**ROM**-eh-ter) is a recording device that measures the amount of air inhaled or exhaled (volume) and the length of time required for each breath (**spir/o** means to breathe, and -**meter** means to measure).

- A **pulse oximeter** (ock-**SIM**-eh-ter) is an external monitor placed on the patient's fingertip or earlobe to measure the oxygen saturation level in the blood (**ox/i** means oxygen, and -**meter** means to measure). This is a noninvasive method of assessing basic respiratory function (Figure 7.18).

- **Phlegm** (**FLEM**) is thick mucus secreted by the tissues lining the respiratory passages.

- **Sputum** (**SPYOU**-tum) is phlegm ejected through the mouth that can be examined for diagnostic purposes. *Sputum cytology* is a procedure in which a sample of mucus is coughed up from the lungs and then examined under a microscope to detect cancer cells.

## Tuberculosis Testing

Two kinds of tests can be used to help detect tuberculosis infection: tuberculin skin testing and blood tests. These tests show whether the patient is infected with TB; however, they do not show whether the infection is latent or active.

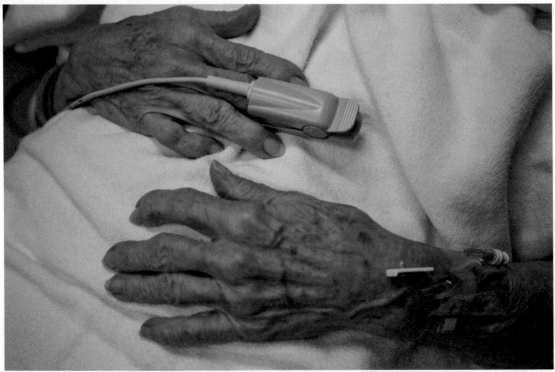

iStockphoto/David Sucsy

**FIGURE 7.18** A pulse oximeter is applied to a finger to provide continuous reassessment of the patient's levels of oxygenation.

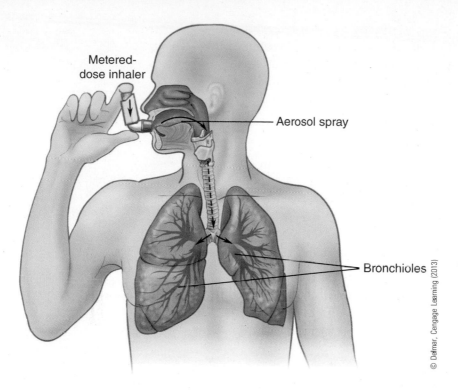

Metered-dose inhaler

Aerosol spray

Bronchioles

© Delmar, Cengage Learning (2013)

**FIGURE 7.19** The metered-dose inhaler delivers medication for inhalation directly into the airways.

■ **Tuberculin skin testing** is a screening test for tuberculosis in which the skin of the arm is injected with a harmless antigen extracted from TB bacteria. The *tuberculin tine test* is performed using an instrument with several small prongs called tines.

■ The **Mantoux PPD skin test** is considered a more accurate skin test for diagnosing tuberculosis. A very small amount of PPD tuberculin (a purified protein derivative) is injected just under the top layer of the skin on the forearm. The site is checked for a reaction 48 to 72 hours later.

A positive result indicates the possibility of exposure to the disease, and this response warrants further testing such as a chest x-ray and sputum cytology.

# ■ TREATMENT PROCEDURES OF THE RESPIRATORY SYSTEM

## Medications and Their Administration

■ An **antitussive** (**an**-tih-**TUSS**-iv), commonly known as *cough medicine*, is administered to prevent or relieve coughing (**anti-** means against, **tuss** means cough, and **-ive** means performs).

■ A **bronchodilator** (**brong**-koh-dye-**LAY**-tor) is a medication that relaxes and expands the bronchial passages into the lungs. Patients with asthma use short-acting bronchodilators as needed as rescue medications, while long-acting bronchodilators are used every day to control the condition.

■ A **metered-dose inhaler** (MDI) administers a specific amount of a medication such as a bronchodilator in aerosol form. A gas propellant mixes with the medicine to push it into the lungs (Figure 7.19).

■ A **nebulizer** (**NEB**-you-lye-zer) is an electronic device that pumps air or oxygen through a liquid medicine to turn it into a mist, which is then inhaled by the patient via a face mask or mouthpiece.

## Asthma Treatment

The goal of asthma treatment is to avoid the substances that trigger symptoms and to control airway inflammation. Most people with asthma take two kinds of medicines.

■ *Controller medicines*, such as inhaled corticosteroids, are long-acting medications taken daily to prevent attacks. These medications help control inflammation and stop the airways from reacting to the factors that trigger the asthma.

■ *Quick-relief*, or *rescue, medicines*, are taken at the first sign of an attack to dilate the airways and make breathing easier. These medications are known as bronchodilators and are discussed under medications. Corticosteroids may also be given intravenously during a severe attack.

## The Nose, Throat, and Larynx

■ **Endotracheal intubation** (**en**-doh-**TRAY**-kee-al **in**-too-**BAY**-shun) (ETT) is the passage of a tube through the mouth into the trachea to establish or maintain an open airway, especially when a patient is on a ventilator (**endo-** means within, **trache** means trachea, and **-al** means pertaining to). *Intubation* is the insertion of a tube, usually for the passage of air or fluids.

■ **Functional endoscopic sinus surgery** (FESS) is a procedure performed using an endoscope in which chronic sinusitis is treated by enlarging the opening between the nose and sinus.

■ A **laryngectomy** (**lar**-in-**JECK**-toh-mee) is the surgical removal of the larynx (**laryng** means larynx, and **-ectomy** means surgical removal).

■ A **laryngotomy** (**lar**-ing-**OT**-oh-mee) is a surgical incision into the larynx, performed when the upper part of the airway is obstructed (**laryng** means larynx, and **-otomy** means surgical incision).

■ **Septoplasty** (**SEP**-toh-**plas**-tee) is the surgical repair or alteration of parts of the nasal septum (**sept/o** means septum, and **-plasty** means surgical repair).

## The Trachea

■ **Tracheostomy** (**tray**-kee-**OS**-toh-mee) is the surgical creation of a stoma into the trachea to insert a temporary or permanent tube to facilitate breathing (**trache** means trachea, and **-ostomy** means surgically creating an opening). The term *tracheostomy* is used to refer to the surgical procedure and to the stoma itself. As used here, a *stoma* means a surgically created opening on a body surface (Figure 7.20).

■ An emergency **tracheotomy** (**tray**-kee-**OT**-oh-mee) is a procedure in which an incision is made into the trachea to gain access to the airway below a blockage (**trache** means trachea, and **-otomy** means surgical incision).

## The Lungs, Pleura, and Thorax

■ A **pneumonectomy** (**new**-moh-**NECK**-toh-mee) is the surgical removal of all or part of a lung (**pneumon** means lung, and **-ectomy** means surgical removal).

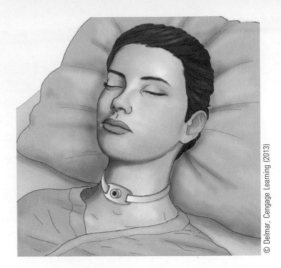

**FIGURE 7.20** A tracheostomy tube creates an open airway for a patient unable to maintain his own airway.

■ A **lobectomy** (loh-**BECK**-toh-mee) is the surgical removal of a lobe of an organ, usually the lung, brain, or liver (**lob** means lobe, and **-ectomy** means surgical removal).

■ **Wedge resection** is a surgery in which a small wedge-shaped piece of cancerous lung tissue is removed, along with a margin of healthy tissue around the cancer.

■ **Thoracentesis** (**thoh**-rah-sen-**TEE**-sis) is the surgical puncture of the chest wall with a needle to obtain fluid from the pleural cavity (**thor/a** means thorax or chest, and **-centesis** means surgical puncture to remove fluid). This procedure is performed to remove liquid (pleural effusion) or air (pneumothorax) from the pleural cavity.

■ A **thoracotomy** (**thoh**-rah-**KOT**-toh-mee) is a surgical incision into the chest walls to open the pleural cavity for biopsy or treatment (**thorac** means chest, and **-otomy** means surgical incision). A thoracotomy is used to gain access to the lungs, heart, esophagus, diaphragm, and other organs.

■ **Video-assisted thoracic surgery** (VATS) is the use of a thoracoscope to view the inside of the pleural cavity through very small incisions. A *thoracoscope* is a specialized endoscope used for treating the thorax. This procedure is used to remove small sections of cancerous tissue and to obtain biopsy specimens to diagnose certain types of pneumonia, infections, or tumors of the chest wall. It is also used to treat repeatedly collapsing lungs.

## Respiratory Therapy

■ **Diaphragmatic breathing**, also known as *abdominal breathing*, is a relaxation technique used to relieve anxiety.

■ A **CPAP machine** (continuous positive airway pressure) is a noninvasive ventilation device used in the treatment of sleep apnea. A face mask is connected to a pump that creates constant air pressure in the nasal passages, holding the airway open. Although this does not cure sleep apnea, it does reduce snoring and prevents dangerous apnea disturbances.

■ A **BiPAP machine** (bilevel positive airway pressure) is like a CPAP machine; however, it can be set at a higher pressure for inhaling and a lower pressure for exhaling. It is used for sleep apnea in patients with neuromuscular diseases or those who find the CPAP machine uncomfortable.

■ An **Ambu bag**, or *bag valve mask*, is an emergency resuscitator used to assist ventilation (Figure 7.21). A flexible air chamber is squeezed to force air through a face mask into the lungs of the patient, a process referred to as "bagging."

■ A **ventilator**, also called a *respirator*, is a mechanical device for artificial respiration that is used to replace or supplement the patient's natural breathing function. The ventilator forces air into the lungs; exhalation takes place passively as the lungs contract.

## Supplemental Oxygen Therapy

**Supplemental oxygen** is administered when the patient is unable to maintain an adequate oxygen saturation level in the blood from breathing normal air. Oxygen is administered by using a compressor either flowing into a hood or tent, or delivered directly to the patient using one of the following devices:

■ A *nasal cannula* is a small tube that divides into two nasal prongs (Figure 7.22).

■ A *rebreather mask* allows the exhaled breath to be partially reused, delivering up to 60% oxygen.

■ A *non-rebreather mask* allows higher levels of oxygen to be added to the air taken in by the patient.

**Hyperbaric oxygen therapy** (**high**-per-**BARE**-ik) (HBOT) involves breathing pure oxygen in a special chamber that allows air pressure to be raised up to three times higher than normal. The lungs and the bloodstream are thus able to absorb more oxygen, which is delivered throughout the body to promote healing and fight infection.

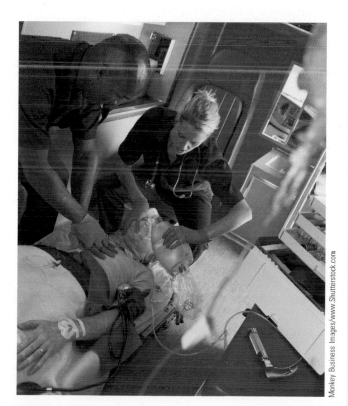

**FIGURE 7.21** Emergency medical technicians use an Ambu bag to assist ventilation.

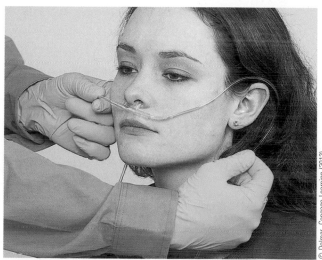

**FIGURE 7.22** One method of delivering supplemental oxygen is through a nasal cannula.

# ABBREVIATIONS RELATED TO THE RESPIRATORY SYSTEM

Table 7.1 presents an overview of the abbreviations related to the terms introduced in this chapter. Note: To avoid errors or confusion, always be cautious when using abbreviations.

**StudyWARE CONNECTION**

For more practice and to test your mastery of this material, go to the StudyWARE™ to play interactive games and complete the quiz for this chapter.

## Workbook Practice

Go to your workbook, and complete the exercises for this chapter.

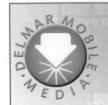

Downloadable audio is available for selected medical terms in this chapter to enhance your learning of medical terminology.

**TABLE 7.1**

**Abbreviations Related to the Respiratory System**

| | |
|---|---|
| acute respiratory distress syndrome = ARDS | **ARDS** = acute respiratory distress syndrome |
| chronic bronchitis = Br | **Br** = chronic bronchitis |
| Cheyne-Stokes breathing = CSB | **CSB** = Cheyne-Stokes breathing |
| chronic obstructive pulmonary disease = COPD | **COPD** = chronic obstructive pulmonary disease |
| cystic fibrosis = CF | **CF** = cystic fibrosis |
| endotracheal intubation = ETT | **ETT** = endotracheal intubation |
| functional endoscopic sinus surgery = FESS | **FESS** = functional endoscopic sinus surgery |
| hyperbaric oxygen therapy = HBOT | **HBOT** = hyperbaric oxygen therapy |
| pulmonary function tests = PFT | **PFT** = pulmonary function tests |
| respiratory failure = RF | **RF** = respiratory failure |
| sudden infant death syndrome = SIDS | **SIDS** = sudden infant death syndrome |
| tuberculosis = TB | **TB** = tuberculosis |
| upper respiratory infection = URI | **URI** = upper respiratory infection |

# LEARNING EXERCISES

## MATCHING WORD PARTS 1

Write the correct answer in the middle column.

| Definition | Correct Answer | Possible Answers |
|---|---|---|
| 7.1. nose | | nas/o |
| 7.2. sleep | | laryng/o |
| 7.3. to breathe | | pharyng/o |
| 7.4. throat, pharynx | | somn/o |
| 7.5. larynx, throat | | spir/o |

## MATCHING WORD PARTS 2

Write the correct answer in the middle column.

| Definition | Correct Answer | Possible Answers |
|---|---|---|
| 7.6. lung | | bronch/o |
| 7.7. oxygen | | ox/o |
| 7.8. pleura | | phon/o |
| 7.9. bronchus | | pleur/o |
| 7.10. sound or voice | | pneum/o |

## MATCHING WORD PARTS 3

Write the correct answer in the middle column.

| Definition | Correct Answer | Possible Answers |
|---|---|---|
| 7.11. windpipe | | -pnea |
| 7.12. sinus | | pulmon/o |

7.13.  lung  _____  **sinus/o**

7.14.  chest  _____  **-thorax**

7.15.  breathing  _____  **trache/o**

## DEFINITIONS

Select the correct answer, and write it on the line provided.

7.16.  The heart, aorta, esophagus, and trachea are located in the _____.

         dorsal cavity        manubrium        mediastinum        pleura

7.17.  The _____ acts as a lid over the entrance to the laryngopharynx.

         Adam's apple        epiglottis        larynx        thyroid cartilage

7.18.  The innermost layer of the pleura is known as the _____.

         parietal pleura        pleural space        pleural cavity        visceral pleura

7.19.  The _____ sinuses are located just above the eyebrows.

         ethmoid        frontal        maxillary        sphenoid

7.20.  The smallest divisions of the bronchial tree are the _____.

         alveoli        alveolus        bronchioles        bronchi

7.21.  During respiration, the exchange of oxygen and carbon dioxide takes place through the walls of

the _____.

         alveoli        arteries        capillaries        veins

7.22.  The term meaning spitting blood or blood-stained sputum is _____.

         effusion        epistaxis        hemoptysis        hemothorax

7.23.  Black lung disease is the lay term for _____.

         anthracosis        asbestosis        pneumoconiosis        silicosis

7.24.  The term _____ means an abnormally rapid rate of respiration.

         apnea        bradypnea        dyspnea        tachypnea

7.25.  The term meaning any voice impairment is _____.

         aphonia        dysphonia        laryngitis        laryngospasm

## MATCHING STRUCTURES

Write the correct answer in the middle column.

| Definition | Correct Answer | Possible Answers |
|---|---|---|
| 7.26. first division of the pharynx | _____ | laryngopharynx |
| 7.27. second division of the pharynx | _____ | larynx |
| 7.28. third division of the pharynx | _____ | nasopharynx |
| 7.29. voice box | _____ | oropharynx |
| 7.30. windpipe | _____ | trachea |

## WHICH WORD?

Select the correct answer, and write it on the line provided.

7.31. The exchange of gases within the cells of the body is known as _____.

external respiration     internal respiration

7.32. The term that describes the lung disease caused by asbestos particles in the lungs

is _____.

asbestosis               silicosis

7.33. The form of pneumonia that can be prevented through vaccination is _____.

bacterial pneumonia     viral pneumonia

7.34. The term commonly known as shortness of breath is _____.

dyspnea                  eupnea

7.35. The emergency procedure to gain access below a blocked airway is known as

a _____.

tracheostomy             tracheotomy

## SPELLING COUNTS

Find the misspelled word in each sentence. Then write the word, spelled correctly, on the line provided.

7.36. The thick mucus secreted by the tissues that line the respiratory passages is called

phlem. _____

7.37. The medical term meaning an accumulation of pus in a body cavity is

empiema. _____

7.38. The medical name for the disease commonly known as whooping cough is

pertusis. _____

7.39. The frenic nerves stimulate the diaphragm and cause it to contract. _____

7.40. An antitussiff is administered to prevent or relieve coughing. _____

## ABBREVIATION IDENTIFICATION

In the space provided, write the words that each abbreviation stands for.

7.41. **ARDS** _____

7.42. **CF** _____

7.43. **FESS** _____

7.44. **SIDS** _____

7.45. **URI** _____

## TERM SELECTION

Select the correct answer, and write it on the line provided.

7.46. Inhaling a foreign substance into the upper respiratory tract can cause _____

pneumonia.

      aspiration           inhalation           inspiration           respiration

7.47. The term meaning abnormally rapid deep breathing is _____.

      dyspnea           hyperpnea           hypopnea           hyperventilation

7.48.  The term meaning the surgical creation of a stoma into the trachea to insert a breathing tube

is _____.

bronchiectasis            thoracotomy            tracheostomy            tracheotomy

7.49.  The diaphragm is relaxed during _____.

exhalation            inhalation            internal respiration            singultus

7.50.  The chronic allergic disorder characterized by episodes of severe breathing difficulty, coughing, and

wheezing is known as _____.

allergic rhinitis            asthma            bronchospasm            laryngospasm

## SENTENCE COMPLETION

Write the correct term on the line provided.

7.51.  The term meaning an absence of spontaneous respiration is _____.

7.52.  The sudden spasmodic closure of the larynx is a/an _____.

7.53.  The term meaning bleeding from the lungs is _____.

7.54.  The term meaning pain in the pleura or in the side is _____.

7.55.  A contraction of the smooth muscle in the walls of the bronchi and bronchioles that tighten and squeeze

the airway shut is known as a/an _____.

## WORD SURGERY

Divide each term into its component word parts. Write these word parts, in sequence, on the lines provided. When necessary, use a slash (/) to indicate a combining vowel. (You may not need all of the lines provided.)

7.56.  **Bronchorrhea** means an excessive discharge of mucus from the bronchi.

_____    _____    _____    _____

7.57.  The **oropharynx** is visible when looking at the back of the mouth.

_____    _____    _____    _____

7.58.  **Polysomnography** measures physiological activity during sleep and is most often performed to detect

nocturnal defects in breathing associated with sleep apnea.

_____    _____    _____    _____

7.59.    **Pneumorrhagia** is bleeding from the lungs.

_____    _____    _____    _____

7.60.    **Rhinorrhea**, also known as a runny nose, is an excessive flow of mucus from the nose.

_____    _____    _____    _____

## TRUE/FALSE

If the statement is true, write **True** on the line. If the statement is false, write **False** on the line.

7.61.    _____ A pulse oximeter is a monitor placed inside the ear to measure the oxygen

saturation level in the blood.

7.62.    _____ In atelectasis, the lung fails to expand because there is a blockage of the air

passages or pneumothorax.

7.63.    _____ Croup is an allergic reaction to airborne allergens.

7.64.    _____ Hypoxemia is the condition of below-normal oxygenation of arterial blood.

7.65.    _____ Emphysema is the progressive loss of lung function in which the chest

sometimes assumes an enlarged barrel shape.

## CLINICAL CONDITIONS

Write the correct answer on the line provided.

7.66.    Baby Jamison was born with _____ _____. This is a genetic

disorder in which the lungs are clogged with large quantities of abnormally thick mucus.

7.67.    Dr. Lee surgically removed a portion of the lung. This procedure is known as

a/an _____.

7.68.    Wendy Barlow required the surgical removal of her larynx. This procedure is known as

a/an _____.

7.69.    During his asthma attacks, Jamaal Nelson uses an inhaler containing a _____. This

medication expands the opening of the passages into his lungs.

7.70.    Each year, Mr. Partin receives a flu shot to prevent _____.

7.71.    When hit during a fight, Marvin Roper's nose started to bleed. The medical term for this condition

is _____.

7.72.    The doctor's examination revealed that Juanita Martinez has an accumulation of blood in the pleural

cavity. This diagnosis is recorded on her chart as a/an _____.

7.73.    Duncan McClanahan had a/an _____ performed to correct damage to the septum

of his nose.

7.74.    Suzanne Holderman is suffering from an inflammation of the bronchial walls. The medical term for

Suzanne's condition is chronic _____.

7.75.    Ted Coleman required the permanent placement of a breathing tube. The procedure for the placement of

this tube is called a/an _____.

## WHICH IS THE CORRECT MEDICAL TERM?

Select the correct answer, and write it on the line provided.

7.76.    An inflammation of the pleura that causes pleurodynia is known as _____.

    atelectasis            emphysema            pleurodynia            pleurisy

7.77.    The substance ejected through the mouth and used for diagnostic purposes in respiratory disorders is

known as _____.

    phlegm            pleural effusion            saliva            sputum

7.78.    The term meaning a bluish discoloration of the skin caused by a lack of adequate oxygen

is _____.

    asphyxia            cyanosis            epistaxis            hypoxia

7.79.    The medical term meaning sudden spasmodic closure of the larynx is _____.

    aphonia            dysphonia            laryngitis            laryngospasm

7.80.    The pattern of alternating periods of rapid breathing, slow breathing, and the absence of breathing is

known as _____.

    anoxia        Cheyne-Stokes respiration        eupnea            tachypnea

## CHALLENGE WORD BUILDING

These terms are *not* found in this chapter; however, they are made up of the following familiar word parts. If you need help in creating the term, refer to your medical dictionary.

| | |
|---|---|
| **bronch/o** | **-itis** |
| **epiglott/o** | **-ologist** |
| **laryng/o** | **-plasty** |
| **pharyng/o** | **-plegia** |
| **pneumon/o** | **-rrhagia** |
| **trache/o** | **-rrhea** |
| | **-scopy** |
| | **-stenosis** |

7.81.   An abnormal discharge from the pharynx is known as _____.

7.82.   Inflammation of the lungs is known as _____.

7.83.   A specialist in the study of the larynx is a/an _____.

7.84.   Bleeding from the larynx is known as _____.

7.85.   Inflammation of both the pharynx and the larynx is known as _____.

7.86.   Abnormal narrowing of the lumen of the trachea is known as _____.

7.87.   The surgical repair of a bronchial defect is a/an _____.

7.88.   Inflammation of the epiglottis is known as _____.

7.89.   The inspection of both the trachea and bronchi through a bronchoscope is a/an _____.

7.90.   Paralysis of the walls of the bronchi is known as _____.

## LABELING EXERCISES

Identify the parts of numbered items on the accompanying figure.

7.91.  _____

7.92.  _____

7.93.  _____

7.94.  _____

7.95.  _____

7.96.  _____ cavity

7.97.  _____

7.98.  _____

7.99.  _____ lung

7.100.  _____ sacs

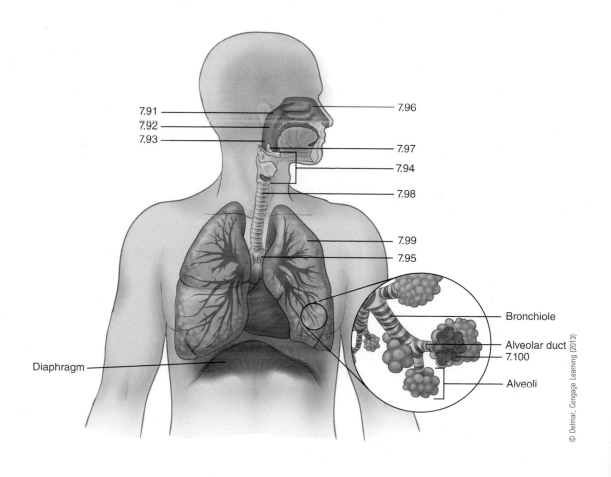

# THE HUMAN TOUCH
## Critical Thinking Exercise

The following story and questions are designed to stimulate critical thinking through class discussion or as a brief essay response. There are no right or wrong answers to these questions.

*Sylvia Gaylord works as a legal aide on the 12th floor of a tall glass-and-steel monument to modern architectural technology. On clear days, the views are spectacular. From her cubicle, Sylvia's eye catches the edge of the beautiful blue and white skyscaper as she reaches for her inhaler. This is the third attack since she returned from lunch 4 hours ago—her asthma is really bad today. But if she leaves work early again, her boss will write her up for it. Sylvia concentrates on breathing normally.*

*Her roommate, Kelly, is a respiratory therapist at the county hospital. Kelly says Sylvia's asthma attacks are probably triggered by the city's high level of air pollution. That can't be true. They both run in the park every morning before work, and Sylvia rarely needs to use her inhaler. The problems start when she gets to work. The wheezing and coughing were so bad today that by the time she got up the elevator and into her cubicle, she could hardly breathe.*

*Last night, the cable news ran a story on the unhealthy air found in some buildings. They called it "sick building syndrome" and reported that certain employees developed allergic reactions just by breathing the air. "Hmmm," she thought, "It seems like more and more people are getting sick in our office. John has had the flu twice. Sid's bronchitis turned into bronchopneumonia, and Hui complains of sinusitis. Could this building have an air quality problem?"*

## Suggested Discussion Topics

1. Discuss which environmental factors might cause an asthma attack.
2. Discuss what Sylvia might do to find out if her building has an air quality problem.
3. What factors did Sylvia and Kelly consider as possible triggers for Sylvia's frequent attack?
4. If Sylvia's inhaler does not control her attack and her condition worsens, what steps should be taken promptly? Why?

# The Digestive System

## Overview of
## STRUCTURES, COMBINING FORMS, AND FUNCTIONS OF THE DIGESTIVE SYSTEM

| Major Structures | Related Combining Forms | Primary Functions |
|---|---|---|
| Mouth | **or/o, stomat/o** | Begins preparation of food for digestion. |
| Pharynx | **pharyng/o** | Transports food from the mouth to the esophagus. |
| Esophagus | **esophag/o** | Transports food from the pharynx to the stomach. |
| Stomach | **gastr/o** | Breaks down food and mixes it with gastric juices. |
| Small Intestine | **enter/o** | Mixes chyme coming from the stomach with digestive juices to complete the digestion and absorption of most nutrients. |
| Large Intestine | **col/o, colon/o** | Absorbs excess water, and prepares solid waste for elimination. |
| Rectum and Anus | **an/o, proct/o, rect/o** | Control the excretion of solid waste. |
| Liver | **hepat/o** | Secretes bile and enzymes to aid in the digestion of fats. |
| Gallbladder | **cholecyst/o** | Stores bile, and releases it into the small intestine as needed. |
| Pancreas | **pancreat/o** | Secretes digestive juices and enzymes into the small intestine as needed. |

# Vocabulary Related to **THE DIGESTIVE SYSTEM**

This list contains essential word parts and medical terms for this chapter. These terms are pronounced in the student StudyWARE™ and Audio CDs that are available for use with this text. These and the other important **primary terms** are shown in boldface throughout the chapter. *Secondary terms*, which appear in *orange* italics, clarify the meaning of primary terms.

## Word Parts

- ☐ **an/o** anus, ring
- ☐ **chol/e** bile, gall
- ☐ **cholecyst/o** gallbladder
- ☐ **col/o, colon/o** colon, large intestine
- ☐ **-emesis** vomiting
- ☐ **enter/o** small intestine
- ☐ **esophag/o** esophagus
- ☐ **gastr/o** stomach, belly
- ☐ **hepat/o** liver
- ☐ **-lithiasis** presence of stones
- ☐ **-pepsia** digest, digestion
- ☐ **-phagia** eating, swallowing
- ☐ **proct/o** anus and rectum
- ☐ **rect/o** rectum, straight
- ☐ **sigmoid/o** sigmoid colon

## Medical Terms

- ☐ **aerophagia** (ay-er-oh-**FAY**-jee-ah)
- ☐ **anastomosis** (ah-**nas**-toh-**MOH**-sis)
- ☐ **anorexia nervosa** (an-oh-**RECK**-see-ah ner-**VOH**-sah)
- ☐ **antiemetic** (an-tih-ee-**MET**-ick)
- ☐ **aphthous ulcers** (**AF**-thus **UL**-serz)
- ☐ **ascites** (ah-**SIGH**-teez)
- ☐ **bariatrics** (bayr-ee-**AT**-ricks)
- ☐ **borborygmus** (bor-boh-**RIG**-mus)
- ☐ **bulimia nervosa** (byou-**LIM**-ee-ah ner-**VOH**-sah)
- ☐ **cachexia** (kah-**KEKS**-eeh-ah)
- ☐ **celiac disease** (**SEE**-lee-ak)
- ☐ **cheilosis** (kee-**LOH**-sis)
- ☐ **cholangiography** (koh-**LAN**-jee-**og**-rah-fee)
- ☐ **cholangitis** (koh-lan-**JIGH**-tis)
- ☐ **cholecystectomy** (koh-luh-sis-**TECK**-toh-mee)
- ☐ **cholecystitis** (koh-luh-sis-**TYE**-tis)
- ☐ **choledocholithotomy** (koh-**led**-oh-koh-lih-**THOT**-oh-mee)

- ☐ **cholelithiasis** (koh-luh-lih-**THIGH**-ah-sis)
- ☐ **cirrhosis** (sih-**ROH**-sis)
- ☐ **colonoscopy** (koh-lun-**OSS**-koh-pee)
- ☐ **colostomy** (koh-**LAHS**-toh-mee)
- ☐ **Crohn's disease**
- ☐ **diverticulitis** (**dye**-ver-tick-you-**LYE**-tis)
- ☐ **diverticulosis** (**dye**-ver-tick-you-**LOH**-sis)
- ☐ **dyspepsia** (dis-**PEP**-see-ah)
- ☐ **dysphagia** (dis-**FAY**-jee-ah)
- ☐ **enteritis** (**en**-ter-**EYE**-tis)
- ☐ **eructation** (eh-ruk-**TAY**-shun)
- ☐ **esophageal varices** (eh-**sof**-ah-**JEE**-al **VAYR**-ih-seez)
- ☐ **esophagogastroduodenoscopy** (eh-**sof**-ah-goh-**gas**-troh-**dew**-oh-deh-**NOS**-koh-pee)
- ☐ **gastroduodenostomy** (**gas**-troh-**dew**-oh-deh-**NOS**-toh-mee)
- ☐ **gastroesophageal reflux disease** (gas-troh-eh-**sof**-ah-**JEE**-al **REE**-flucks)
- ☐ **gastrostomy tube** (gas-**TROS**-toh-mee)
- ☐ **hematemesis** (hee-mah-**TEM**-eh-sis)
- ☐ **Hemoccult test** (**HEE**-moh-kult)
- ☐ **hepatitis** (hep-ah-**TYE**-tis)
- ☐ **herpes labialis** (**HER**-peez **lay**-bee-**AL**-iss)
- ☐ **hiatal hernia** (high-**AY**-tal **HER**-nee-ah)
- ☐ **hyperemesis** (**high**-per-**EM**-eh-sis)
- ☐ **ileus** (**ILL**-ee-us)
- ☐ **inguinal hernia** (**ING**-gwih-nal **HER**-nee-ah)
- ☐ **jaundice** (**JAWN**-dis)
- ☐ **leukoplakia** (loo-koh-**PLAY**-kee-ah)
- ☐ **melena** (meh-**LEE**-nah)
- ☐ **morbid obesity** (**MOR**-bid oh-**BEE**-sih-tee)
- ☐ **nasogastric intubation** (**nay**-zoh-**GAS**-trick in-too-**BAY**-shun)
- ☐ **obesity** (oh-**BEE**-sih-tee)
- ☐ **palatoplasty** (**PAL**-ah-toh-**plas**-tee)
- ☐ **peptic ulcers** (**UL**-serz)
- ☐ **peristalsis** (pehr-ih-**STAL**-sis)
- ☐ **polyp** (**POL**-up)
- ☐ **proctologist** (prock-**TOL**-oh-jist)
- ☐ **regurgitation** (ree-**gur**-jih-**TAY**-shun)
- ☐ **salmonellosis** (sal-moh-nel-**LOH**-sis)
- ☐ **sigmoidoscopy** (sig-moi-**DOS**-koh-pee)
- ☐ **stomatitis** (stoh-mah-**TYE**-tis)
- ☐ **trismus** (**TRIZ**-mus)
- ☐ **ulcerative colitis** (**UL**-ser-**ay**-tiv koh-**LYE**-tis)
- ☐ **volvulus** (**VOL**-view-lus)
- ☐ **xerostomia** (**zeer**-oh-**STOH**-mee-ah)

# STRUCTURES OF THE DIGESTIVE SYSTEM

The digestive system consists primarily of the **gastrointestinal tract** (**gas**-troh-in-**TESS**-tih-nal), which is also known as the *GI tract* (**gastr/o** means stomach, **intestin** means intestine, and **-al** means pertaining to). These organs work in cooperation with *accessory organs* (Figure 8.1).

■ The *upper GI tract* consists of the mouth, pharynx (throat), esophagus, and stomach. This transports food from the entry into the body until digestion begins in the stomach.

■ The *lower GI tract*, which is sometimes referred to as the *bowels*, is made up of the small and large intestines plus the rectum and anus. Here digestion is completed, and waste material is prepared for expulsion from the body.

■ The accessory organs of the digestive system include the liver, gallbladder, and pancreas.

## The Oral Cavity

The major structures of the **oral cavity**, also known as the *mouth*, are the lips, hard and soft palates, salivary glands, tongue, teeth, and the periodontium (Figure 8.2).

### The Lips

The **lips**, which are also known as the *labia*, surround the opening to the oral cavity (singular, *labium*). The term *labia* is also used to describe parts of the female genitalia (see Chapter 14).

■ During eating, the lips, tongue, and cheeks hold the food in the mouth.

■ The lips also have important roles in breathing, speaking, and the expression of emotions.

## The Palate

The **palate** (**PAL**-at), which forms the roof of the mouth, consists of three major parts (Figure 8.2).

■ The **hard palate** is the anterior portion of the palate. This area is covered with specialized mucous membrane. *Rugae* are irregular ridges or folds in this mucous membrane (singular, *ruga*).

■ The **soft palate** is the flexible posterior portion of the palate. During swallowing, it has the important role of closing off the nasal passage to prevent food and liquid from moving upward into the nasal cavity.

■ The **uvula** (**YOU**-view-lah) is the third part, and it hangs from the free edge of the soft palate. During swallowing, it moves upward with the soft palate. It also plays an important role in snoring and in the formation of some speech sounds.

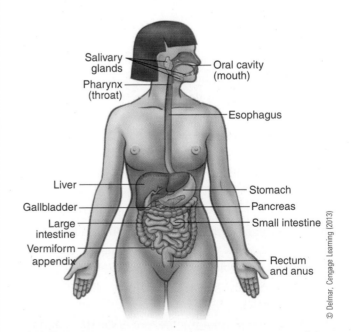

Salivary glands
Oral cavity (mouth)
Pharynx (throat)
Esophagus
Liver
Stomach
Gallbladder
Pancreas
Large intestine
Small intestine
Vermiform appendix
Rectum and anus

© Delmar, Cengage Learning (2013)

**FIGURE 8.1** Major structures and accessory organs of the digestive system.

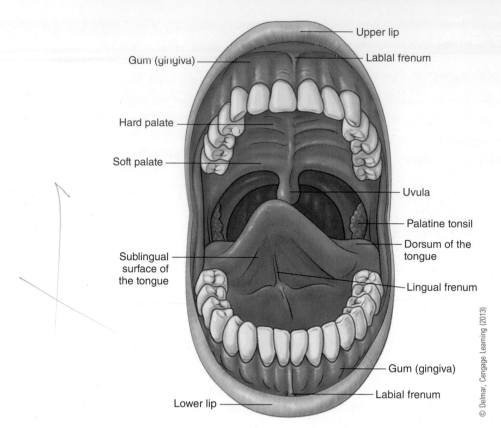

Upper lip
Gum (gingiva)
Labial frenum
Hard palate
Soft palate
Uvula
Palatine tonsil
Dorsum of the tongue
Sublingual surface of the tongue
Lingual frenum
Gum (gingiva)
Labial frenum
Lower lip

© Delmar, Cengage Learning (2013)

**FIGURE 8.2** Structures of the tongue and oral cavity.

## The Tongue

The **tongue** is very strong, flexible, and muscular. The posterior portion of the tongue is attached. The anterior end of the tongue moves freely and is flexible. It is the structure of the tongue that makes it so important for chewing, speaking, and swallowing (Figure 8.2).

■ The upper surface of the tongue is the *dorsum*. This surface has a tough protective covering and in some areas, small bumps known as **papillae** (pah-**PILL**-ee) (singular, *papilla*). These papillae contain *taste buds*, which are the sensory receptors for the sense of taste.

■ The *sublingual surface* of the tongue and the tissues that lie under the tongue are covered with delicate highly vascular tissues. *Sublingual* means under the tongue. *Highly vascular* means containing many blood vessels.

■ The presence of this rich blood supply under the tongue makes it suitable for administering certain medications sublingually by placing them under the tongue, where they are quickly absorbed into the bloodstream.

■ The *lingual frenum* is a band of tissue that attaches the tongue to the floor of the mouth. This frenum limits the motion of the tongue.

## Soft Tissues of the Oral Cavity

■ The term **periodontium** (**pehr**-ee-oh-**DON**-shee-um) describes the structures that surround, support, and are attached to the teeth (**peri**- means surrounding, **odonti** means the teeth, and -**um** is the noun ending). This consists of the bone of the dental arches and the soft tissues that surround and support the teeth.

■ The **gingiva** (**JIN**-jih-vah), also known as *masticatory mucosa* or the *gums*, is the specialized mucous membrane that covers the bone of the dental arches and surrounds the neck of the teeth (plural *gingivae*).

## The Dental Arches

The **dental arches** are the bony structures of the oral cavity (Figure 8.3 A & B). These arches hold the teeth firmly in position to facilitate chewing and speaking.

■ The *maxillary arch* is commonly known as the upper jaw and consists of bones of the lower surface of the skull. This arch does not move.

■ The *mandibular arch*, commonly know as the lower jaw, is a separate bone and is the only movable component part of the joint.

- The **temporomandibular joint** (**tem**-poh-roh-man-**DIB**-you-lar), commonly known as the *TMJ*, is formed at the back of the mouth where the maxillary and mandibular arches come together.

## The Teeth

The term **dentition** (den-**TISH**-un) refers to the natural teeth arranged in the upper and lower jaws. Human dentition consists of four types of teeth (Figure 8.3). These are the:

- *Incisors* and *canines* (also known as *cuspids*). These teeth are used for biting and tearing.

- *Premolars*, which are also known as *bicuspids*, and *molars*. These teeth are used for chewing and grinding.

## Primary and Permanent Dentition

- The primary dentition is also known as the *deciduous dentition*, or *baby teeth*. These 20 teeth erupt during early childhood, are normally lost in late childhood, and are replaced by the permanent teeth. The primary dentition consists of 8 incisors, 4 canines, and 8 molars, but no premolars.

- The permanent dentition consists of 32 teeth designed to last a lifetime. Of these teeth, 20 replace primary teeth and 12 erupt at the back of the mouth. The permanent dentition includes 8 incisors, 4 canines, 8 premolars, and 12 molars.

- The term **occlusion**, as used in dentistry, describes any contact between the chewing surfaces of the upper and lower teeth.

## Structures and Tissues of the Teeth

The *crown* is the portion of a tooth that is visible in the mouth. It is covered with *enamel*, which is the hardest substance in the body (Figure 8.4).

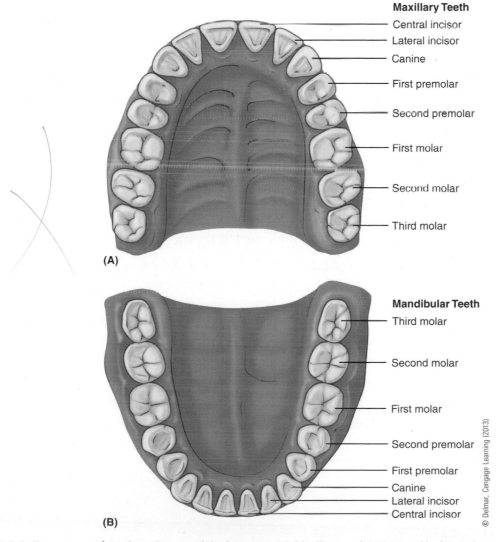

**Maxillary Teeth**
- Central incisor
- Lateral incisor
- Canine
- First premolar
- Second premolar
- First molar
- Second molar
- Third molar

**(A)**

**Mandibular Teeth**
- Third molar
- Second molar
- First molar
- Second premolar
- First premolar
- Canine
- Lateral incisor
- Central incisor

**(B)**

© Delmar, Cengage Learning (2013)

**FIGURE 8.3** Four types of teeth make up adult dentition. (A) Maxillary arch. (B) Mandibular arch.

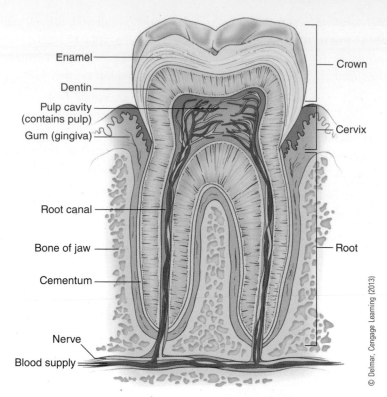

Enamel — Crown

Dentin

Pulp cavity
(contains pulp)

Gum (gingiva) — Cervix

Root canal

Bone of jaw — Root

Cementum

Nerve

Blood supply

© Delmar, Cengage Learning (2013)

**FIGURE 8.4** Structures and tissues of the tooth.

- The *roots* of the tooth hold it securely in place within the dental arch. The roots are protected by *cementum*. This substance is hard, but it is not as strong as enamel.

- The *cervix*, also known as the neck of the tooth, is where the crown and root meet.

- *Dentin* makes up the bulk of the tooth. The portion that is above the gum line is covered with enamel. The root area is covered with cementum.

- The *pulp cavity* is the area within the crown and roots of the tooth that is surrounded by the dentin to protect the delicate pulp of the tooth. In the roots, the pulp continues in the space known as the *root canals*.

- The *pulp* itself consists of a rich supply of blood vessels and nerves that provide nutrients and innervation to the tooth.

## Saliva and Salivary Glands

**Saliva** is a colorless liquid that maintains the moisture in the mouth. It helps maintain the health of the teeth, and it begins the digestive process by lubricating food during chewing and swallowing.

The three pairs of **salivary glands** (**SAL**-ih-ver-ee) secrete saliva that is carried by ducts into the mouth (Figure 8.5).

- The *parotid glands* are located on the face, slightly in front of each ear. The ducts for these glands are on the inside of the cheek near the upper molars.

- The *sublingual glands* and their ducts are located on the floor of the mouth under the tongue.

- The *submandibular glands* and their ducts are located on the floor of the mouth near the mandible.

## The Pharynx

The **pharynx** (**FAR**-inks), which is the common passageway for both respiration and digestion, is discussed in Chapter 7.

- The pharynx plays an important role in *deglutition*, which is commonly known as swallowing.

- The *epiglottis* (**ep**-ih-**GLOT**-is) is a lid-like structure that closes off the entrance to the trachea (windpipe) to prevent food and liquids from moving from the pharynx during swallowing. This is discussed further in Chapter 7.

**StudyWARE CONNECTION**

Watch the **Swallowing Safeguards** animation in the StudyWARE™.

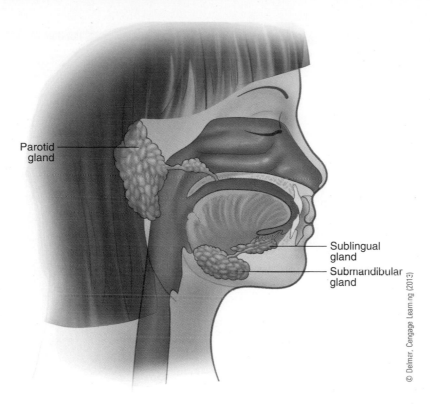

**FIGURE 8.5** The salivary glands.

## The Esophagus

The **esophagus** (eh-**SOF**-ah-gus) is the muscular tube through which ingested food passes from the pharynx to the stomach (Figure 8.1).

- The **lower esophageal sphincter**, also known as the *cardiac sphincter*, is a muscular ring between the esophagus and stomach. During swallowing, it relaxes to allow food to enter the stomach (Figure 8.6).

- This sphincter normally opens to allow the flow of food into the stomach and closes to prevent the stomach contents from regurgitating into the esophagus. *Regurgitating* means to flow backward.

## The Stomach

The **stomach** is a sac-like organ composed of the *fundus* (upper, rounded part), *body* (main portion), and *antrum* (lower part) (Figure 8.6).

- **Rugae** (**ROO**-gay) are the folds in the mucosa lining of the stomach. These folds allow flexibility of the stomach increasing and decreasing in size. Glands located within these folds produce gastric juices.

- **Gastric juices** aid in the beginning of food digestion. Mucus produced by glands in the stomach create a protective coating on the lining of the stomach.

- The **pyloric sphincter** (pye-**LOR**-ick) is the ring-like muscle at the base of the stomach that controls the flow of partially digested food from the stomach to the duodenum of the small intestine.

- The **pylorus** (pye-**LOR**-us) is the narrow passage that connects the stomach with the small intestine.

## The Small Intestine

The **small intestine** extends from the pyloric sphincter to the first part of the large intestine. This coiled organ is up to 20 feet in length and consists of three sections where food is digested and the nutrients are absorbed into the bloodstream (see Figure 8.1).

1. The **duodenum** (**dew**-oh-**DEE**-num) is the first portion of the small intestine. The duodenum extends from the pylorus of the stomach to the jejunum.

2. The **jejunum** (jeh-**JOO**-num), which is the middle portion of the small intestine, extends from the duodenum to the ileum.

3. The **ileum** (**ILL**-ee-um), which is the last and longest portion of the small intestine, extends from the jejunum to the cecum of the large intestine.

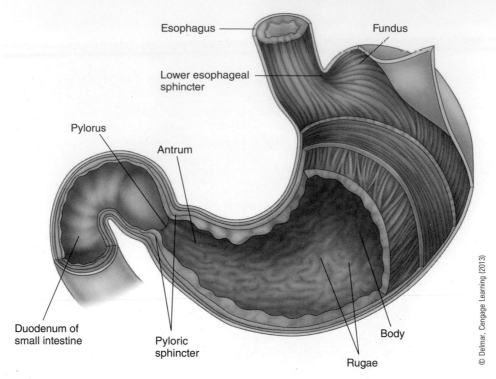

Esophagus

Fundus

Lower esophageal sphincter

Pylorus

Antrum

Duodenum of small intestine

Pyloric sphincter

Body

Rugae

© Delmar, Cengage Learning (2013)

**FIGURE 8.6** Structures of the stomach.

## The Large Intestine

The **large intestine** extends from the end of the small intestine to the anus. It is about twice as wide as the small intestine; however, it is only one-fourth as long. It is here that the waste products of digestion are processed in preparation for excretion through the anus. The major parts of the large intestine are the cecum, colon, rectum, and anus (Figure 8.7).

## The Cecum

The **cecum** (**SEE**-kum) is a pouch that lies on the right side of the abdomen. It extends from the end of the ileum to the beginning of the colon.

- The **ileocecal sphincter** (**ill**-ee-oh-**SEE**-kull) is the ring-like muscle that controls the flow from the ileum of the small intestine into the cecum of the large intestine (Figure 8.7).

- The **vermiform appendix**, commonly called the *appendix*, hangs from the lower portion of the cecum. The term *vermiform* refers to a worm-like shape. The appendix, which consists of lymphoid tissue, is discussed in Chapter 6.

## The Colon

The **colon**, which is the longest portion of the large intestine, is subdivided into four parts (Figure 8.7):

- The **ascending colon** travels upward from the cecum to the undersurface of the liver. *Ascending* means upward.

- The **transverse colon** passes horizontally across the abdominal cavity from right to left toward the spleen. *Transverse* means across.

- The **descending colon** travels down the left side of the abdominal cavity to the sigmoid colon. *Descending* means downward.

- The **sigmoid colon** (**SIG**-moid) is an S-shaped structure that continues from the descending colon above and joins the rectum below. *Sigmoid* means curved like the letter *S*.

## The Rectum and Anus

- The **rectum** is the widest division of the large intestine. It makes up the last 4 inches of the large intestine and ends at the anus.

- The **anus** is the lower opening of the digestive tract. The flow of waste through the anus is controlled by the *internal anal sphincter* and the *external anal sphincter*.

- The term **anorectal** (**ah**-noh-**RECK**-tal) refers to the anus and rectum as a single unit (**an/o** means anus, **rect** means rectum, and **-al** means pertaining to).

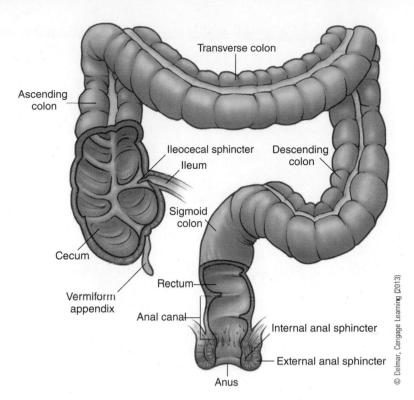

**FIGURE 8.7** Structures of the large intestine.

## Accessory Digestive Organs

The **accessory organs** of the digestive system are so named because they play a key role in the digestive process, but are not part of the gastrointestinal tract (Figure 8.8). The accessory digestive organs are the liver, gallbladder, and pancreas.

### The Liver

The **liver** is the largest organ in the body (Figure 8.8). It has several important functions related to removing toxins from the blood and turning food into the fuel and nutrients the body needs. The term **hepatic** means pertaining to the liver (**hepat** means liver, and **-ic** means pertaining to).

■ The liver removes excess *glucose*, which is commonly known as blood sugar, from the bloodstream and stores it as glycogen. *Glycogen* is a form of starch that is stored in the liver. When the blood sugar level is low, the liver converts glycogen back into glucose and releases it for use by the body. Glucose and glycogen are discussed further in Chapter 13.

■ **Bilirubin** (bill-ih-**ROO**-bin) is a yellow to green fluid, commonly known as bile, that is manufactured by the liver and is necessary for the digestion of fat. Excessive amounts of bilirubin in the body can lead to jaundice and other diseases.

■ **Bile**, which aids in the digestion of fats, is a digestive juice secreted by the liver. Bile travels from the liver to the gallbladder, where it is concentrated and stored.

### The Biliary Tree

The **biliary tree** (**BILL**-ee-air-ee) provides the channels through which bile is transported from the liver to the small intestine. *Biliary* means pertaining to bile.

■ Small ducts in the liver join together like branches to form the biliary tree. The trunk, which is just outside the liver, is known as the *common hepatic duct*.

■ The bile travels from the liver through the common hepatic duct to the gallbladder where it enters and exits through the narrow *cystic duct*.

■ The cystic duct leaving the gallbladder rejoins the common hepatic duct to form the *common bile duct*. The common bile duct joins the *pancreatic duct*, and together they enter the duodenum of the small intestine.

### The Gallbladder

The **gallbladder** is a pear-shaped organ about the size of an egg located under the liver. It stores and concentrates bile for later use (Figures 8.8 and 8.9).

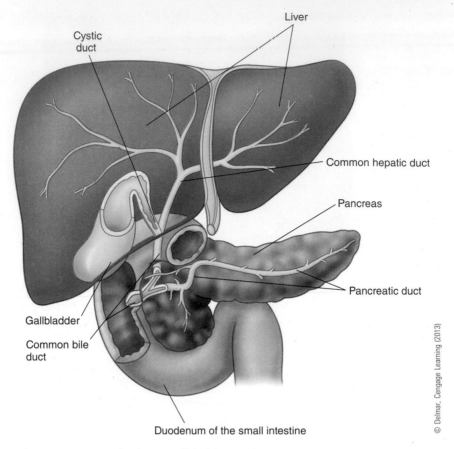

**FIGURE 8.8** Accessory digestive organs: the liver, gallbladder, and pancreas.

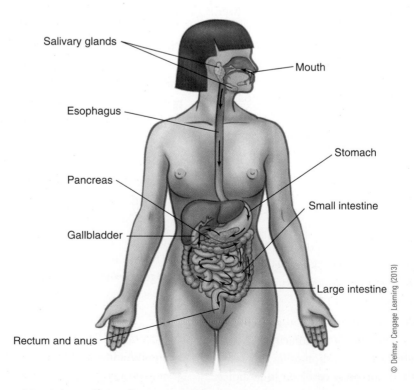

**FIGURE 8.9** The pathway of food through the digestive system.

- When bile is needed, the gallbladder contracts, forcing the bile out through the biliary tree.

- The term **cholecystic** (**koh**-luh-**SIS**-tick) means pertaining to the gallbladder (**cholecyst** means gallbladder, and **-ic** means pertaining to).

## The Pancreas

The **pancreas** (**PAN**-kree-as) is a soft, 6-inch long oblong gland that is located behind the stomach (Figures 8.8 and 8.9). This gland has important roles in both the digestive and endocrine systems. The digestive functions are discussed here. The endocrine functions, plus the pathology and procedures related to the pancreas, are discussed in Chapter 13.

- The pancreas produces and secretes *pancreatic juices* that aid in digestion and contain digestive enzymes and sodium bicarbonate to help neutralize stomach acids. *Pancreatic* means pertaining to the pancreas.

- The pancreatic juices leave the pancreas through the *pancreatic duct* that joins the *common bile duct* just before the entrance into the duodenum.

## ■ DIGESTION

**Digestion** is the process by which complex foods are broken down into nutrients in a form the body can use. The flow of food through the digestive system is shown in Figure 8.9.

- *Digestive enzymes* are responsible for the chemical changes that break foods down into simpler forms of nutrients for use by the body.

- A *nutrient* is a substance, usually from food, that is necessary for normal functioning of the body. The primary nutrients are *carbohydrates*, *fats*, and *proteins*. *Vitamins* and *minerals* are essential nutrients, which are required only in small amounts.

## Metabolism

The term **metabolism** (meh-**TAB**-oh-lizm) includes all of the processes involved in the body's use of nutrients (**metabol** means change, and **-ism** means condition). It consists of two parts: anabolism and catabolism.

- **Anabolism** (an-**NAB**-oh-lizm) is the building up of body cells and substances from nutrients. Anabolism is the opposite of catabolism.

- **Catabolism** (kah-**TAB**-oh-lizm) is the breaking down of body cells or substances, releasing energy and carbon dioxide. Catabolism is the opposite of anabolism.

## Absorption

**Absorption** (ab-**SORP**-shun) is the process by which completely digested nutrients are transported to the cells throughout the body.

- The mucosa that lines the small intestine is covered with finger-like projections called **villi** (**VILL**-eye) (singular, *villus*). Each villus contains blood vessels and lacteals. The blood vessels absorb nutrients directly from the digestive system into the bloodstream for delivery to the cells of the body.

- The *lacteals*, which are specialized structures of the lymphatic system, absorb fats and fat-soluble vitamins that cannot be transported directly by the bloodstream. Instead they absorb these nutrients and transport them via lymphatic vessels. As these nutrients are being transported, they are filtered by the lymph nodes in preparation for their delivery to the bloodstream. (Lacteals are discussed in Chapter 6.)

## The Role of the Mouth, Salivary Glands, and Esophagus

- **Mastication** (**mass**-tih-**KAY**-shun), also known as *chewing*, breaks food down into smaller pieces, mixes it with saliva, and prepares it to be swallowed.

- A **bolus** (**BOH**-lus) is a mass of food that has been chewed and is ready to be swallowed. The *term* bolus is also used in relation to the administration of medication and is discussed in Chapter 15.

- During swallowing, food travels from the mouth into the pharynx and on into the esophagus.

- In the esophagus, food moves downward through the action of gravity and peristalsis. **Peristalsis** (pehr-ih-**STAL**-sis) is a series of wave-like contractions of the smooth muscles in a single direction that moves the food forward into the digestive system.

## The Role of the Stomach

- The gastric juices of the stomach contain hydrochloric acid and digestive enzymes to begin the digestive process. Few nutrients enter the bloodstream through the walls of the stomach.

- The churning action of the stomach works with the gastric juices by converting the food into chyme.

**Chyme** (**KYM**) is the semifluid mass of partly digested food that passes out of the stomach, through the pyloric sphincter, and into the small intestine.

## The Role of the Small Intestine

The conversion of food into usable nutrients is completed as the chyme is moved through the small intestine by peristaltic action.

■ In the duodenum, chyme is mixed with pancreatic juice and bile. The bile breaks apart large fat globules so enzymes in the pancreatic juices can digest the fats. This action is called *emulsification* and must be completed before the nutrients can be absorbed into the body.

■ The jejunum secretes large amounts of digestive enzymes and continues the process of digestion.

■ The primary function of the ileum is the absorption of nutrients from the digested food.

## The Role of the Large Intestine

The role of the entire large intestine is to receive the waste products of digestion and store them until they are eliminated from the body.

■ Food waste enters the large intestine in liquid form. Excess water is reabsorbed into the body through the walls of the large intestine, helping maintain the body's fluid balance, and the remaining waste forms into feces.

■ **Feces** (**FEE**-seez), also known as *solid body wastes*, are expelled through the rectum and anus.

■ **Defecation** (**def**-eh-**KAY**-shun), also known as a *bowel movement (BM)*, is the evacuation or emptying of the large intestine.

■ The large intestine contains billions of bacteria, most of them harmless, which help break down organic waste material. This process produces gas.

■ **Borborygmus** (**bor**-boh-**RIG**-mus) is the rumbling noise caused by the movement of gas in the intestine.

■ **Flatulence** (**FLAT**-you-lens), also known as *flatus*, is the passage of gas out of the body through the rectum.

**StudyWARE CONNECTION**

Watch the **Digestion** animation in the StudyWARE™.

## MEDICAL SPECIALTIES RELATED TO THE DIGESTIVE SYSTEM

■ **Bariatrics** (**bayr**-ee-**AT**-ricks) is the branch of medicine concerned with the prevention and control of obesity and associated diseases.

■ A **dentist** holds a doctor of dental surgery (DDS) or doctor of medical dentistry (DMD) degree and specializes in diagnosing and treating diseases and disorders of teeth and tissues of the oral cavity.

■ A **gastroenterologist** (**gas**-troh-**en**-ter-**OL**-oh-jist) is a physician who specializes in diagnosing and treating diseases and disorders of the stomach and intestines (**gastr/o** means stomach, **enter** means small intestine, and **-ologist** means specialist).

■ An **oral or maxillofacial surgeon** (mack-**sill**-oh-**FAY**-shul) specializes in surgery of the face and jaws to correct deformities, treat diseases, and repair injuries.

■ An **orthodontist** (**or**-thoh-**DON**-tist) is a dental specialist who prevents or corrects malocclusion of the teeth and related facial structures (**orth** means straight or normal, **odont** means the teeth, and **-ist** means specialist).

■ A **periodontist** (**pehr**-ee-oh-**DON**-tist) is a dental specialist who prevents or treats disorders of the tissues surrounding the teeth (**peri-** means surrounding, **odont** means the teeth, and **-ist** means specialist).

■ A **proctologist** (prock-**TOL**-oh-jist) is a physician who specializes in disorders of the colon, rectum, and anus (**proct** means anus and rectum, and **-ologist** means specialist).

## PATHOLOGY OF THE DIGESTIVE SYSTEM

### Tissues of the Oral Cavity

■ **Aphthous ulcers** (**AF**-thus **UL**-serz), also known as *canker sores* or *mouth ulcers*, are gray-white pits with a red border in the soft tissues lining the mouth. Although the exact cause is unknown, the appearance of these very common sores is associated with stress, certain foods, or fever.

■ An *ulcer* is an open lesion of the skin or mucous membrane resulting in tissue loss around the edges (see Chapter 12).

- **Cheilosis** (kee-**LOH**-sis), also known as *cheilitis*, is a disorder of the lips characterized by crack-like sores at the corners of the mouth (**cheil** means lips, and **-osis** means abnormal condition or disease).

- **Herpes labialis** (**HER**-peez **lay**-bee-**AL**-iss), also known as *cold sores* or *fever blisters*, are blister-like sores on the lips and adjacent facial tissue that are caused by the *oral herpes simplex virus type 1* (HSV-1). Most adults have been infected by this extremely common virus, and in some, it becomes reactivated periodically, causing cold sores.

- **Leukoplakia** (**loo**-koh-**PLAY**-kee-ah) is an abnormal white precancerous lesion (sore) that develops on the tongue or the inside of the cheek (**leuk/o** means white, and **-plakia** means plaque). These lesions develop in response to chronic irritation in the mouth such as constant rubbing against a broken tooth. Occasionally, leukoplakia patches occur on the genitals, in the digestive system, or in the urinary tract.

- **Stomatitis** (stoh-mah-**TYE**-tis) is an inflammation of the mucosa of the mouth (**stomat** means mouth or oral cavity, and **-itis** means inflammation). *Note:* the word *stoma*, which occurs in the later section "Ostomies," refers to an artificial mouth-like opening between an organ and the body's surface.

- **Stomatomycosis** (stoh-mah-toh-my-**KOH**-sis) is any disease of the mouth due to a fungus (**stomat/o** means mouth or oral cavity, **myc** means fungus, and **-osis** means abnormal condition or disease).

- **Oral thrush** is a type of stomatomycosis that develops when the fungus *Candida albicans* grows out of control.

The symptoms are creamy white lesions on the tongue or inner cheeks. This condition occurs most often in infants, older adults with weakened immune systems, or individuals who have been taking antibiotics.

- The term **trismus** (**TRIZ**-mus) describes any restriction to the opening of the mouth caused by trauma, surgery, or radiation associated with the treatment of oral cancer. This condition causes difficulty in speaking and affects the patient's nutrition due to impaired ability to chew and swallow.

- **Xerostomia** (zeer-oh-**STOH**-mee-ah), also known as *dry mouth*, is the lack of adequate saliva due to diminished secretions by the salivary glands (**xer/o** means dry, **stom** means mouth or oral cavity, and **-ia** means pertaining to). This condition can be due to medications or radiation of the salivary glands, and can cause discomfort, difficulty in swallowing, changes in the taste of food, and dental decay.

## Cleft Lip and Cleft Palate

- A **cleft lip**, also known as a *harelip*, is a birth defect in which there is a deep groove of the lip running upward to the nose as a result of the failure of this portion of the lip to close during prenatal development.

- A **cleft palate** is the failure of the palate to close during the early development of the fetus. This opening can involve the upper lip, hard palate, and/or soft palate. If not corrected, this opening between the nose and mouth makes it difficult for the child to eat and speak. Cleft lip and cleft palate can occur singly or together, and usually can be corrected surgically (Figure 8.10).

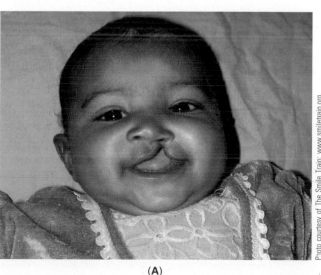
(A)

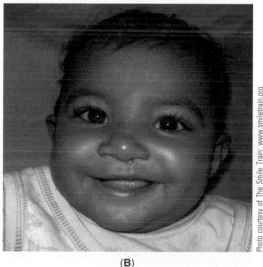
(B)

**FIGURE 8.10** A child with a cleft palate (A) before and (B) after treatment.

## Dental Diseases and Conditions

- **Bruxism** (**BRUCK**-sizm) is the involuntary grinding or clenching of the teeth that usually occurs during sleep and is associated with tension or stress. It can also occur habitually during the day. Bruxism wears away tooth structure, damages periodontal tissues, and injures the temporomandibular joint.

- **Dental caries** (**KAYR**-eez), also known as *tooth decay* or a *cavity*, is an infectious disease caused by bacteria that destroy the enamel and dentin of the tooth. If the decay process is not arrested, the pulp can be exposed and become infected.

- **Dental plaque** (**PLACK**), which is a major cause of dental caries and periodontal disease, forms as soft deposits in sheltered areas near the gums and between the teeth. Dental plaque consists of bacteria and bacterial by-products. In contrast, the *plaque* associated with heart conditions consists of deposits of cholesterol that form within blood vessels.

- **Edentulous** (ee-**DEN**-too-lus) means without teeth. This term describes the situation after the natural permanent teeth have been lost.

- **Halitosis** (hal-ih-**TOH**-sis), also known as *bad breath*, is an unpleasant odor coming from the mouth that can be caused by dental diseases or respiratory or gastric disorders (**halit** means breath, and **-osis** means abnormal condition or disease).

- **Malocclusion** (**mal**-oh-**KLOO**-zhun) is any deviation from the normal positioning of the upper teeth against the lower teeth.

### Periodontal Disease

**Periodontal disease**, also known as *periodontitis*, is an inflammation of the tissues that surround and support the teeth (**peri-** means surrounding, **odont** means tooth or teeth, and **-al** means pertaining to). This progressive disease is classified according to the degree of tissue involvement. In severe cases, the gums and bone surrounding the teeth are involved.

- **Dental calculus** (**KAL**-kyou-luhs), also known as *tartar*, is dental plaque that has calcified (hardened) on the teeth. These deposits irritate the surrounding tissues and cause increasingly serious periodontal diseases. The term *calculus* is also used to describe hard deposits, such as gallstones or kidney stones, that form in other parts of the body.

- **Gingivitis** (**jin**-jih-**VYE**-tis) is the earliest stage of periodontal disease, and the inflammation affects only the gums (**gingiv** means gums, and **-itis** means inflammation).

- **Acute necrotizing ulcerative gingivitis** (ANUG), also known as *trench mouth*, is caused by the abnormal growth of bacteria in the mouth. As this condition progresses, the inflammation, bleeding, deep ulceration, and the death of gum tissue become more severe. *Necrotizing* means causing ongoing tissue death.

## The Esophagus

- **Dysphagia** (dis-**FAY**-jee-ah) is difficulty in swallowing (**dys-** means difficult, and **-phagia** means swallowing).

- **Gastroesophageal reflux disease** (gas-troh-eh-**sof**-ah-**JEE**-al **REE**-flucks), also known as *GERD*, is the upward flow of acid from the stomach into the esophagus (**gastr/o** means stomach, **esophag** means esophagus, and **-eal** means pertaining to). *Reflux* means a backward or return flow. When this occurs, the stomach acid irritates and damages the delicate lining of the esophagus.

- **Barrett's esophagus** is a condition that occurs when the cells in the epithelial tissue of the esophagus are damaged by chronic acid exposure. Some patients with chronic GERD develop this complication, which increases the risk of esophageal cancer.

- **Pyrosis** (pye-**ROH**-sis), also known as *heartburn*, is the burning sensation caused by the return of acidic stomach contents into the esophagus (**pyr** means fever or fire, and **-osis** means abnormal condition or disease).

- **Esophageal varices** (eh-**sof**-ah-**JEE**-al **VAYR**-ih-seez) are enlarged and swollen veins at the lower end of the esophagus (singular, *varix*). Severe bleeding occurs if one of these veins ruptures.

- A **hiatal hernia** (high-**AY**-tal **HER**-nee-ah) is an anatomical abnormality in which a portion of the stomach protrudes upward into the chest, through an opening in the diaphragm (**hiat** means opening, and **-al** means pertaining to). A *hernia* is the protrusion of a part or structure through the tissues that normally contain it. This condition can cause GERD and pyrosis (Figure 8.11).

## The Stomach

- **Gastritis** (gas-**TRY**-tis) is a common inflammation of the stomach lining that is often caused by the bacterium *Helicobacter pylori* (**gastr** means stomach, and **-itis** means inflammation).

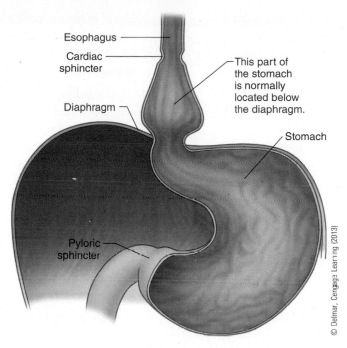

**FIGURE 8.11** In a hiatal hernia, part of the stomach protrudes through the esophageal opening in the diaphragm.

- **Gastroenteritis** (**gas**-troh-en-ter-**EYE**-tis) is an inflammation of the mucous membrane lining the stomach and intestines (**gastr/o** means stomach, **enter** means small intestine, and **-itis** means inflammation).

- **Gastrorrhea** (**gas**-troh-**REE**-ah) is the excessive secretion of gastric juice or mucus in the stomach (**gastr/o** is stomach, and **-rrhea** means flow or discharge).

## Peptic Ulcers

**Peptic ulcers** (**UL**-serz) are sores that affect the mucous membranes of the digestive system (**pept** means digestion, and **-ic** means pertaining to). Peptic ulcers are caused by the bacterium *Helicobacter pylori* or by medications, such as aspirin, that irritate the mucous membranes (Figure 8.12). The condition of having peptic ulcers is referred to as *peptic ulcer disease.*

- *Gastric ulcers* are peptic ulcers that occur in the stomach.

- *Duodenal ulcers* are peptic ulcers that occur in the upper part of the small intestine.

- A *perforating ulcer* is a complication of a peptic ulcer in which the ulcer erodes through the entire thickness of the organ wall.

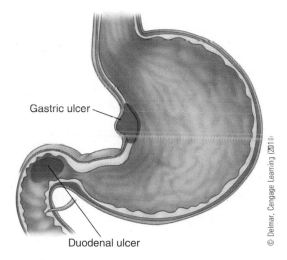

**FIGURE 8.12** The locations of peptic ulcers, gastric and duodenal.

## Eating Disorders

- **Anorexia** (**an**-oh-**RECK**-see-ah) is the loss of appetite for food, especially when caused by disease.

- **Anorexia nervosa** (**an**-oh-**RECK**-see-ah ner-**VOH**-sah) is an eating disorder characterized by a false perception of body appearance. This leads to an intense fear of gaining weight and refusal to maintain a normal body weight. Voluntary starvation and excessive exercising often cause the patient to become emaciated. *Emaciated* means abnormally thin.

- **Bulimia nervosa** (byou-**LIM**-ee-ah ner-**VOH**-sah) is an eating disorder characterized by frequent episodes of binge eating followed by compensatory behaviors such as self-induced vomiting or the misuse of laxatives, diuretics, or other medications. The term *bulimia* means continuous, excessive hunger.

- **Cachexia** (kah-**KEKS**-eeh-ah) is a condition of physical wasting away due to the loss of weight and muscle mass that occurs in patients with diseases such as advanced cancer or AIDS. Although these patients are eating enough, the wasting happens because their bodies are unable to absorb the nutrients.

- **Pica** (**PYE**-kah) is an abnormal craving or appetite for nonfood substances, such as dirt, paint, or clay, that lasts for at least one month. Pica is not the same as the short-lasting abnormal food cravings that are sometimes associated with pregnancy.

## Nutritional Conditions

- **Dehydration** is a condition in which fluid loss exceeds fluid intake and disrupts the body's normal electrolyte balance (**de-** means removal, **hydra** means water, and **-tion** means the process of).

- **Malnutrition** is a lack of proper food or nutrients in the body due to a shortage of food, poor eating habits, or the inability of the body to digest, absorb, and distribute these nutrients. **Mal-** is a prefix meaning bad or poor.

- **Malabsorption** (**mal**-ab-**SORP**-shun) is a condition in which the small intestine cannot absorb nutrients from food that passes through it.

## *Obesity*

**Obesity** (oh-**BEE**-sih-tee) is an excessive accumulation of fat in the body. The term *obese* is usually used to refer to individuals who are more than 20 to 30% over the established weight standards for their height, age, and gender. The term *gender* refers to the differences between men and women.

- **Morbid obesity** (**MOR**-bid oh-**BEE**-sih-tee), also known as *severe obesity*, is the condition of weighing two times or more than the ideal weight or having a body mass index value greater than 40. As used here, the term *morbid* means a diseased state.

- The **body mass index** (BMI) is a number that shows body weight adjusted for height. The results fall into

one of these categories: underweight, normal, overweight, or obese. A high BMI is one of many factors related to developing chronic diseases such as heart disease, cancer, or diabetes.

- **Obesity** is frequently present as a comorbidity with conditions such as hypertension (Chapter 5) or diabetes (Chapter 13). *Comorbidity* describes the presence of more than one disease or health condition in an individual at a given time.

## Indigestion and Vomiting

- **Aerophagia** (**ay**-er-oh-**FAY**-jee-ah) is the excessive swallowing of air while eating or drinking, and is a common cause of gas in the stomach (**aer/o** means air, and **-phagia** means swallowing).

- **Dyspepsia** (dis-**PEP**-see-ah), also known as *indigestion*, is pain or discomfort in digestion (**dys-** means painful, and **-pepsia** means digestion).

- **Emesis** (**EM**-eh-sis), also known as *vomiting*, is the reflex ejection of the stomach contents outward through the mouth. Emesis is used either as a standalone term or as the suffix **-emesis**.

- **Eructation** (eh-ruk-**TAY**-shun) is the act of belching or raising gas orally from the stomach.

- **Hematemesis** (**hee**-mah-**TEM**-eh-sis) is the vomiting of blood (**hemat** means blood, and **-emesis** means vomiting). The substance that is vomited often resembles coffee grounds.

- **Hyperemesis** (**high**-per-**EM**-eh-sis) is extreme, persistent vomiting that can cause dehydration (**hyper-** means excessive, and **-emesis** means vomiting). During the early stages of pregnancy, this is known as *morning sickness*.

- **Nausea** (**NAW**-see-ah) is the urge to vomit.

- **Regurgitation** (ree-**gur**-jih-**TAY**-shun) is the return of swallowed food into the mouth.

## Intestinal Disorders

- **Celiac disease** (**SEE**-lee-ak) is an inherited autoimmune disorder, also known as *gluten intolerance*, characterized by a severe reaction to foods containing gluten. *Gluten* is a class of proteins found in grains such as wheat, barley, rye, and possibly oats. This disorder damages the villi of the small intestine and can lead to the failure of the body to absorb these substances properly.

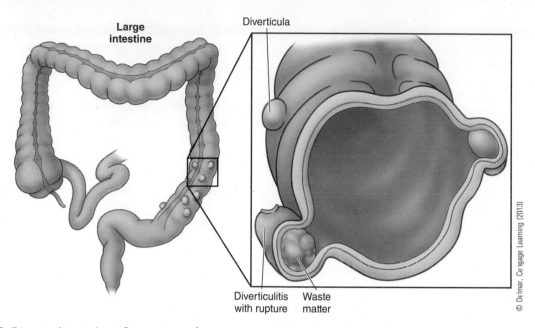

**Large intestine**

Diverticula

Diverticulitis with rupture    Waste matter

© Delmar, Cengage Learning (2013)

**FIGURE 8.13** Diverticulitis is the inflammation of one or more diverticula in the colon.

- **Colorectal carcinoma**, commonly known as *colon cancer*, often first manifests itself in polyps in the colon (Figure 6.13).

- A **polyp** (**POL**-up) is a mushroom-like growth from the surface of a mucous membrane. Not all polyps are malignant.

- **Diverticulosis** (dye-ver-tick-you-**LOH**-sis) is the chronic presence of an abnormal number of diverticula in the colon (**diverticul** means diverticulum, and **-osis** means abnormal condition or disease). Diverticulosis, which often has no symptoms, is believed to be related to a low-fiber diet.

- A **diverticulum** (dye-ver-**TICK**-you-lum) is a small pouch, or sac, found in the lining or wall of a tubular organ such as the colon (plural, *diverticula*).

- **Diverticulitis** (dye-ver-tick-you-**LYE**-tis), which sometimes develops as a result of diverticulosis, is the inflammation or infection of one or more diverticulum in the colon (**diverticul** means diverticulum, and **-itis** means inflammation). Symptoms of this condition can include sudden abdominal pain, cramping, and nausea (Figure 8.13).

- **Enteritis** (en-ter-**EYE**-tis) is an inflammation of the small intestine caused by eating or drinking substances contaminated with viral and bacterial pathogens (**enter** means small intestine, and **-itis** means inflammation).

- **Ischemic colitis** (is-**KEY**-mick koh-**LYE**-tis) occurs when part of the large intestine is partially or completely deprived of blood. If this lack of blood lasts for more than a day, this shortage of blood leads to inflammation or permanent damage of the affected area.

## Ileus

**Ileus** (**ILL**-ee-us) is the partial or complete blockage of the small or large intestine. This condition is also known as *paralytic ileus*, and it is caused by the stopping of the normal peristalsis of this area of the intestine. Symptoms of ileus can include severe pain, cramping, abdominal distention, vomiting, and the failure to pass gas or stools.

*Postoperative ileus* is a temporary impairment (stoppage) of bowel action that is considered to be a normal response to abdominal surgery. It is often present for 24 to 72 hours, depending on which part of the digestive system was treated.

## Irritable Bowel Syndrome

**Irritable bowel syndrome** (IBS), which is also known as *spastic colon*, is a common condition of unknown cause with symptoms that can include intermittent cramping, abdominal pain, bloating, constipation, and diarrhea. This condition, which is usually aggravated by stress and by eating certain foods, is *not* caused by pathogens (bacteria or viruses) or by structural changes.

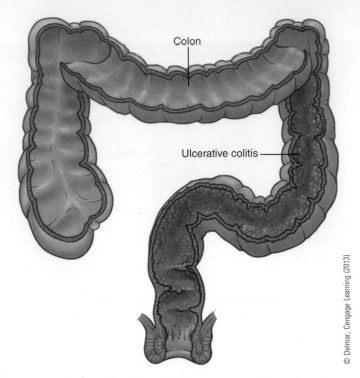

Colon

Ulcerative colitis

© Delmar, Cengage Learning (2013)

**FIGURE 8.14** Ulcerative colitis causes ulcers and irritation in the rectum and large intestine.

## Inflammatory Bowel Diseases

**Inflammatory bowel disease** (IBD) is the general name for diseases that cause inflammation and swelling in the intestines. The two most common inflammatory bowel diseases are ulcerative colitis and Crohn's disease.

■ These conditions are grouped together because both are chronic and incurable, and can affect the large and small intestines. They also have similar symptoms, which include abdominal pain, weight loss, fatigue, fever, rectal bleeding, and diarrhea.

■ These conditions tend to occur at intervals of active disease known as *flares* alternating with periods of remission. Flares of these disorders are treated with medication and surgery to remove diseased portions of the intestine.

## Ulcerative Colitis

**Ulcerative colitis** (**UL**-ser-**ay**-tiv koh-**LYE**-tis) is a chronic condition of unknown cause in which repeated episodes of inflammation in the rectum and large intestine cause ulcers (lesions in the mucous membrane) and irritation (**col** means colon, and **-itis** means inflammation) (Figure 8.14).

■ Ulcerative colitis usually starts in the rectum and progresses upward to the lower part of the colon; however, it can affect the entire large intestine.

■ Ulcerative colitis affects only the innermost lining and not the deep tissues of the colon.

## Crohn's Disease

**Crohn's disease** (CD) is a chronic autoimmune disorder that can occur anywhere in the digestive tract; however, it is most often found in the ileum and in the colon.

In contrast to *ulcerative colitis*, Crohn's disease generally penetrates every layer of tissue in the affected area. This can result in scarring and thickening of the walls of the affected structures. The most common complication of Crohn's disease is blockage of the intestine due to swelling and scarring.

## Intestinal Obstructions

An **intestinal obstruction** is the partial or complete blockage of the small or large intestine caused by a physical obstruction. This blockage can result from many causes such as scar tissue or a tumor.

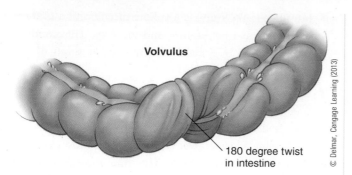

**FIGURE 8.15** Volvulus is the twisting of the bowel on itself.

- *Intestinal adhesions* abnormally hold together parts of the intestine that normally should be separate. This condition, which is caused by inflammation or trauma, can lead to intestinal obstruction.

- In a *strangulating obstruction*, the blood flow to a segment of the intestine is blocked. This can lead to gangrene or perforation. *Gangrene* is tissue death that is associated with a loss of normal circulation. As used here, *perforation* describes a hole through the wall of a structure.

- **Volvulus** (**VOL**-view-lus) is the twisting of the intestine on itself, causing an obstruction. *Volvulus* is a Latin word meaning rolled up or twisted. This condition can cause necrosis of the affected segment of the bowel (Figure 8.15).

- **Intussusception** (**in**-tus-sus-**SEP**-shun) is the telescoping of one part of the small intestine into the opening of an immediately adjacent part (**intussuscept** means to take up or to receive within, and **-ion** means condition). This rare but serious condition is sometimes found in children between three months and six years of age.

- An **inguinal hernia** (**ING**-gwih-nal **HER**-nee-ah) is the protrusion of a small loop of bowel through a weak place in the lower abdominal wall or groin (**inguin** means groin, and **-al** means pertaining to). This condition can be caused by obesity, pregnancy, heavy lifting, or straining to pass a stool.

- A **strangulated hernia** occurs when a portion of the intestine is constricted inside the hernia, causing ischemia (insufficient oxygen) in this tissue by cutting off its blood supply.

## Infectious Diseases of the Intestines

Infectious diseases of the intestines can be transmitted through contaminated food and water or through poor sanitation practices. The more common of these infectious diseases include:

- *Clostridium difficile* (klos-**TRID**-ee-um dif-us-**SEEL**), also known as *C. diff*, is a bacterial infection common to older adults in hospitals or long-term care facilities, typically following the use of antibiotics that wipe out competing bacteria. This disease causes diarrhea and can lead to inflammation of the colon. Infection control measures such as hand-scrubbing or wearing gloves can help prevent its spread.

- **Dysentery** (**DIS**-en-**ter**-ee), which is bacterial infection, occurs most frequently in hot countries where it is spread through food or water contaminated by human feces.

- *E. coli*, which is caused by the bacterium *Escherichia coli*, is transmitted through contaminated foods that have not been cooked properly.

- **Salmonellosis** (**sal**-muh-nel-**LOH**-sis), also referred to as *salmonella*, is transmitted by feces, either through direct contact with animals, or by eating contaminated raw or undercooked meats and eggs or unpasteurized milk and cheese products.

## Anorectal Disorders

- An **anal fissure** is a small crack-like sore in the skin of the anus that can cause severe pain during a bowel movement. As used here, a *fissure* is a groove or crack-like sore of the skin.

- **Bowel incontinence** (in-**KON**-tih-nents) is the inability to control the excretion of feces. (*Urinary incontinence* is discussed in Chapter 9.)

- **Constipation** is defined as having a bowel movement fewer than three times per week. With constipation, stools are usually hard, dry, small in size, and difficult to eliminate.

- **Diarrhea** (**dye**-ah-**REE**-ah) is an abnormally frequent flow of loose or watery stools that can lead to dehydration (**dia-** means through, and **-rrhea** means flow or discharge).

- **Hemorrhoids** (**HEM**-oh-roids) occur when a cluster of veins, muscles, and tissues slip near or through the anal opening. These veins can become inflamed, resulting in pain, fecal leakage, itching, and bleeding.

- A **rectocele** (**RECK**-toh-seel) is a bulging of the front wall of the rectum into the vagina, usually as the result of childbirth or pregnancy (**rect/o** means rectum, and **-cele** means hernia).

## Abnormal Stools

- **Hematochezia** (hee-**mat**-oh-**KEE**-zee-uh) is the flow of bright red blood in the stool. This bright red color usually indicates that the blood is coming from the lower part of the gastrointestinal tract.

- **Melena** (meh-**LEE**-nah), in contrast to *hematochezia*, is the passage of black, tarry, and foul-smelling stools (**melan** means black or dark, and **-a** is a noun ending). This appearance of the stools is caused by the presence of digested blood and often indicates an injury or disorder in the upper part of the gastrointestinal tract.

- **Steatorrhea** (**stee**-at-oh-**REE**-ah) is the presence of an excess of fat in the stool (**steat/o** means fat and **-rrhea** means flow or discharge). This condition, which results in frothy, foul-smelling feces, is usually caused by pancreatic disease, the removal of the gallbladder, or malabsorption disorders.

## The Liver

Liver disorders are a major concern because the functioning of the liver is essential to the digestive process.

- **Ascites** (ah-**SIGH**-teez) is an abnormal accumulation of serous fluid in the peritoneal cavity. This condition is usually the result of severe liver disease. As used here, the term *serous* means a substance having a watery consistency.

- **Hepatomegaly** (hep-ah-toh-**MEG**-ah-lee) is the abnormal enlargement of the liver (**hepat/o** means liver, and **-megaly** means enlargement).

- **Jaundice** (**JAWN**-dis) is a yellow discoloration of the skin, mucous membranes, and the eyes. This condition is caused by greater-than-normal amounts of bilirubin in the blood.

- **Hepatitis** (hep-ah-**TYE**-tis) is an inflammation of the liver usually caused by a viral infection (**hepat** means liver, and **-itis** means inflammation). Viral hepatitis is the leading cause of liver cancer and the most common reason for liver transplants. The three most common varieties of viral hepatitis are shown in Table 8.1.

## Cirrhosis

**Cirrhosis** (sih-**ROH**-sis) is a chronic degenerative disease of the liver characterized by scarring (**cirrh** means yellow or orange, and **-osis** means abnormal condition or disease). *Degenerative* means progressive deterioration resulting in the loss of tissue or organ function.

- Cirrhosis is often caused by excessive alcohol abuse or by viral hepatitis B or C.

- The progress of cirrhosis is marked by the formation of areas of scarred liver tissue that are filled with fat. The liver damage causes abnormal conditions throughout the other body systems (Figure 8.16).

## Nonalcoholic Fatty Liver Disease

The term **nonalcoholic fatty liver disease** (NAFLD) describes the accumulation of fat in the liver of people who drink little or no alcohol. Those with this condition, which usually has no signs or symptoms, is most common in middle-aged individuals who are obese, have type 2 diabetes, have high cholesterol, or have a combination of these.

### TABLE 8.1
### The ABCs of Hepatitis

| | |
|---|---|
| **HAV** | **Hepatitis A virus** is the most prevalent type of hepatitis. This condition is caused by the highly contagious HAV virus and is transmitted mainly through contamination of food and water with infected fecal matter. A vaccine is available to provide immunity against HAV. |
| **HBV** | **Hepatitis B virus** is a bloodborne disease that is transmitted through contact with blood and other body fluids that are contaminated with this virus. A vaccine is available to provide immunity against HBV. |
| **HCV** | **Hepatitis C virus** is a bloodborne disease that is spread through contact with blood and other body fluids that are contaminated with this virus. HCV is described as a silent epidemic because it can be present in the body for years, and destroy the liver, before any symptoms appear. There is no vaccine available to prevent this form of hepatitis. |

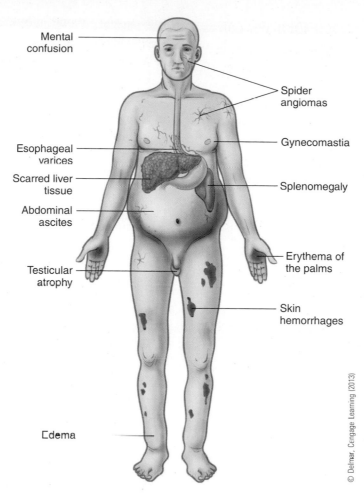

Mental confusion

Spider angiomas

Gynecomastia

Esophageal varices

Scarred liver tissue

Splenomegaly

Abdominal ascites

Testicular atrophy

Erythema of the palms

Skin hemorrhages

Edema

© Delmar, Cengage Learning (2013)

**FIGURE 8.16** Clinical conditions associated with cirrhosis of the liver.

**Nonalcoholic steatohepatitis** (**stee**-ah-toh-hep-ah-**TYE**-tis) (NASH) is a more serious form of this condition since it consists of fatty accumulations plus liver-damaging inflammation (**steat/o** means fat, **hepat** means liver, and **-itis** mean inflammation). In some cases, this will progress to cirrhosis, irreversible liver scarring, or liver cancer.

## The Gallbladder

- **Cholangitis** (**koh**-lan-**JIGH**-tis) is an acute inflammation of the bile duct characterized by pain in the upper-right quadrant of the abdomen, fever, and jaundice (**cholang** means bile duct, and **-itis** means inflammation). The most common cause is a bacterial infection.

- **Cholecystitis** (**koh**-luh-sis-**TYE**-tis) is inflammation of the gallbladder, usually associated with gallstones

blocking the flow of bile (**cholecyst** means gallbladder, and **-itis** means inflammation).

- A **gallstone**, also known as a *cholelith*, is a hard deposit formed in the gallbladder and bile ducts due to the concretion of bile components (plural, *calculi*). The formation of stones is discussed further in Chapter 9.

- **Cholelithiasis** (**koh**-leh-lih-**THIGH**-ah-sis) is the presence of gallstones in the gallbladder or bile ducts (**chole** means bile or gall, and **-lithiasis** means presence of stones).

- Pain caused by the passage of a gallstone through the bile duct is called *biliary colic*.

## The Pancreas

Disorders of the pancreas are discussed in Chapter 13.

# ◼ DIAGNOSTIC PROCEDURES OF THE DIGESTIVE SYSTEM

- **Abdominal computed tomography** (CT) is a radiographic procedure that produces a detailed cross-section of the tissue structure within the abdomen, showing, for example, the presence of a tumor or obstruction. CT scans are discussed in Chapter 15.

- An **abdominal ultrasound** is a noninvasive test used to visualize internal organs by using very-high-frequency sound waves.

- **Cholangiography** (koh-**LAN**-jee-**og**-rah-fee) is a radiographic examination of the bile ducts with the use of a contrast medium (**cholangi/o** means bile duct, and **-graphy** means the process of recording). This test is used to identify obstructions in the liver or bile ducts that slow or block the flow of bile from the liver. The resulting record is a *cholangiogram*.

- An **enema** (**EH**-neh-ma) is the placement of a solution into the rectum and colon to empty the lower intestine through bowel activity. An enema is sometimes part of the preparation for an endoscopic examination; however, enemas are also used to treat severe constipation and as a means of injecting medication into the body.

- An **esophagogastroduodenoscopy** (eh-**sof**-ah-goh-**gas**-troh-**dew**-oh-deh-**NOS**-koh-pee) is an endoscopic procedure that allows direct visualization of the upper GI tract (**esophag/o** means esophagus, **gastr/o** means stomach, **duoden/o** means duodenum, and **-scopy** means visual examination). This includes the esophagus, stomach, and upper duodenum.

- An **upper GI series** and a **lower GI series** are radiographic studies to examine the digestive system. A contrast medium is required to make these structures visible. A *barium swallow* is used for the upper GI series, and a *barium enema* is used for the lower GI series.

- **Stool samples** are specimens of feces that are examined for content and characteristics. For example, fatty stools might indicate the presence of pancreatic disease. Cultures of the stool sample can be examined in the laboratory for the presence of bacteria or *O & P*. This abbreviation stands for ova (parasite eggs) and parasites.

## Endoscopic Procedures

An **endoscope** (**EN**-doh-**skope**) is an instrument used for visual examination of internal structures (**endo-** means within, and **-scope** means an instrument for visual examination).

- An **anoscopy** (ah-**NOS**-koh-pee) is the visual examination of the anal canal and lower rectum (**an/o** means anus, and **-scopy** means visual examination).

- A **capsule endoscopy** is the use of a tiny video camera in a capsule that the patient swallows (Figure 8.17). For approximately eight hours, as it passes through the small intestine, this camera transmits images of the walls of the small intestine. The images are detected by sensor devices attached to the patient's abdomen and transmitted to a data recorder worn on the patient's belt.

## Screening for Colorectal Carcinoma

The following diagnostic tests are used for the early detection of polyps that may be cancerous.

- **Colonoscopy** (koh-lun-**OSS**-koh-pee) is the direct visual examination of the inner surface of the entire colon from the rectum to the cecum (**colon/o** means colon, and **-scopy** means visual examination). A *virtual colonoscopy* uses x-rays and computers to produce two- and three-dimensional images of the colon.

- **Sigmoidoscopy** (sig-moi-**DOS**-koh-pee) is the endoscopic examination of the interior of the rectum, sigmoid colon, and possibly a portion of the descending colon (**sigmoid/o** means sigmoid colon, and **-scopy** is the visual examination).

- A **Hemoccult test** (**HEE**-moh-kult), also known as the *fecal occult blood test*, is a laboratory test for hidden blood in the stools (**hem** means blood, and **-occult** means hidden). This test kit is used to obtain the specimens at home, and these are then evaluated in a laboratory. *Note:* the term Hemoccult is capitalized because it is the name of the manufacturer.

# ◼ TREATMENT PROCEDURES OF THE DIGESTIVE SYSTEM

## Medications

- **Antacids,** which neutralize the acids in the stomach, are taken to relieve the discomfort of conditions such as pyrosis or to help peptic ulcers heal.

- **Proton pump inhibitors** decrease the amount of acid produced by the stomach. These medications are used to treat the symptoms of GERD.

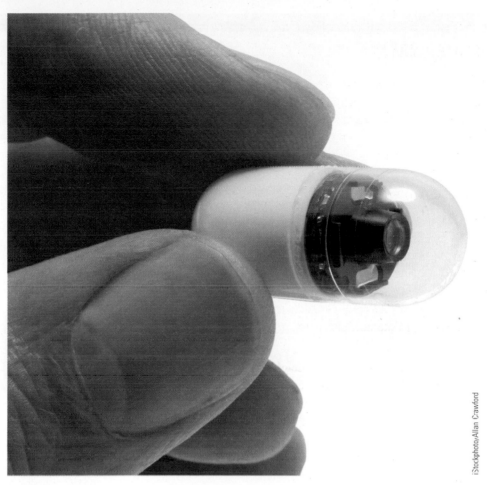

iStockphoto/Allan Crawford

**FIGURE 8.17** The capsule endoscopy camera is swallowed by the patient so that it can transmit images from the small intestine to a sensor device.

- An **antiemetic** (**an**-tih-ee-**MET**-ick) is a medication that is administered to prevent or relieve nausea and vomiting (**anti-** means against, **emet** means vomit, and **-ic** means pertaining to).

- **Laxatives** are medications or foods given to stimulate bowel movements. *Bulk-forming laxatives*, such as bran, treat constipation by helping fecal matter retain water and remain soft as it moves through the intestines.

- **Intravenous fluids** (**in**-trah-**VEE**-nus) (IV) are administered to combat the effects of dehydration (**intra-** means within, **ven/o** means vein, and **-us** is the noun ending).

- **Oral rehydration therapy** (ORT) is a treatment in which a solution of electrolytes is administered in a liquid preparation to counteract the dehydration that can accompany severe diarrhea, especially in young children (**re-** means back or again, **hydra** means water, and **-tion** is the process of).

## The Oral Cavity and Esophagus

- A **dental prophylaxis** (**proh**-fih-**LACK**-sis) is the professional cleaning of the teeth to remove plaque and calculus. The term *prophylaxis* also refers to a treatment intended to prevent a disease or stop it from spreading. Examples include vaccination to provide immunity against a specific disease.

- A **gingivectomy** (**jin** -jih-**VECK**-toh-mee) is the surgical removal of diseased gingival tissue (**gingiv** means gingival tissue, and **-ectomy** means surgical removal).

- **Maxillofacial surgery** (mack-**sill**-oh-**FAY**-shul) is specialized surgery of the face and jaws to correct deformities, treat diseases, and repair injuries.

- **Palatoplasty** (**PAL**-ah-toh-**plas**-tee) is surgical repair of a cleft palate, also used to refer to the repair of a cleft lip (**palat/o** means palate, and **-plasty** means surgical repair) (Figure 8.10).

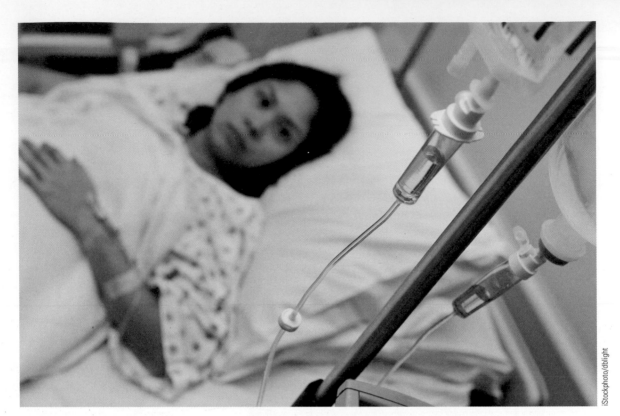

**FIGURE 8.18** Fluids are administered intravenously to combat the effects of dehydration.

## The Stomach

- A **gastrectomy** (gas-**TRECK**-toh-mee) is the surgical removal of all or a part of the stomach (**gastr** means stomach, and **-ectomy** means surgical removal).

- **Nasogastric intubation** (**nay**-zoh-**GAS**-trick **in**-too-**BAY**-shun) is the placement of a feeding tube through the nose and into the stomach (**nas/o** means nose, **gastr** means stomach, and **-ic** means pertaining to). This tube, which is placed temporarily, provides nutrition for patients who cannot take sufficient nutrients by mouth (Figure 8.19).

- A **gastrostomy tube** (gas-**TROS**-toh-mee) is a surgically placed feeding tube from the exterior of the body directly into the stomach (**gastr** means stomach, and **-ostomy** means surgically creating an opening). This is also known as a *G-tube* and it is permanently placed, to provide nutrition for patients who cannot swallow or take sufficient nutrients by mouth (Figure 8.19).

- **Total parenteral nutrition** (pah-**REN**-ter-al) (TPN) is administered to patients who cannot or should not get their nutrition through eating. All of the patient's nutritional requirements are met through a specialized solution administered intravenously. *Parenteral* means not in or through the digestive system.

## Bariatric Surgery

**Bariatric surgery** is performed to treat morbid obesity by restricting the amount of food that can enter the stomach and be digested. These procedures limit food intake and force dietary changes that enable weight reduction.

- *Gastric bypass surgery* makes the stomach smaller, usually by stapling a section to create a small pouch, and causes food to bypass the first part of the small intestine. This procedure, which is the most common bariatric surgery, is not reversible.

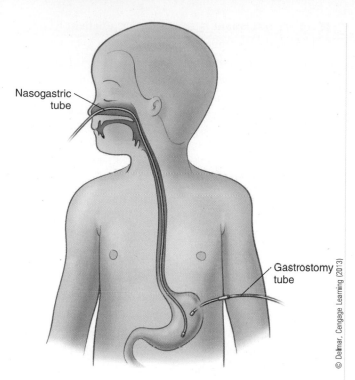

**FIGURE 8.19** Nasogastric and gastrostomy tubes can be used to supply nutrition to a child who cannot eat by mouth.

■ The *lap-band adjustable gastric banding* (LAGB) procedure involves placing a band around the exterior of the stomach to restrict the amount of food that can enter (Figure 8.20). This procedure has the advantage of being reversible through the removal of the band.

## The Intestines

■ A **colectomy** (koh-**LECK**-toh-mee) is the surgical removal of all or part of the colon (**col** means colon, and **-ectomy** means surgical removal).

■ A **colotomy** (koh-**LOT**-oh-mee) is a surgical incision into the colon (**col** means colon, and **-otomy** means a surgical incision).

■ A **diverticulectomy** (**dye**-ver-**tick**-you-**LECK**-toh-mee) is the surgical removal of a diverticulum (**diverticul** means diverticulum, and **-ectomy** means surgical removal).

■ A **gastroduodenostomy** (**gas**-troh-**dew**-oh-deh-**NOS**-toh-mee) is the establishment of an anastomosis between the upper portion of the stomach, and the duodenum (**gastr/o** means stomach, **duoden** means first part of the small intestine, and **-ostomy** means surgically creating an opening). This procedure is performed to treat stomach cancer or to remove a malfunctioning pyloric valve.

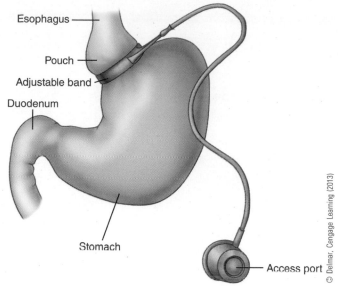

**FIGURE 8.20** Lap-band adjustable gastric banding is one type of bariatric surgery.

■ An **anastomosis** (ah-**nas**-toh-**MOH**-sis) is a surgical connection between two hollow, or tubular, structures (plural, *anastomoses*).

■ An **ileectomy** (**ill**-ee-**ECK**-toh-mee) is the surgical removal of the ileum (**ile** means the ileum, and **-ectomy** means surgical removal. Note: This term is spelled with a double *e*.)

## Ostomies

An **ostomy** (**OSS**-toh-mee) is a surgical procedure to create an artificial opening between an organ and the body surface. This artificial opening is also known as a *stoma*. Ostomy can be used alone as a noun to describe a procedure or as a suffix with the word part that describes the organ involved.

■ An **ileostomy** (**ill**-ee-**OS**-toh-mee) is the surgical creation of an artificial excretory opening between the ileum, at the end of the small intestine, and the outside of the abdominal wall (**ile** means small intestine, and **-ostomy** means surgically creating an opening).

■ A **colostomy** (koh-**LAHS**-toh-mee) is the surgical creation of an artificial excretory opening between the colon and the body surface (**col** means colon, and **-ostomy** means surgically creating an opening). The segment of the intestine below the ostomy is usually removed, and the fecal matter flows through the stoma into a disposable bag. A colostomy can be temporary to divert feces from an area that needs to heal (Figure 8.21).

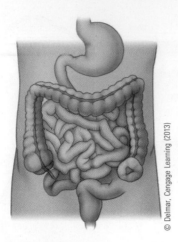

© Delmar, Cengage Learning (2013)

**FIGURE 8.21** Colostomy sites are named for portion of the bowel removed. Shown here is a sigmoid colostomy. The stoma is located at the end of the remaining intestine, which is shown in brown. The portion that has been removed is shown in blue.

## The Rectum and Anus

■ A **hemorrhoidectomy** (**hem**-oh-roid-**ECK**-toh-mee) is the surgical removal of hemorrhoids (**hemorrhoid** means piles, and **-ectomy** means surgical removal). *Rubber band ligation* is often used instead of surgery. Rubber bands cut off the circulation at the base of the hemorrhoid, causing it to eventually fall off. *Ligation* means the tying off of blood vessels or ducts.

■ **Proctopexy** (**PROCK**-toh-**peck**-see) is the surgical fixation of a prolapsed rectum to an adjacent tissue or organ (**proct/o** means rectum, and **-pexy** means surgical fixation). *Prolapse* means the falling or dropping down of an organ or internal part.

## The Liver

■ A **hepatectomy** (hep-ah-**TECK**-toh-mee) is the surgical removal of all or part of the liver (**hepat** means liver, and **-ectomy** means surgical removal).

■ A **liver transplant** is an option for a patient whose liver has failed for a reason other than liver cancer. Because liver tissue regenerates, a *partial liver transplant*, in which only part of the organ is donated, can be adequate. A partial liver can be donated by a living donor whose blood and tissue types match.

## The Gallbladder

■ A **choledocholithotomy** (koh-**led**-oh-koh-lih-**THOT**-oh-mee) is an incision into the common bile duct for the removal of a gallstone (**choledoch/o** means the common bile duct, **lith** means stone, and **-otomy** means surgical incision).

■ A **cholecystectomy** (koh-luh-sis-**TECK**-toh-mee) is the surgical removal of the gallbladder (**chole-** means gallbladder, **cyst** means bladder, and **-ectomy** means surgical removal). An *open cholecystectomy* is performed through an incision in the right side of the upper abdomen. A *laparoscopic cholecystectomy*, also known as a *lap choley*, is the surgical removal of the gallbladder using a laparoscope and other instruments inserted through three or four small incisions in the abdominal wall.

## ■ ABBREVIATIONS RELATED TO THE DIGESTIVE SYSTEM

Table 8.2 presents an overview of the abbreviations related to the terms introduced in this chapter. Note: To avoid errors or confusion, always be cautious when using abbreviations.

## TABLE 8.2
## Abbreviations Related to the Digestive System

| | |
|---|---|
| **body mass index** = BMI | **BMI** = body mass index |
| **colonoscopy** = COL | **COL** = colonoscopy |
| **esophagogastroduodenoscopy** = EGD | **EGD** = esophagogastroduodenoscopy |
| **gastroesophageal reflux disease** = GERD | **GERD** = gastroesophageal reflux disease |
| **gastrointestinal** = GI | **GI** = gastrointestinal |
| **inguinal hernia** = IH | **IH** = inguinal hernia |
| **inflammatory bowel disease** = IBD | **IBD** = inflammatory bowel disease |
| **irritable bowel syndrome** = IBS | **IBS** = irritable bowel syndrome |
| **nasogastric tube** = NG tube | **NG tube** = nasograstric tube |
| **peptic ulcer disease** = PUD | **PUD** = peptic ulcer disease |
| **total parenteral nutrition** = TPN | **TPN** = total parenteral nutrition |
| **ulcerative colitis** = UC | **UC** = ulcerative colitis |

**StudyWARE CONNECTION**

For more practice and to test your mastery of this material, go to the StudyWARE™ to play interactive games and complete the quiz for this chapter.

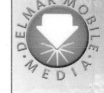

*Downloadable audio is available for selected medical terms in this chapter to enhance your learning of medical terminology.*

## ☐ Workbook Practice

Go to your workbook, and complete the exercises for this chapter.

# LEARNING EXERCISES

## MATCHING WORD PARTS 1

Write the correct answer in the middle column.

| | Definition | Correct Answer | Possible Answers |
|---|---|---|---|
| 8.1. | anus | | chol/e |
| 8.2. | bile, gall | | an/o |
| 8.3. | large intestine | | col/o |
| 8.4. | swallowing | | enter/o |
| 8.5. | small intestine | | -phagia |

## MATCHING WORD PARTS 2

Write the correct answer in the middle column.

| | Definition | Correct Answer | Possible Answers |
|---|---|---|---|
| 8.6. | stomach | | cholecyst/o |
| 8.7. | liver | | esophag/o |
| 8.8. | gallbladder | | gastr/o |
| 8.9. | esophagus | | hepat/o |
| 8.10. | presence of stones | | -lithiasis |

## MATCHING WORD PARTS 3

Write the correct answer in the middle column.

| | Definition | Correct Answer | Possible Answers |
|---|---|---|---|
| 8.11. | sigmoid colon | sigmoid/o | -pepsia |
| 8.12. | anus and rectum | proct/o | -emesis |

| | | |
|---|---|---|
| 8.13. | digestion | _pepsia_ (handwritten) | **proct/o** |
| 8.14. | vomiting | _emesis_ (handwritten) | **rect/o** |
| 8.15. | rectum | _rect/o_ (handwritten) | **sigmoid/o** |

## DEFINITIONS

Select the correct answer, and write it on the line provided.

8.16.   The visual examination of the anal canal and lower rectum is known as _____.

   anoscopy          colonoscopy          proctoscopy          sigmoidoscopy

8.17.   The term _____ means any disease of the mouth due to a fungus.

   salmonellosis          stomatomycosis          stomatitis          steatorrhea

8.18.   The _____ is the last and longest portion of the small intestine.

   cecum          ileum          jejunum          pylorus

8.19.   The inability to control the excretion of feces is called _____.

   bowel incontinence          constipation          anal fissure          hematochezia

8.20.   The liver secretes _____, which is stored in the gallbladder for later use.

   bile          glycogen          insulin          pepsin

8.21.   The _____ travels upward from the cecum to the undersurface of the liver.

   ascending colon          descending colon          sigmoid colon          transverse colon

8.22.   The process of the building up of body cells and substances from nutrients is known

   as _____.

   anabolism          catabolism          defecation          mastication

8.23.   The receptors of taste are located on the dorsum of the _____.

   hard palate          rugae          tongue          uvula

8.24.   The bone and soft tissues that surround and support the teeth are known as

   the _____.

   dentition          gingiva          occlusion          periodontium

8.25.    The condition characterized by the telescoping of one part of the intestine into another

is _____.

borborygmus          flatus          (intussusception)          volvulus

## MATCHING STRUCTURES

Write the correct answer in the middle column.

| Definition | Correct Answer | Possible Answers |
|---|---|---|
| 8.26.   connects the small and large intestine | _cecum_ | cecum |
| 8.27.   S-shaped structure of the large intestine | | duodenum |
| 8.28.   widest division of the large intestine | | jejunum |
| 8.29.   middle portion of the small intestine | | rectum |
| 8.30.   first portion of the small intestine | | sigmoid colon |

## WHICH WORD?

Select the correct answer, and write it on the line provided.

8.31.    The medical term meaning vomiting blood is _____.

(hematemesis)          hyperemesis

8.32.    The _____ virus is transmitted mainly through contamination of food and water

with infected fecal matter.

(hepatitis A)          hepatitis B

8.33.    _____ is characterized by a severe reaction to foods containing gluten.

(celiac disease)          Crohn's disease

8.34. The medical term meaning inflammation of the small intestine is _____.

colitis        (enteritis)

8.35. The _____ hangs from the free edge of the soft palate.

rugae        (uvula)

## SPELLING COUNTS

Find the misspelled word in each sentence. Then write that word, spelled correctly, on the line provided.

8.36. An ilectomy is the surgical removal of the last portion of the ileum. _Ileostomy_

8.37. The bacterial infection disentary occurs mostly in hot countries and is spread through food or water contaminated by human feces. _dysentery_

8.38. The chronic degenerative disease of the liver characterized by scarring is known as serosis. _serous_

8.39. A proctoplexy is the surgical fixation of the rectum to some adjacent tissue or organ. _Proctopexy_

8.40. The lack of adequate saliva due to the absence of or diminished secretions by the salivary glands is known as zerostomia. _Xerostomia_

## ABBREVIATION IDENTIFICATION

In the space provided, write the words that each abbreviation stands for.

8.41. **UC** _____

8.42. **COL** _____ _____

8.43. **GERD** _____

8.44. **IBS** _____

8.45. **PUD** _____

## TERM SELECTION

Select the correct answer, and write it on the line provided.

8.46.    The surgical removal of all or part of the stomach is a _____.

   (gastrectomy)        gastritis        gastroenteritis        gastrotomy

8.47.    The medical term meaning difficulty in swallowing is _____.

   anorexia        dyspepsia        (dysphagia)        pyrosis

8.48.    The involuntary grinding or clenching of the teeth is called _____.

   (bruxism)        edentulous        malocclusion        dental caries

8.49.    The chronic degeneration of the liver often caused by excessive alcohol abuse is

   called _____.

   (cirrhosis)        hepatitis C        hepatitis A        hepatomegaly

8.50    The pigment manufactured by the liver and necessary for the digestion of fat is

   called _____.

   bile        bilirubin        hydrochloric acid        (pancreatic juice)

## SENTENCE COMPLETION

Write the correct term or terms on the lines provided.

8.51.    The excessive swallowing of air while eating or drinking is known as _Aerophagia_

8.52.    The return of swallowed food to the mouth is known as _Regurgitation_.

8.53.    A yellow discoloration of the skin caused by greater-than-normal amounts of bilirubin in the blood is

   called _Jandice_.

8.54.    The _Pyloric sphincter_ is the ring-like muscle that controls the flow from the stomach to the

   small intestine.

8.55.    The medical term for the solid body wastes that are expelled through the rectum

   is _feces, bowl movements and stool faces_

## WORD SURGERY

Divide each term into its component word parts. Write these word parts, in sequence, on the lines provided. When necessary use a slash (/) to indicate a combining vowel. (You may not need all of the lines provided.)

8.56. An **esophagogastroduodenoscopy** is an endoscopic procedure that allows direct visualization of the upper GI tract.

_esoph/a_      _gogastr/o_      _denp_      _scopy_

8.57. A **periodontist** is a dental specialist who prevents or treats disorders of the tissues surrounding the teeth.

_peri/o_      _dontist_      _____      _____

8.58. A **sigmoidoscopy** is the endoscopic examination of the interior of the rectum, sigmoid colon, and possibly a portion of the descending colon.

_sigmp_      _id/o_      _scopy_      _____

8.59. An **antiemetic** is a medication that is administered to prevent or relieve nausea and vomiting.

_antie_      _metic_      _____      _____

8.60. A **gastroduodenostomy** is the establishment of an anastomosis between the upper portion of the stomach and the duodenum.

_gastr/o_      _dup_      _denp_      _stomy_

## TRUE/FALSE

If the statement is true, write **True** on the line. If the statement is false, write **False** on the line.

8.61. _____T_____ Cholangitis is an acute infection of the bile duct characterized by pain in the upper right quadrant of the abdomen, fever, and jaundice.

8.62. _____F_____ Cholangiography is an endoscopic diagnostic procedure.

8.63. _____T_____ Acute necrotizing ulcerative gingivitis is caused by the abnormal growth of bacteria in the mouth.

8.64. _____F_____ Bruxism means to be without natural teeth.

8.65. _____T_____ A choledocholithotomy is an incision in the common bile duct for the removal of gallstones.

## CLINICAL CONDITIONS

Write the correct answer on the line provided.

8.66. James Ridgeview was diagnosed as having _____, which is the partial or complete blockage of the small or large intestine.

8.67. Chang Hoon suffers from _____. This condition is an abnormal accumulation of serous fluid in the peritoneal cavity.

8.68. Rita Martinez is a dentist. She described her patient Mr. Espinoza as being _____, which means that he was without natural teeth.

8.69. Baby Kilgore was vomiting almost continuously. The medical term for this excessive vomiting is _____.

8.70. A/An _____ was performed on Mr. Schmidt to create an artificial excretory opening between his colon and body surface.

8.71. After eating, Mike Delahanty often complained about heartburn. The medical term for this condition is _____.

8.72. After the repeated passage of black, tarry, and foul-smelling stools, Catherine Baldwin was diagnosed as having _____. This condition is caused by the presence of digested blood in the stools.

8.73. Alberta Roberts was diagnosed as having an inflammation of one or more diverticula. The medical term for this condition is _____.

8.74. Carlotta Hansen has blister-like sores on her lips and adjacent facial tissue. She says they are cold sores; however, the medical term for this condition is _____ .

8.75. Lisa Wilson saw her dentist because she was concerned about bad breath. Her dentist refers to this condition as _____.

## WHICH IS THE CORRECT MEDICAL TERM?

Select the correct answer, and write it on the line provided.

8.76. The _____ test detects hidden blood in the stools.

anoscopy          colonoscopy          enema          Hemoccult

8.77.    A/An _____ is a surgical connection between two hollow or tubular structures.

    (anastomosis)          ostomy          stoma          sphincter

8.78.    The eating disorder characterized by voluntary starvation and excessive exercising because of an intense

    fear of gaining weight is known as_____.

    anorexia          (anorexia nervosa)          bulimia          bulimia nervosa

8.79.    The hardened deposit that forms on the teeth and irritate the surrounding tissues is known as

    dental _____.

    (calculus)          caries          decay          plaque

8.80.    The surgical removal of all or part of the liver is known as _____.

    anoplasty          palatoplasty          proctopexy          (hepatectomy)

## CHALLENGE WORD BUILDING

These terms are *not* found in this chapter; however, they are made up of the following familiar word parts. If you need help in creating the term, refer to your medical dictionary.

| | |
|---|---|
| col/o | -algia |
| enter/o | -ectomy |
| esophag/o | -itis |
| gastr/o | -megaly |
| hepat/o | -ic |
| proct/o | -pexy |
| sigmoid/o | -rrhaphy |

8.81.    Surgical suturing of a stomach wound is known as _____.

8.82.    Pain in the esophagus is known as _____.

8.83.    The surgical removal of all or part of the sigmoid colon is a/an _____.

8.84.    Pain in and around the anus and rectum is known as _____.

8.85.    The surgical fixation of the stomach to correct displacement is a/an _____.

8.86.    Inflammation of the sigmoid colon is known as _____.

8.87.   The surgical removal of all or part of the esophagus and stomach is a/an _____.

8.88.   The term meaning relating to the liver and intestines is _____.

8.89.   Abnormal enlargement of the liver is known as _____.

8.90.   Inflammation of the stomach, small intestine, and colon is known as _____.

## LABELING EXERCISES

Identify the numbered items on the accompanying figure.

8.91.   _____ glands

8.92.   _____

8.93.   _____

8.94.   _____

8.95.   _____

8.96.   _____

8.97.   _____ intestine

8.98.   vermiform _____

8.99.   _____ intestine

8.100.  _____ and anus

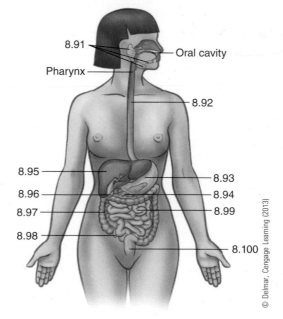

© Delmar, Cengage Learning (2013)

# THE HUMAN TOUCH
## Critical Thinking Exercise

The following story and questions are designed to stimulate critical thinking through class discussion or as a brief essay response. There are no right or wrong answers to these questions.

*"Stick the landing, and our team walks away with the gold!" Coach Schaefer meant to be supportive as she squeezed Claire's shoulder. "What you mean is beat Leia's score for the Riverview team, and we'll win," Claire thought sarcastically. She watched as Leia's numbers were shown from her last vault. A 6.8 out of a possible 7. "Great, just great! She chooses a less difficult vault, but with that toothpick body she gets more height than I ever will!" She wondered if Leia was naturally that thin, or did she use the secret method—you can't gain weight if the food doesn't stay in your stomach.*

*All season it had been that way. Everyone seemed to be watching the rivalry between West High's Claire and Riverview's "tiny-mighty" Leia. Claire was pretty sure that her 10-pound weight loss had improved both her floor routine and her tricky dismount off the beam. "I'm less than a half point behind, so Coach should be happy," she thought. But just last week, Coach Schaefer had a long talk with her when she got dizzy and fell off the balance beam. Coach had asked Claire the one question she hoped she'd never have to answer: "Just what have you been doing to lose the weight?"*

*Claire felt her hands sweat. "Just stick the landing," she told herself, but her body had a different agenda. Starved for fuel, her muscles failed, she fell, and the gold slipped out of reach.*

## Suggested Discussion Topics

1. What do you think Claire is doing to lose weight?
2. What effects would anorexia or bulimia nervosa have on the long-term health of a young woman?
3. Athletes sometimes abuse their bodies through dieting or drugs to achieve peak performances. What should the groups that oversee competitive athletics do about this practice?
4. Imagine you have a daughter. How would you know if she had an eating disorder? How could you help her?

## CHAPTER 9

# The Urinary System

## Overview of
## STRUCTURES, COMBINING FORMS, AND FUNCTIONS OF THE URINARY SYSTEM

| Major Structures | Related Combining Forms | Primary Functions |
| --- | --- | --- |
| Kidneys | **nephr/o, ren/o** | Filter the blood to remove waste products, maintain electrolyte concentrations, and remove excess water to maintain the fluid volume within the body. |
| Renal Pelvis | **pyel/o** | Collects urine produced by the kidneys. |
| Urine | **ur/o, urin/o** | Liquid waste products to be excreted. |
| Ureters | **ureter/o** | Transport urine from the kidneys to the bladder. |
| Urinary Bladder | **cyst/o** | Stores urine until it is excreted. |
| Urethra | **urethr/o** | Transports urine from the bladder through the urethral meatus, where it is excreted. |
| Prostate | **prostat/o** | A gland of the male reproductive system that surrounds the male urethra. Disorders of this gland can disrupt the flow of urine. |

# Vocabulary Related to THE URINARY SYSTEM

This list contains essential word parts and medical terms for this chapter. These terms are pronounced in the student StudyWARE™ and Audio CDs that are available for use with this text. These and the other important **primary terms** are shown in boldface throughout the chapter. *Secondary terms*, which appear in *orange* italics, clarify the meaning of primary terms.

## Word Parts

- [ ] **-cele** hernia, tumor, swelling
- [ ] **cyst/o** urinary bladder, cyst, sac of fluid
- [ ] **dia-** through, between, apart, complete
- [ ] **-ectasis** stretching, dilation, enlargement
- [ ] **glomerul/o** glomerulus
- [ ] **lith/o** stone, calculus
- [ ] **-lysis** breakdown, separation, setting free, destruction, loosening
- [ ] **nephr/o** kidney
- [ ] **-pexy** surgical fixation
- [ ] **pyel/o** renal pelvis, bowl of kidney
- [ ] **-tripsy** to crush
- [ ] **ur/o** urine, urinary tract
- [ ] **ureter/o** ureter
- [ ] **urethr/o** urethra
- [ ] **-uria** urination, urine

## Medical Terms

- [ ] **ablation** (ab-**LAY**-shun)
- [ ] **anuria** (ah-**NEW**-ree-ah)
- [ ] **benign prostatic hyperplasia** (bee-**NINE** pros-**TAT**-ick **high**-per-**PLAY**-zee-ah)
- [ ] **chronic kidney disease**
- [ ] **cystitis** (sis-**TYE**-tis)
- [ ] **cystocele** (**SIS**-toh-seel)
- [ ] **cystolith** (**SIS**-toh-lith)
- [ ] **cystopexy** (**SIS**-toh-**peck**-see)
- [ ] **cystoscopy** (sis-**TOS**-koh-pee)
- [ ] **dialysis** (dye-**AL**-ih-sis)
- [ ] **diuresis** (**dye**-you-**REE**-sis)
- [ ] **end-stage renal disease**
- [ ] **enuresis** (**en**-you-**REE**-sis)
- [ ] **epispadias** (ep-ih-**SPAY**-dee-as)
- [ ] **extracorporeal shockwave lithotripsy** (**ecks**-trah-kor-**POUR**-ee-al **LITH**-oh-**trip**-see)
- [ ] **glomerulonephritis** (gloh-**mer**-you-loh-neh-**FRY**-tis)
- [ ] **hemodialysis** (**hee**-moh-dye-**AL**-ih-sis)
- [ ] **hydronephrosis** (**high**-droh-neh-**FROH**-sis)
- [ ] **hydroureter** (high-droh-**YOUR**-eh-ter)

- [ ] **hyperproteinuria** (**high**-per-**proh**-tee-in-**YOU**-ree-ah)
- [ ] **hypoproteinemia** (**high**-poh-**proh**-tee-in-**EE**-mee-ah)
- [ ] **hypospadias** (**high**-poh-**SPAY**-dee-as)
- [ ] **incontinence** (in-**KON**-tih-nents)
- [ ] **interstitial cystitis** (in-ter-**STISH**-al sis-**TYE**-tis)
- [ ] **intravenous pyelogram** (**in**-trah-**VEE**-nus **PYE**-eh-loh-**gram**)
- [ ] **nephrolith** (**NEF**-roh-lith)
- [ ] **nephrolithiasis** (**nef**-roh-lih-**THIGH**-ah-sis)
- [ ] **nephrolysis** (neh-**FROL**-ih-sis)
- [ ] **nephrons** (**NEF**-ronz)
- [ ] **nephropathy** (neh-**FROP**-ah-thee)
- [ ] **nephroptosis** (**nef**-rop-**TOH**-sis)
- [ ] **nephropyosis** (**nef**-roh-pye-**OH**-sis)
- [ ] **nephrostomy** (neh-**FROS**-toh-me)
- [ ] **nephrotic syndrome** (neh-**FROT**-ick)
- [ ] **neurogenic bladder** (new-roh-**JEN**-ick)
- [ ] **nocturia** (nock-**TOO**-ree-ah)
- [ ] **nocturnal enuresis** (nock-**TER**-nal **en**-you-**REE**-sis)
- [ ] **oliguria** (**ol**-ih-**GOO** ree-ah)
- [ ] **percutaneous nephrolithotomy** (**per**-kyou-**TAY**-nee-us **nef**-roh-lih-**THOT**-oh-mee)
- [ ] **peritoneal dialysis** (**pehr**-ih-toh-**NEE**-al dye-**AL**-ih-sis)
- [ ] **polycystic kidney disease** (**pol**-ee-**SIS**-tick)
- [ ] **polyuria** (**pol**-ee-**YOU**-ree-ah)
- [ ] **prostatism** (**PROS**-tah-tizm)
- [ ] **pyeloplasty** (**PYE**-eh-loh-**plas**-tee)
- [ ] **pyelotomy** (**pye**-eh-**LOT**-oh-mee)
- [ ] **suprapubic catheterization** (**soo**-prah-**PYOU**-bick **kath**-eh-ter-eye-**ZAY**-shun)
- [ ] **uremia** (you-**REE**-mee-ah)
- [ ] **ureterectasis** (you-**reh**-ter-**ECK**-tah-sis)
- [ ] **ureterolith** (you-**REE**-ter-oh-**lith**)
- [ ] **ureterorrhagia** (you-**ree**-ter-oh-**RAY**-jee-ah)
- [ ] **ureterorrhaphy** (you-**reet**-eh-**ROAR**-ah-fee)
- [ ] **urethritis** (**you**-reh-**THRIGH**-tis)
- [ ] **urethropexy** (you-**REE**-throh-**peck**-see)
- [ ] **urethrorrhagia** (you-**ree**-throh-**RAY**-jee-ah)
- [ ] **urethrostenosis** (**you**-ree-throh-steh-**NOH**-sis)
- [ ] **urethrotomy** (**you**-reh-**THROT**-oh-mee)
- [ ] **urinary catheterization** (**kath**-eh-ter-eye-**ZAY**-shun)
- [ ] **vesicovaginal fistula** (**ves**-ih-koh-**VAJ**-ih-nahl **FIS**-tyou-lah)
- [ ] **voiding cystourethrography** (**sis**-toh-you-ree-**THROG**-rah-fee)
- [ ] **Wilms tumor**

# ■ FUNCTIONS OF THE URINARY SYSTEM

The urinary system performs many functions that are important in maintaining homeostasis. *Homeostasis* is the process through which the body maintains a constant internal environment (**home/o** means constant, and **-stasis** means control). These functions include:

- Maintaining the proper balance of water, salts, and acids in the body by filtering the blood as it flows through the kidneys.

- Constantly filtering the blood to remove urea, creatinine, uric acid, and other waste materials from the bloodstream. **Urea** (you-REE-ah) is the major waste product of protein metabolism. *Creatinine* is a waste product of muscle metabolism.

- Converting these waste products and excess fluids into **urine** in the kidneys and excrete them from the body via the urinary bladder.

# ■ STRUCTURES OF THE URINARY SYSTEM

The urinary system, also referred to as the *urinary tract*, consists of two kidneys, two ureters, one bladder, and a urethra (Figures 9.1 and 9.4). The adrenal glands, which are part of the endocrine system, are located on the top of the kidneys.

The urinary tract is located in close proximity to the reproductive organs, so these two body systems are sometime referred to together as the *genitourinary tract*.

## The Kidneys

The **kidneys** constantly filter the blood to remove waste products and excess water. These are excreted as urine, which is 95% water and 5% urea and other body wastes.

About 200 quarts of blood are processed every day, producing an average of 2 quarts of urine. The kidneys also help the body maintain the proper level of fluid, produce hormones that control blood pressure and make red blood cells, and activate vitamin D to maintain healthy bones.

- The term **renal** (REE-nal) means pertaining to the kidneys (**ren** means kidney or kidneys, and **-al** means pertaining to).

- The two bean-shaped kidneys are located in the retroperitoneal space, with one on each side of the vertebral column below the diaphragm and the lower edge of the rib cage. *Retroperitoneal* means behind the peritoneum, which is the membrane that lines the abdominal cavity.

- The **renal cortex** (REE-nal KOR-tecks) is the outer region of the kidney. This layer of tissue contains more than one million microscopic units called nephrons. The term *cortex* means the outer portion of an organ.

- The **medulla** (meh-DULL-ah) is the inner region of the kidney, and it contains most of the urine-collecting tubules. A *tubule* is a small tube.

### Nephrons

The **nephrons** (NEF-ronz) are the microscopic functional units of each kidney. It is here that urine is produced through the processes of filtration, reabsorption, and secretion (Figure 9.2). *Reabsorption* is the return to the blood of some of the substances that were removed during filtration.

- Each nephron contains a **glomerulus** (gloh-MER-you-lus), which is a cluster of capillaries (plural, *glomeruli*), surrounded by a cup-shaped membrane called the Bowman's capsule, and a **renal tubule**.

- Blood enters the kidney through the **renal artery** and flows into the nephrons.

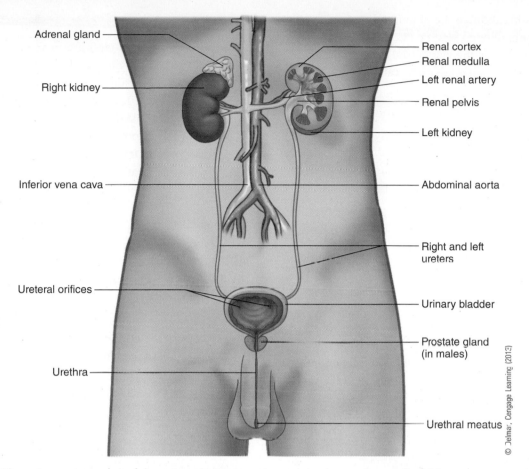

**FIGURE 9.1** The primary structures of the urinary system, as shown here in a male, are the kidneys, ureters, urinary bladder, and urethra. The adrenal gland, positioned on top of each kidney, is a structure of the endocrine system. The prostrate gland, which is part of the male reproductive system, surrounds the urethra.

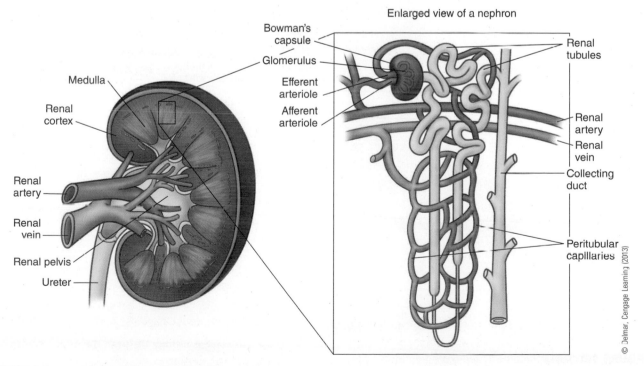

**FIGURE 9.2** A nephron and its associated structures.

- After passing through the filtration system of the glomerulus, the filtered blood containing protein and blood cells leaves the kidney and returns to the bloodstream through the **renal vein**.

- The remaining filtrate flows into the renal tubules, where elements, including some water, sugar, and salts, are returned to the bloodstream via a nearby capillary.

- Remaining waste products are continuously converted into urine, which is transported to the renal pelvis and collected in preparation for entry into the ureters.

- If waste products are not efficiently removed from the bloodstream, the body cannot maintain homeostasis, with a stable balance of salts and other substances.

## The Renal Pelvis

The **renal pelvis** is the funnel-shaped area inside each kidney that is surrounded by the renal cortex and medulla. This is where the newly formed urine from the nephrons collects before it flows into the ureters.

## The Ureters

The **ureters** (you **REE**-ters) are two narrow tubes, each about 10 to 12 inches long, which transport urine from the kidney to the bladder. *Peristalsis*, which is a series of wave-like contractions, moves urine down each ureter to the bladder. (Peristalsis is also part of the digestive process, as described in Chapter 8.)

Urine drains from the ureters into the bladder through the **ureteral orifices** in the wall of the urinary bladder (Figure 9.1). *Orifice* means opening.

## The Urinary Bladder

The **urinary bladder** is an oval, hollow muscular organ that is a reservoir for urine before it is excreted from the body (Figure 9.3).

- The bladder is located in the anterior portion of the pelvic cavity behind the pubic symphysis. The average adult bladder stores more than one pint of urine.

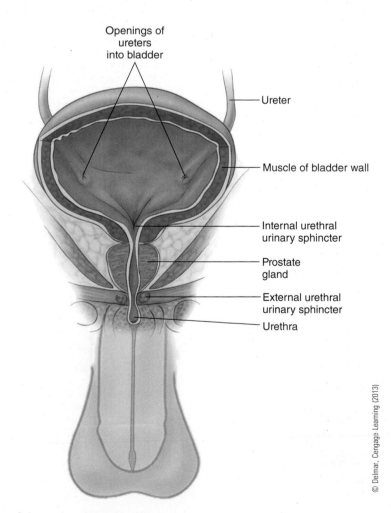

Openings of ureters into bladder

Ureter

Muscle of bladder wall

Internal urethral urinary sphincter

Prostate gland

External urethral urinary sphincter

Urethra

© Delmar, Cengage Learning (2013)

**FIGURE 9.3** The structures of the male urinary bladder.

- Like the stomach, the bladder is lined with *rugae*. These folds allow it to expand when full and contract when empty.

## The Urethra

The **urethra** (you-**REE**-thrah) is the tube extending from the bladder to the exterior of the body. Caution: the spellings of *ureter* and *urethra* are very similar! You may find it helpful to remember that the ureter comes first, both anatomically and alphabetically.

- There are two *urinary sphincters*, one located at either end of the urethra. These muscular rings control the flow of urine from the bladder into the urethra, and out of the urethra through the urethral meatus. A *sphincter* is a ring-like muscle that closes a passageway (Figure 9.3).

- The **urethral meatus** (you-**REE**-thrahl mee-**AY**-tus), also known as the *urinary meatus*, is the external opening of the urethra. The term *meatus* means the external opening of a canal.

- The **female urethra** is approximately 1.5 inches long, and the urethral meatus is located between the clitoris and the opening of the vagina (see Chapter 14). In the female, the urethra conveys only urine.

- The **male urethra** is approximately 8 inches long, and the urethral meatus is located at the tip of the penis (Figure 9.1). This urethra transports both urine and semen.

- The **prostate gland** (**PROS**-tayt), which is part of the male reproductive system, surrounds the urethra (Figure 9.3). Most disorders of the prostate affect the male's ability to urinate. For more information about the role of the prostate gland in reproduction, see Chapter 14.

## ◼ THE EXCRETION OF URINE

**Urination**, also known as *voiding* or *micturition*, is the normal process of excreting urine.

- As the bladder fills up with urine, pressure is placed on the base of the urethra, resulting in the urge to **urinate** or *micturate*.

- Urination requires the coordinated contraction of the bladder muscles and relaxation of the sphincters. This action forces the urine through the urethra and out through the urethral meatus.

**StudyWARE CONNECTION**

Watch the **Urine Formation** animation in the StudyWARE™.

## ◼ MEDICAL SPECIALTIES RELATED TO THE URINARY SYSTEM

- A **nephrologist** (neh-**FROL**-oh-jist) is a physician who specializes in diagnosing and treating diseases and disorders of the kidneys (**nephr** means kidney, and **-ologist** means specialist).

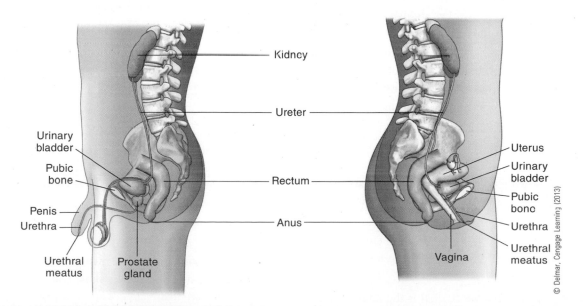

Kidney

Ureter

Urinary bladder

Pubic bone

Penis

Urethra

Urethral meatus

Prostate gland

Rectum

Anus

Uterus

Urinary bladder

Pubic bone

Urethra

Urethral meatus

Vagina

© Delmar, Cengage Learning (2013)

**FIGURE 9.4** Cross sections of the male and female urinary systems.

- A **urologist** (you-**ROL**-oh-jist) is a physician who specializes in diagnosing and treating diseases and disorders of the urinary system of females and the genitourinary system of males (**ur** means urine, and **-ologist** means specialist).

# PATHOLOGY OF THE URINARY SYSTEM

## Nephropathy

The term **nephropathy** (neh-**FROP**-ah-thee) means any disease of the kidney (**nephr/o** means kidney, and **-pathy** means disease). This definition includes both degenerative and inflammatory conditions. *Diabetic nephropathy* is kidney disease resulting from late-stage diabetes mellitus.

## Renal Failure

**Renal failure**, also known as *kidney failure*, is the inability of one or both of the kidneys to perform their functions. The body cannot replace damaged nephrons, and when too many nephrons have been destroyed, the result is kidney failure.

- **Uremia** (you-**REE**-mee-ah), also known as *uremic poisoning*, is a toxic condition resulting from renal failure in which kidney function is compromised and urea and other waste products normally secreted in the urine are retained in the blood (**ur** means urine, and **-emia** means blood condition).

- **Acute renal failure** (ARF) has sudden onset and is characterized by uremia. It can be fatal if not reversed promptly. This condition can be caused by the kidneys not receiving enough blood to filter due to dehydration or a sudden drop in blood volume or blood pressure because of injury, burns, or a severe infection.

- **Chronic kidney disease** (CKD), also known as *chronic renal disease*, or *kidney failure*, is the progressive loss of renal function over months or years. This common condition, which can be life-threatening, may result from diabetes mellitus, hypertension, or a family history of kidney disease.

- The buildup of waste in the blood from chronic kidney disease can be a contributing factor in heart attacks and strokes.

- **End-stage renal disease** (ESRD) is the final stage of chronic kidney disease, and this condition is fatal unless the functions of the failed kidneys are successfully replaced by dialysis, or with a successful kidney transplant.

## Nephrotic Syndrome

*a group of disorder all together*

**Nephrotic syndrome** (neh-**FROT**-ick), also known as *nephrosis*, is a group of conditions in which excessive amounts of protein are lost through the urine. This condition, which is usually caused by damage to the kidney's glomeruli, results in abnormally low levels of protein in the blood (**nephr/o** means kidney, and **-tic** means pertaining to).

- **Edema** (eh-**DEE**-mah) is excessive fluid accumulation in body tissues that can be symptomatic of nephrotic syndrome and other kidney diseases. This swelling can be in the area around the eyes, the abdomen, or the legs and feet.

- **Hyperproteinuria** (high-per-**proh**-tee-in-**YOU**-ree-ah) is the presence of abnormally high concentrations of protein in the *urine* (**hyper-** means excessive, **protein** means protein, and **-uria** means urine).

- **Hypoproteinemia** (high-poh-**proh**-tee-in-**EE**-mee-ah) is the presence of abnormally low concentrations of protein in the *blood* (**hypo-** means deficient or decreased, **protein** means protein, and **-emia** means blood condition). This condition is often associated with hyperproteinuria.

- Causes of nephrotic syndrome include diabetes mellitus, infection, and kidney disorders. *Minimal change disease*, so called because the nephrons look normal under a regular microscope, is the most common cause of nephrotic syndrome in children.

## Additional Kidney Conditions

- **Hydronephrosis** (high-droh-neh-**FROH**-sis) is the dilation (swelling) of one or both kidneys (**hydr/o** means water, **nephr** means kidney, and **-osis** means abnormal condition or disease). This condition can be caused by problems associated with the backing up of urine due to an obstruction such as a nephrolith (kidney stone) or a stricture (narrowing) in the ureter (Figure 9.5).

- **Nephritis** (neh-**FRY**-tis) is an inflammation of the kidney or kidneys (**nephr** means kidney, and **-itis** means inflammation). The most common causes of nephritis are toxins, infection, or an autoimmune disease.

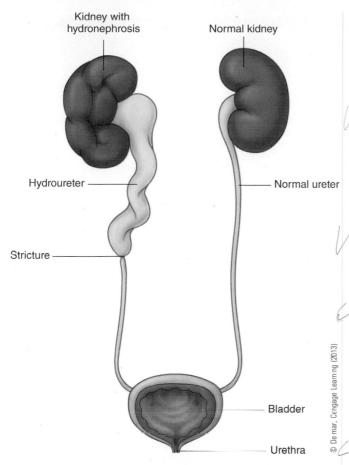

Kidney with hydronephrosis

Normal kidney

Hydroureter

Normal ureter

Stricture

Bladder

Urethra

© Delmar, Cengage Learning (2013)

**FIGURE 9.5** A stricture of the ureter can cause both hydronephrosis and hydroureter.

Pain

■ **Glomerulonephritis** (gloh-**mer**-you-loh-neh-**FRY**-tis) is a type of nephritis caused by inflammation of the glomeruli that causes red blood cells and proteins to leak into the urine (**glomerul/o** means glomeruli, **nephr** means kidney, and **-itis** means inflammation).

■ **Nephroptosis** (**nef**-rop-**TOH**-sis), also known as a *floating kidney*, is the prolapse, or dropping down, of a kidney into the pelvic area when the patient stands. (**nephr/o** means kidney, and **-ptosis** means droop or sag). *Prolapse* means slipping or falling out of place.

■ **Nephropyosis** (**nef**-roh-pye-**OH**-sis), also known as *pyonephrosis*, is suppuration of the kidney (**nephr/o** means kidney, **py** means pus, and **-osis** means abnormal condition or disease). *Suppuration* means the formation or discharge of pus.

■ **Polycystic kidney disease** (PKD) (**pol**-ee-**SIS**-tick) is a genetic disorder characterized by the growth of numerous fluid-filled cysts in the kidneys (**poly-** means many, **cyst** means cyst, and **-ic** means pertaining to). These cysts, which slowly replace much of the mass of the kidney, reduce the kidney function, and this eventually leads to kidney failure (Figure 9.6).

■ **Renal colic** (**REE**-nal **KOLL**-ick) is an acute pain in the kidney area that is caused by blockage during the passage of a nephrolith (kidney stone). *Colic* means spasms of pain in the abdomen. Renal colic pain sometimes comes in waves due to the peristaltic movement of the ureters.

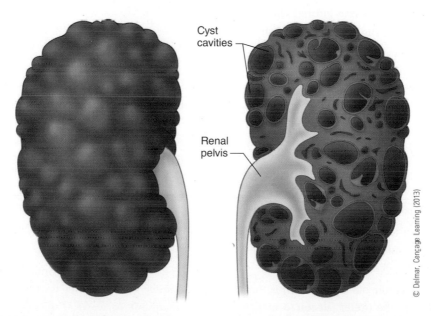

Cyst cavities

Renal pelvis

© Delmar, Cengage Learning (2013)

**FIGURE 9.6** Polycystic kidney disease: On the left is the exterior of a kidney with polycystic disease. On the right is a cross-section view of a kidney with polycystic disease.

■ A **Wilms tumor** is a rare type of malignant tumor of the kidney that occurs in young children. There is a high cure rate for this condition when treated promptly.

## Stones

A **stone**, also known as *calculus*, is an abnormal mineral deposit that has formed within the body and is named for the organ or tissue where it is located (plural, *calculi*). These stones vary in size from small sand-like granules that pass through the body unnoticed to stones the size of marbles that can become lodged, causing acute pain.

■ In the urinary system, stones form when waste products in the urine separate and crystallize (Figure 9.7). Normally urine contains chemicals to prevent this from happening; however, dehydration and other factors may also disrupt this balance.

■ The term **nephrolithiasis** (**nef**-roh-lih-**THIGH**-ah-sis) describes the presence of stones in the kidney (**nephr/o** means kidney, and **-lithiasis** means the presence of stones). As these stones travel with the flow of urine, they are named for the location where they become lodged.

■ A **nephrolith** (**NEF**-roh-lith), also known as a *kidney stone* or a *renal calculus*, is found in the kidney (**nephr/o** means kidney, and **-lith** means stone).

■ A **ureterolith** (you-**REE**-ter-oh-**lith**) is a stone located anywhere along the ureter (**ureter/o** means ureter, and **-lith** means stone).

■ A **cystolith** (**SIS**-toh-lith) is a stone located within the urinary bladder (**cyst/o** means bladder, and **-lith** means stone).

## The Ureters

■ **Hydroureter** (**high**-droh-**YOUR**-eh-ter) is the condition of the distention (swelling) of the ureter with urine that cannot flow because the ureter is blocked (**hydr/o** means water, and **-ureter** means ureter) (Figure 9.5). Hydroureter always accompanies hydronephrosis, discussed earlier.

■ **Ureterectasis** (you-**reh**-ter-**ECK**-tah-sis) is the distention (enlargement) of a ureter (**ureter** means ureter, and **-ectasis** means enlargement).

■ **Ureterorrhagia** (you-**ree**-ter-oh-**RAY**-jee-ah) is the discharge of blood from the ureter (**ureter/o** means ureter, and **-rrhagia** means bleeding).

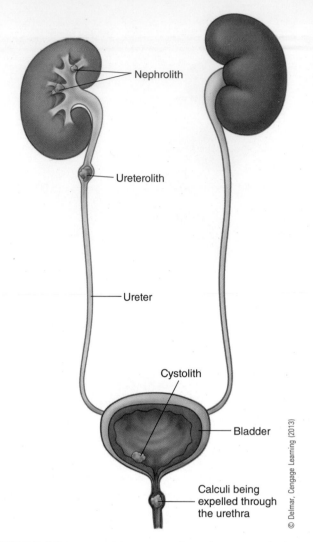

**FIGURE 9.7** Potential locations of renal stones (calculi) as they move through the urinary system.

## The Urinary Bladder

■ **Cystalgia** (sis-**TAL**-jee-ah) and *cystodynia* both mean pain in the bladder (**cyst** means bladder, and **-algia** means pain).

■ A **cystocele** (**SIS**-toh-seel), also known as a *prolapsed bladder*, is a hernia of the bladder through the vaginal wall (**cyst/o** means bladder, and **-cele** means hernia). This sometimes occurs as a result of pregnancy or childbirth.

■ **Interstitial cystitis** (**in**-ter-**STISH**-al sis-**TYE**-tis) is a chronic inflammation within the walls of the bladder. The symptoms of this condition are similar to those of cystitis; however, they do not respond to traditional treatment. *Interstitial* means relating to spaces within a tissue or organ.

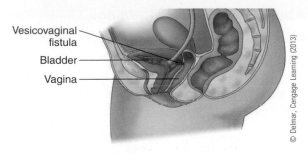

**FIGURE 9.8** A vesicovaginal fistula allows urine to flow into the vagina.

- A **vesicovaginal fistula** (**ves**-ih-koh-**VAJ**-ih-nahl **FIS**-tyou-lah) is an abnormal opening between the bladder and vagina that allows constant involuntary flow of urine from the bladder into the vagina (**vesic/o** means bladder, **vagin** means vagina, and **-al** means pertaining to). A *fistula* is an abnormal passage between two internal organs (Figure 9.8). A vesicovaginal fistula may be caused by prolonged labor during childbirth or surgery such as a hysterectomy.

### Neurogenic Bladder

**Neurogenic bladder** (new-roh-**JEN**-ick) is a urinary problem caused by interference with the normal nerve pathways associated with urination (**neur/o** means nerve, and **-genic** means created by). Normal urinary function depends on nerves to sense when the bladder is full, and to control the muscles that either retain the urine or allow the bladder to empty.

- Depending on the type of neurological disorder causing the problem, the bladder may empty spontaneously, resulting in incontinence, which is discussed in a later section.

- In contrast, the problem can prevent the bladder from emptying at all or from emptying completely. This can result in urinary retention with overflow leakage.

- Some of the causes of this condition are a tumor of the nervous system, trauma, neuropathy, or an inflammatory condition such as multiple sclerosis. *Neuropathy* is any disease or damage to a nerve.

## The Prostate Gland    *increase size*

- **Benign prostatic hyperplasia (BPH)**, (bee-**NINE** pros-**TAT**-ick **high**-per-**PLAY**-zee-ah), also known as *benign prostatic hypertrophy* or *enlarged prostate*, is an enlargement of the prostate gland that most often occurs in men older than age 50 (Figure 9.9). This condition can make urination difficult and causes other urinary tract problems for men. *Hyperplasia* is an increase in cell numbers typically associated with tumor growth; however, in this case, it is not caused by cancer or infection.

- **Prostatism** (**PROS**-tah-tizm) is a disorder resulting from the compression or obstruction of the urethra due to benign prostatic hyperplasia (**prostat** means prostate gland, and **-ism** means condition of). This can produce difficulties with urination and with urinary retention.

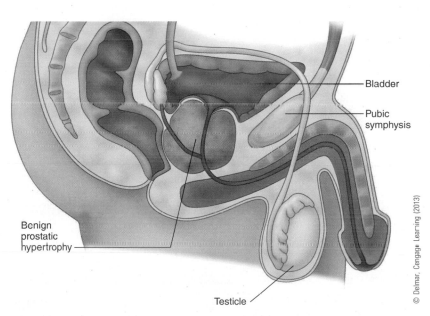

**FIGURE 9.9** In benign prostatic hyperplasia, the enlarged prostate presses against the bladder and slows the flow of urine through the urethra.

- **Prostate cancer** is one of the most common cancers among men. The disease can grow slowly with no symptoms, or it can grow aggressively and spread throughout the body.
- **Prostatitis** (**pros**-tah-**TYE**-tis) is a group of disorders characterized by the inflammation of the prostate gland (**prostat** means prostate gland, and **-itis** means inflammation).
    - The most common type is *chronic nonbacterial prostatitis*, with no single known cause.
    - *Bacterial prostatitis* usually results from bacteria transported in the urine.

## The Urethra

- **Urethrorrhagia** (you-**ree**-throh-**RAY**-jee-ah) is bleeding from the urethra (**urethr/o** means urethra, and **-rrhagia** means bleeding).
- **Urethrorrhea** (you-**ree**-throh-**REE**-ah) is an abnormal discharge from the urethra (**urethr/o** means urethra, and **-rrhea** means flow or discharge). This condition is associated with some sexually transmitted diseases (see Chapter 14).
- **Urethrostenosis** (you-**ree**-throh-steh-**NOH**-sis), or *urethral stricture*, is narrowing of the urethra (**urethr/o** means urethra, and **-stenosis** means tightening or narrowing). This condition occurs almost exclusively in men and is caused by scarring from infection or injury.

## Abnormal Urethral Openings

- **Epispadias** (ep-ih-**SPAY**-dee-as) is a congenital abnormality of the urethral opening. In the male with epispadias, the urethral opening is located on the upper surface of the penis. In the female with epispadias, the urethral opening is in the region of the clitoris.
- **Hypospadias** (**high**-poh-**SPAY**-dee-as) is a congenital abnormality of the urethral opening. In the male with hypospadias, the urethral opening is on the ventral surface (underside) of the penis. In the female with hypospadias, the urethra opens into the vagina.

## Urinary Tract Infections

A **urinary tract infection (UTI)** usually begins in the bladder; however, such an infection can affect all parts of the urinary system. These common infections are caused by bacteria, most often *E. coli*, entering the urinary system through the urethra. They occur more frequently in women because the urethra is short and located near the opening to the rectum.

- **Cystitis** (sis-**TYE**-tis) is an inflammation of the bladder (**cyst** mean bladder, and **-itis** means inflammation) (Figure 9.10A). See also *interstitial cystitis* in the earlier section on the urinary bladder.
- **Pyelitis** (pye-eh-**LYE**-tis) is an inflammation of the renal pelvis (**pyel** means renal pelvis, and **-itis** means inflammation) (Figure 9.10B).

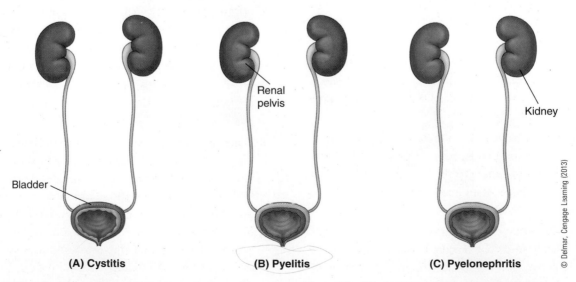

Renal pelvis

Kidney

Bladder

© Delmar, Cengage Learning (2013)

**(A) Cystitis**    **(B) Pyelitis**    **(C) Pyelonephritis**

**FIGURE 9.10** Infections of the urinary tract, indicated in green: (A) cystitis; (B) pyelitis; and (C) pyelonephritis.

- **Pyelonephritis** (pye-eh-loh-neh-**FRY**-tis) is an inflammation of both the renal pelvis and of the kidney (**pyel/o** means renal pelvis, **nephr** means kidney, and **-itis** means inflammation). This is usually caused by a bacterial infection that has spread upward from the bladder (Figure 9.10C).

- **Urethritis** (**you**-reh-**THRIGH**-tis) is an inflammation of the urethra (**urethr** means urethra, and **-itis** means inflammation).

## Urination

- **Anuria** (ah-**NEW**-ree-ah) is the absence of urine formation by the kidneys (**an-** means without, and **-uria** means urine). This condition is often caused by a failure in kidney function, or a urinary tract obstruction.

- **Diuresis** (dye-you-**REE**-sis) is the increased output of urine (**diur** means increasing the output of urine, and **-esis** means an abnormal condition).

- **Dysuria** (dis-**YOU**-ree-ah) is difficult, or painful urination (**dys-** means painful, and **-uria** means urination). This condition is frequently associated with urinary tract infections.

- **Enuresis** (en-you-**REE**-sis) is the involuntary discharge of urine (**en-** means into, and **-uresis** means urination).

- **Nocturnal enuresis** (nock-**TER**-nal **en**-you-**REE**-sis) is urinary incontinence during sleep. It is also known as *bed-wetting*. *Nocturnal* means pertaining to night.

- **Nocturia** (nock-**TOO**-ree-ah) is frequent and excessive urination during the night (**noct** means night, and **-uria** means urination).

- **Oliguria** (ol-ih-**GOO**-ree-ah) means scanty urination (**olig** means scanty, and **-uria** means urination). This can be caused by dehydration, renal failure, or a urinary tract obstruction. Oliguria is the opposite of polyuria.

- **Polyuria** (pol-ee-**YOU**-ree-ah) means excessive urination and is a common symptom of diabetes (**poly-** means many, and **-uria** means urination). Polyuria is the opposite of oliguria.

- **Urinary hesitancy** is difficulty in starting a urinary stream. This condition is most common in older men with enlarged prostate glands. In younger people, the inability to urinate when another person is present is known as *bashful bladder syndrome*.

- **Urinary retention**, also known as *ischuria*, is the inability to completely empty the bladder when attempting to urinate. This condition is also more common in men and is frequently associated with an enlarged prostate gland.

## Incontinence

**Incontinence** (in-**KON**-tih-nents) is the inability to control the excretion of urine, feces, or both.

- **Urinary incontinence** is the inability to control the voiding of urine.

- **Overflow incontinence** is continuous leaking from the bladder either because it is full or because it does not empty completely. It is usually caused by a blocked urethra and is prevalent in older men with enlarged prostates.

- **Stress incontinence** is the inability to control the voiding of urine under physical stress such as running, lifting, sneezing, laughing, or coughing. This condition occurs much more often in women than in men.

- **Overactive bladder** (OAB), also known as *urge incontinence*, occurs when the muscles of the bladder contract involuntarily even though the bladder is not actually full enough to indicate the need to urinate. The urinary sphincters' relaxation in response to this urgent need to urinate may result in urinary frequency or accidental urination. This is a common condition in adults older than 40 and may be caused by excessive consumption of caffeine or alcohol, urinary tract infections, neurological diseases, or bladder or prostate problems.

## ■ DIAGNOSTIC PROCEDURES OF THE URINARY SYSTEM

- **Urinalysis** (**you**-rih-**NAL**-ih-sis) is the examination of urine to determine the presence of abnormal elements (**urin** means urine, and **-analysis** means a study of the parts). These tests, which are used to diagnose diseases as well as to detect the presence of substances such as illegal drugs, are discussed further in Chapter 15.

- A **bladder ultrasound** is the use of a handheld ultrasound transducer to look for stones or for elevation of the bladder by an enlarged prostate, and to measure the residual amount of urine remaining in the bladder after urination. A normal bladder holds between 300 and 400 mL of urine. When more than this amount is still present after urination, the bladder is described as being *distended*, or enlarged.

■ **Urinary catheterization** (**kath**-eh-ter-eye-**ZAY**-shun) is the insertion of a tube into the bladder to procure a sterile specimen for diagnostic purposes. It is also used to drain urine from the bladder when the patient is unable to urinate for other reasons. Another use is to place medication into the bladder. (See the later section "Treatment Procedures for the Urinary Bladder.")

■ **Cystoscopy** (sis-**TOS**-koh-pee) is the visual examination of the urinary bladder with the use of a specialized type of endoscope known as a cystoscope (**cyst/o** means bladder, and **-scopy** means visual examination) (Figure 9.11). An *endoscope* is an instrument used for visual examination of internal structures. A specialized cystoscope is also used for treatment procedures such as the removal of tumors or the reduction of an enlarged prostate gland.

■ **Voiding cystourethrography** (**sis**-toh-you-ree-**THROG**-rah-fee) is a diagnostic procedure in which a fluoroscope is used to examine the flow of urine from the bladder and through the urethra (**cyst/o** means bladder, **urethr/o** means urethra, and **-graphy** means the process of producing a picture or record). This procedure is often performed after cystography.

■ **Computed tomography**, also known as a *CAT scan*, is more commonly used as a primary tool for evaluation of the urinary system because it can be rapidly performed and provides additional imaging of the abdomen, which may reveal other potential sources for the patient's symptoms. *Nephrotomography* is the use of a CAT scan to examine the kidneys.

**StudyWARE CONNECTION**

Watch the **Cystoscopy** animation in the StudyWARE™.

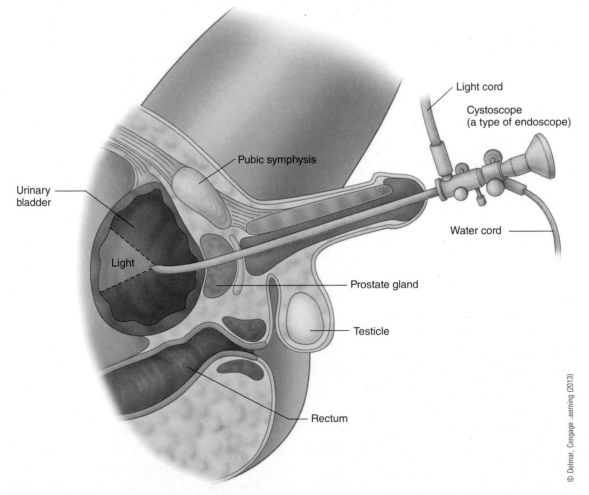

Light cord

Cystoscope (a type of endoscope)

Pubic symphysis

Urinary bladder

Light

Water cord

Prostate gland

Testicle

Rectum

© Delmar, Cengage Learning (2013)

**FIGURE 9.11** Use of a cystoscope to examine the interior of the bladder in a male.

## Radiographic Examinations of the Urinary System

- **Cystography** (sis-**TOG**-rah-fee) is a radiographic, or x-ray, examination of the bladder after a contrast medium is instilled via a urethral catheter (**cyst/o** means bladder, and **-graphy** means the process of creating a picture or record). The resulting film is a *cystogram*.

- An **intravenous pyelogram** (**in**-trah-**VEE**-nus **PYE**-eh-loh-**gram**) (IVP), also known as *excretory urography*, is a radiographic study of the kidneys and ureters (**pyel/o** means renal pelvis, and **-gram** means a picture or record). A contrast medium is administered intravenously to clearly define these structures in the resulting image. This examination is used to diagnose changes in the urinary tract resulting from nephroliths, infections, enlarged prostate, tumors, and internal injuries after an abdominal trauma (Figure 9.12).

- A **KUB** (Kidneys, Ureters, Bladder) is a radiographic study without the use of a contrast medium. This study, also referred to as a *flat-plate of the abdomen*, is used to detect bowel obstructions and nephroliths. Despite its name, a KUB x-ray does not show the ureters.

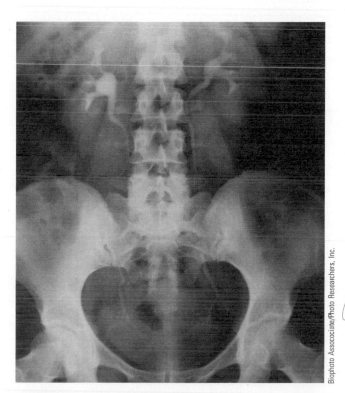

**FIGURE 9.12** This normal, intravenous pyelogram shows the urinary tract, including the ureters, a kidney, and the bladder.

- **Retrograde urography** is a radiograph of the urinary system taken after a contrast medium has been placed in the urethra through a sterile catheter and caused to flow upward through the urinary tract (**ur/o** means urine, and **-graphy** means the process of creating a picture or record). *Retrograde* means moving backward.

## Diagnostic Procedures of the Prostate Gland

- A **digital rectal examination** is performed on men by using a lubricated, gloved finger placed in the rectum to palpate the prostate gland to detect prostate enlargement and to look for indications of prostate cancer or tumors of the rectum. In this context, the term *digital* means using a finger. *Palpate* means the use of touch to examine a body part.

- The **prostate-specific antigen (PSA)** blood test is used to screen for prostate cancer. This test measures the amount of prostate-specific antigen that is present in a blood specimen. The *prostate-specific antigen* is a protein produced by the cells of the prostate gland to help liquefy semen. The higher a man's PSA level, the more likely cancer is present.

## ■ TREATMENT PROCEDURES OF THE URINARY SYSTEM

### Medications

- **Diuretics** (**dye**-you-**RET**-icks) are medications administered to increase urine secretion, primarily to rid the body of excess water and salt. Some foods and drinks, such as coffee, tea, and alcoholic beverages, also have a diuretic effect.

- Other drugs used to treat urinary tract problems include *antibiotics* for urinary tract infections and *antispasmodics* to block the signals that cause urinary incontinence.

### Dialysis

**Dialysis** (dye-**AL**-ih-sis) is a procedure to remove waste products, such as urea, creatinine, as well as excess water from the blood of a patient whose kidneys no longer function (**dia-** means complete or through, and **-lysis** means separation). The two types of dialysis in common use are *hemodialysis* and *peritoneal dialysis*. Patients can sometimes choose the type of long-term dialysis they prefer.

Biophoto Associate/Photo Researchers, Inc.

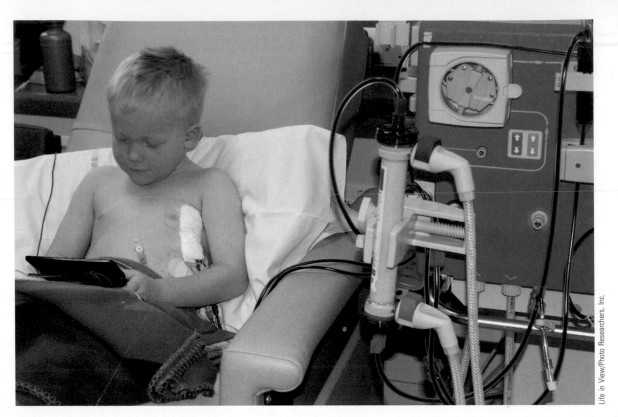

Life in View/Photo Researchers, Inc.

**FIGURE 9.13** In a hemodialysis unit, waste is filtered from the patient's blood. The filtered blood is then returned to the patient's body.

## Hemodialysis

**Hemodialysis** (**hee**-moh-dye-**AL**-ih-sis) is the process by which waste products are filtered directly from the patient's blood (**hem/o** means blood, **dia** means complete or through, and **-lysis** means separation). Treatment is performed on an external hemodialysis unit commonly referred to as an *artificial kidney* (Figure 9.13). Hemodialysis is the most common type of dialysis.

- A shunt implanted in the patient's arm is connected to the hemodialysis unit, and arterial blood flows through the filters of the unit. A *shunt* is an artificial passage that allows the blood to flow between the body and the hemodialysis unit.

- The filters contain *dialysate*, which is a sterilized solution made up of water and electrolytes. This solution cleanses the blood by removing waste products and excess fluids.

- *Electrolytes* are the salts that conduct electricity and are found in the body fluid, tissue, and blood.

- The cleansed blood is returned to the body through a vein.

- These treatments each take several hours and must be repeated about three times a week.

## Peritoneal Dialysis

In **peritoneal dialysis** (**pehr**-ih-toh-**NEE**-al dye-**AL**-ih-sis) the lining of the peritoneal cavity acts as the filter to remove waste from the blood. The dialysate, which is a sterile solution containing glucose, flows into the peritoneal cavity around the intestine through a catheter implanted in the abdominal wall. This fluid is left in for a period of time to absorb waste products and then drained out through the tube.

The process is normally repeated several times during the day and can be done using an automated system. This type of dialysis has some advantages: for example, it can be done at home by the patient. However, it is considered less effective than hemodialysis (Figure 9.14).

- *Continuous ambulatory peritoneal dialysis* provides ongoing dialysis as the patient goes about his or her daily activities. In this procedure, a dialysate solution is instilled from a plastic container worn under the patient's clothing. About every 4 hours, the used solution is drained back into this bag and the bag is discarded. A new bag is then attached, the solution is instilled, and the process continues.

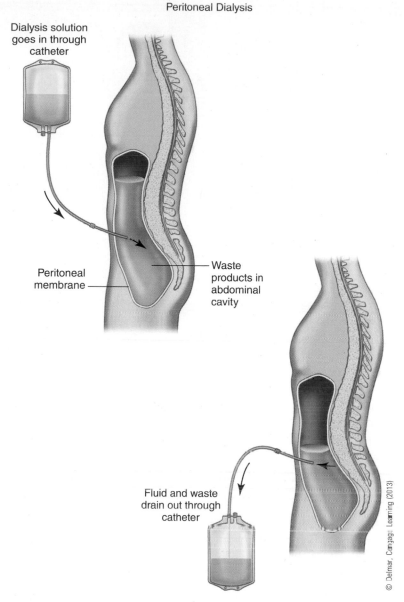

Peritoneal Dialysis

Dialysis solution goes in through catheter

Peritoneal membrane

Waste products in abdominal cavity

Fluid and waste drain out through catheter

© Delmar, Cengage Learning (2013)

**FIGURE 9.14** Peritoneal dialysis removes waste through a fluid exchange in the peritoneal cavity.

■ *Continuous cycling peritoneal dialysis* uses a machine to cycle the dialysate fluid during the night while the patient sleeps.

## The Kidneys

■ **Nephrolysis** (neh-**FROL**-ih-sis) is the surgical freeing of a kidney from adhesions (**nephr/o** means kidney, and **-lysis** means setting free). An *adhesion* is a band of fibers that holds structures together abnormally.

■ Note: The suffix **-lysis** means setting free; however, it also means destruction. Therefore, the term *nephrolysis* can also describe a pathologic condition in which there is destruction of renal cells.

■ A **nephropexy** (**NEF**-roh-**peck**-see), also known as *nephrorrhaphy*, is the surgical fixation of nephroptosis, or a floating kidney (**nephr/o** means kidney, and **-pexy** means surgical fixation).

■ A **nephrostomy** (neh-**FROS**-toh-mee) is the placement of a catheter to maintain an opening from the pelvis of one or both kidneys to the exterior of the body (**nephr** means kidney, and **-ostomy** means creating an opening). In a kidney affected by hydronephrosis, this allows urine from the kidney to be drained directly through the lower back. Nephrostomy tubes are also used to gain access to the kidneys for diagnostic procedures.

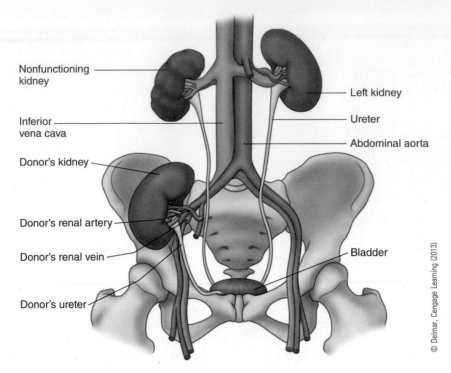

Nonfunctioning kidney

Inferior vena cava

Donor's kidney

Donor's renal artery

Donor's renal vein

Donor's ureter

Left kidney

Ureter

Abdominal aorta

Bladder

© Delmar, Cengage Learning (2013)

**FIGURE 9.15** In a kidney transplant, the nonfunctioning kidney is usually not removed. Instead, the donor kidney and its associated structures are sutured into place at a lower point in the abdomen.

■ **Pyeloplasty** (**PYE**-eh-loh-**plas**-tee) is the surgical repair of the ureter and renal pelvis (**pyel/o** means the renal pelvis, and -**plasty** means surgical repair). Hydronephrosis can cause damage to the ureter and renal pelvis.

■ A **pyelotomy** (pye-eh-**LOT**-oh-mee) is a surgical incision into the renal pelvis (**pyel** means the renal pelvis, and -**otomy** means surgical incision). This procedure is performed to correct obstructions such as a stone lodged in the junction between the renal pelvis and the ureter.

■ **Renal transplantation**, commonly known as a *kidney transplant*, is the grafting of a donor kidney, from either a living or nonliving donor, into the body to replace the recipient's failed kidneys. Kidney donors need to be genetically similar to the recipient, although a tissue match increases the success rate. A single transplanted kidney is capable of adequately performing all kidney functions and frees the patient from the need for dialysis (Figure 9.15).

## Treatment of Nephroliths

Most small nephroliths (kidney stones) pass out of the urinary tract naturally over a period of two days to three weeks. This process can be quite painful and is sometimes accompanied by vomiting due to the pain. Larger stones may require surgical intervention.

■ **Extracorporeal shockwave lithotripsy** (**ecks**-trah-kor-**POUR**-ee-al **LITH**-oh-**trip**-see) (ESWL) is the most common kidney stone treatment (**lith/o** means stone, and -**tripsy** means to crush). High-energy ultrasonic waves traveling through water or gel are used to break up the stone into fragments, which are then excreted in the urine. *Extracorporeal* means situated or occurring outside the body (Figure 9.16).

■ Lithotripsy is also used to break up calculi in the ureter, bladder, or urethra.

■ A **percutaneous nephrolithotomy** (**per**-kyou-**TAY**-nee-us **nef**-roh-lih-**THOT**-oh-mee) is the surgical removal of a nephrolith through a small incision in the back (**nephr/o** means kidney, **lith** means stone, and -**otomy** means surgical incision). A small tube is temporarily inserted through the incision into the kidney. First urine is removed; then the stone is crushed and the pieces are removed. This procedure is used if ESWL has not been successful, if an infection is present, or if the stone is particularly large. *Percutaneous* means performed through the skin.

## The Ureters

■ A **ureterectomy** (**you**-reh-ter-**ECK**-toh-mee) is the surgical removal of a ureter (**ureter** means ureter, and -**ectomy** means surgical removal).

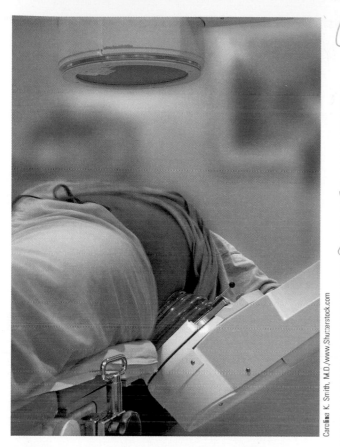

**FIGURE 9.16** Extracorporeal shockwave lithotripsy uses shock waves traveling through water or a gel to destroy kidney stones.

- **Ureteroplasty** (you-**REET**-er-oh-**plas**-tee) is the surgical repair of a ureter (**ureter/o** means ureter, and **-plasty** means surgical repair).

- **Ureterorrhaphy** (you-**reet**-eh-**ROAR**-ah-fee) is the surgical suturing of a ureter (**ureter/o** means ureter, and **-rrhaphy** means surgical suturing).

- **Ureteroscopy** (you-**reet**-eh-**ROS**-koh-pee) is a treatment for a nephrolith lodged in the ureter (**ureter/o** means ureter, and **-scopy** means visual examination). A specialized instrument called a *ureteroscope* is inserted through the urethra and bladder into the ureter. If possible, the nephrolith is removed intact through the scope. If the stone is too large, a laser is used to break it up and the pieces are then removed.

## The Urinary Bladder

- A **cystectomy** (sis-**TECK**-toh-mee) is the surgical removal of all or part of the urinary bladder. This procedure is usually performed to treat bladder cancer (**cyst** means bladder, and **-ectomy** means surgical removal).

- A **neobladder** (**NEE**-oh-**blad**-er) is a replacement for the missing bladder created by using about 20 inches of the small intestine. It allows patients to avoid having an abdominal stoma.

- An **ileal conduit** (**ill**-ee-al **KON**-doo-it), or *ileostomy*, is the use of a small piece of intestine to convey urine to the ureters and to a stoma in the abdomen (**ile** means ileum or small intestine, and **-al** means pertaining to).

- **Cystopexy** (**sis**-toh-**peck**-see) is the surgical fixation of the bladder to the abdominal wall (**cyst/o** means bladder, and **-pexy** means surgical fixation).

- **Cystorrhaphy** (sis-**TOR**-ah-fee) is the surgical suturing of a wound or defect in the bladder (**cyst/o** means bladder, and **-rrhaphy** means surgical suturing).

- A **lithotomy** (lih-**THOT**-oh-mee) is a surgical incision for the removal of a nephrolith from the bladder (**lith** means stone, and **-otomy** means surgical incision). Although this surgery is no longer common, its name is still used to describe a physical examination position for procedures involving the pelvis and lower abdomen (see Chapter 15).

## Urinary Catheterization

**Urinary catheterization**, also known as *cathing*, is performed to withdraw urine for diagnostic purposes, to allow urine to drain freely, or to place a fluid such as a chemotherapy solution into the bladder (Figure 9.16). Note that the term *catheterization* may also refer to inserting a tube into the heart (see Chapter 5).

- An **indwelling catheter** remains inside the body for a prolonged time based on need (Figure 9.17A). *Indwelling* means residing within. This can be either a urethral or a suprapubic catheter.

- **Urethral catheterization** is performed by inserting a plastic tube called a *catheter* though the urethra and into the bladder.

- **Suprapubic catheterization** (soo-prah-**PYOU**-bick **kath**-eh-ter-eye-**ZAY**-shun) is the placement of a catheter into the bladder through a small incision made through the abdominal wall just above the pubic bone (Figure 9.17B).

- A **Foley catheter** is the most common type of indwelling catheter. This device is made of a flexible tube with a balloon filled with sterile water at the end to hold it in place in the bladder. It is commonly used on postsurgical patients.

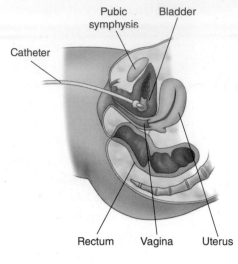

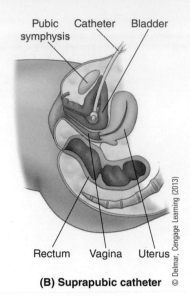

**(A) Indwelling catheter**    **(B) Suprapubic catheter**

© Delmar, Cengage Learning (2013)

**FIGURE 9.17** Types of urinary catheterization.

■ An **intermittent catheter**, also known as a *short-term catheter*, is inserted as needed several times a day to drain urine from the bladder.

## The Urethra

■ A **meatotomy** (**mee**-ah-**TOT**-oh-mee) is a surgical incision made in the urethral meatus to enlarge the opening (**meat** means meatus, and **-otomy** means surgical incision).

■ **Urethropexy** (you-**REE**-throh-**peck**-see) is the surgical fixation of the urethra to nearby tissue (**urethr/o** means urethra, and **-pexy** means surgical fixation). This procedure is usually performed to correct urinary stress incontinence.

■ A **urethrotomy** (**you**-reh-**THROT**-oh-mee) is a surgical incision into the urethra for relief of a stricture (**urethr** means urethra, and **-otomy** means surgical incision). A *stricture* is an abnormal narrowing of a bodily passage.

## Prostate Treatment

■ **Ablation** (ab-**LAY**-shun) is the term used to describe some types of treatment of prostate cancer. This treatment involves the removal of a body part or the destruction of its function through the use of surgery, hormones, drugs, heat, chemicals, electrocautery, or other methods. *Electrocautery* is the use of high-frequency electrical current to destroy tissue.

■ A **prostatectomy** (**pros**-tah-**TECK**-toh-mee) is the surgical removal of part or all of the prostate gland (**prostat** means prostate, and **-ectomy** means surgical removal). This procedure is performed to treat prostate cancer or to reduce an enlarged prostate gland; however, this treatment can lead to erectile difficulties.

■ A *radical prostatectomy* is the surgical removal of the entire prostate gland in cases where it is extremely enlarged or when cancer is suspected.

■ A **transurethral prostatectomy**, also known as a *TURP*, is the removal of excess tissue from an enlarged prostate gland with the use of a resectoscope. A *resectoscope* is a specialized endoscopic instrument that resembles a cystoscope (Figure 9.18).

■ **Retrograde ejaculation** is when an orgasm results in semen flowing backward into the bladder instead of out through the penis. This is a common side effect of the transurethral prostatectomy. *Retrograde* means moving backward.

■ *Radiation therapy* and *hormone therapy* are additional treatments used to control prostate cancer. *Watchful waiting* is often the prescribed course of action in older patients because this disease normally progresses slowly.

## Urinary Incontinence Treatment

■ **Kegel exercises**, which were named for Dr. Arnold Kegel, are a series of pelvic muscle exercises used to strengthen the muscles of the pelvic floor. They are used to control urinary stress incontinence in both sexes, in men to treat prostate pain and swelling, and in women to condition the muscles so that they will recover quickly after childbirth.

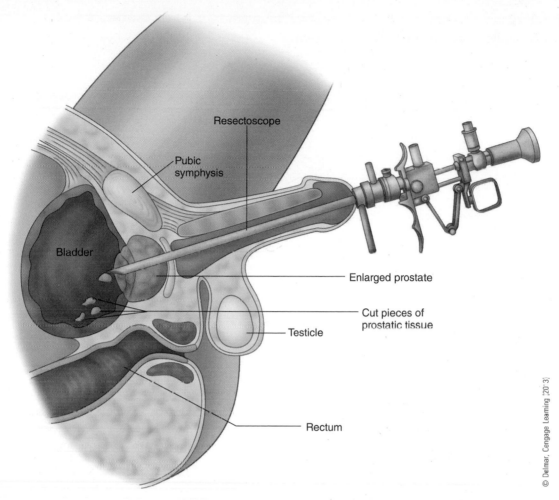

Resectoscope

Pubic
symphysis

Bladder

Enlarged prostate

Cut pieces of
prostatic tissue

Testicle

Rectum

© Delmar, Cengage Learning '20 '3)

**FIGURE 9.18** A transurethral prostatectomy (TURP) being performed with the use of a resectoscope.

■ **Bladder retraining** is behavioral therapy in which the patient learns to urinate on a schedule, with increasingly longer time intervals as the bladder increases its capacity. The goal is to reestablish voluntary bladder control and to break the cycle of frequency and urgency that results from urge incontinence.

# ■ ABBREVIATIONS RELATED TO THE URINARY SYSTEM

Table 9.1 presents an overview of the abbreviations related to the terms introduced in this chapter. Note: To avoid errors or confusion, always be cautious when using abbreviations.

## TABLE 9.1
## Abbreviations Related to the Urinary System

| | |
|---|---|
| **acute renal failure** = ARF | **ARF** = acute renal failure |
| **benign prostatic hyperplasia** = BPH | **BPH** = benign prostatic hyperplasia |
| **catheterization** = cath | **cath** = catheterization |
| **chronic kidney disease** = CKD | **CKD** = chronic kidney disease |
| **cystoscopy** = cysto | **cysto** = cystoscopy |
| **digital rectal examination** = DRE | **DRE** = digital rectal examination |
| **end-stage renal disease** = ESRD | **ESRD** = end-stage renal disease |
| **intravenous pyelogram** = IVP | **IVP** = intravenous pyelogram |
| **polycystic kidney disease** = PKD | **PKD** = polycystic kidney disease |
| **transurethral resection of the prostate** = TURP | **TURP** = transurethral resection of the prostate |
| **urinary tract infection** = UTI | **UTI** = urinary tract infection |

**StudyWARE CONNECTION**

For more practice and to test your mastery of this material, go to the StudyWARE™ to play interactive games and complete the quiz for this chapter.

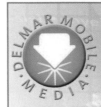

Downloadable audio is available for selected medical terms in this chapter to enhance your learning of medical terminology.

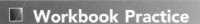

## ☐ Workbook Practice

Go to your workbook, and complete the exercises for this chapter.

## MATCHING WORD PARTS 1

Write the correct answer in the middle column.

| Definition | | Correct Answer | Possible Answers |
|---|---|---|---|
| 9.1. | bladder | _____ | -cele |
| 9.2. | glomerulus | _____ | cyst/o |
| 9.3. | hernia, tumor, cyst | _____ | glomerul/o |
| 9.4. | kidney | _____ | lith/o |
| 9.5. | stone, calculus | _____ | nephr/o |

## MATCHING WORD PARTS 2

Write the correct answer in the middle column.

| Definition | | Correct Answer | Possible Answers |
|---|---|---|---|
| 9.6. | urine, urinary tract | _ur/o_ | -tripsy |
| 9.7. | renal pelvis | _pyel/o_ | pyel/o |
| 9.8. | setting free, separation | _-lysis_ | -ur/o |
| 9.9. | surgical fixation | _pexy_ | -pexy |
| 9.10. | to crush | _tripsy_ | -lysis |

## MATCHING WORD PARTS 3

Write the correct answer in the middle column.

| Definition | | Correct Answer | Possible Answers |
|---|---|---|---|
| 9.11. | complete, through | _dia-_ | -uria |
| 9.12. | enlargement, stretching | _-ectasis_ | urethr/o |

9.13.   ureter          _____ureter_____          **ureter/o**

9.14.   urethra          _____urethr/o_____          **-ectasis**

9.15.   urination, urine          _____uria_____          **dia-**

## DEFINITIONS

Select the correct answer, and write it on the line provided.

9.16.   Urine is carried from the kidneys to the urinary bladder by the _____.

glomeruli          nephrons          urethras          (ureters)

9.17.   A stone in the urinary bladder is known as a _____.

cholelith          (cystolith)          nephrolith          ureterolith

9.18.   The increased output of urine is known as _____.

anuria          (diuresis)          dysuria          oliguria

9.19.   Before entering the ureters, urine collects in the _____.

glomeruli          renal cortex          (renal pelvis)          urinary bladder

9.20.   Urine leaves the bladder through the _____.

prostate          kidney          ureter          (urethra)

9.21.   Urine is produced in microscopic functional units of each kidney called _____.

uremia          ~~ureters~~          urethra          (nephrons)

9.22.   In the male, the _____ carries both urine and semen.

prostate gland          renal pelvis          ureter          (urethra)

9.23.   A specialist who treats the genitourinary system of males is a/an _____.

gynecologist          nephrologist          neurologist          (urologist)

9.24.   In _____, the urethral opening is on the upper surface of the penis.

(epispadias)          hyperspadias          hypospadias          ~~urethritis~~

9.25.   The term _____ describes treatment in which a body part is removed or its

function is destroyed. This type of procedure is frequently used to treat prostate cancer.

(ablation)          adhesion          lithotomy          meatotomy

## MATCHING STRUCTURES

Write the correct answer in the middle column.

| Definition | Correct Answer | Possible Answers |
|---|---|---|
| 9.26. the opening through which urine leaves the body | _____ | urethral meatus |
| 9.27. the portion of a nephron that is active in filtering urine | _____ | urethra |
| 9.28. the outer region of the kidney | _____ | ureters |
| 9.29. the tube from the bladder to the outside of the body | _____ | renal cortex |
| 9.30. the tubes that carry urine from the kidney to the bladder | _____ | glomerulus |

## WHICH WORD?

Select the correct answer, and write it on the line provided.

9.31.   A surgical incision into the renal pelvis is _____.

pyelotomy          pyeloplasty

9.32.   The discharge of blood from the ureter is _____.

ureterorrhagia          urethrorrhagia

9.33.   The term meaning excessive urination is _____.

incontinence          polyuria

9.34.   The term meaning inflammation of the bladder is _____.

cystitis          pyelitis

9.35.   The major waste product of protein metabolism is _____.

urea          urine

## SPELLING COUNTS

Find the misspelled word in each sentence. Then write that word, spelled correctly, on the line provided.

9.36.   A Willms tumor is a malignant tumor of the kidney that occurs in children. _____

9.37.   Being unable to control excretory functions is known as incontinance. _____

9.38.   The process of withdrawing urine from the bladder is known as urinary

cathaterization. _____

9.39.   Keagel exercises are a series of pelvic muscle exercises used to strengthen the muscles of the pelvic floor

to control urinary stress incontinence. _____

9.40.   A vesicovaginel fistula is an abnormal opening between the bladder and

vagina. _____

## ABBREVIATION IDENTIFICATION

In the space provided, write the words that each abbreviation stands for.

9.41.   **BPH** _____

9.42.   **ESRD** _____

9.43.   **ESWL** _____

9.44.   **IVP** _____

9.45.   **OAB** _____

## TERM SELECTION

Select the correct answer, and write it on the line provided.

9.46.   The absence of urine formation by the kidneys is known as _____.

      anuria        nocturia        oliguria        polyuria

9.47.   The surgical suturing of the bladder is known as _____.

      cystorrhaphy        cystorrhagia        cystorrhexis        nephrorrhaphy

9.48.   The term meaning the freeing of a kidney from adhesions is _____.

      nephrolithiasis        nephrolysis        anuria        pyelitis

9.49.   The term meaning scanty urination is _____.

      diuresis        dysuria        enuresis        oliguria

9.50.    The process of artificially filtering waste products from the patient's blood is known

as _____.

         diuresis            hemodialysis          homeostasis          hydroureter

## SENTENCE COMPLETION

Write the correct term or terms on the lines provided.

9.51.    An inflammation of the kidney, most commonly caused by toxins, infection, or an autoimmune disease is

called _____.

9.52.    A stone located anywhere along the ureter is known as a _____.

9.53.    The placement of a catheter into the bladder through a small incision made through the abdominal wall

just above the pubic bone is known as _____.

9.54.    The surgical fixation of the bladder to the abdominal wall is a/an _____.

9.55.    A/An _____ (TURP) is the removal of excess tissue from the prostate with the use

of a resectoscope.

## WORD SURGERY

Divide each term into its component word parts. Write these word parts, in sequence, on the lines provided.
When necessary, use a slash (/) to indicate a combining vowel. (You may not need all of the lines provided.)

9.56.    **Hyperproteinuria** is abnormally high concentrations of protein in the urine.

_____  _____  _____  _____

9.57.    **Hydronephrosis** is the dilation of one or both kidneys.

_____  _____  _____  _____

9.58.    Voiding **cystourethrography** is a diagnostic procedure in which a fluoroscope is used to examine the

flow of urine from the bladder and through the urethra.

_____  _____  _____  _____

9.59.    A percutaneous **nephrolithotomy** is the surgical removal of a kidney stone through a small incision in

the back.

_____  _____  _____  _____

9.60.    **Ureterorrhaphy** means the surgical suturing of a ureter.

_____  _____  _____  _____

## TRUE/FALSE

If the statement is true, write **True** on the line. If the statement is false, write **False** on the line.

9.61. _____ Stress incontinence is the inability to control the voiding of urine under physical stress such as

running, sneezing, laughing, or coughing.

9.62. _____ Prostatism is a malignancy of the prostate gland.

9.63. _____ Urethrorrhea is bleeding from the urethra.

9.64. _____ Renal colic is an acute pain in the kidney area that is caused by blockage during the passage of

a kidney stone.

9.65. _____ Acute renal failure has sudden onset and is characterized by uremia.

## CLINICAL CONDITIONS

Write the correct answer on the line provided.

9.66. Mr. Baldridge suffers from excessive urination during the night. The medical term for

this is _____.

9.67. Rosita LaPinta inherited _____ kidney disease. These cysts slowly reduce the

kidney function, and this eventually leads to kidney failure.

9.68. Doris Volk has a chronic bladder condition involving inflammation within the wall of the bladder. This is

known as _____.

9.69. John Danielson has an enlarged prostate gland. This caused narrowing of the urethra, which is known

as _____.

9.70. Norman Smith was born with the opening of the urethra on the upper surface of the penis. This is

known as _____.

9.71. Henry Wong's kidneys failed. He is being treated with _____

_____, which involves the removal of waste from his blood through a fluid

exchange in the abdominal cavity.

9.72. Roberta Gridley is scheduled for surgical repair of damage to the ureter. This procedure is

a/an _____.

9.73. When Lenny Nowicki's _____ blood test showed a very high PSA level, his physician was concerned about the possibility of prostate cancer.

9.74. Dr. Morita's patient was diagnosed as having _____. This is a type of kidney disease caused by inflammation of the glomeruli that causes red blood cells and proteins to leak into the urine.

9.75. Mrs. Franklin describes her condition as a floating kidney. The medical term for this condition, in which there is a dropping down of the kidney, is _____.

## WHICH IS THE CORRECT MEDICAL TERM?

Select the correct answer, and write it on the line provided.

9.76. Acute renal failure has sudden onset and is characterized by _____. This condition can be caused by many factors, including a sudden drop in blood volume or blood pressure due to injury or surgery.

      anuria        dysuria        enuresis        uremia

9.77. The term _____ means urinary incontinence during sleep. It is also known as bed-wetting.

      nocturnal enuresis    overactive bladder    stress incontinence    urinary incontinence

9.78. The term meaning the distention of the ureter is _____.

      ureteritis      ureterectasis      ureterolith      urethrostenosis

9.79. The presence of abnormally *low* concentrations of protein in the blood is known as _____.

      hyperplasia      hyperproteinuria      hypocalcemia      hypoproteinemia

9.80. A specialist in diagnosing and treating diseases and disorders of the kidneys is a/an _____.

      gynecologist      nephrologist      proctologist      urologist

## CHALLENGE WORD BUILDING

These terms are *not* found in this chapter; however, they are made up of the following familiar word parts. If you need help in creating the term, refer to your medical dictionary.

| | |
|---|---|
| cyst/o | -cele |
| nephr/o | -itis |
| pyel/o | -lysis |
| ureter/o | -malacia |
| urethr/o | -ostomy |
| | -otomy |
| | -plasty |
| | -ptosis |
| | -rrhexis |
| | -sclerosis |

9.81.  The creation of an artificial opening between the urinary bladder and the exterior of the body is

a/an _____.

9.82.  A surgical incision into the kidney is a/an _____.

9.83.  Abnormal hardening of the kidney is known as _____.

9.84.  Prolapse of the bladder into the urethra is known as _____.

9.85.  A prolapse of the female urethra is a/an _____.

9.86.  The procedure to separate adhesions around a ureter is a/an _____.

9.87.  Abnormal softening of the kidney is known as _____.

9.88.  Inflammation of the renal pelvis and kidney is known as _____.

9.89.  The surgical creation of an outside excretory opening from the urethra is

a/an _____.

9.90.  The surgical repair of the bladder is a/an _____.

## LABELING EXERCISES

Identify the numbered items on the accompanying figure.

9.91. ___Adrenal___ gland

9.92. exterior view of the right ___kidney___

9.93. inferior ___vena cava___

9.94. ___Urethra___

9.95. renal ___Cortex___

9.96. renal ___medulla___

9.97. abdominal ___aorta___

9.98. right and left ___ureters___

9.99. urinary ___bladder___

9.100. urethral ___meatus___

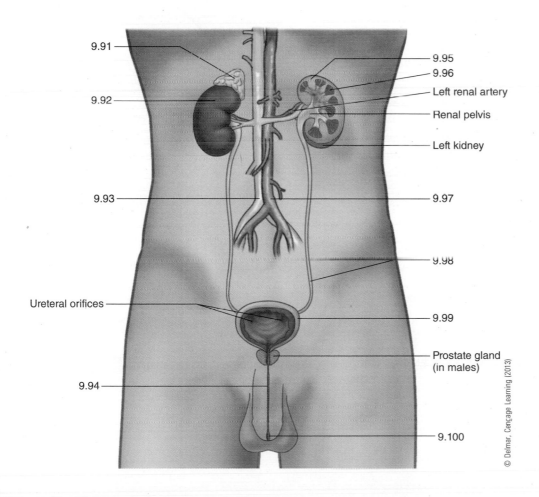

© Delmar, Cengage Learning (2013)

# THE HUMAN TOUCH
## Critical Thinking Exercise

The following story and questions are designed to stimulate critical thinking through class discussion or as a brief essay response. There are no right or wrong answers to these questions.

*"Mom, they want me to play for the National Women's Hockey League!" Josie yelled as she ran into the living room. She had just finished practice, and the scouts had told her afterward how impressed they were with her moves. Finally, her lifelong dream of winning an Olympic gold medal for Canada might actually come true! She'd had to make some sacrifices, like living at home after high school, but it looked like that would all pay off. As soon as she saw the looks on the faces of her parents, her smile disappeared.*

*"Honey, we just got back from the doctor. It turns out that your brother's recurrent bouts of pyelonephritis have led to irreversible renal damage. The nephrologist is recommending that Xavier have a kidney transplant," her mom explained with a pained look. "We know that he has a better chance if he has a related donor, but he could always go on hemodialysis and wait for a cadaver donor ..."*

*Josie saw her dreams of a hockey career fade away. After Xavier's third bout with nephrotic syndrome, the whole family had been tested for compatibility in case he needed a transplant. Josie was the only one with a positive cross-match. The doctors had explained to her then what it would mean if she decided to donate one of her kidneys, but Josie had brushed it off, assuming that her brother would get better. Now the voices of the doctors came back to her. "No contact sports after a nephrectomy," she heard them say, "there's too big a risk of rupturing the remaining kidney."*

*Josie was faced with the toughest decision of all: she loved Xavier, but hockey was her life.*

## Suggested Discussion Topics

1. Discuss the long-term repercussions of being a living organ donor.
2. Imagine that you are Josie's mom or dad and one of your children has the opportunity to save the life of another one of your children. Would you encourage him or her to donate an organ?
3. If Josie decides to donate her kidney and then later chooses to continue playing hockey, what advice should her parents give her?
4. What options might be open to Josie's brother other than having his sister donate a kidney?

# The Nervous System

## Overview of
## STRUCTURES, COMBINING FORMS, AND FUNCTIONS OF THE NERVOUS SYSTEM

| Major Structures | Related Combining Forms | Primary Functions |
| --- | --- | --- |
| Brain | **cerebr/o, encephal/o** | Coordinates all body activities by receiving and transmitting messages throughout the body. |
| Spinal Cord | **myel/o** | Transmits nerve impulses between the brain, arms and legs, and lower part of the body. |
| Nerves | **neur/i, neur/o** | Receive and transmit messages to and from all parts of the body. |
| Sensory Organs and Receptors | | Receive external stimulation and transmit these stimuli to the sensory neurons. |
|   Eyes (sight) | | See Chapter 11. |
|   Ears (hearing) | | See Chapter 11. |
|   Nose (smell) | | See Chapter 7. |
|   Skin (touch) | | See Chapter 12. |
|   Tongue (taste) | | See Chapter 8. |

## Vocabulary Related to THE NERVOUS SYSTEM

This list contains essential word parts and medical terms for this chapter. These terms are pronounced in the student StudyWARE™ and Audio CDs that are available for use with this text. These and the other important **primary terms** are shown in boldface throughout the chapter. *Secondary terms*, which appear in *orange* italics, clarify the meaning of primary terms.

### Word Parts

- [ ] **caus/o** burning, burn
- [ ] **cerebr/o** cerebrum, brain
- [ ] **concuss/o** shaken together, violently agitated
- [ ] **contus/o** bruise
- [ ] **encephal/o** brain
- [ ] **-esthesia** sensation, feeling
- [ ] **esthet/o** feeling, nervous sensation, sense of perception
- [ ] **-graphy** the process of producing a picture or record
- [ ] **mening/o** membranes, meninges
- [ ] **myel/o** spinal cord, bone marrow
- [ ] **neur/i, neur/o** nerve, nerve tissue
- [ ] **phobia** abnormal fear
- [ ] **psych/o** mind
- [ ] **radicul/o** root or nerve root
- [ ] **tropic** having an affinity for

### Medical Terms

- [ ] **acrophobia** (ack-roh-**FOH**-bee-ah)
- [ ] **Alzheimer's disease** (**ALTZ**-high-merz)
- [ ] **amyotrophic lateral sclerosis** (ah-**my**-oh-**TROH**-fick skleh-**ROH**-sis)
- [ ] **anesthetic** (an-es-**THET**-ick)
- [ ] **anesthetist** (ah-**NES**-theh-tist)
- [ ] **anxiety disorders**
- [ ] **autism** (**AW**-tizm)
- [ ] **Bell's palsy** (**PAWL**-zee)
- [ ] **carotid ultrasonography** (kah-**ROT**-id ul-trah-son-**OG**-rah-fee)
- [ ] **causalgia** (kaw-**ZAL**-jee-ah)
- [ ] **cerebral contusion** (**SER**-eh-bral kon-**TOO**-zhun)
- [ ] **cerebral palsy** (seh-**REE**-bral **PAWL**-zee)
- [ ] **cerebrovascular accident** (**ser**-eh-broh-**VAS**-kyou-lar)
- [ ] **cervical radiculopathy** (rah-**dick**-you-**LOP**-ah-thee)
- [ ] **claustrophobia** (**klaws**-troh-**FOH**-bee-ah)

- [ ] **cognition** (kog-**NISH**-un)
- [ ] **coma** (**KOH**-mah)
- [ ] **concussion** (kon-**KUSH**-un)
- [ ] **cranial hematoma** (hee-mah-**TOH**-mah)
- [ ] **delirium** (deh-**LEER**-ee-um)
- [ ] **delirium tremens** (deh-**LEER**-ee-um **TREE**-mens)
- [ ] **delusion** (dih-**LOO**-zhun)
- [ ] **dementia** (dih-**MEN**-shah)
- [ ] **dura mater** (**DOO**-rah **MAH**-ter)
- [ ] **dyslexia** (dis-**LECK**-see-ah)
- [ ] **echoencephalography** (**eck**-oh-en-**sef**-ah-**LOG**-rah-fee)
- [ ] **electroencephalography** (ee-**leck**-troh-en-**sef**-ah-**LOG**-rah-fee)
- [ ] **encephalitis** (**en**-sef-ah-**LYE**-tis)
- [ ] **epidural anesthesia** (**ep**-ih-**DOO**-ral an-es-**THEE**-zee-ah)
- [ ] **epilepsy** (**EP**-ih-**lep**-see)
- [ ] **factitious disorder** (fack-**TISH**-us)
- [ ] **Guillain-Barré syndrome** (gee-**YAHN**-bah-**RAY SIN**-drohm)
- [ ] **hallucination** (hah-**loo**-sih-**NAY**-shun)
- [ ] **hemorrhagic stroke** (**hem**-oh-**RAJ**-ick)
- [ ] **hydrocephalus** (high-droh-**SEF**-ah-lus)
- [ ] **hyperesthesia** (**high**-per-es-**THEE**-zee-ah)
- [ ] **hypochondriasis** (**high**-poh-kon-**DRY**-ah-sis)
- [ ] **ischemic stroke** (iss-**KEE**-mick)
- [ ] **lethargy** (**LETH**-ar-jee)
- [ ] **meningitis** (**men**-in-**JIGH**-tis)
- [ ] **meningocele** (meh-**NING**-goh-**seel**)
- [ ] **migraine headache** (**MY**-grayn)
- [ ] **multiple sclerosis** (skleh-**ROH**-sis)
- [ ] **myelitis** (my-eh-**LYE**-tis)
- [ ] **myelography** (my-eh-**LOG**-rah-fee)
- [ ] **narcolepsy** (**NAR**-koh-**lep**-see)
- [ ] **neurotransmitters** (**new**-roh-trans-**MIT**-erz)
- [ ] **obsessive-compulsive disorder**
- [ ] **panic attack**
- [ ] **paresthesia** (**pair**-es-**THEE**-zee-ah)
- [ ] **Parkinson's disease**
- [ ] **peripheral neuropathy** (new-**ROP**-ah-thee)
- [ ] **post-traumatic stress disorder**
- [ ] **Reye's syndrome** (**RIZE SIN**-drome)
- [ ] **schizophrenia** (**skit**-soh-**FREE**-nee-ah)
- [ ] **sciatica** (sigh-**AT**-ih-kah)
- [ ] **seizure** (**SEE**-zhur)
- [ ] **shaken baby syndrome**
- [ ] **syncope** (**SIN**-koh-pee)
- [ ] **trigeminal neuralgia** (try-**JEM**-ih-nal new- **RAL**-jee-ah)

# FUNCTIONS OF THE NERVOUS SYSTEM

The nervous system, with the brain as its center, coordinates and controls all bodily activities. When the brain ceases functioning, the body dies.

# STRUCTURES OF THE NERVOUS SYSTEM

The major structures of the nervous system are the nerves, brain, spinal cord, and sensory organs. The sensory organs, which are the eyes, ears, nose, skin, and tongue, are discussed in other chapters.

## Divisions of the Nervous System

For descriptive purposes, the nervous system is divided into two primary parts: the central and peripheral nervous systems (Figure 10.1).

- The **central nervous system** (CNS) includes the brain and spinal cord. The functions of the central nervous system are to receive and process information, and to regulate all bodily activity.

- The **peripheral nervous system** (PNS) includes the 12 pairs of cranial nerves extending from the brain and the 31 pairs of peripheral spinal nerves extending outward from the spinal cord. The function of the peripheral nervous system is to transmit nerve signals to and from the central nervous system.

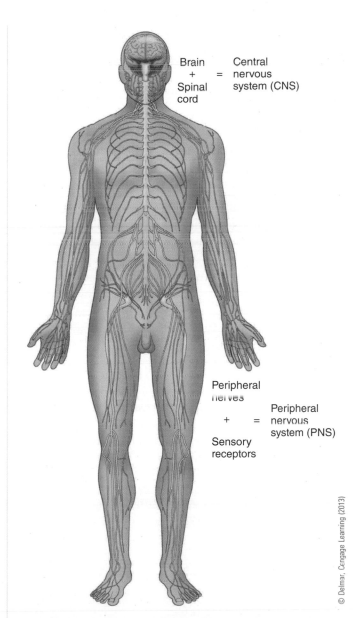

**FIGURE 10.1** The structural organization of the central and peripheral nervous systems.

## The Nerves

A **nerve** is one or more bundles of *neurons* that connect the brain and the spinal cord with other parts of the body. A **tract** is a bundle or group of nerve fibers located within the brain or spinal cord.

- *Ascending nerve tracts* carry nerve impulses *toward* the brain.

- *Descending nerve tracts* carry nerve impulses *away from* the brain.

- A **ganglion** (**GANG**-glee-on) is a nerve center made up of a cluster of nerve cell bodies outside the central nervous system (plural, *ganglia* or *ganglions*). Note: The term *ganglion* also describes a benign, tumor-like cyst.

- The term **innervation** (**in**-err-**VAY**-shun) means the supply of nerves to a specific body part.

- A **plexus** (**PLECK**-sus) is a network of intersecting spinal nerves (plural, *plexuses*) (Figure 10.8A). This term also describes a network of intersecting blood or lymphatic vessels.

- **Receptors** are sites in the sensory organs (eyes, ears, skin, nose, and taste buds) that receive external stimulation. The receptors send the stimulus through the sensory neurons to the brain for interpretation.

- A **stimulus** is anything that excites (activates) a nerve and causes an impulse (plural, *stimuli*). An *impulse* is a wave of excitation transmitted through nerve fibers and neurons.

## The Reflexes

A **reflex** (**REE**-flecks) is an automatic, involuntary response to some change, either inside or outside the body. Examples of reflex actions include:

- Changes in the heart rate, breathing rate, and blood pressure

- Coughing and sneezing

- Responses to painful stimuli

    Deep tendon reflexes are discussed in Chapter 4.

## The Neurons

**Neurons** (**NEW**-ronz) are the basic cells of the nervous system that allow different parts of the body to communicate with each other.

- The body has billions of neurons carrying nerve impulses throughout the body via an electrochemical process. In the brain, this process creates patterns of neuron electrical activity known as *brain waves*. Different types of brain waves are produced during periods of intense activity, rest, and sleep.

- The three types of neurons are described according to their function. The system of naming the neurons is summarized in Table 10.1. The memory aid **A-C-E** will help you remember their names, and **S-A-M** will help you remember their functions.

## Neuron Parts

Each neuron consists of a cell body, several dendrites, a single axon, and terminal end fibers (Figure 10.2).

- The **dendrites** (**DEN**-drytes) are the root-like processes that receive impulses and conduct them to the cell body. A *process* is a structure that extends out from the cell body.

- The **axon** (**ACK**-son) is a process that conducts impulses away from the nerve cell. An axon can be more than 3 feet long. Many, but not all, axons are protected by a myelin sheath, which is a white fatty tissue covering.

## TABLE 10.1
### Types of Neurons and Their Functions

| Types of Neurons | Neuron functions |
|---|---|
| **"ACE"** | **"SAM"** |
| **Afferent neurons** (**AF**-er-ent) *Afferent* means toward. | Also known as *sensory neurons*, these neurons emerge from sensory organs and the skin to carry the impulses from the sensory organs *toward* the brain and spinal cord. |
| **Connecting neurons** | Also known as *associative neurons*, these neurons link afferent and efferent neurons. |
| **Efferent neurons** (**EF**-er-ent) *Efferent* means away from. | Also known as *motor neurons*, these neurons carry impulses *away from* the brain and spinal cord and toward the muscles and glands. |

- **Terminal end fibers** are the branching fibers at the end of the axon that lead the nervous impulse from the axon to the synapse.

- A **synapse** (**SIN**-apps) is the space between two neurons or between a neuron and a receptor organ. A single neuron can have a few or several hundred synapses.

## Neurotransmitters

**Neurotransmitters** (**new**-roh-trans-**MIT**-erz) are chemical substances that make it possible for messages to cross from the synapse of a neuron to the target receptor. There are between 200 and 300 known neurotransmitters, and each has a specialized function. Examples of neurotransmitters and their roles follow:

- *Acetylcholine* is released at some synapses in the spinal cord and at neuromuscular junctions; it influences muscle action.

- *Dopamine* is released within the brain. It is believed to be involved in mood and thought disorders and in abnormal movement disorders such as Parkinson's disease.

- *Endorphins* are naturally occurring substances that are produced by the brain to help relieve pain.

- *Norepinephrine* affects alertness and arousal, increasing blood pressure and heart rate, and releasing stores of glucose in response to stress. It is also a hormone released by the adrenal gland as part of the body's fight-or-flight response (see Chapter 13).

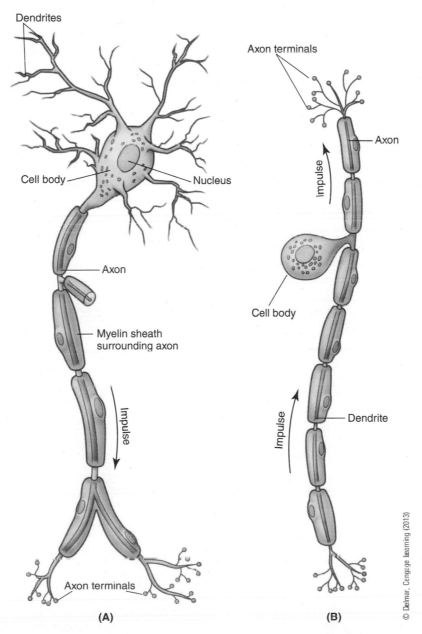

© Delmar, Cengage Learning (2013)

**FIGURE 10.2** The structure of two types of neurons. (A) Efferent (motor) neurons. (B) Afferent (sensory) neurons.

■ *Serotonin*, which is released in the brain, has roles in sleep, hunger, and pleasure recognition. It is also sometimes linked to mood disorders.

## Glial Cells

**Glial cells** (**GLEE**-ul) provide support and protection for neurons, and their four main functions are (1) to surround neurons and hold them in place, (2) to supply nutrients and oxygen to neurons, (3) to insulate one neuron from another, and (4) to destroy and remove dead neurons.

## The Myelin Sheath

A **myelin sheath** (**MY**-eh-lin) is the protective covering made up of glial cells. This white sheath forms the white matter of the brain and covers some parts of the spinal cord and the axon of most peripheral nerves (Figure 10.2).

■ The portion of the nerve fibers that are myelinated are known as *white matter*. The term *myelinated* means having a myelin sheath. It is the color of this covering that makes these fibers white.

■ The portion of the nerve fibers that are unmyelinated are known as *gray matter*. The term *unmyelinated* means lacking a myelin sheath. It is the lack of the myelin sheath that creates the gray color of the brain and spinal cord.

## ■ THE CENTRAL NERVOUS SYSTEM

The **central nervous system** is made up of the brain and spinal cord. These structures are protected externally by the bones of the cranium and the vertebrae of the spinal column, which are discussed in Chapter 3. Within these bony structures, the brain and spinal cord are further protected by the meninges and the cerebrospinal fluid (Figure 10.3).

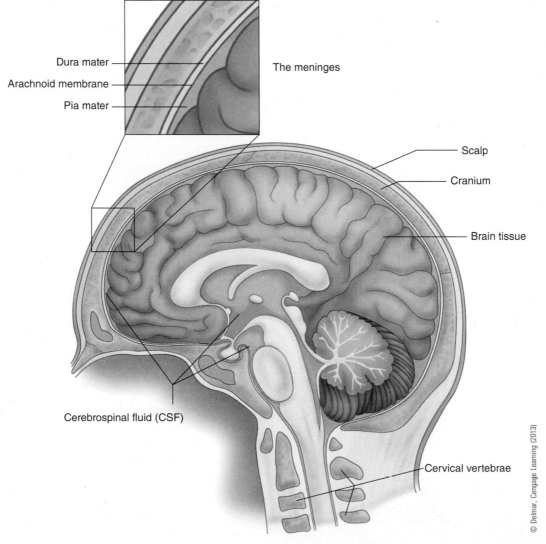

Dura mater
Arachnoid membrane
Pia mater

The meninges

Scalp

Cranium

Brain tissue

Cerebrospinal fluid (CSF)

Cervical vertebrae

© Delmar, Cengage Learning (2013)

**FIGURE 10.3** A cross-section of the brain showing the meninges and the protective coverings. The cerebrospinal fluid is shown in purple.

## The Meninges

The **meninges** (meh-**NIN**-jeez) are the system of membranes that enclose the brain and spinal cord (singular *meninx*). The meninges consist of three layers of connective tissue. These are the dura mater, arachnoid membrane, and the pia mater (Figure 10.3).

### The Dura Mater

The **dura mater** (**DOO**-rah **MAH**-ter) is the thick, tough, outermost membrane of the meninges. *Dura* means hard, and *mater* means mother.

■ The inner surface of the cranium (skull) is lined with the dura mater.

■ The inner surface of the vertebral column is known as the *epidural space*. This space, which is located between the walls of the vertebral column and the dura mater of the meninges, contains fat and supportive connective tissues to cushion the dura mater.

■ In both the skull and vertebral column, the *subdural space* is located between the dura mater and the arachnoid membrane.

### The Arachnoid Membrane

The **arachnoid membrane** (ah-**RACK**-noid), which resembles a spiderweb, is the second layer of the meninges and is located between the dura mater and the pia mater. *Arachnoid* means having to do with spiders.

■ The arachnoid membrane is loosely attached to the other meninges to allow space for fluid to flow between the layers.

■ The *subarachnoid space*, which is located below the arachnoid membrane and above the pia mater, contains cerebrospinal fluid.

### The Pia Mater

The **pia mater** (**PEE**-ah **MAH**-ter), which is the third layer of the meninges, is located nearest to the brain and spinal cord. It consists of delicate connective tissue that contains a rich supply of blood vessels. *Pia* means tender or delicate, and *mater* means mother.

## Cerebrospinal Fluid

**Cerebrospinal fluid** (**ser**-eh-broh-**SPY**-nal), also known as *spinal fluid*, is produced by special capillaries within the four ventricles located in the middle region of the cerebrum (Figures 10.3 and 10.4). Cerebrospinal fluid is a clear, colorless, and watery fluid that flows throughout the brain and around the spinal cord. The functions of this fluid are to:

■ Cool and cushion these organs from shock or injury

■ Nourish the brain and spinal cord by transporting nutrients and chemical messengers to these tissues

## The Parts of the Brain

The brain parts are shown in Figures 10.4 through 10.6. The body functions that are controlled by these brain parts are summarized in Table 10.2. Notice that the functions most essential to the support of life are located within the most protected portions of the brain.

## The Cerebrum

The **cerebrum** (seh-**REE**-brum) is the largest and uppermost portion of the brain. It is responsible for all thought, judgment, memory, and emotion, as well as for controlling and integrating motor and sensory functions. Note that *cerebrum* and *cerebellum* are similar words, but refer to very different parts of the brain. Memory aid: The cere*bel*lum is *bel*ow the cerebrum.

■ The term **cerebral** (**see**-**EE**-bral) means pertaining to the cerebrum or to the brain (**cerebr** means brain, and **-al** means pertaining to).

■ The **cerebral cortex**, which is made up of gray matter, is the outer layer of the cerebrum and is made up of elevated folds and deep fissures (Figure 10.6).

  ■ *Gyri* (singular *gyrus*) are the elevated folds of gray matter in the cerebral cortex.

  ■ *Sulci* are the fissures of the cerebral cortex. As used here, a *fissure* is a normally occurring deep groove. Skin fissures, which are crack-like sores, are discussed in Chapter 12.

### The Cerebral Hemispheres

The cerebrum is divided to create two **cerebral hemispheres** that are connected at the lower midpoint by the *corpus callosum* (Figure 10.5).

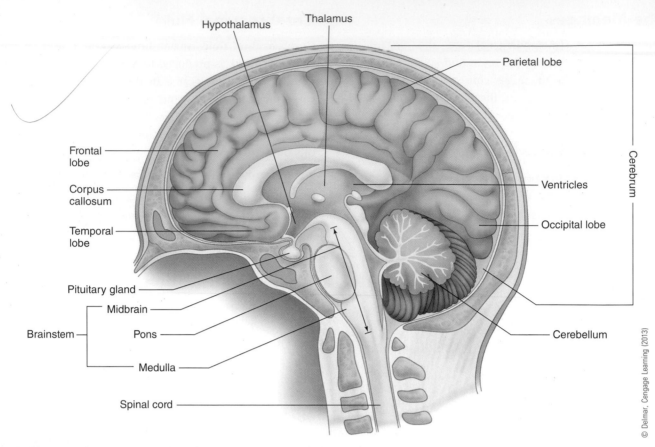

**FIGURE 10.4** A cross-section showing the major parts of the brain.

© Delmar, Cengage Learning (2013)

## TABLE 10.2

### Brain Parts and Their Functions

| Brain Part | Functions |
|---|---|
| The **cerebrum**, which is the largest and uppermost part of the brain, consists of four lobes. | Controls the highest level of thought, including judgment, memory, association, and critical thinking. It also processes sensations and controls all voluntary muscle activity. |
| The **thalamus** is located below the cerebrum. | Relays sensory stimuli from the spinal cord and midbrain to the cerebral cortex. The thalamus suppresses some stimuli and magnifies others. |
| The **hypothalamus** is located below the thalamus | Controls vital bodily functions (Table 10.3). |
| The **cerebellum** is located in the lower back of the cranium below the cerebrum. | Coordinates muscular activity and balance for smooth and steady movements. |
| The **brainstem** is located in the base of the brain and forms the connection between the brain and spinal cord. It consists of the:<br>• midbrain<br>• pons<br>• medulla oblongata | Controls the functions necessary for survival (breathing, digestion, heart rate, and blood pressure), and for arousal (being awake and alert). |

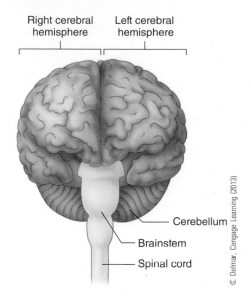

Right cerebral hemisphere    Left cerebral hemisphere

Cerebellum

Brainstem

Spinal cord

© Delmar, Cengage Learning (2013)

**FIGURE 10.5** An anterior view showing how the brain is divided into right and left hemispheres.

- The *left cerebral hemisphere* controls the majority of functions on the right side of the body. An injury to the left hemisphere produces sensory and motor deficits on the right side of the body.

- The *right cerebral hemisphere* controls most of the functions on the left side of the body. An injury to the right hemisphere produces sensory and motor deficits on the left side of the body.

- The crossing of nerve fibers that makes this arrangement possible occurs in the brainstem (Figure 10.4).

## The Cerebral Lobes

Each cerebral hemisphere is subdivided to create pairs of **cerebral lobes**. Each lobe is named for the bone of the cranium that covers it (Figure 10.6).

- The *frontal lobe* controls skilled motor functions, memory, and behavior.

- The *parietal lobe* receives and interprets nerve impulses from sensory receptors in the tongue, skin, and muscles.

- The *occipital lobe* controls eyesight.

- The *temporal lobe* controls the senses of hearing and smell, and the ability to create, store, and access new information.

## The Thalamus

The **thalamus** (**THAL**-ah-mus), which is located below the cerebrum, produces sensations by relaying impulses to and from the cerebrum and the sense organs of the body.

## The Hypothalamus

The **hypothalamus** (**high**-poh-**THAL**-ah-mus) is located below the thalamus (Figure 10.4). The seven major regulatory functions of the hypothalamus are summarized in Table 10.3.

## The Cerebellum

The **cerebellum** (**ser**-eh-**BELL**-um) is the second-largest part of the brain. It is located at the back of

## TABLE 10.3

### Regulatory Functions of the Hypothalamus

1. Regulates and integrates the autonomic nervous system, including controlling heart rate, blood pressure, respiratory rate, and digestive tract activity.

2. Regulates emotional responses, including fear and pleasure.

3. Regulates body temperature.

4. Regulates food intake by controlling hunger sensations.

5. Regulates water balance by controlling thirst sensations.

6. Regulates sleep-wakefulness cycles.

7. Regulates the pituitary gland and endocrine system activity (see Chapter 13).

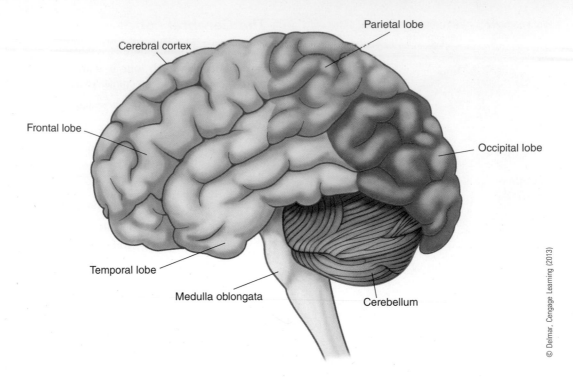

Cerebral cortex

Parietal lobe

Frontal lobe

Occipital lobe

Temporal lobe

Medulla oblongata

Cerebellum

© Delmar, Cengage Learning (2013)

**FIGURE 10.6** A left lateral view of the exterior of the brain showing the four lobes of the cerebrum plus the medulla oblongata and the cerebellum. The cerebral cortex is the outer layer of the cerebrum.

the head below the posterior portion of the cerebrum (Figures 10.4 through 10.6).

- The cerebellum receives incoming messages regarding movement within joints, muscle tone, and positions of the body. From here, messages are relayed to the different parts of the brain that control the motions of skeletal muscles.

- The general functions of the cerebellum are to produce smooth and coordinated movements, to maintain equilibrium, and to sustain normal postures.

## The Brainstem

The **brainstem** is the stalk-like portion of the brain that connects the cerebral hemispheres with the spinal cord. It is made up of three parts: the midbrain, pons, and medulla oblongata (Figure 10.4).

- The **midbrain** and **pons** (**PONZ**) provide conduction pathways to and from the higher and lower centers in the brain. They also control reflexes for movements of the eyes and head in response to visual and auditory stimuli. (*Pons* is the Latin word for bridge.)

- The **medulla oblongata** (meh-**DULL**-ah ob-long-**GAH**-tah), which is located at the lowest part of the brainstem, is connected to the spinal cord. It controls basic survival

functions, including the muscles that make possible respiration, heart rate, and blood pressure, as well as reflexes for coughing, sneezing, swallowing, and vomiting.

## The Spinal Cord

The **spinal cord** is a long, fragile tube-like structure that begins at the end of the brainstem and continues down almost to the bottom of the spinal column (Figure 10.1).

- The spinal cord contains all the nerves that affect the limbs and lower part of the body, and serves as the pathway for impulses traveling to and from the brain.

- The spinal cord is surrounded and protected by cerebrospinal fluid and the meninges.

## ■ THE PERIPHERAL NERVOUS SYSTEM

The **peripheral nervous system** consists of the 12 pairs of cranial nerves that extend from the brain, plus 31 pairs of spinal nerves that extend from the spinal cord. *Peripheral* means pertaining to body parts that are away from the center of the body.

Three types of specialized peripheral nerves transmit signals to and from the central nervous system. These are autonomic, sensory, and somatic nerve fibers.

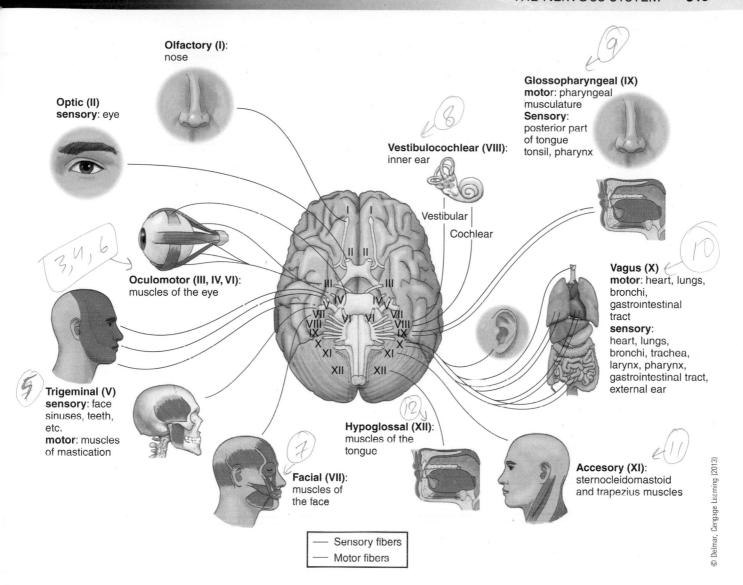

**FIGURE 10.7** Cranial nerves are identified with Roman numerals and are named for the area or function they serve.

- *Autonomic nerve fibers* carry instructions to the organs and glands from the autonomic nervous system.

- *Sensory nerve fibers* receive external stimuli, such as how something feels, and transmit this information to the brain where it is interpreted.

- *Somatic nerve fibers*, which are also known as *motor nerve fibers*, convey information that controls the body's voluntary muscular movements.

## The Cranial Nerves

The 12 pairs of **cranial nerves** originate from the undersurface of the brain. The two nerves of a pair are identical in function and structure, and each nerve of a pair serves half of the body. These cranial nerves are identified by Roman numerals and are named for the area or function they serve (Figure 10.7).

## The Peripheral Spinal Nerves

The 31 pairs of **peripheral spinal nerves** are grouped together and named based on the region of the body they innervate.

- Within each region, the nerves are referred to by number. The cervical nerves are C1–C8, the thoracic nerves are T1–T12, the lumbar nerves are L1–L5, and the sacral nerves are S1–S5 (Figure 10.8B).

- Spinal nerves sometimes join with others to form a plexus to innervate a certain area. The lumbar plexus, as shown in Figure 10.8A, is made up of the first four lumbar nerves (L1–L4) and serves the lower back.

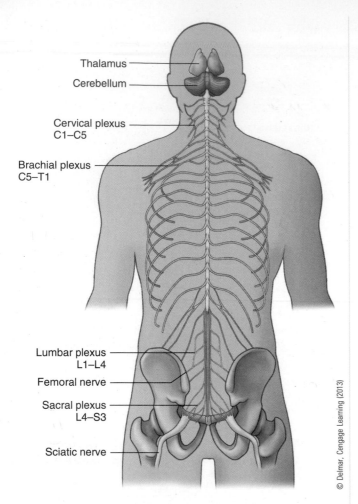

**FIGURE 10.8A** Most spinal cord plexuses are named for the corresponding vertebrae.

## ◼ THE AUTONOMIC NERVOUS SYSTEM

The **autonomic nervous system** is organized into two divisions, one comprising *sympathetic nerves* and the other *parasympathetic nerves*. The autonomic nervous system controls the involuntary actions of the body such as the functioning of internal organs. To maintain homeostasis within the body, each division balances the activity of the other division. *Homeostasis* is the process of maintaining the constant internal environment of the body (See Chapter 2).

- The **sympathetic nerves** prepare the body for emergencies and stress by increasing the breathing rate, heart rate, and blood flow to muscles. These nerves become aroused as part of the *fight-or-flight response*, which is the body's natural reaction to real or imaginary danger.

- The **parasympathetic nerves** return the body to normal after a response to stress. They also maintain

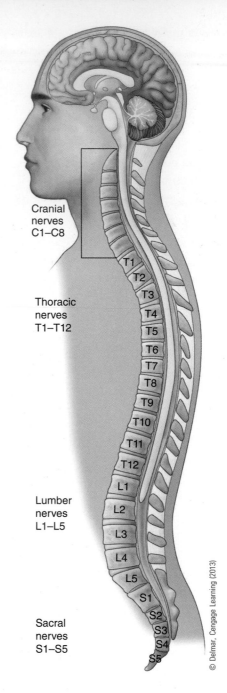

**FIGURE 10.8B** Within each spinal region, the nerves are referred to by number.

normal body functions during ordinary circumstances that are not emotionally or physically stressful.

## ◼ MEDICAL SPECIALTIES RELATED TO THE NERVOUS SYSTEM

- An **anesthesiologist** (**an**-es-**thee**-zee-**OL**-oh-jist) is a physician who specializes in administering anesthetic agents before and during surgery (**an-** means without, **esthesi** means feeling, and **-ologist** means specialist).

- An **anesthetist** (ah-**NES**-theh-tist) is a medical professional who specializes in administering anesthesia, but is not a physician, for example, a nurse anesthetist (**an-** means without, **esthet** means feeling, and **-ist** means specialist).

- A **neurologist** (new-**ROL**-oh-jist) is a physician who specializes in diagnosing and treating diseases and disorders of the nervous system (**neur** means nerve, and **-ologist** means specialist).

- A **neurosurgeon** is a physician who specializes in surgery of the nervous system.

- A **psychiatrist** (sigh-**KYE**-ah-trist) is a physician (MD) who specializes in diagnosing and treating chemical dependencies, emotional problems, and mental illness (**psych** means mind, and **-iatrist** means specialist). A psychiatrist can prescribe medications.

- A **psychologist** (sigh-**KOL**-oh-jist) has a doctoral degree (PhD or PsyD), but is not a medical doctor (MD). This specialist evaluates and treats emotional problems and mental illness (**psych** means mind, and **-ologist** means specialist).

## ■ PATHOLOGY OF THE NERVOUS SYSTEM

### The Head and Meninges

- **Cephalalgia** (**sef**-ah-**LAL**-jee-ah), also known as a *headache*, is pain in the head (**cephal** means head, and **-algia** means pain).

- A **migraine headache** (**MY**-grayn), which may be preceded by a warning aura, is characterized by throbbing pain on one side of the head. Migraine headaches primarily affect women and are sometimes accompanied by nausea, vomiting, and sensitivity to light or sound. A *warning aura* is a visual disturbance perceived by the patient preceding a migraine headache or epileptic seizure.

- **Cluster headaches** are intensely painful headaches that affect one side of the head and may be associated with tearing of the eyes and nasal congestion. These headaches, which primarily affect men, are named for their repeated occurrence in groups or clusters.

- An **encephalocele** (en-**SEF**-ah-loh-**seel**), also known as a *craniocele*, is a congenital herniation of brain tissue through a gap in the skull (**encephal/o** means

brain, and **-cele** means hernia). *Congenital* means present at birth, and *herniation* means protrusion of a structure from its normal position. Compare this with a *meningocele*.

- A **meningocele** (meh-**NING**-goh-**seel**) is the congenital herniation of the meninges through a defect in the skull or spinal column (**mening/o** means meninges, and **-cele** means hernia). Compare this with an *encephalocele*.

- **Hydrocephalus** (high-droh-**SEF**-ah-lus) is a condition in which excess cerebrospinal fluid accumulates in the ventricles of the brain (**hydr/o** means water, **cephal** means head, and **-us** is a singular noun ending). This condition can occur at birth or develop later on in life from obstructions related to meningitis, brain tumors, or other causes.

- A **meningioma** (meh-**nin**-jee-**OH**-mah) is a common, slow-growing and usually benign tumor of the meninges (**mening/i** means meninges, and **-oma** means tumor).

- **Meningitis** (**men**-in-**JIGH**-tis), also referred to as *infectious meningitis*, is an inflammation of the meninges of the brain and spinal cord (**mening** means meninges, and **-itis** means inflammation). This condition, which can be caused by a bacterial or viral infection elsewhere in the body, is characterized by intense headache and flu-like symptoms. Bacterial meningitis, which is less common, is sometimes fatal. Compare with *encephalitis*.

### Disorders of the Brain

- The term **cognition** (kog-**NISH**-un) describes the mental activities associated with thinking, learning, and memory. *Mild cognitive impairment* is a memory disorder, usually associated with recently acquired information, which may be an early predictor of Alzheimer's disease.

- **Dementia** (dih-**MEN**-shah) is a slowly progressive decline in mental abilities, including memory, thinking, and judgment, that is often accompanied by personality changes. *Senile dementia* is dementia of the aged.

- **Vascular dementia** is a form of dementia caused by a stroke or other restriction of the flow of blood to the brain. Although Alzheimer's disease is the primary cause of dementia, vascular dementia accounts for about 10 to 20% of all cases.

- **Encephalitis** (**en**-sef-ah-**LYE**-tis), which is an inflammation of the brain, can be caused by a viral infection such as rabies (**encephal** means brain, and -**itis** means inflammation). Compare with meningitis.

- **Reye's syndrome** (**RIZE**) (RS) is a potentially serious or deadly disorder in children that is characterized by vomiting and confusion. This syndrome sometimes follows a viral illness in which the child was treated with aspirin.

- **Tetanus** (**TET**-ah-nus), also known as *lockjaw*, is an acute and potentially fatal infection of the central nervous system caused by a toxin produced by the tetanus bacteria. Tetanus can be prevented through immunization. In unimmunized people, this condition is typically acquired through a deep puncture wound.

- **Tourette syndrome** (tuh **RET**) (TS) is a complex neurological disorder characterized by involuntary tics, grunts, and compulsive utterances that sometimes include obscenities.

## Neurodegenerative Diseases

The term **neurodegenerative disease** (**new**-roh-deh-**JEN**-er-ah-tiv) is an umbrella term for disorders in which there is a progressive loss of the structure or functions of the neurons.

- **Alzheimer's disease** (**ALTZ**-high-merz) is a group of disorders involving the parts of the brain that control thought, memory, and language (Figure 10.9). It is the leading cause of dementia and is marked by progressive deterioration that affects both the memory and reasoning capabilities of an individual.

- *Huntington's disease* is a genetic disorder that is classified as a neurodegenerative disease (See Chapter 2).

- **Parkinson's disease** (PD) is a chronic, degenerative central nervous disorder characterized by fine muscle tremors, rigidity, and a slow or shuffling gait. *Gait* describes the manner of walking. This slow or shuffling gait is caused by gradual progressive loss of control over movements due to inadequate levels of the neurotransmitter dopamine in the brain.

## Brain Injuries

- **Amnesia** (am-**NEE**-zee-ah) is a memory disturbance characterized by a total or partial inability to recall past experiences. This condition can be caused by a brain injury, illness, or a psychological disturbance.

- A **concussion** (kon-**KUSH**-un) is a violent shaking up or jarring of the brain (**concuss** means shaken together, and -**ion** means condition or state of). A concussion may result in a temporary loss of awareness and function. Compare with a cerebral contusion.

- A **cerebral contusion** (**SER**-eh-bral kon-**TOO**-zhun) is the bruising of brain tissue as the result of a head injury that causes the brain to bounce against the rigid bone of the skull (**contus** means bruise, and -**ion** means condition). Compare with concussion.

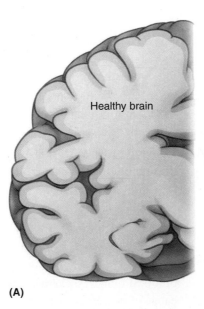

(A)

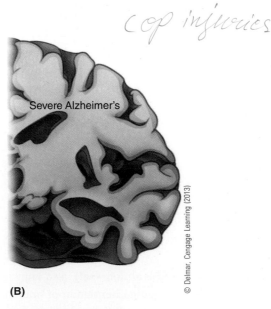

(B)

© Delmar, Cengage Learning (2013)

**FIGURE 10.9** (A) A healthy brain and (B) the brain of a patient with Alzheimer's disease.

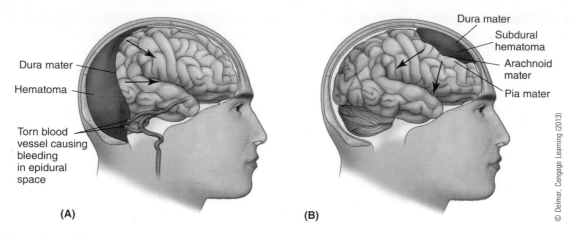

**FIGURE 10.10** Cranial hematomas. (A) Epidural hematoma. (B) Subdural hematoma.

■ A **cranial hematoma** (**hee**-mah-**TOH**-mah) is a collection of blood trapped in the tissues of the brain (**hemat** means blood, and **-oma** means tumor). Named for their location, the types of cranial hematomas include an *epidural hematoma* located above the dura mater or a *subdural hematoma*, which is located below the dura mater (Figure 10.10). Cranial hematomas may be caused by a major or even minor head injury.

## Traumatic Brain Injury

A **traumatic brain injury** is a blow to the head or a penetrating head injury that damages the brain. Not all blows to the head result in damage to the brain. When an injury does occur, it can range from mild, with only a brief change in mental status, to severe, with longer lasting effects.

■ The term *coup* describes an injury occurring within the skull near the point of impact, such as hitting the windshield in an auto accident. A *contrecoup*, also described as a *counterblow*, is an injury that occurs beneath the skull opposite to the area of impact (Figure 10.11).

■ **Shaken baby syndrome** describes the results of a child being violently shaken by someone. This action can cause brain injury, blindness, fractures, seizures, paralysis, and death.

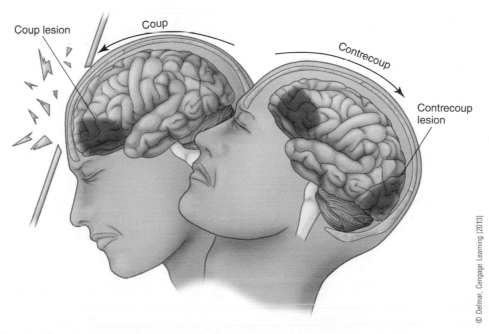

**FIGURE 10.11** Coup and contrecoup brain injuries.

## Levels of Consciousness

**Levels of consciousness** (LOC) describe the measurement of response to arousal and stimulus. *Altered levels of consciousness (ALOC)* refer to a decrease in consciousness due to injury, disease, or substances such as medication, drugs, or alcohol.

- Being **conscious** is the state of being awake, alert, aware, and responding appropriately.

- Being **unconscious** is a state of being unaware and unable to respond to any stimuli, including pain.

- **Lethargy** (**LETH**-ar-jee) is a lowered level of consciousness marked by listlessness, drowsiness, and apathy. As used here, *apathy* means indifference and a reduced level of activity. The term *lethargic* refers to a person who is at this level of consciousness.

- A **stupor** (**STOO**-per) is an unresponsive state from which a person can be aroused only briefly despite vigorous, repeated attempts.

- **Syncope** (**SIN**-koh-pee), also known as *fainting*, is the brief loss of consciousness caused by the decreased flow of blood to the brain.

- A **coma** (**KOH**-mah) is a profound (deep) state of unconsciousness marked by the absence of spontaneous eye movements, no response to painful stimuli, and the lack of speech. The term *comatose* refers to a person who is in a coma.

- A **persistent vegetative state** is a type of coma in which the patient exhibits alternating sleep and wake cycles; however, due to severe damage to certain areas of the brain, the person is unconscious even when appearing to be awake.

### Delirium

**Delirium** (deh-**LEER**-ee-um) is an acute condition of confusion, disorientation, disordered thinking and memory, agitation, and hallucinations.

This condition is usually caused by a treatable physical condition, such as a high fever. An individual suffering from this condition is described as being *delirious*.

### Brain Tumors

A **brain tumor** is an abnormal growth located inside the skull (Figure 10.12).

- An invasive *malignant brain tumor* destroys brain tissue. When this cancer originates in the brain, it is considered to be the primary site. If this cancer metastasizes (spreads) to the brain from another body system, it is considered to be a secondary site.

- A *benign brain tumor* does not invade the brain tissue; however, because this growth is surrounded by rigid bone, as the tumor enlarges, it can damage the brain tissue by placing pressure against the tissues and by increasing the intracranial pressure.

- **Intracranial pressure** is the amount of pressure inside the skull (**intra-** means within, **crani** means cranium, and **-al** means pertaining to). Elevated intracranial pressure can be due to a tumor, an injury, or improper drainage of cerebrospinal fluid.

## Strokes

A stroke, or CVA, is properly known as a **cerebrovascular accident** (ser-eh-broh-**VAS**-kyou-lar). This condition is damage to the brain that occurs when the blood flow to the brain is disrupted because a blood vessel is either blocked or has ruptured. Strokes are currently the third-leading cause of death and the primary cause of long-term disability.

The location of the disruption determines the symptoms that will be present.

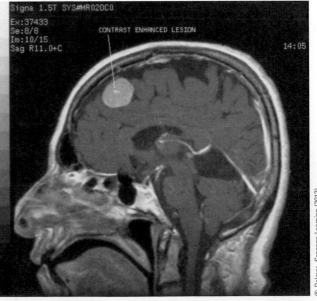

**FIGURE 10.12** A brain tumor visualized by magnetic resonance imaging (MRI).

© Delmar, Cengage Learning (2013)

- Damage to the right side of the brain produces symptoms on the left side of the body.

- Damage to the left side of the brain produces symptoms on the right side of the body (Figure 10.13).

## Ischemic Stroke

An **ischemic stroke** (iss-**KEE**-mick), which is the most common type of stroke in older people, occurs when the flow of blood to the brain is blocked by the narrowing or blockage of a carotid artery. *Ischemic* means pertaining to the disruption of the blood supply (see Chapter 5).

One type of ischemic stroke is a *thrombotic stroke*, which occurs when a blood clot forms in a carotid artery

and blocks it. The other is an *embolic stroke*, which occurs when a blood clot or other debris forms in a blood vessel somewhere other than the brain and travels through the bloodstream to lodge in the narrower brain arteries.

- A **transient ischemic attack** (TIA), sometimes referred to as a mini-stroke, is the temporary interruption in the blood supply to the brain. *Transient* means passing quickly. Symptoms of a TIA include numbness, blurred vision, dizziness, or loss of balance. A TIA passes in less than an hour; however, this incident is often a warning sign that the individual is at risk for a more serious and debilitating stroke.

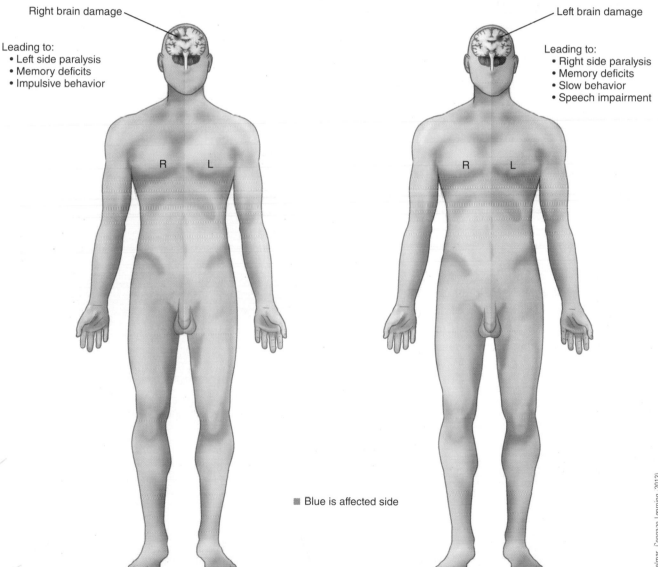

Right brain damage

Leading to:
- Left side paralysis
- Memory deficits
- Impulsive behavior

Left brain damage

Leading to:
- Right side paralysis
- Memory deficits
- Slow behavior
- Speech impairment

R L

R L

■ Blue is affected side

© Delmar, Cengage Learning 2013

**FIGURE 10.13** The location of the damage caused by a cerebrovascular accident depends upon which side of the brain is affected.

■ **Aphasia** (ah-**FAY**-zee-ah), which is often caused by brain damage associated with a stroke, is the loss of the ability to speak, write, and/or comprehend the written or spoken word (**a-** means without, and **-phasia** means speech).

## Hemorrhagic Stroke

A **hemorrhagic stroke** (**hem**-oh-**RAJ**-ick), also known as a *bleed*, occurs when a blood vessel in the brain leaks. A bleed also occurs when an aneurysm within the brain ruptures. An *aneurysm* is a localized, weak, balloon-like enlargement of an artery wall. This type of stroke is less common than ischemic strokes and is often fatal. A hemorrhagic stroke affects the area of the brain damaged by the leaking blood (Figures 10.14 and 10.15).

**Arteriovenous malformation** (ar-**tee**-ree-oh-**VEE**-nus) (AVM) is one of the causes of hemorrhagic strokes. This abnormal connection between the arteries and veins in the brain is usually congenital and can rupture suddenly at any age (**arteri/o** means artery, **ven** means vein, and **-ous** means pertaining to).

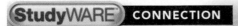

**StudyWARE** CONNECTION

Watch an animation on **Strokes** in the StudyWARE™.

## Sleep Disorders

■ **Insomnia** is the prolonged or abnormal inability to sleep. This condition is usually a symptom of another problem such as depression, pain, or excessive caffeine (**in-** means without, **somn** means sleep, and **-ia** means abnormal condition).

■ **Narcolepsy** (**NAR**-koh-**lep**-see) is a sleep disorder consisting of sudden and uncontrollable brief episodes of falling asleep during the day (**narc/o** means stupor, and **-lepsy** means seizure).

■ **Sleep deprivation** is a sufficient lack of restorative sleep over a cumulative period so as to cause physical or psychiatric symptoms and affect routine performance or tasks.

■ **Somnambulism** (som-**NAM**-byou-lizm), also known as *sleepwalking* or *noctambulism*, is the condition of walking or performing some other activity without awakening (**somn** means sleep, **ambul** means to walk, and **-ism** means condition of).

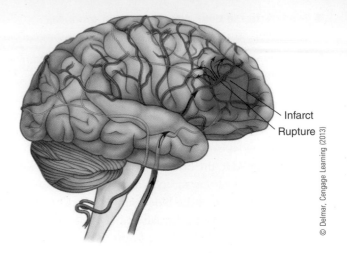

**FIGURE 10.14** In a hemorrhagic stroke, the rupture of a blood vessel causes decreased blood flow to an area of the brain tissue. An *infarct* is a localized area of dead tissue caused by a lack of blood.

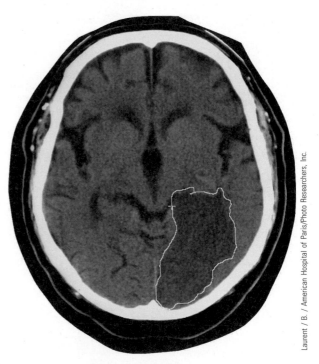

**FIGURE 10.15** Magnetic resonance image of a brain with the area of a bleed visible in the lower right.

## The Spinal Cord

■ **Myelitis** (**my**-eh-**LYE**-tis) is an inflammation of the spinal cord (**myel** means spinal cord and bone marrow, and **-itis** means inflammation). The term *myelitis* also means inflammation of bone marrow.

- A **myelosis** (**my**-eh-**LOH**-sis) is a tumor of the spinal cord (**myel** means spinal cord and bone marrow, and **-osis** means abnormal condition). *Myelosis* also means an abnormal proliferation of bone marrow tissue.

- **Poliomyelitis** (**poh**-lee-oh-**my**-eh-**LYE**-tis), also known as *polio*, is a highly contagious viral infection of the brainstem and spinal cord that sometimes leads to paralysis (**poli/o** means gray matter, **myel** means spinal cord and bone marrow, and **-itis** means inflammation). There is no known cure for polio; however, it can be prevented through vaccination.

- *Post-polio syndrome* is the recurrence later in life of some polio symptoms in individuals who have had childhood poliomyelitis and have recovered from it.

- **Spinal cord injuries** are discussed in Chapter 4.

## Pinched Nerves

**Radiculitis** (rah-**dick**-you-**LYE**-tis), also known as a *pinched nerve*, is an inflammation of the root of a spinal nerve that causes pain and numbness radiating down the affected limb (**radicul** means root or nerve root, and **-itis** means inflammation). This term usually applies to that portion of the root that lies between the spinal cord and the intervertebral canal of the spinal column. Figure 3.18 in Chapter 3 shows one cause of this condition.

- **Cervical radiculopathy** (rah-**dick**-you-**LOP**-ah-thee) is nerve pain caused by pressure on the spinal nerve roots in the neck region (**radicul/o** means nerve root, and **-pathy** means disease).

- **Lumbar radiculopathy** is nerve pain in the lower back caused by muscle spasms or by nerve root irritation from the compression of vertebral disks such as a herniated disk.

## Multiple Sclerosis

**Multiple sclerosis** (skleh-**ROH**-sis) is a progressive auto-immune disorder characterized by inflammation that causes demyelination of the myelin sheath. This scars the brain, spinal cord, and optic nerves and disrupts the transmission of nerve impulses. This damage leaves the patient with varying degrees of pain plus physical and cognitive problems.

- *Demyelination* is the loss of patches of the protective myelin sheath.

- The disease is characterized by periods of *exacerbations*, which are episodes of worsening symptoms that are also referred to as *flares*. Between these episodes, the patient may be in remission. *Remission* is a time during which the symptoms ease, but the disease has not been cured.

## Nerves

- **Amyotrophic lateral sclerosis** (ah-**my**-oh-**TROH**-fick), also known as *Lou Gehrig's disease*, is a rapidly progressive neurological disease that attacks the nerve cells responsible for controlling voluntary muscles. Patients affected with this condition become progressively weaker until they are completely paralyzed and die.

- **Bell's palsy** is the temporary paralysis of the seventh cranial nerve that causes paralysis only of the affected side of the face. In addition, paralysis symptoms can include the inability to close the eye, pain, tearing, drooling, hypersensitivity to sound in the affected ear, and impairment of taste.

- **Guillain-Barré syndrome** (gee-**YAHN**-bah-**RAY**), also known as *infectious polyneuritis*, is an inflammation of the myelin sheath of peripheral nerves, characterized by rapidly worsening muscle weakness that can lead to temporary paralysis. This condition is an autoimmune reaction that can occur after certain viral infections or an immunization.

- **Neuritis** (new-**RYE**-tis) is an inflammation of a nerve accompanied by pain and sometimes loss of function (**neur/o** means nerve, and **-itis** means inflammation).

- **Sciatica** (sigh-**AT**-ih-kah) is inflammation of the sciatic nerve that results in pain, burning, and tingling along the course of the affected sciatic nerve through the thigh, leg, and foot (Figure 10.8A).

- **Trigeminal neuralgia** (try-**JEM**-ih-nal new-**RAL**-jee-ah) is characterized by severe lightning-like pain due to an inflammation of the fifth cranial nerve. These sudden, intense, brief attacks of sharp pain affect the cheek, lips, and gums only on the side of the face innervated by the affected nerve.

## Cerebral Palsy

**Cerebral palsy** (seh-**REE**-bral **PAWL**-zee) is a condition characterized by poor muscle control, spasticity, speech defects, and other neurologic deficiencies due to damage that affects the cerebrum. *Spasticity* is a condition in which certain muscles are continuously contracted. *Palsy* means paralysis of a body part that is often accompanied by loss of feeling and uncontrolled body movements, such as shaking.

- Cerebral palsy occurs most frequently in premature or low-birth-weight infants.

- Cerebral palsy is usually caused by an injury that occurs during pregnancy, birth, or soon after birth.

## Epilepsy and Seizures

**Epilepsy** (**EP**-ih-**lep**-see) is a chronic neurological condition characterized by recurrent episodes of seizures of varying severity. Also known as a *seizure disorder*, epilepsy can usually be controlled with medication.

A **seizure** (**SEE**-zhur) is a sudden surge of electrical activity in the brain that affects how a person feels or acts for a short time. Some seizures can hardly be noticed, whereas others cause a brief loss of consciousness. Seizures are symptoms of different disorders that can affect the brain and also can be caused by extreme high fever, brain injury, or brain lesions.

- A **tonic-clonic seizure**, also called a *grand mal seizure*, involves the entire body. In the tonic phase of the seizure, the body becomes rigid, and in the clonic phase, there is uncontrolled jerking.

- An **absence seizure**, also called a *petit mal seizure*, is a brief disturbance in brain function in which there is a loss of awareness often described as a staring episode.

## Abnormal Sensations

- **Causalgia** (kaw-**ZAL**-jee-ah) is persistent, severe burning pain that usually follows an injury to a sensory nerve (**caus** means burning, and **-algia** means pain).

- **Hyperesthesia** (**high**-per-es-**THEE**-zee-ah) is a condition of abnormal and excessive sensitivity to touch, pain, or other sensory stimuli (**hyper-** means excessive, and **-esthesia** means sensation or feeling).

- **Paresthesia** (**pair**-es-**THEE**-zee-ah) refers to a burning or prickling sensation that is usually felt in the hands, arms, legs, or feet, but can also occur in other parts of the body (**par-** means abnormal, and **-esthesia** means sensation or feeling). These sensations may constitute the first symptoms of peripheral neuropathy or may be a drug side effect.

- **Peripheral neuropathy** (new-**ROP**-ah-thee) is a disorder of the peripheral nerves that carry information to and from the brain and spinal cord (**neur/o** means nerve, and **-pathy** means disease). This produces pain, the loss of sensation, and the inability to control muscles, particularly in the arms or legs.

  - *Neuropathy* is any disease or damage to a nerve.

  - *Mononeuropathy* is damage to a singular peripheral nerve, as in carpal tunnel syndrome (see Chapter 4).

  - *Polyneuropathy* is when multiple peripheral nerves are damaged. Diabetes is a common cause of polyneuropathy, along with trauma, vitamin deficiencies, and alcoholism.

- **Restless legs syndrome** (RLS) is a neurological disorder characterized by uncomfortable feelings in the legs, producing a strong urge to move them. The sensation is usually most noticeable at night or when trying to rest.

## ■ DIAGNOSTIC PROCEDURES OF THE NERVOUS SYSTEM

- **Magnetic resonance imaging** (MRI) and **computed tomography** (CT) are important neuroimaging tools because they facilitate the examination of the soft tissue structures of the brain and spinal cord (Figures 10.12 and 10.15). These diagnostic techniques are discussed further in Chapter 15.

- A **functional MRI** (fMRI) detects changes in blood flow in the brain when the patient is asked to perform a specific task. This gives a clearer picture of the brain tissue relevant to accomplishing this task.

- **Carotid ultrasonography** (kah-**ROT**-id **ul**-trah-son-**OG**-rah-fee) is an ultrasound study of the carotid artery (**ultra-** means beyond, **son/o** means sound, and **-graphy** means the process of producing a picture or record). This diagnostic test is performed to detect plaque buildup in the artery to predict or diagnose an ischemic stroke.

- **Echoencephalography** (**eck**-oh-en-**sef**-ah-**LOG**-rah-fee) is the use of ultrasound imaging to create a detailed visual image of the brain for diagnostic purposes (**ech/o** means sound, **encephal/o** means brain, and **-graphy** means the process of producing a picture or record).

■ **Electroencephalography** (ee-**leck**-troh-en-**sef**-ah-**LOG**-rah-fee) is the process of recording the electrical activity of the brain through the use of electrodes attached to the scalp (**electr/o** means electric, **encephal/o** means brain, and **-graphy** means the process of producing a picture or record). The resulting record is an *electroencephalogram*. This electrical activity may also be displayed on a monitor as brain waves.

■ **Myelography** (**my**-eh-**LOG**-rah-fee) is a radiographic study of the spinal cord after the injection of a contrast medium through a lumbar puncture (**myel/o** means spinal cord, and **-graphy** means the process of producing a picture or record). The resulting record is a *myelogram*.

■ A **lumbar puncture**, also known as a *spinal tap*, is the process of obtaining a sample of cerebrospinal fluid by inserting a needle into the subarachnoid space of the lumbar region to withdraw fluid. Changes in the composition of the cerebrospinal fluid can be an indication of injury, infection, or disease.

## ■ TREATMENT PROCEDURES OF THE NERVOUS SYSTEM

### Sedative and Hypnotic Medications

■ A **hypnotic** depresses the central nervous system and usually produces sleep.

■ An **anticonvulsant** (**an**-tih-kon-**VUL**-sant) is administered to prevent seizures such as those associated with epilepsy.

■ **Barbiturates** (bar-**BIT**-you-raytz) are a class of drugs whose major action is a calming or depressed effect on the central nervous system.

  ■ *Amobarbital* is a barbiturate used as a sedative and hypnotic.

  ■ *Phenobarbital* is a barbiturate used as a sedative and as an anticonvulsant.

■ A **sedative** depresses the central nervous system to produce calm and diminished responsiveness without producing sleep. *Sedation* is the effect produced by a sedative.

### Anesthesia

**Anesthesia** (an-es-**THEE**-zee-ah) is the absence of normal sensation, especially sensitivity to pain, that is induced by the administration of an anesthetic agent (**an-** means without, and **-esthesia** means feeling).

■ An **anesthetic** (**an**-es-**THET**-ick) is the medication used to induce anesthesia. The anesthetic may be topical, local, regional, or general (**an-** means without, **esthet** means feeling, and **-ic** means pertaining to).

■ **Epidural anesthesia** (ep-ih-**DOO**-ral **an**-es-**THEE**-zee-ah) is regional anesthesia produced by injecting medication into the epidural space of the lumbar or sacral region of the spine. When administered during childbirth, it numbs the nerves from the uterus and birth passage without stopping labor (Figure 10.16).

■ *General anesthesia* involves the total loss of body sensation and consciousness induced by anesthetic agents administered primarily by inhalation or intravenous injection.

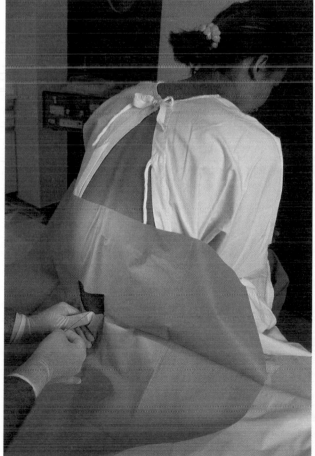

Laurent/B./American Hospital of Paris/Photo Researchers, Inc.

**FIGURE 10.16** Epidural anesthesia administered during childbirth numbs the nerves from the uterus and birth passage without stopping labor.

- *Local anesthesia* causes the loss of sensation in a limited area by injecting an anesthetic solution near that area.

- *Regional anesthesia*, the temporary interruption of nerve conduction, is produced by injecting an anesthetic solution near the nerves to be blocked.

- **Spinal anesthesia** is regional anesthesia produced by injecting medication into the subarachnoid space. As with epidural anesthesia, the patient remains conscious. Spinal anesthesia provides numbness from the toes to the waist or lower chest.

- *Topical anesthesia* numbs only the tissue surface and is applied as a liquid, ointment, or spray.

## The Brain

- **Deep brain stimulation** (DBS) is a neurosurgical procedure used in the treatment of dystonia, tremors, and Parkinson's disease. A device to stimulate the brain with mild electrical signals is implanted in the brain and is connected to a stimulator implanted near the collar bone. *Dystonia* is the impairment of voluntary muscle movement (see Chapter 4).

- **Gamma knife surgery** is a type of radiation treatment for brain tumors performed without a knife or an incision. The surgeon uses gamma radiation to destroy diseased tissue while preserving the healthy tissue around the tumor. *Gamma radiation,* which is characterized by high energy and a short wavelength, is also used in nuclear medicine (see Chapter 15).

- **Electroconvulsive therapy** (ECT) (ee-**leck**-troh-kon-**VUL**-siv), also known as *electroshock therapy,* is a procedure in which small amounts of electric current are passed through the brain, deliberately triggering a brief seizure in order to reverse symptoms of certain mental illnesses.

- **Light therapy** is exposure to daylight or to specific wavelengths of light in order to counteract seasonal affective disorder (SAD).

- A **lobectomy** (loh-**BECK**-toh-mee) is surgical removal of a portion of the brain to treat brain cancer or seizure disorders that cannot be controlled with medication.

- A **thalamotomy** (**thal**-ah-**MOT**-oh-mee) is a surgical incision into the thalamus (**thalam** means thalamus, and **-otomy** means surgical incision). This procedure, which destroys brain cells, is primarily performed to quiet the tremors of Parkinson's disease.

## Nerves

- **Neuroplasty** (**NEW**-roh-**plas**-tee) is the surgical repair of a nerve or nerves (**neur/o** means nerve, and **-plasty** means surgical repair).

- **Neurorrhaphy** (new-**ROR**-ah-fee) is surgically suturing together the ends of a severed nerve (**neur/o** means nerve, and **-rrhaphy** means surgical suturing).

- **Neurotomy** (new-**ROT**-oh-mee) is the surgical division or dissection (cutting) of a nerve (**neur** means nerve, and **-otomy** means a surgical incision).

## ◼ MENTAL HEALTH

Although described as being disorders of mental health, the causes of the following conditions also include congenital abnormalities, physical changes, substance abuse, medications, or any combination of these factors.

## Anxiety Disorders

**Anxiety disorders** are mental conditions characterized by excessive, irrational dread of everyday situations or fear that is out of proportion to the real danger in a situation. Without treatment, an anxiety disorder can become chronic.

- A **generalized anxiety disorder** (GAD) is characterized by chronic, excessive worrying. Physical symptoms associated with this condition can include muscle tension, sleep disturbance, irritability, trouble concentrating, and restlessness.

- **Obsessive-compulsive disorder** (OCD) is characterized by recurrent *obsessions* (repetitive, intrusive, distressing thoughts or impulses) and/or *compulsions* (repeatedly feeling compelled to do things, like wash or pray). OCD makes someone feel he or she must do compulsive behaviors, such as repeated cleaning or checking, to prevent harm or stop the obsession. Performing compulsions provides only temporary relief, but not performing them temporarily increases anxiety.

- **Panic disorder** is characterized by a fear of panic attacks. Panic disorder can cause people to develop *agoraphobia* or other *phobias* (see following section on phobias).

- A **panic attack** is an unexpected, sudden experience of fear in the absence of danger, accompanied by physical symptoms such as heart palpitations, shortness of breath, chest tightness, dizziness, sweating, nausea, feelings of unreality, choking sensations, or a combination of these. A panic attack is simply unneeded activation of the body's fight-or-flight response.

- **Post-traumatic stress disorder** (PTSD) may develop after an event involving actual or threatened death or injury to the individual or someone else, during which the person felt intense fear, helplessness, or horror (**post-** means after, **trauma** means injury, and **-tic** means pertaining to). War, natural disasters, or other life-threatening experiences can cause PTSD. Symptoms include emotional numbing, hyperarousal, anxiety, sleep disorders, and persistent reliving of the event (Figure 10.17).

## Phobias

A **phobia** (**FOH**-bee-ah) is a persistent irrational fear of a specific thing or situation, strong enough to cause sig-nificant distress, to interfere with functioning, and to lead to the avoidance of the thing or situation that causes this reaction. There are countless types of phobias, and they are named by adding **-phobia** to the name of the object.

- **Acrophobia** (**ack**-roh-**FOH**-bee-ah) is an excessive fear of heights (**acr/o** means top, and **-phobia** means abnormal fear).

- **Agoraphobia** (**ag**-oh-rah-**FOH**-bee-ah) is an excessive fear of environments where the person fears a panic attack might occur. In order to avoid these situations, someone suffering from agoraphobia might not even be able to leave home (**agor/a** means marketplace, and **-phobia** means abnormal fear).

- **Claustrophobia** (**klaws**-troh-**FOH**-bee-ah) is an abnormal fear of being in small or enclosed spaces (**claustr/o** means barrier, and **-phobia** means abnormal fear).

- **Social phobia,** also called *social anxiety disorder*, is an excessive fear of social situations where the person fears negative evaluation by others and embarrassing himself in front of others.

## Developmental Disorders

- An **attention deficit/hyperactivity disorder** (ADHD) is characterized by a short attention span and impulsive behavior that is inappropriate for the child's developmental age. *Hyperactivity* is restlessness or a continuing excess of movement. The term *attention deficit disorder (ADD)* is sometimes used if hyperactivity is not present. These conditions may persist into adulthood.

- **Dyslexia** (dis-**LECK**-see-ah), also known as a *developmental reading disorder*, is a learning disability characterized by substandard reading achievement due to the inability of the brain to process symbols.

- **Learning disabilities** are disorders found in children of normal intelligence who have difficulties in learning specific skills such as processing language or grasping mathematical concepts.

- **Mental retardation/intellectual disability** (MR/ID) is a diagnosis of significant below-average intellectual and adaptive functioning present from birth or early infancy. Note: the traditional term *mental retardation* is gradually being replaced by *intellectual disability*; however, during this transition both are used.

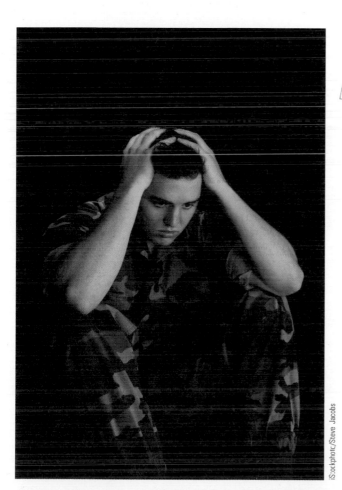

iStockphoto/Steve Jacobs

**FIGURE 10.17** Post-traumatic stress disorder may develop after military service as a result of actual or threatened death or injury to the individual or someone else.

## Autism Spectrum Disorders

**Autistic spectrum disorders** (aw-**TIS**-tic) (ASD) describes a group of conditions in which a young child has difficulty developing normal social relationships and communication skills, may compulsively follow repetitive routines, and has narrowly focused, intense interests that are sometimes unusual.

■ **Autism** (**AW**-tizm) is a subgroup of autistic spectrum disorders. Children with autism have significant developmental delays, including speech and language. Most children with autism have very minimal verbal skills and lack normal social relationships (Figure 10.18).

■ *Asperger's syndrome* is another subgroup of the autism disorders spectrum. Individuals with Asperger's syndrome usually have normal or above-average intelligence but are impaired in social interactions and nonverbal communication.

## Dissociative Disorders

**Dissociative disorders** occur when normal thought is separated from consciousness.

■ **Dissociative identity disorder**, formerly known as *multiple personality disorder*, is a mental illness characterized by the presence of two or more distinct personalities, each with its own characteristics, which appear to exist within the same individual.

## Factitious Disorders

A **factitious disorder** (fack-**TISH**-us) is a condition in which an individual acts as if he or she has a physical or mental illness when he or she is not really sick. The term *factitious* means artificial, self-induced, or not naturally occurring. Visible symptoms are self-inflicted and seem motivated by a desire for attention and sympathy rather than for external benefits like malingering (see the later section "Somatoform Disorders").

■ A **factitious disorder by proxy** is a form of child abuse. Although seeming very concerned about the child's well-being, the mentally ill parent will falsify an illness in a child by making up or inducing symptoms, and then seeking medical treatment, even surgery, for the child.

## Impulse Control Disorders

**Impulse control disorders** are a group of psychiatric disorders characterized by a failure to resist an impulse despite potential negative consequences. In addition to

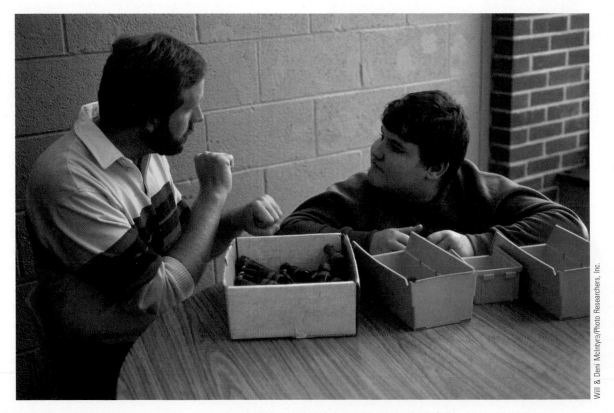

Will & Deni McIntyre/Photo Researchers, Inc.

**FIGURE 10.18** A therapist works with a boy with autism to develop communication skills.

the examples listed below, this disorder includes compulsive shopping and gambling. The suffix **-mania** means madness.

- *Kleptomania* is a disorder characterized by repeatedly stealing objects neither for personal use nor for their monetary value.

- *Pyromania* is a disorder characterized by repeated, deliberate fire setting.

- *Trichotillomania* is a disorder characterized by the repeated pulling out of one's own hair.

## Mood Disorders

- A **bipolar disorder** is a condition characterized by cycles of severe mood changes shifting from highs (manic behavior) and severe lows (depression) that affect a person's attitude, energy, and ability to function.

- **Manic behavior** includes an abnormally elevated mood state, including inappropriate elation, increased irritability, severe insomnia, poor judgment, and inappropriate social behavior.

- **Depression** is a common mood disorder characterized by lethargy and sadness, as well as the loss of interest or pleasure in normal activities. Severe depression may lead to feelings of worthlessness and thoughts of death or suicide. *Suicide* is the intentional taking of one's own life.

- **Dysthymia** (dis-THIGH-mee-ah), also known as *dysthymic disorder*, is a low-grade chronic depression with symptoms that are milder than those of severe depression but are present on a majority of days for 2 or more years (**dys-** means bad, **thym** means mind, and **-ia** means condition).

- **Seasonal affective disorder** (SAD) is a seasonal bout of depression associated with the decrease in hours of daylight during winter months.

## Personality Disorders

A **personality disorder** is a chronic pattern of inner experience and behavior that causes serious problems with relationships and work. This pattern is pervasive and inflexible, has an onset in adolescence or early adulthood, is stable over time, and leads to distress or impairment.

- An *antisocial personality disorder* is a pattern of disregard for and violation of the rights of others. This pattern brings the individual into continuous conflict with society.

- A *borderline personality disorder* is characterized by impulsive actions, often with the potential for self-harm, as well as mood instability and chaotic relationships.

- A *narcissistic personality disorder* is a pattern of extreme preoccupation with the self and complete lack of empathy for others. *Empathy* is the ability to understand another person's mental and emotional state without becoming personally involved.

## Psychotic Disorders *away from reality*

A **psychotic disorder** (sigh-KOT-ick) is characterized by the loss of contact with reality and deterioration of normal social functioning.

- **Catatonic behavior** (kat-ah-TON-ick) is marked by a lack of responsiveness, stupor, and a tendency to remain in a fixed posture (Figure 10.19).

- A **delusion** (dee-LOO-zhun) is a false personal belief that is maintained despite obvious proof or evidence to the contrary. The belief is not one ordinarily accepted by other members of the individual's culture or religious faith.

- A **hallucination** (hah-loo-sih-NAY-shun) is a sensory perception (i.e., sight, touch, sound, smell, or taste) experienced in the absence of external stimulation.

- **Schizophrenia** (skit-soh-FREE-nee-ah) is a psychotic disorder usually characterized by withdrawal from reality, illogical patterns of thinking, delusions, and hallucinations, and accompanied in varying degrees by other emotional, behavioral, or intellectual disturbances (Figure 10.19).

## Somatoform Disorders

A **somatoform disorder** (soh-MAT-oh-form) is characterized by physical complaints or concerns about one's body that are out of proportion to any physical findings or disease.

- A **conversion disorder** is characterized by serious temporary or ongoing changes in function, such as paralysis or blindness, that are triggered by psychological factors rather than by any physical cause.

- **Hypochondriasis** (high-poh-kon-DRY-ah-sis) is characterized by fearing that one has a serious illness despite appropriate medical evaluation and reassurance. A person exhibiting this syndrome is known as a *hypochondriac*.

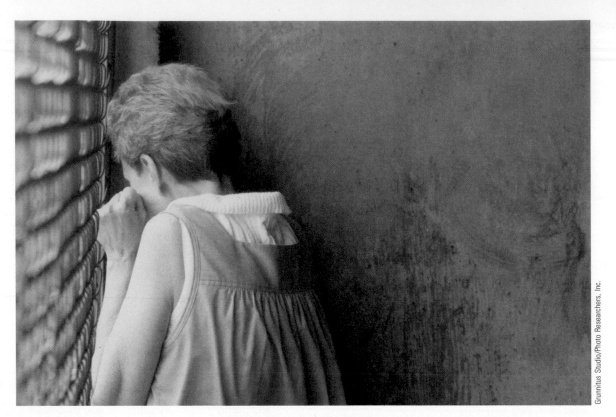

Grumitus Studio/Photo Researchers, Inc.

**FIGURE 10.19** Schizophrenia is marked by withdrawal from reality and may include catatonic behavior.

■ **Malingering** (mah-**LING**-ger-ing) is characterized by the intentional creation of false or grossly exaggerated physical or psychological symptoms. In contrast to a factitious disorder, this condition is motivated by incentives such as avoiding work.

## Substance-Related Disorders

**Substance abuse** is the addictive use of tobacco, alcohol, medications, or illegal drugs. This abuse leads to significant impairment in functioning, danger to one's self or others, and recurrent legal and/or interpersonal problems.

■ **Alcoholism** (**AL**-koh-hol-izm) is chronic alcohol dependence with specific signs and symptoms upon withdrawal. *Withdrawal* is a psychological or physical syndrome (or both) caused by the abrupt cessation (stopping) of the use of alcohol or a drug in an addicted individual.

■ **Delirium tremens** (deh-**LEER**-ee-um **TREE**-mens) (DTs) is a disorder involving sudden and severe mental changes or seizures caused by abruptly stopping the use of alcohol.

■ **Drug abuse** is the excessive use of illegal or recreational drugs, or the misuse of prescription drugs. A *recreational drug* is one normally used for personal pleasure or satisfaction rather than medical purposes.

■ **A drug overdose** is the accidental or intentional use of an illegal drug or prescription medicine in an amount higher than what is safe or normal.

## Medications to Treat Mental Disorders

A **psychotropic drug** (sigh-koh-**TROP**-pick) acts primarily on the central nervous system, where it produces temporary changes affecting the mind, emotions, and behavior (**psych/o** means mind, and **-tropic** means having an affinity for). These drugs are used as medications to control pain, and to treat narcolepsy and attention disorders.

■ An **antidepressant** is administered to prevent or relieve depression. Some of these medications are also used to treat obsessive-compulsive and generalized anxiety disorders and to help relieve chronic pain.

■ An **antipsychotic drug** (**an**-tih-sigh-**KOT**-ick) or *neuroleptic* is administered to treat symptoms of severe disorders of thinking and mood that are associated with neurological and psychiatric illnesses such as schizophrenia, mania, and delusional disorders (**anti-** means against, **psych/o** means mind, and **-tic** means pertaining to).

■ An **anxiolytic drug** (ang-zee-oh-**LIT**-ick), also known as an *antianxiety drug* or *tranquilizer*, is administered to temporarily relieve anxiety and to reduce tension (**anxi/o** means anxiety, and **-lytic** means to destroy).

■ **Mood-stabilizing drugs**, such as lithium, are used to treat mood instability and bipolar disorders.

■ A **stimulant** works by increasing activity in certain areas of the brain to increase concentration and wakefulness. Drug therapies using stimulants have been effective in treating ADHD and narcolepsy. The overuse of stimulants, including caffeine, can cause sleeplessness and palpitations.

## Psychological Therapies to Treat Mental Disorders

Mental disorders are often treated with individual or group therapy by a qualified psychotherapist.

■ **Psychoanalysis** (**sigh**-koh-ah-**NAL**-ih-sis) is based on the idea that mental disorders have underlying causes stemming from childhood and can only be overcome by gaining insight into one's feelings and patterns of behavior.

■ **Behavioral therapy** focuses on changing behavior by identifying problem behaviors, replacing them with appropriate behaviors and using rewards or other consequences to make the changes.

■ **Cognitive therapy** focuses on changing cognitions or thoughts that are affecting a person's emotions and actions. These are identified and then are challenged through logic, gathering evidence, testing in action, or a combination of these. The goal is to change problematic beliefs.

■ **Hypnotherapy** is the use of hypnosis to produce an altered state of focused attention in which the patient may be more willing to believe and act on suggestions. It is used for pain relief, anxiety reduction, and behavioral modification.

## ABBREVIATIONS RELATED TO THE NERVOUS SYSTEM

Table 10.4 presents an overview of the abbreviations related to the terms introduced in this chapter. Note: To avoid errors or confusion, always be cautious when using abbreviations.

## TABLE 10.4
## Abbreviations Related to the Nervous System

| | |
|---|---|
| Alzheimer's disease = AD | **AD** = Alzheimer's disease |
| amyotrophic lateral sclerosis = ALS | **ALS** = amyotrophic lateral sclerosis |
| attention-deficit hyperactivity disorder = ADHD | **ADHD** = attention-deficit hyperactivity disorder |
| cerebral palsy = CP | **CP** = cerebral palsy |
| cerebrospinal fluid = CSF | **CSF** = cerebrospinal fluid |
| electroencephalography = EEG | **EEG** = electroencephalography |
| intracranial pressure = ICP | **ICP** = intracranial pressure |
| levels of consciousness or loss of consciousness = LOC | **LOC** = levels of consciousness or loss of consciousness |
| lumbar puncture = LP | **LP** = lumbar puncture |
| multiple sclerosis = MS | **MS** = multiple sclerosis |
| obsessive-compulsive disorder = OCD | **OCD** = obsessive-compulsive disorder |
| post-traumatic stress disorder = PTSD | **PTSD** = post-traumatic stress disorder |
| seizure = Sz | **Sz** = seizure |
| transient ischemic attack = TIA | **TIA** = transient ischemic attack |

**StudyWARE** CONNECTION

For more practice and to test your mastery of this material, go to the StudyWARE™ to play interactive games and complete the quiz for this chapter.

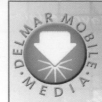

Downloadable audio is available for selected medical terms in this chapter to enhance your learning of medical terminology.

## ☐ Workbook Practice

Go to your workbook, and complete the exercises for this chapter.

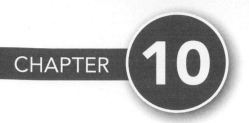
# LEARNING EXERCISES

## MATCHING WORD PARTS 1

Write the correct answer in the middle column.

| Definition | Correct Answer | Possible Answers |
|---|---|---|
| 10.1. feeling | *esthet/o* | psych/o |
| 10.2. brain | *encephal* | encephal/o |
| 10.3. bruise | *contus/o* | contus/o |
| 10.4. mind | *psych/o* | concuss/o |
| 10.5. shaken together | *concuss/o* | esthet/o |

## MATCHING WORD PARTS 2

Write the correct answer in the middle column.

| Definition | Correct Answer | Possible Answers |
|---|---|---|
| 10.6. brain covering | *mening/o* | -esthesia |
| 10.7. process of producing a picture | *-graphy* | -graphy |
| 10.8. sensation, feeling | *-esthesia* | radicul/o |
| 10.9. spinal cord | *myel/o* | mening/o |
| 10.10. nerve root | *radicul/o* | myel/o |

## MATCHING WORD PARTS 3

Write the correct answer in the middle column.

| Definition | Correct Answer | Possible Answers |
|---|---|---|
| 10.11. abnormal fear | *Phobia* | -tropic |
| 10.12. burning sensation | *caus/o* | phobia |

10.13. brain _____cerebr/o_____ **neur/o**

10.14. nerve, nerves _____neur/o_____ **cerebr/o**

10.15. having an affinity for _____tropic_____ **caus/o**

## DEFINITIONS

Select the correct answer, and write it on the line provided.

10.16. The space between two neurons or between a neuron and a receptor organ is known

as a _____.

    dendrite      ganglion      plexus      synapse

10.17. The white protective covering over some parts of the spinal cord and the axon of most peripheral nerves

is the _____.

    myelin sheath      neuroglia      neurotransmitter      pia mater

10.18. The _____ are the root-like structures of a nerve that receive impulses and conduct

them to the cell body.

    axons      dendrites      ganglions      neurotransmitters

10.19. The _____ is the layer of the meninges that is located nearest to the brain and

spinal cord.

    arachnoid membrane      dura mater      meninx      pia mater

10.20. Seven vital body functions are regulated by the _____.

    cerebral cortex      cerebellum      hypothalamus      thalamus

10.21. The _____ nerves are the division of the autonomic nervous system that prepare

the body for emergencies and stress.

    afferent      parasympathetic      peripheral      sympathetic

10.22. A _____ is a network of intersecting nerves.

    ganglion      plexus      synapse      tract

10.23.  Cranial nerves are part of the _____ nervous system.

      autonomic          central          cranial          (peripheral)

10.24.  The _____ relays sensory stimuli from the spinal cord and midbrain to the cerebral cortex.

      cerebellum          hypothalamus          medulla oblongata          thalamus

10.25.  The _____ neurons carry impulses away from the brain and spinal cord.

      afferent          associative          efferent          (sensory)

## MATCHING STRUCTURES

Write the correct answer in the middle column.

| Definition | Correct Answer | Possible Answers |
|---|---|---|
| 10.26. connects the brain and spinal cord | _____ | medulla oblongata |
| 10.27. controls vital body functions | _____ | hypothalamus |
| 10.28. coordinates muscular activity | _____ | cerebrum |
| 10.29. controls basic survival functions | _____ | cerebellum |
| 10.30. uppermost layer of the brain | _____ | brainstem |

## WHICH WORD?

Select the correct answer, and write it on the line provided.

10.31.  A physician who specializes in administering anesthetic agents is an _____.

      anesthetist          anesthesiologist

10.32.  A _____ is a profound state of unconsciousness marked by the absence of spontaneous eye movements, no response to painful stimuli, and the lack of speech.

      coma          stupor

10.33.  An _____ drug is also known as a tranquilizer.

      antipsychotic          anxiolytic

10.34. A/An _____ is a sensory perception that has no basis in external stimulation.

      delusion          hallucination

10.35. An excessive fear of heights is _____.

      acrophobia        agoraphobia

## SPELLING COUNTS

Find the misspelled word in each sentence. Then write that word, spelled correctly, on the line provided.

10.36. A migrane headache is characterized by throbbing pain on one side of the

      head. _____

10.37. Alzhiemer's disease is a group of disorders involving the parts of the brain that control thought, memory,

      and language. _____

10.38. An anasthetic is the medication used to induce anesthesia. _____

10.39. Epalepsy is a chronic neurological condition characterized by recurrent episodes of seizures of varying

      severity. _____

10.40. Siatica is a nerve inflammation that results in pain, burning, and tingling through the thigh, leg, and

      foot. _____

## ABBREVIATION IDENTIFICATION

In the space provided, write the words that each abbreviation stands for.

10.41. **CP** _____

10.42. **CSF** _____

10.43. **OCD** _____

10.44. **PTSD** _____

10.45. **TIA** _____

## TERM SELECTION

Select the correct answer, and write it on the line provided.

10.46.  The acute condition that is characterized by confusion, disorientation, disordered thinking and memory,

agitation, and hallucinations is known as _____.

       delirium              dementia              lethargy              stupor

10.47.  The term meaning inflammation of the spinal cord is _____. This term also means

inflammation of bone marrow.

       encephalitis           myelitis           myelosis           radiculitis

10.48.  The medical term meaning an abnormal fear of being in small or enclosed spaces

is _____.

       acrophobia          claustrophobia        kleptomania        pyromania

10.49.  The condition known as _____ is characterized by severe lightning-like pain due to

an inflammation of the fifth cranial nerve.

       Bell's palsy          Guillain-Barré syndrome       Lou Gehrig's disease       trigeminal neuralgia

10.50.  The medical term for the condition also known as a developmental reading disorder

is _____.

       autism          dissociative disorder       dyslexia        mental retardation

## SENTENCE COMPLETION

Write the correct term or terms on the lines provided.

10.51.  A _____ is the bruising of brain tissue as the result of a head injury.

10.52.  The mental conditions characterized by excessive, irrational dread of everyday situations or fear that is

out of proportion to the real danger in a situation are known as _____.

10.53.  A low-grade chronic depression with symptoms that are milder than those of severe depression but are

present on a majority of days for two or more years is known as _____.

10.54. A/An _____ disorder is a condition in which an individual acts as if he or she has

a physical or mental illness when he or she is not really sick.

10.55. A/An _____ drug is administered to treat symptoms of severe disorders of thinking

and mood that are associated with neurological and psychiatric illnesses such as schizophrenia, mania,

and delusional disorders.

## WORD SURGERY

Divide each term into its component word parts. Write these word parts, in sequence, on the lines provided. When necessary, use a slash (/) to indicate a combining vowel. (You may not need all of the lines provided.)

10.56. An **anesthetic** is the medication used to induce anesthesia.

_____    _____    _____    _____

10.57. **Somnambulism** is commonly known as sleepwalking.

_____    _____    _____    _____

10.58. **Electroencephalography** is the process of recording the electrical activity of the brain through the use of

electrodes attached to the scalp.

_____    _____    _____    _____

10.59. **Paresthesia** refers to a burning or prickling sensation that is usually felt in the hands, arms, legs, or feet.

_____    _____    _____    _____

10.60. **Poliomyelitis** is a contagious viral infection of the brainstem and spinal cord, which sometimes leads to

paralysis.

_____    _____    _____    _____

## TRUE/FALSE

If the statement is true, write **True** on the line. If the statement is false, write **False** on the line.

10.61. _____ A hemorrhagic stroke occurs when a blood vessel in the brain leaks.

10.62. _____ An absence seizure is a brief disturbance in brain function in which there is

a loss of awareness.

10.63. _____ A sedative is administered to prevent the seizures associated with epilepsy.

10.64. _____ A patient in a persistent vegetative state sleeps through the night and is

awake and conscious during the day.

10.65. _____ A psychotropic drug acts primarily on the central nervous system where it

produces temporary changes affecting the mind, emotions, and behavior.

## CLINICAL CONDITIONS

Write the correct answer on the line provided.

10.66.  Harvey Ikeman has mood shifts from highs to severe lows that affect his attitude, energy, and ability to

function. Harvey's doctor describes this condition as a/an _____ disorder.

10.67.  In the auto accident, Anthony DeNicola hit his head on the windshield. The paramedics were concerned

that this jarring of the brain had caused a/an _____.

10.68.  Georgia Houghton suffered a _____ attack (TIA), and her doctors were concerned

that this was a warning of an increased stroke risk.

10.69.  To control her patient's tremors caused by Parkinson's disease, Dr. Wang performed

a/an _____. This is a surgical incision into the thalamus.

10.70.  Mary Beth Cawthorn was diagnosed as having _____. This progressive autoim-

mune disease is characterized by inflammation that causes demyelination of the myelin sheath.

10.71.  After several months of being unable to sleep well, Wayne Ladner visited his doctor about this problem.

His doctor recorded this condition as being _____.

10.72.  After her stroke, Rosita Valladares was unable to understand written or spoken words. This condition is

known as _____.

10.73.  Jill Beck said she fainted. The medical term for this brief loss of consciousness caused by the decreased

blood flow to the brain is _____.

10.74.  The Baily baby was born with _____. This condition is an abnormally increased

amount of cerebrospinal fluid in the ventricles of the brain.

10.75.  The MRI indicated that Mrs. Hoshi had a collection of blood trapped in the tissues of her brain. This

condition, which was caused by a head injury, is called a cranial _____.

## WHICH IS THE CORRECT MEDICAL TERM?

Select the correct answer, and write it on the line provided.

10.76.  Persistent, severe burning pain that usually follows an injury to a sensory nerve is known

as ＿＿＿＿＿＿＿＿＿＿＿.

causalgia          hyperesthesia          hypoesthesia          paresthesia

10.77.  The classification of drug that depresses the central nervous system and usually produces sleep is known

as a/an ＿＿＿＿＿＿＿＿＿＿＿.

anesthetic          barbiturate          hypnotic          sedative

10.78.  A/An ＿＿＿＿＿＿＿＿＿＿＿ disorder is characterized by serious temporary or ongoing changes in

function, such as paralysis or blindness, that are triggered by psychological factors rather than by any

physical cause.

anxiety          conversion          factitious          panic

10.79.  During childbirth, ＿＿＿＿＿＿＿＿＿＿＿ anesthesia is administered to numb the nerves from the

uterus and birth passage without stopping labor.

epidural          local          regional          topical

10.80.  The condition known as ＿＿＿＿＿＿＿＿＿＿＿ is a rapidly progressive neurological disease that

attacks the nerve cells responsible for controlling voluntary muscles.

amyotrophic lateral sclerosis          cerebral palsy          epilepsy          multiple sclerosis

## CHALLENGE WORD BUILDING

These terms are *not* found in this chapter; however, they are made up of the following familiar word parts. If you need help in creating the term, refer to your medical dictionary.

| poly- | encephal/o | -algia |
|---|---|---|
| | mening/o | -itis |
| | myel/o | -malacia |
| | neur/o | -oma |
| | | -pathy |

10.81.   Based on word parts, the term meaning inflammation of the nerves and spinal cord

is _____my_____.

10.82.   Abnormal softening of the meninges is known as _____.

10.83.   A benign neoplasm made up of nerve tissue is a/an _____.

10.84.   Based on word parts, the term meaning any degenerative disease of the brain

is _____.

10.85.   Pain affecting many nerves is known as _____.

10.86.   Abnormal softening of nerve tissue is known as _____.

10.87.   Inflammation of the meninges and the brain is known as _____.

10.88.   Based on word parts, the term meaning any pathological condition of the spinal cord

is _____.

10.89.   Abnormal softening of the brain is known as _____.

10.90.   Inflammation of the meninges, brain, and spinal cord is known as _____.

## LABELING EXERCISES

Identify the numbered items on the accompanying figures.

10.91. _Cerebral_ cortex

10.92. _Frontal_ lobe

10.93. _Temporal_ lobe

10.94. _Parietal_ lobe

10.95. _Occipital_ lobe

10.96. _Ventricles_

10.97. _Hypothalamus_

10.98. _Medulla oblongata_

10.99. _Spinal_ cord

10.100. _Cerebellum_

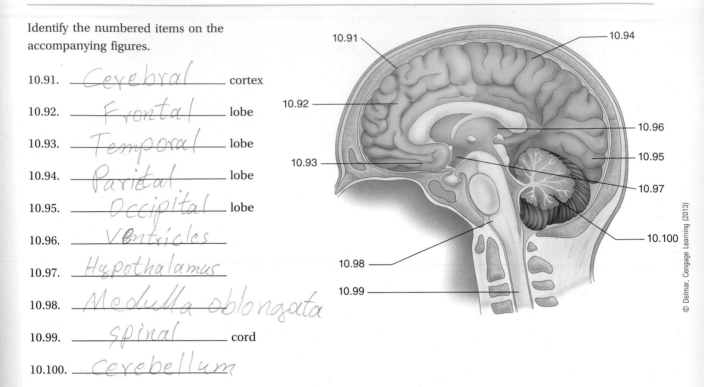

© Delmar, Cengage Learning (2013)

# THE HUMAN TOUCH

## Critical Thinking Exercise

The following story and questions are designed to stimulate critical thinking through class discussion or as a brief essay response. There are no right or wrong answers to these questions.

*Calle Washington read the information Dr. Thakker gave her with numb disbelief. "Multiple sclerosis (MS) is a neurological disorder characterized by demyelination of nerve fibers in the brain and spinal column. This disease may be progressively debilitating with symptoms that could include numbness, paralysis, ataxia, pain, and blindness. Some patients do experience life-threatening complications. This disease attacks young adults. It affects more women than men."*

*"Well, I sure fit the profile," thought Calle bitterly. She took a deep breath, trying to quiet the fluttering in her stomach. How could this happen now? Everything was so perfect. Her wedding gown was getting its last alterations, and the tickets for their honeymoon in Jamaica were in the desk drawer. Gabe was putting the final touches on the house where they planned on raising their family. She couldn't expect Gabe to waste his future caring for someone in a wheelchair, could she? Suddenly, her fairy tale life was turning into a nightmare.*

*Calle occasionally feels off balance. If she lost her balance suddenly, would this put the children she worked with at the day care center at risk? What would happen once her fellow teachers at the day care center noticed that? She would not risk hurting one of the children, but if she lost her job she would lose her health insurance. Dr. Thakker had said there were new drugs for MS, but he had also mentioned that they were very expensive. And what about the children that she and Gabe both wanted? Could she still have a baby and take care of it?*

*"Maybe I should take out an ad that says '25-year-old female seeks cure for deadly disease before marrying Prince Charming,'" she thought, trying to laugh through her tears ...*

## Suggested Discussion Topics

1. Which symptoms of Calle's condition might affect her job? She has been working with the youngest children. Should she consider resigning, or could she ask for a different assignment?

2. Calle and Gabe decide to go ahead with the wedding. If they have children, is there a risk that Calle will transmit this condition? If Calle cannot have children, what other options would enable them to have the family they both want?

3. After their marriage, Calle will be covered by her husband's health insurance. Calle is ethical in completing her application for this coverage and mentions the MS diagnosis. But she has questions. Where could Calle get information as to whether or not the insurance company will ever cover her for this disease? Will her coverage begin immediately?

4. Calle is an excellent teacher and the children love her. In the past, her coworkers have commented, **"I wish I could learn to be as good at this as you are."** Even with multiple sclerosis, could Calle have a future in training other teachers? What other positive steps might she contemplate taking?

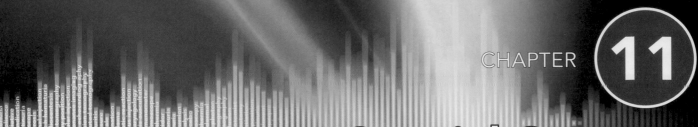

## CHAPTER 11

# Special Senses: The Eyes and Ears

## Overview of
## STRUCTURES, COMBINING FORMS, AND FUNCTIONS OF THE EYES AND EARS

| Major Structures | Related Combining Forms | Primary Functions |
|---|---|---|
| Eyes | opt/i, opt/o, optic/o, ophthalm/o | Receptor organs for the sense of sight. |
| Iris | ir/i, ir/o, irid/o, irit/o | Controls the amount of light entering the eye. |
| Lens | phac/o, phak/o | Focuses rays of light on the retina. |
| Retina | retin/o | Converts light images into electrical impulses and transmits them to the brain. |
| Lacrimal Apparatus | dacryocyst/o, lacrim/o | Accessory structures of the eyes that produce, store, and remove tears. |
| Ears | acous/o, acoust/o, audi/o, audit/o, ot/o | Receptor organs for the sense of hearing; also helps maintain balance. |
| Outer Ear | pinn/i | Transmits sound waves to the middle ear. |
| Middle Ear | myring/o, tympan/o | Transmits sound waves to the inner ear. |
| Inner Ear | labyrinth/o | Receives sound vibrations and transmits them to the brain. |

# Vocabulary Related to **THE SPECIAL SENSES**

This list contains essential word parts and medical terms for this chapter. These terms are pronounced in the student StudyWARE™ and Audio CDs that are available for use with this text. These and the other important **primary terms** are shown in boldface throughout the chapter. *Secondary terms*, which appear in *orange* italics, clarify the meaning of primary terms.

## Word Parts

- [ ] **blephar/o** eyelid
- [ ] **-cusis** hearing
- [ ] **irid/o** iris, colored part of eye
- [ ] **kerat/o** horny, hard, cornea
- [ ] **myring/o** tympanic membrane, eardrum
- [ ] **ophthalm/o** eye, vision
- [ ] **-opia** vision condition
- [ ] **opt/o** eye, vision
- [ ] **ot/o** ear, hearing
- [ ] **phak/o** lens of eye
- [ ] **presby/o** old age
- [ ] **retin/o** retina, net
- [ ] **scler/o** sclera, white of eye, hard
- [ ] **trop/o** turn, change
- [ ] **tympan/o** tympanic membrane, eardrum

## Medical Terms

- [ ] **adnexa** (ad-**NECK**-sah)
- [ ] **amblyopia** (**am**-blee-**OH**-pee-ah)
- [ ] **ametropia** (**am**-eh-**TROH**-pee-ah)
- [ ] **anisocoria** (**an**-ih-so-**KOH**-ree-ah)
- [ ] **astigmatism** (ah-**STIG**-mah-tizm)
- [ ] **audiometry** (aw-dee-**OM**-eh-tree)
- [ ] **cataract** (**KAT**-ah-rakt)
- [ ] **chalazion** (kah-**LAY**-zee-on)
- [ ] **cochlear implant** (**KOCK**-lee-ar)
- [ ] **conjunctivitis** (kon-**junk**-tih-**VYE**-tis)
- [ ] **dacryoadenitis** (**dack**-ree-oh-ad-eh-**NIGH**-tis)
- [ ] **diplopia** (dih-**PLOH**-pee-ah)
- [ ] **ectropion** (eck-**TROH**-pee-on)
- [ ] **emmetropia** (em-eh-**TROH**-pee-ah)
- [ ] **entropion** (en-**TROH**-pee-on)
- [ ] **esotropia** (es-oh-**TROH**-pee-ah)
- [ ] **exotropia** (eck-soh-**TROH**-pee-ah)
- [ ] **fluorescein angiography** (**flew**-oh-**RES**-ee-in an-jee-**OG**-rah-fee)

- [ ] **glaucoma** (glaw-**KOH**-mah)
- [ ] **hemianopia** (**hem**-ee-ah-**NOH**-pee-ah)
- [ ] **hordeolum** (hor-**DEE**-oh-lum)
- [ ] **hyperopia** (**high**-per-**OH**-pee-ah)
- [ ] **infectious myringitis** (**mir**-in-**JIGH**-tis)
- [ ] **iridectomy** (**ir**-ih-**DECK**-toh-mee)
- [ ] **iritis** (eye-**RYE**-tis)
- [ ] **keratitis** (**ker**-ah-**TYE**-tis)
- [ ] **labyrinthectomy** (**lab**-ih-rin-**THECK**-toh-mee)
- [ ] **laser trabeculoplasty** (trah-**BECK**-you-loh-**plas**-tee)
- [ ] **mastoidectomy** (**mas**-toy-**DECK**-toh-mee)
- [ ] **mydriasis** (mih-**DRY**-ah-sis)
- [ ] **myopia** (my-**OH**-pee-ah)
- [ ] **myringotomy** (**mir**-in-**GOT**-oh-mee)
- [ ] **nyctalopia** (**nick**-tah-**LOH**-pee-ah)
- [ ] **nystagmus** (nis-**TAG**-mus)
- [ ] **ophthalmoscopy** (ahf-thal-**MOS**-koh-pee)
- [ ] **optometrist** (op-**TOM**-eh-trist)
- [ ] **otitis media** (oh-**TYE**-tis **MEE**-dee-ah)
- [ ] **otomycosis** (**oh**-toh-my-**KOH**-sis)
- [ ] **otopyorrhea** (**oh**-toh-**pye**-oh-**REE**-ah)
- [ ] **otorrhea** (**oh**-toh-**REE**-ah)
- [ ] **otosclerosis** (**oh**-toh-skleh-**ROH**-sis)
- [ ] **papilledema** (**pap**-ill-eh-**DEE**-mah)
- [ ] **periorbital edema** (**pehr**-ee-**OR**-bih-tal eh-**DEE**-mah)
- [ ] **photophobia** (**foh**-toh-**FOH**-bee-ah)
- [ ] **presbycusis** (**pres**-beh-**KOO**-sis)
- [ ] **presbyopia** (**pres**-bee-**OH**-pee-ah)
- [ ] **ptosis** (**TOH**-sis)
- [ ] **radial keratotomy** (**ker**-ah-**TOT**-oh-mee)
- [ ] **retinopexy** (**RET**-ih-noh-**peck**-see)
- [ ] **scleritis** (skleh-**RYE**-tis)
- [ ] **sensorineural hearing loss** (sen-suh-ree-**NOOR**-al)
- [ ] **stapedectomy** (**stay**-peh-**DECK**-toh-mee)
- [ ] **strabismus** (strah-**BIZ**-mus)
- [ ] **tarsorrhaphy** (tahr-**SOR**-ah-fee)
- [ ] **tinnitus** (tih-**NIGH**-tus)
- [ ] **tonometry** (toh-**NOM**-eh-tree)
- [ ] **tympanometry** (**tim**-pah-**NOM**-eh-tree)
- [ ] **vertigo** (**VER**-tih-go)
- [ ] **vitrectomy** (vih-**TRECK**-toh-mee)
- [ ] **xerophthalmia** (**zeer**-ahf-**THAL**-mee-ah)

## LEARNING GOALS

On completion of this chapter, you should be able to:

1. Describe the functions and structures of the eyes and their accessory structures.

2. Recognize, define, spell, and pronounce the primary terms related to the structures and function, pathology, and the diagnostic and treatment procedures of the eyes and vision.

3. Describe the functions and structures of the ears.

4. Recognize, define, spell, and pronounce the primary terms related to the structures and function, pathology, and the diagnostic and treatment procedures of the ears and hearing.

## ■ FUNCTIONS OF THE EYES

The eyes are the receptor organs of sight, and their functions are to receive images and transmit them to the brain.

The abbreviations relating to the eyes, with the Latin words from which they originate, are shown in Table 11.1.

### TABLE 11.1
### Abbreviations Relating to the Eyes

| OD | Right eye (*oculus dexter*) |
|----|------------------------------|
| OS | Left eye (*oculus sinister*) |
| OU | Each eye (*oculus uterque*) or both eyes (*oculi uterque*) |

*Oculus* means eye, and the plural is *oculi*. Note: **The Joint Commission on Accreditation of Healthcare Organizations** recommends writing out these terms instead of using abbreviations.

## ■ STRUCTURES OF THE EYES

The structures of the eye include the eyeball and the adnexa that are attached to or surround the eyeball (Figure 11.1).

### The Adnexa of the Eyes

The **adnexa of the eyes**, also known as *adnexa oculi*, are the structures outside the eyeball. These include the orbit, eye muscles, eyelids, eyelashes, conjunctiva, and lacrimal apparatus. **Adnexa** (ad-**NECK**-sah) means the accessory or adjoining anatomical parts of an organ. The term *adnexa* is plural.

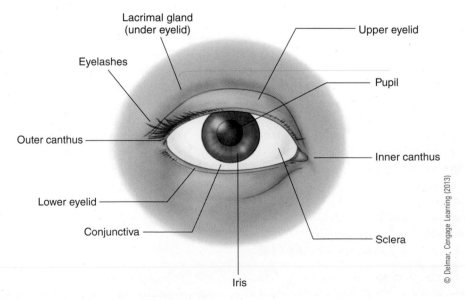

© Delmar, Cengage Learning (2013)

**FIGURE 11.1** Major structures of the adnexa and eyeball.

## The Orbit

The **orbit**, also known as the *eye socket*, is the bony cavity of the skull that contains and protects the eyeball and its associated muscles, blood vessels, and nerves.

## Muscles of the Eye

Six major **eye muscles**, which are arranged in three pairs, are attached to each eye (Figure 11.2). These are the:

- Superior and inferior oblique muscles
- Superior and inferior rectus muscles
- Lateral and medial rectus muscles

These muscles make a wide range of very precise eye movements possible. *Oblique* describes an angle that is slanted but is not perpendicular or parallel. *Rectus* means straight.

**Binocular vision** (**bin-** means two, **ocul** means eye, and **-ar** means pertaining to) occurs when the muscles of both eyes work together in coordination to make normal depth perception possible. *Depth perception* is the ability to see things in three dimensions.

## The Eyelids, Eyebrows, and Eyelashes

The **upper** and **lower eyelids**, together with the **eyebrows** and **eyelashes,** help protect the eyeball from foreign matter, excessive light, and injuries due to other causes (Figure 11.1).

- The **canthus** (**KAN**-thus) is the angle where the upper and lower eyelids meet (**canth** means corner of the eye, and **-us** is a singular noun ending) (plural, *canthi*).

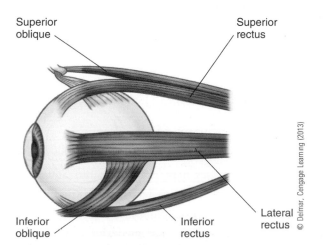

Superior oblique

Superior rectus

Inferior oblique

Inferior rectus

Lateral rectus

© Delmar, Cengage Learning (2013)

**FIGURE 11.2** Six muscles, arranged as three pairs, make major eye movement possible. The medial rectus muscle is not visible here.

- The edges of the eyelids contain oil-producing sebaceous glands. These glands are discussed in Chapter 12.

- The **cilia** (**SIL**-ee-ah), which are small hairs, make up the eyebrows and eyelashes. Cilia are also present in the nose to prevent foreign matter from being inhaled.

- The **tarsus** (**TAHR**-suhs), also known as the *tarsal plate*, is the framework within the upper and lower eyelids that provides the necessary stiffness and shape (**tars** means edge of the eyelid, and **-us** is a singular noun ending) (plural, *tarsi*). Note: *Tarsus* also refers to the seven tarsal bones of the foot's instep.

## The Conjunctiva

The **conjunctiva** (**kon**-junk-**TYE**-vah) is the transparent mucous membrane that lines the underside of each eyelid and continues to form a protective covering over the exposed surface of the eyeball (plural, *conjunctivae*) (Figure 11.1).

## The Lacrimal Apparatus

The **lacrimal apparatus** (**LACK**-rih-mal), also known as the *tear apparatus*, consists of the structures that produce, store, and remove tears. *Lacrimation* is the secretion of tears.

- The **lacrimal glands**, which secrete lacrimal fluid (tears), are located on the underside of the upper eyelid just above the outer corner of each eye (Figure 11.1).

- The function of **lacrimal fluid**, commonly known as *tears*, is to maintain moisture on the anterior surface of the eyeball. Blinking distributes the lacrimal fluid across the eye.

- The **lacrimal canal** consists of a duct at the inner corner of each eye. These ducts collect tears and empty them into the lacrimal sacs. Crying is the overflowing of tears from the lacrimal canals.

- The **lacrimal sac**, also known the *tear sac*, is an enlargement of the upper portion of the lacrimal duct.

- The **lacrimal duct**, also known as the *nasolacrimal duct*, is the passageway that drains excess tears into the nose.

## The Eyeball

The **eyeball**, also known as the *globe*, is a 1-inch sphere with only about one sixth of its surface visible (Figure 11.3).

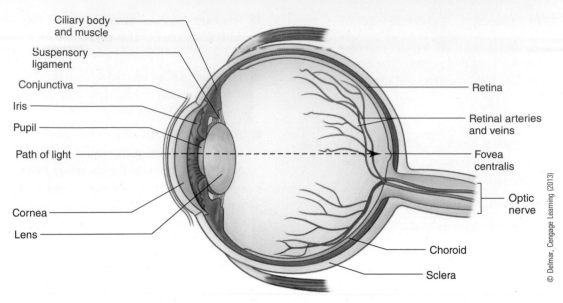

Ciliary body and muscle

Suspensory ligament

Conjunctiva

Iris

Pupil

Path of light

Cornea

Lens

Retina

Retinal arteries and veins

Fovea centralis

Optic nerve

Choroid

Sclera

© Delmar, Cengage Learning (2013)

**FIGURE 11.3** The structures of the eyeball shown in cross-section.

- The term **optic** (**OP**-tik) means pertaining to the eye or sight (**opt** means sight, and **-ic** means pertaining to).

- **Ocular** (**OCK**-you-lar) means pertaining to the eye (**ocul** means eye, and **-ar** means pertaining to).

- **Extraocular** (**eck**-strah-**OCK**-you-lar) means outside the eyeball (**extra-** means on the outside, **ocul** means eye, and **-ar** means pertaining to).

- **Intraocular** (**in**-trah-**OCK**-you-lar) means within the eyeball (**intra-** means within, **ocul** means eye, and **-ar** means pertaining to).

## Walls of the Eyeball

The walls of the eyeball are made up of three layers: the sclera, choroid, and retina (Figure 11.4).

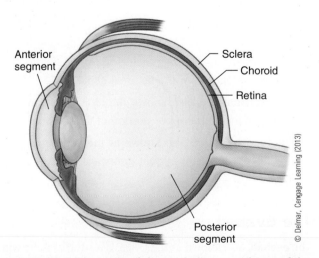

Anterior segment

Sclera

Choroid

Retina

Posterior segment

© Delmar, Cengage Learning (2013)

**FIGURE 11.4** The walls of the eyeball are made up of the sclera, choroid, and retina.

- The **sclera** (**SKLEHR**-ah), also known as the *white of the eye*, maintains the shape of the eye and protects the delicate inner layers of tissue. This tough, fibrous tissue forms the outer layer of the eye, except for the part covered by the cornea. Note: The combining form **scler/o** means the white of the eye, and it also means hard.

- The **choroid** (**KOH**-roid), also known as the *choroid coat*, is the opaque middle layer of the eyeball that contains many blood vessels and provides the blood supply for the entire eye. *Opaque* means that light cannot pass through this substance.

- The **retina** (**RET**-ih-nah) is the sensitive innermost layer that lines the posterior segment of the eye. The retina receives nerve impulses and transmits them to the brain via the *optic nerve*. This is also known as the *second cranial nerve* and is discussed in Chapter 10 (Figure 11.4).

## Segments of the Eyeball

The interior of the eyeball is divided into the anterior and posterior segments (Figures 11.4 and 11.5).

### Anterior Segment of the Eye

The **anterior segment** makes up the front one-third of the eyeball. This segment is divided into anterior and posterior chambers (Figures 11.5A and 11.6).

- The **anterior chamber** is located behind the cornea and in front of the iris. The **posterior chamber** is located behind the iris and in front of the ligaments holding the lens in place. Note: Don't confuse the posterior *chamber* with the posterior *segment*.

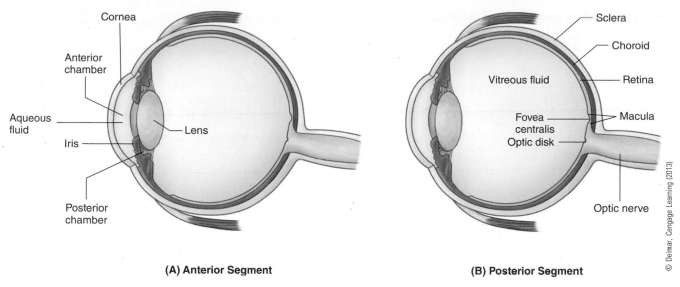

**(A) Anterior Segment**   **(B) Posterior Segment**

**FIGURE 11.5** The segments of the eyeball. (A) The anterior segment is divided into anterior and posterior chambers. (B) The posterior segment.

■ **Aqueous humor** (**AH**-kwee-uhs), which is also known as *aqueous fluid*, fills both of these chambers. The term *aqueous* means watery or containing water. As used here, the term *humor* describes any clear body liquid or semifluid substance.

■ The aqueous humor helps the eye maintain its shape and nourishes the intraocular structures. This fluid is constantly filtered and drained through the *trabecular meshwork* and the *canal of Schlemm* (Figure 11.6).

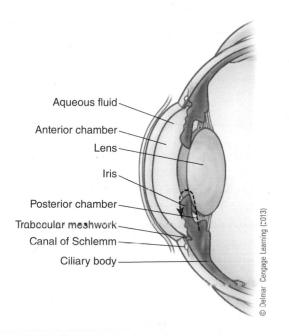

**FIGURE 11.6** The flow of aqueous humor in the anterior segment of the eye.

■ **Intraocular pressure** (IOP) is a measurement of the fluid pressure inside the eye. This pressure is regulated by the rate at which aqueous humor enters and leaves the eye.

## Posterior Segment of the Eye

The **posterior segment**, which makes up the remaining two-thirds of the eyeball, is lined with the retina and filled with **vitreous** (**VIT**-ree-us) **humor**. Also known as *vitreous gel*, this is a soft, clear, jelly-like mass that contains millions of fine fibers. These fibers, which are attached to the surface of the retina, help the eye maintain its shape (Figures 11.3, 11.4, and 11.5B).

## Structures of the Retina

■ The **rods** and **cones** of the retina receive images that have passed through the lens of the eye. These images are converted into nerve impulses and transmitted to the brain via the optic nerve. *Rods* are the black and white receptors, and *cones* are the color receptors.

■ The **macula** (**MACK**-you-lah), also known as the *macula lutea*, is the clearly defined light-sensitive area in the center of the retina that is responsible for sharp central vision. Note that the term *macula* means a small spot. A macula, also known as a macule, can also refer to a small, discolored spot on the skin, such as a freckle (see Chapter 12).

■ The **fovea centralis** (**FOH**-vee-ah sen-**TRAH**-lis) is a pit in the middle of the macula. Color vision is best in this area because it contains a high concentration of cones and no rods.

- The **optic disk**, also known as the *blind spot*, is a small region in the eye where the nerve endings of the retina enter the optic nerve. This is called the blind spot, because it does not contain any rods or cones to convert images into nerve impulses.

- The **optic nerve** transmits these nerve impulses from the retina to the brain.

## The Uvea

The **uvea** (**YOU**-vee-ah) is the pigmented layer of the eye. It has a rich blood supply and consists of the choroid, ciliary body, and iris (Figure 11.3).

### The Ciliary Body

The **ciliary body** (**SIL**-ee-ehr-ee), which is located within the choroid, is a set of muscles and suspensory ligaments that adjust the thickness of the lens to refine the focus of light rays on the retina (Figure 11.6).

- The ciliary body produces the aqueous humor that fills the anterior segment of the eye.

- To focus on nearby objects, these muscles adjust the lens to make it *thicker*.

- To focus on distant objects, these muscles stretch the lens so it is *thinner*.

### The Iris

The **iris** is the colorful circular structure that surrounds the pupil (Figure 11.3). The muscles within the iris control the amount of light that is allowed to enter the eye through the pupil.

- To *decrease* the amount of light entering the eye, the muscles of the iris contract, making the opening of the pupil smaller.

- To *increase* the amount of light entering the eye, the muscles of the iris relax, or *dilate*, making the opening of the pupil larger. See *dilation* under the section on diagnostic procedures. Note that the term *dilate* refers to expanding any opening of the body, for example, the dilating pores of the skin or of the cervix during childbirth (see Chapter 14).

### The Cornea, Pupil, and Lens

- The **cornea** (**KOR**-nee-ah) is the transparent outer surface of the eye covering the iris and pupil. It is the primary structure focusing light rays entering the eye (Figure 11.3).

- The **pupil** is the black circular opening in the center of the iris that permits light to enter the eye.

- The **lens** is the clear, flexible, curved structure that focuses images on the retina. The lens is contained within a clear capsule located behind the iris and pupil.

## Normal Action of the Eyes

- **Accommodation** (ah-**kom**-oh-**DAY**-shun) is the process whereby the eyes make adjustments for seeing objects at various distances. These adjustments include contraction (narrowing) and dilation (widening) of the pupil, movement of the eyes, and changes in the shape of the lens.

- **Convergence** (kon-**VER**-jens) is the simultaneous inward movement of the eyes toward each other. This occurs in an effort to maintain single binocular vision as an object comes nearer.

- **Emmetropia** (em-eh-**TROH**-pee-ah) is the normal relationship between the refractive power of the eye and the shape of the eye that enables light rays to focus correctly on the retina (**emmetr** means in proper measure, and **-opia** means vision condition).

- **Refraction**, also *refractive power*, is the ability of the lens to bend light rays so they focus on the retina. Normal refraction is shown in Figure 11.10A.

- **Visual acuity** (ah-**KYOU**-ih-tee) is the ability to distinguish object details and shape at a distance. *Acuity* means sharpness (Figure 11.8A).

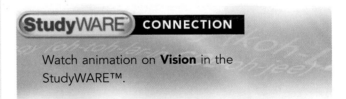

Watch animation on **Vision** in the StudyWARE™.

## ■ MEDICAL SPECIALTIES RELATED TO THE EYES

- An **ophthalmologist** (ahf-thal-**MOL**-oh-jist) is a physician who specializes in diagnosing and treating the full spectrum of diseases and disorders of the eyes, from vision correction to eye surgery (**ophthalm** means eye, and **-ologist** means specialist).

- An **optometrist** (op-**TOM**-eh-trist) holds a doctor of optometry degree and provides primary eye care, including diagnosing eye diseases and conditions, and measuring the accuracy of vision to determine whether corrective lenses are needed (**opt/o** means vision, and **-metrist** means one who measures).

- An **optician** (op-**TISH**-uhn) is a health care practitioner who designs, fits, and dispenses lenses for vision correction.

# PATHOLOGY OF THE EYES AND VISION

## The Eyelids

- **Ptosis** (**TOH**-sis) is the drooping of the upper eyelid that is usually due to paralysis (**ptosis** means drooping or sagging). The term *blepharoptosis* has the same meaning (**blephar/o** means eyelid, and -**ptosis** means droop or sag).

- A **chalazion** (kah-**LAY**-zee on) is a nodule or cyst, usually on the upper eyelid, caused by obstruction in a sebaceous gland (plural, *chalazia*). A chalazion is a type of granuloma (see Chapter 12). Compare with a *hordeolum*.

- **Ectropion** (eck-**TROH**-pee-on) is the eversion of the edge of an eyelid (**ec-** means out, **trop** means turn, and -**ion** means condition). *Eversion* means turning outward. This usually affects the lower lid, thereby exposing the inner surface of the eyelid to irritation and preventing tears from draining properly (Figure 11.7A). Ectropion is the opposite of *entropion*.

- **Entropion** (en-**TROH**-pee-on) is the inversion of the edge of an eyelid (**en-** means in, **trop** means turn, and -**ion** means condition). *Inversion* means turning inward. This usually affects the lower eyelid and causes the eyelashes to rub against the cornea (Figure 11.7B). Entropion is the opposite of *ectropion*.

- A **hordeolum** (hor-**DEE**-oh-lum), also known as a *stye*, is a pus-filled and often painful lesion on the eyelid resulting from an acute infection in a sebaceous gland. Compare with a *chalazion*.

- **Periorbital edema** (pehr-ee-**OR**-bih-tal eh-**DEE**-mah) is swelling of the tissues surrounding the eye or eyes (**peri-** means surrounding, **orbit** means eyeball, and -**al** means pertaining to). This can give the face a bloated appearance and cause the eyes to be partially covered by the swollen eyelids. This swelling is associated with conditions such as allergic reaction (see Chapter 6), nephrotic syndrome (see Chapter 9), or cellulitis (see Chapter 12).

## Additional Adnexa Pathology

- **Conjunctivitis** (kon-**junk**-tih-**VYE**-tis), also known as *pinkeye*, is an inflammation of the conjunctiva that is usually caused by an infection or allergy (**conjunctiv** means conjunctiva, and -**itis** means inflammation).

- **Dacryoadenitis** (dack-ree-oh-ad-eh-**NIGH**-tis) is an inflammation of the lacrimal gland caused by a bacterial, viral, or fungal infection (**dacry/o** means tear, **aden** means gland, and -**itis** means inflammation). Signs and symptoms of this condition include sudden severe pain, redness, and pressure in the orbit of the eye.

- **Subconjunctival hemorrhage** (sub-kon-junk-**TIH**-val HEM-or-idj) is bleeding between the conjunctiva and the sclera. This condition, which is usually caused by an injury, creates a red area over the white of the eye.

- **Xerophthalmia** (zeer-ahf-**THAL**-mee-ah), also known as *dry eye*, is drying of eye surfaces, including the conjunctiva (**xer** means dry, **ophthalm** means eye, and -**ia** means abnormal condition). This condition is often associated with aging. It can also be due to systemic diseases such as rheumatoid arthritis or to a lack of vitamin A.

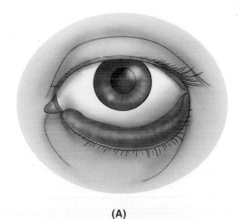
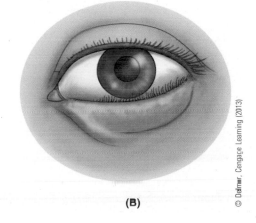

© Delmar, Cengage Learning (2013)

(A)  (B)

**FIGURE 11.7** Disorders of the eyelid. (A) Ectropion. (B) Entropion.

## Uvea, Cornea, Iris, and Sclera

- **Uveitis** (you-vee-**EYE-tis**) is an inflammation of the uvea causing swelling and irritation (**uve** means uvea, and **-itis** means inflammation). It can potentially lead to blindness.

- **Iritis** (eye-**RYE**-tis) is the most common form of uveitis. This inflammation of the uvea affects primarily structures in the front of the eye (**ir** means iris, and **-itis** means inflammation). This condition has a sudden onset and may last 6 to 8 weeks.

- A **corneal abrasion** (ah-**BRAY**-zhun) is an injury, such as a scratch or irritation, to the outer layers of the cornea (**corne** means cornea, and **-al** means pertaining to). Compare with *corneal ulcer*.

- A **corneal ulcer** is a pitting of the cornea caused by an infection or injury. Although these ulcers heal with treatment, they can leave a cloudy scar that impairs vision. Compare with *corneal abrasion*.

- **Diabetic retinopathy** is damage to the retina as a complication of uncontrolled diabetes. This is discussed in the section "Diabetic Complications" in Chapter 13.

- **Keratitis** (ker-ah-**TYE**-tis) is an inflammation of the cornea (**kerat** means cornea, and **-itis** means inflammation). This condition can be due to many causes, including bacterial, viral, or fungal infections. Note: **kerat/o** also means hard.

- **Scleritis** (skleh-**RYE**-tis) is an inflammation of the sclera (**scler** means white of the eye, and **-itis** means inflammation). This condition is usually associated with infections, chemical injuries, or autoimmune diseases.

## The Eye

- **Anisocoria** (an-ih-so-**KOH**-ree-ah) is a condition in which the pupils are unequal in size (**anis/o** means unequal, **cor** means pupil, and **-ia** means abnormal condition). This condition can be congenital or caused by a head injury, aneurysm, or pathology of the central nervous system.

- A **cataract** (**KAT**-ah-rakt) is the loss of transparency of the lens that causes a progressive loss of visual clarity. The formation of most cataracts is associated with aging; however, this condition can be congenital or due to an injury or disease (Figure 11.8B).

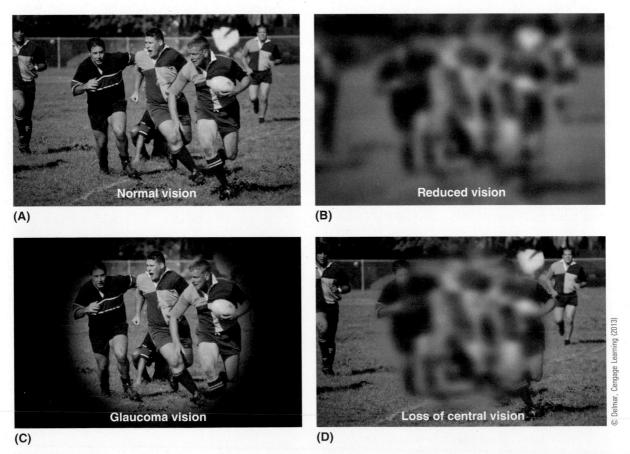

(A)    Normal vision

(B)    Reduced vision

(C)    Glaucoma vision

(D)    Loss of central vision

© Delmar, Cengage Learning (2013)

**FIGURE 11.8** Normal vision and pathologic vision changes. (A) Normal vision. (B) Vision reduced by cataracts. (C) The loss of peripheral vision due to untreated glaucoma. (D) The loss of central vision due to macular degeneration.

- **Floaters**, also known as *vitreous floaters*, are particles of cellular debris that float in the vitreous humor and cast shadows on the retina. Floaters occur normally with aging or in association with retinal detachment, retinal tears, or intraocular inflammation.

- **Photopsia** (foh-**TOP**-see-ah) is the presence of what appears to be flashes of light, or *flashers* (**phot** means light, and **-opsia** means view of). These are often caused by damage to the eye or migraine headaches.

- **Miosis** (mye-**OH**-sis) is the contraction of the pupil, normally in response to exposure to light, but also possibly due to the use of prescription or illegal drugs (**mio-** means smaller, and **-sis** means abnormal condition).

- **Mydriasis** (mih-**DRY**-ah-sis), the dilation of the pupil, is the opposite of miosis (**mydrias** means the dilation of the pupil, and **-is** means abnormal condition). The causes of mydriasis include diseases, trauma (injury), or drugs.

- **Nystagmus** (nis-**TAG**-mus) is an involuntary, constant, rhythmic movement of the eyeball that can be congenital or caused by a neurological injury or drug use.

- **Papilledema** (**pap**-ill-eh-**DEE**-mah), also known as *choked disk*, is swelling and inflammation of the optic nerve at the point of entrance into the eye through the optic disk (**papill** means nipplelike, and **-edema** means swelling). This swelling is caused by increased intracranial pressure and can be due to a tumor pressing on the optic nerve.

- **Retinal detachment,** also known as a *detached retina*, and **retinal tears** are the separation of some or all of the light-sensitive retina from the choroid. If not treated, the entire retina can detach, causing blindness. These conditions can be caused by a head trauma, aging, or from the vitreous humor separating from the retina (Figure 11.9).

- **Retinitis pigmentosa** (**ret**-ih-**NIGH**-tis pig-men-**TOH**-sah) is a progressive degeneration of the retina that affects night and peripheral vision. It can be detected by the presence of dark pigmented spots in the retina.

## Glaucoma

**Glaucoma** (glaw-**KOH**-mah) is a group of diseases characterized by increased intraocular pressure that causes damage to the retinal nerve fibers and the optic nerve (Figure 11.8C). This increase in pressure is caused by a blockage in the flow of fluid out of the eye. If untreated, this pressure can cause the loss of peripheral vision and eventually blindness.

- **Open-angle glaucoma**, also known as *chronic glaucoma*, is by far the most common form of this condition. The trabecular meshwork gradually becomes blocked, causing a buildup of pressure. Symptoms of this condition are not noticed by the patient until the optic nerve has been damaged; however, it can be detected earlier through regular eye examinations, including tonometry and visual field testing. See the later section "Diagnostic Procedures for Vision and the Eyes."

- In **closed-angle glaucoma**, also known as *acute glaucoma*, the opening between the cornea and iris narrows so that fluid cannot reach the trabecular meshwork. This narrowing can cause a sudden increase in the intraocular pressure that produces severe pain, nausea, redness of the eye, and blurred vision. Without immediate treatment, blindness can occur in as little as two days.

## Macular Degeneration

**Macular degeneration** (**MACK**-you-lar) is a gradually progressive condition in which the macula at the center of the retina is damaged, resulting in the loss of central vision, but not in total blindness (**macul** means spot, and **-ar** mean pertaining to) (Figure 11.8D).

- *Age-related macular degeneration* occurs most frequently in older people and is the leading cause of legal blindness in those older than age 60.

- *Dry macular degeneration*, which accounts for 90% of these cases, is caused by the slow deterioration of the cells of the macula.

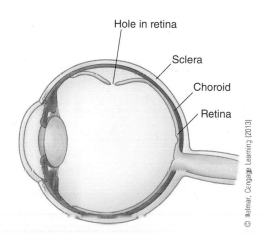

Hole in retina

Sclera

Choroid

Retina

© Delmar, Cengage Learning (2013)

**FIGURE 11.9** A retinal detachment.

■ *Wet macular degeneration* is damage to the macula that develops as a complication as the disease progresses. This damage is caused by the formation of new blood vessels that produce small hemorrhages that usually result in rapid and severe vision loss.

## Functional Defects

■ **Diplopia** (dih-**PLOH**-pee-ah), also known as *double vision*, is the perception of two images of a single object (**dipl** means double, and **-opia** means vision condition). It is sometimes a symptom of a serious underlying disorder such as multiple sclerosis or a brain tumor.

■ **Hemianopia** (**hem**-ee-ah-**NOH**-pee-ah) is blindness in one-half of the visual field (**hemi-** means half, **an-** means without, and **-opia** means vision).

■ **Monochromatism** (**mon**-oh-**KROH**-mah-tizm), also known as *color blindness*, is the inability to distinguish certain colors in a normal manner (**mon/o** means one, **chromat** means color, and **-ism** means condition). This is a genetic condition caused by deficiencies in or the absence of certain types of cones in the retina.

■ **Nyctalopia** (**nick**-tah-**LOH**-pee-ah), also known as *night blindness*, is a condition in which an individual with normal daytime vision has difficulty seeing at night (**nyctal** means night, and **-opia** means vision condition).

■ **Photophobia** (**foh**-toh-**FOH**-bee-ah) means excessive sensitivity to light and can be the result of migraines, excessive wearing of contact lenses, drug use, or inflammation (**phot/o** means light, and **-phobia** means abnormal fear).

■ **Presbyopia** (**pres**-bee-**OH**-pee-ah) is the condition of common changes in the eyes that occur with aging (**presby** means old age, and **-opia** means vision condition). With age, near vision declines noticeably as the lens becomes less flexible and the muscles of the ciliary body become weaker. The result is that the eyes are no longer able to focus the image properly on the retina.

### Strabismus

**Strabismus** (strah-**BIZ**-mus) is a disorder in which the eyes point in different directions or are not aligned correctly, because the eye muscles are unable to focus together.

■ **Esotropia** (**es**-oh-**TROH**-pee-ah), also known as *cross-eyes*, is strabismus characterized by an inward deviation of one or both eyes (**eso-** means inward, **trop** means turn, and **-ia** means abnormal condition). Esotropia is the opposite of exotropia.

■ **Exotropia** (**eck**-soh-**TROH**-pee-ah), also known as *walleye*, is strabismus characterized by the outward deviation of one eye relative to the other (**exo-** means outward, **trop** means turn, and **-ia** means abnormal condition). Exotropia is the opposite of esotropia.

## Refractive Disorders

A **refractive disorder** is a focusing problem that occurs when the lens and cornea do not bend light so that it focuses properly on the retina (Figure 11.10).

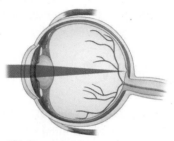

**(A)** Normal vision
Light rays focus on the retina.

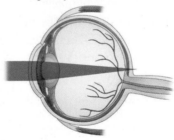

**(B)** Hyperopia (farsightedness)
Light rays focus beyond the retina.

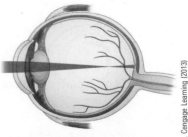

**(C)** Myopia (nearsightedness)
Light rays focus in front of the retina.

© Delmar, Cengage Learning (2013)

**FIGURE 11.10** Refraction. (A) Normal vision. (B) Hyperopia. (C) Myopia.

- **Ametropia** (**am**-eh-**TROH**-pee-ah) is any error of refraction in which images do not focus properly on the retina (**ametr** means out of proportion, and **-opia** means vision condition). Astigmatism, hyperopia, and myopia are all forms of ametropia.

- **Astigmatism** (ah-**STIG**-mah-tizm) is a condition in which the eye does not focus properly because of uneven curvatures of the cornea.

- **Hyperopia** (**high**-per-**OH**-pee-ah), also known as *far-sightedness*, is a defect in which light rays focus beyond the retina (**hyper-** means excessive, and **-opia** means vision condition). This condition can occur in childhood, but usually causes difficulty after age 40 (Figure 11.10B). *Hyperopia* is the opposite of myopia.

- **Myopia** (my-**OH**-pee-ah), also known as *nearsightedness*, is a defect in which light rays focus in front of the retina (**my** is from the Greek word for short-sighted, and **-opia** means vision condition). This condition occurs most commonly around puberty (Figure 11.10C). *Myopia* is the opposite of hyperopia.

## Blindness

**Blindness** is the inability to see. Although some sight remains, *legal blindness* is the point at which, under law, an individual is considered to be blind. A commonly used standard is that a person is legally blind when his or her best-corrected vision is reduced to 20/200 or less. See the earlier section "Normal Action of the Eyes."

- **Amblyopia** (**am**-blee-**OH**-pee-ah) is a dimness of vision or the partial loss of sight, especially in one eye, without detectable disease of the eye (**ambly** means dim or dull, and **-opia** means vision condition).

- **Scotoma** (skoh-**TOH**-mah), also known as *blind spot*, is an abnormal area of diminished vision surrounded by an area of normal vision.

## ■ DIAGNOSTIC PROCEDURES FOR VISION AND THE EYES

### Diagnostic Procedures for Vision

- A **Snellen chart** (SC) is used to measure visual acuity. The results for each eye are recorded as a fraction with 20/20 being considered normal.
  - The *first number* indicates the standard distance from the chart, which is 20 feet.

- The *second number* indicates the deviation from the norm based on the ability to read progressively smaller lines of letters on the chart.

- **Refraction** is an examination procedure to determine an eye's refractive error so that the best corrective lenses can be prescribed. This term also refers to the ability of the lens to bend light rays so they focus on the retina.

- A **diopter** (dye-**AHP**-tur) is the unit of measurement of a lens' refractive power.

- The **cover test** is an examination of how the two eyes work together and is used to assess binocular vision. One eye at a time is covered while the patient focuses on an object across the room.

- **Visual field testing**, also known as *perimetry*, is performed to determine losses in peripheral vision. *Peripheral* means occurring away from the center. Blank sections in the visual field can be symptomatic of glaucoma or an optic nerve disorder.

### Diagnostic Procedures for the Eyes

- **Ophthalmoscopy** (**ahf**-thal-**MOS**-koh-pee), also known as *funduscopy*, is the use of an ophthalamoscope to visually examine the fundus (back part) of the eye (Figure 15.8). This examination includes the retina, optic disk, choroid, and blood vessels.

- **Dilation** (dye-**LAY**-shun) of the eyes is required in preparation for the ophthalmoscopic examination of the interior of the eye. Artificial enlargement of the pupils is achieved through the use of mydriatic drops.

- **Mydriatic drops** (**mid**-ree-**AT**-ick) are placed into the eyes to produce temporary paralysis, forcing the pupils to remain dilated even in the presence of bright light.

- **Slit-lamp ophthalmoscopy** (**ahf**-thal-**MOS**-koh-pee) is a diagnostic procedure in which a narrow beam of light is focused onto parts of the eye to permit the ophthalmologist to examine the structures at the front of the eye, including the cornea, iris, and lens (Figure 11.11). Often fluorescein staining is used to help detect foreign bodies or an infected or injured area of the eye.

- **Fluorescein staining** (**flew**-oh-**RES**-ee-in) is the application of fluorescent dye to the surface of the eye via eye drops or a strip applicator. This dye causes a corneal abrasion to temporarily appear bright green.

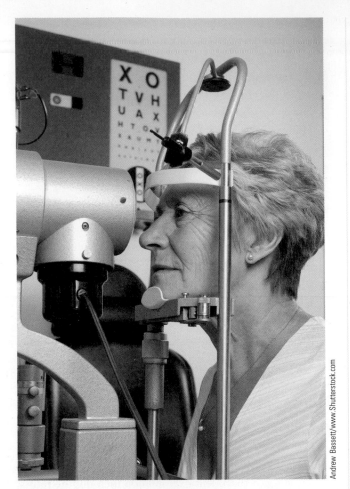

Andrew Bassett/www.Shutterstock.com

**FIGURE 11.11** Slit-lamp ophthalmoscopy is used to examine the structures at the front of the eye, including the cornea, iris, and lens. A Snellen chart is on the wall above the patient.

- **Fluorescein angiography** (**flew**-oh-**RES**-ee-in **an**-jee-**OG**-rah-fee) is a radiographic study of the blood vessels in the retina of the eye following the intravenous injection of a fluorescein dye as a contrast medium. The resulting *angiograms* are used to determine whether there is proper circulation in the retinal vessels.

- **PERRLA** is an acronym meaning **P**upils are **E**qual, **R**ound, **R**esponsive to **L**ight and **A**ccommodation. This is a diagnostic observation, and any abnormality here could indicate a head injury or damage to the brain.

- **Tonometry** (toh-**NOM**-eh-tree) is the measurement of intraocular pressure (**ton/o** means tension, and **-metry** means to measure). Abnormally high pressure can be an indication of glaucoma.

## ■ TREATMENT PROCEDURES OF THE EYES AND VISION

### The Orbit and Eyelids

- An **orbitotomy** (**or**-bih-**TOT**-oh-mee) is a surgical incision into the orbit (**orbit** means bony socket, and **-otomy** means surgical incision). This procedure is performed for biopsy, abscess drainage, or removal of a tumor or foreign object.

- **Tarsorrhaphy** (tahr-**SOR**-ah-fee) is the partial or complete suturing together of the upper and lower eyelids to protect the eye when the lids are paralyzed and unable to close normally (**tars/o** means eyelid, and **-rrhaphy** means surgical suturing).

- Cosmetic procedures relating to the eyelids are discussed in Chapter 12.

### The Conjunctiva and Eyeball

- A **corneal transplant**, also known as *keratoplasty*, is the surgical replacement of a scarred or diseased cornea with clear corneal tissue from a donor.

- **Enucleation** (ee-**new**-klee-**AY**-shun) is the removal of the eyeball, leaving the eye muscles intact (**e-** means out of, **nucle** means nucleus, and **-ation** means action).

- An **ocular prosthesis** (pros-**THEE-sis**), also known as an *artificial eye*, may be fitted to wear over a malformed eye or to replace an eyeball that is either congenitally missing or has been surgically removed. A *prosthesis* is an artificial substitute for a diseased or missing body replacement part.

- An **iridectomy** (ir-ih-**DECK**-toh-mee) is the surgical removal of a portion of the tissue of the iris (**irid** means iris, and **-ectomy** means surgical removal). This procedure is most frequently performed to treat closed-angle glaucoma.

- A **radial keratotomy** (ker-ah-**TOT**-oh-mee) is a surgical procedure to treat myopia (**kerat** means cornea, and **-otomy** means surgical incision). During the surgery, incisions are made in the cornea to cause it to flatten. These incisions allow the sides of the cornea to bulge outward and thereby flatten the central portion of the cornea. This brings the focal point of the eye closer to the retina and improves distance vision. Compare with *LASIK*, in the section "Laser Treatments."

- A **scleral buckle** (**SKLER**-al) is a silicone band or sponge used to repair a detached retina. The detached layers are brought closer together by attaching this band onto the sclera, or outer wall, of the eyeball, creating an indentation or buckle effect inside the eye.

- **Vitrectomy** (vih-**TRECK**-toh-mee) is the removal of the vitreous humor and its replacement with a clear solution (**vitr** means vitreous humor, and **-ectomy** means removal). This procedure is sometimes performed to treat a retinal detachment or when diabetic retinopathy causes blood to leak and cloud the vitreous humor.

## Cataract Surgery

- **Lensectomy** (len-**SECK**-toh-mee) is the general term used to describe the surgical removal of a cataract-clouded lens (**lens** means lens, and **-ectomy** means surgical removal).

- **Phacoemulsification** (**fack**-koh-ee-**mul**-sih-fih-**KAY**-shun) is the use of ultrasonic vibration to shatter and remove the lens clouded by a cataract. This is performed through a very small opening, and the same opening is used to slide the intraocular lens into place (**intra-** means within, **ocul** means eye, and **-ar** mean pertaining to).

- An **intraocular lens** (IOL) is a surgically implanted replacement for a natural lens that has been removed (**intra-** means within, **ocul** means eye, and **-ar** means pertaining to).

## Corrective Lenses

Refractive errors in the eye can often be corrected with lenses that alter the angle of light rays before they reach the cornea. *Concave lenses* (curved inward) are used for myopia, or nearsightedness, and *convex lenses* (curved outward) for hyperopia (farsightedness).

- Corrective lenses can combine two or three different refractive powers, one above the other, to allow for better distance vision when looking up and near vision when looking down. *Bifocals* are lenses with two powers. *Trifocals* are lenses with three powers.

- Strabismus is sometimes treated with corrective lenses or an eye patch covering the stronger eye and thus strengthening the muscles in the weaker eye.

- *Contact lenses* are refractive lenses that float directly on the tear film in front of the eye. Rigid gas-permeable lenses cover the central part of the cornea, and disposable soft lenses cover the entire cornea.

## Laser Treatments of the Eyes

In the treatment of eye disorders, lasers have many uses. More details on how lasers work can be found in Chapter 12.

- A **laser iridotomy** (**ir**-ih-**DOT**-oh-mee) uses a focused beam of light to create a hole in the iris of the eye (**irid** means iris, and **-otomy** means surgical incision). This procedure is performed to treat closed-angle glaucoma by creating an opening that allows the aqueous humor to flow between the anterior and posterior chambers of the anterior segment of the eye.

- A **laser trabeculoplasty** (trah-**BECK**-you-loh-**plas**-tee) is used to treat open-angle glaucoma by creating openings in the trabecular meshwork to allow the fluid to drain properly.

- **LASIK** is the acronym for **Laser-Assisted in Situ Ker**-atomileusis (**kerat/o** means cornea, and **-mileusis** means carving). *In situ* means in its original place. LASIK is used to treat vision conditions, such as myopia, that are caused by the shape of the cornea. During this procedure, a flap is opened in the surface of the cornea and then a laser is used to change the shape of a deep corneal layer. Compare with *radial keratotomy*.

- **Photocoagulation** (**foh**-toh-koh-**AG**-you-lay-shun) is the use of a laser to treat some forms of wet macular degeneration by sealing leaking or damaged blood vessels. This technique is also used to repair small retinal tears by intentionally forming scar tissue to seal the holes.

- **Retinopexy** (**RET**-ih-noh-**peck**-see) is used to reattach the detached area in a retinal detachment (**retin/o** means retina, and **-pexy** means surgical fixation).

- In *pneumatic retinopexy*, a gas bubble is injected into the vitreous cavity to put pressure on the area of repair while it heals. The bubble gradually dissipates.

- Lasers are used to remove clouded tissue that can have formed in the posterior portion of the lens capsule after cataract extraction.

## ■ FUNCTIONS OF THE EARS

The ears are the receptor organs of hearing, and their functions are to receive sound impulses and transmit them to the brain. The inner ear also helps maintain balance.

The abbreviations relating to the ears, with the Latin words from which they originated, are shown in Table 11.2. (Note: **The Joint Commission on Accreditation of Healthcare Organizations** recommends writing out these terms instead of using abbreviations.)

## TABLE 11.2
### Abbreviations Relating to the Ears

| AD | Right ear (*auris dexter*) |
|---|---|
| AS | Left ear (*auris sinister*) |
| AU | Each ear (*auris uterque*) or both ears (*auris unitas*) |

- The term **auditory** (**AW**-dih-**tor**-ee) means pertaining to the sense of hearing (**audit** means hearing or sense of hearing, and **-ory** means pertaining to).

- **Acoustic** (ah-**KOOS**-tick) means pertaining to sound or hearing (**acous** means hearing or sound, and **-tic** means pertaining to).

## ▇ STRUCTURES OF THE EARS

The ear is divided into three separate regions: the outer ear, the middle ear, and the inner ear (Figure 11.12).

### The Outer Ear

- The **pinna** (**PIN**-nah), also known as the *auricle* or the *outer ear*, is the external portion of the ear. The pinna captures sound waves and transmits them into the external auditory canal.

- The **external auditory canal** transmits these sound waves to the tympanic membrane (eardrum) of the middle ear.

- **Cerumen** (seh-**ROO**-men), also known as *earwax*, is secreted by ceruminous glands that line the auditory canal. This sticky yellow-brown substance has protective functions because it traps small insects, dust, debris, and some bacteria to prevent them from entering the middle ear.

### The Middle Ear

The **middle ear**, which is located between the outer ear and the inner ear, transmits sound across the space between these two parts (Figure 11.13).

- The **tympanic membrane** (tim-**PAN**-ick), also known as the *eardrum*, is located between the outer and middle ear (Figure 11.13). The word parts **myring/o** and **tympan/o** both mean tympanic membrane. When sound waves reach the eardrum, this membrane transmits the sound by vibrating.

- The **mastoid process** is the temporal bone containing hollow air space that surrounds the middle ear.

### *The Auditory Ossicles*

The **auditory ossicles** (**OSS**-ih-kulz) are three small bones located within the middle ear (Figure 11.12). The role of these bones is to transmit the sound waves from the eardrum to the inner ear by vibration. These bones are named for the Latin terms that describe their shapes. They are the:

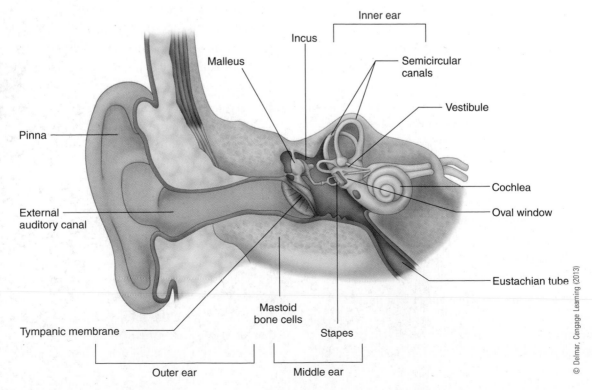

**FIGURE 11.12** Structures of the ear shown in cross-section.

© Delmar, Cengage Learning (2013)

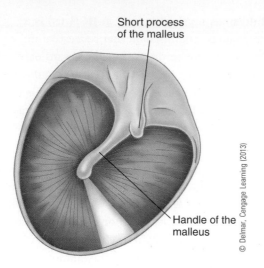

Short process
of the malleus

Handle of the
malleus

© Delmar, Cengage Learning (2013)

**FIGURE 11.13** Schematic of the normal tympanic membrane as viewed from the external auditory canal.

- **Malleus** (**MAL**-ee-us), also known as the *hammer*
- **Incus** (**ING**-kus), also known as the *anvil*
- **Stapes** (**STAY**-peez), also known as the *stirrup*

### The Eustachian Tubes

The **eustachian tubes** (you-**STAY**-shun), also known as the *auditory tubes*, are narrow tubes that lead from the middle ear to the nasal cavity and the throat. The purpose of these tubes is to equalize the air pressure within the middle ear with that of the outside atmosphere.

### The Inner Ear

The **inner ear** contains the sensory receptors for hearing and balance. The structures of the inner ear are known as the **labyrinth** (**LAB**-ih-rinth) (Figure 11.12).

- The **oval window**, which is located under the base of the stapes, is the membrane that separates the middle ear from the inner ear. Vibrations enter the inner ear through this structure.
- The **cochlea** (**KOCK**-lee-ah) is the snail-shaped structure of the inner ear and is where sound vibrations are converted into nerve impulses. Located within the cochlea are the cochlear duct, the organ of Corti, the semicircular canals, and the acoustic nerves. *Cochlea* comes from the Greek term for snail.
- The **organ of Corti** receives the vibrations from the cochlear duct and relays them to the auditory nerve fibers. These fibers transmit the sound impulses to the

auditory center of the brain's cerebral cortex, where they are heard and interpreted.

- The three **semicircular canals** contain the liquid *endolymph* and sensitive hair-like cells. The bending of these hair-like cells in response to the movements of the head sets up impulses in nerve fibers to help maintain equilibrium. *Equilibrium* is the state of balance.
- The **acoustic nerves** (cranial nerve VIII) transmit this information to the brain, and the brain sends messages to muscles in all parts of the body to ensure that equilibrium is maintained. These nerves are discussed in Chapter 10.

## Normal Action of the Ears

- **Air conduction** is the process by which sound waves enter the ear through the pinna and then travel down the external auditory canal until they strike the tympanic membrane, which is located between the outer ear and middle ear.
- **Bone conduction** occurs as the eardrum vibrates and causes the auditory ossicles of the middle ear to vibrate. The vibration of these bones transmits the sound waves through the middle ear to the oval window of the inner ear.
- **Sensorineural conduction** (sen-suh-ree-**NOOR**-al) occurs when these sound vibrations reach the inner ear. The structures of the inner ear receive the sound waves and relay them to the auditory nerve for transmission to the brain.

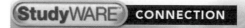

Watch an animation on **Hearing** in the StudyWARE™.

## ■ MEDICAL SPECIALTIES RELATED TO THE EARS

- An **audiologist** (aw-dee-**OL**-oh-jist) specializes in the measurement of hearing function and in the rehabilitation of persons with hearing impairments (**audi** means hearing, and -**ologist** means specialist).

## ■ PATHOLOGY OF THE EARS AND HEARING

### The Outer Ear

- **Impacted cerumen** is an accumulation of earwax that forms a solid mass by adhering to the walls of the external auditory canal. *Impacted* means lodged or wedged firmly in place.

- **Otalgia** (oh-**TAL**-gee-ah), also known as an *earache*, is pain in the ear (**ot** means ear, and **-algia** means pain).

- **Otitis** (oh-**TYE**-tis) means any inflammation of the ear (**ot** means ear, and **-itis** means inflammation). The second part of the term gives the location of the inflammation. For example, *otitis externa* is an inflammation of the external auditory canal.

- **Otomycosis** (oh-toh-my-**KOH**-sis), also known as *swimmer's ear*, is a fungal infection of the external auditory canal (**ot/o** means ear, **myc** means fungus, and **-osis** means abnormal condition).

- **Otopyorrhea** (oh-toh-**pye**-oh-**REE**-ah) is the flow of pus from the ear (**ot/o** means ear, **py/o** means pus, and **-rrhea** means flow or discharge).

- **Otorrhea** (oh-toh-**REE**-ah) is any discharge from the ear (**ot/o** means ear, and **-rrhea** means discharge). In rare cases this could include leakage of cerebrospinal fluid.

- **Otorrhagia** (oh-toh-**RAY**-jee-ah) is bleeding from the ear (**ot/o** means ear, and **-rrhagia** means bleeding).

### The Middle Ear

- **Barotrauma** (bar-oh-**TRAW**-mah) is a pressure-related ear condition (**bar/o** means pressure, and **-trauma** means injury). These conditions can be caused by pressure changes when flying, driving in the mountains, scuba diving, or when the eustachian tube is blocked.

- A **cholesteatoma** (koh-**les**-tee-ah-**TOH**-mah) also known as a *pearly tumor*, is a destructive epidermal cyst in the middle ear and/or the mastoid process made up of epithelial cells and cholesterol (**cholesteat** refers to cholesterol, and **-oma** means tumor). It can be congenital or a serious complication of chronic otitis media (see below).

- **Mastoiditis** (mas-toy-**DYE**-tis) is an inflammation of any part of the mastoid bone cells (**mastoid** means mastoid process, and **-itis** means inflammation). This condition may develop when acute otitis media that cannot be controlled with antibiotics spreads to the mastoid process.

- **Infectious myringitis** (mir-in-**JIGH**-tis) is a contagious inflammation that causes painful blisters on the eardrum (**myring** means eardrum, and **-itis** means inflammation). This condition is associated with a middle ear infection. It is not to be confused with *infectious meningitis*, which is an inflammation of the brain and spinal cord (see Chapter 10).

- **Otitis media** (oh-**TYE**-tis **MEE**-dee-ah) is an inflammation of the middle ear.
  - *Acute otitis media* is usually associated with an upper respiratory infection and is most commonly seen in young children. This condition can lead to a ruptured eardrum due to the buildup of pus or fluid in the middle ear.
  - *Serous otitis media* is a fluid buildup in the middle ear without symptoms of an infection. This condition can follow acute otitis media or can be caused by obstruction of the eustachian tube.

- **Otosclerosis** (oh-toh-skleh-**ROH**-sis) is the ankylosis of the bones of the middle ear, resulting in a conductive hearing loss (**ot/o** means ear, and **-sclerosis** means abnormal hardening). *Ankylosis* means fused together. This condition is treated with a stapedectomy.

### The Inner Ear

- **Labyrinthitis** (lab-ih-rin-**THIGH**-tis) is an inflammation of the labyrinth that can result in vertigo and deafness (**labyrinth** means labyrinth, and **-itis** means inflammation).

- **Vertigo** (**VER**-tih-goh) is a sense of whirling, dizziness, and loss of balance that are often combined with nausea and vomiting. Although it is a symptom of many disorders, recurrent vertigo is sometimes associated with inner ear problems such as Ménière's disease.

- **Ménière's disease** (men-**YEHRS**) is a rare chronic disorder in which the amount of fluid in the inner ear increases intermittently, producing attacks of vertigo, a fluctuating hearing loss (usually in one ear), and tinnitus.

- **Tinnitus** (tih-**NITE**-us), also commonly pronounced (**TIN**-uh-tus), is a condition of a ringing, buzzing, or roaring sound in one or both ears. It is often associated with hearing loss and is more likely to occur when there has been prolonged exposure to loud noises.

# Hearing Loss

- An **acoustic neuroma** (new-**ROH-mah**) is a brain tumor that develops adjacent to the cranial nerve running from the brain to the inner ear (**acous** means hearing, and **-tic** means pertaining to; **neur** means nerve, and **-oma** means tumor). This is one of the most common types of brain tumors and can cause hearing loss, vertigo, and tinnitus.

- **Deafness** is the complete or partial loss of the ability to hear. It can range from the inability to hear sounds of a certain pitch or intensity, to a complete loss of hearing.

- **Presbycusis** (**pres**-beh-**KOO**-sis) is a gradual loss of sensorineural hearing that occurs as the body ages (**presby** means old age, and **-cusis** means hearing).

- A **conductive hearing loss** occurs when sound waves are prevented from passing from the air to the fluid-filled inner ear. Causes of this hearing loss include a buildup of earwax, infection, fluid in the middle ear, a punctured eardrum, otosclerosis, and scarring. This type of hearing loss can often be treated.

- **Sensorineural hearing loss** (**sen**-suh-ree-**NOOR**-al), also known as *nerve deafness*, develops when the auditory nerve or hair cells in the inner ear are damaged. This is usually due to age, noise exposure, or an acoustic neuroma. The source of this hearing loss can be located in the inner ear, in the nerve from the inner ear to the brain, or in the brain.

## Noise-Induced Hearing Loss

A **noise-induced hearing loss** (NIHL) is a type of nerve deafness caused by repeated exposure to extremely loud noises such as a gunshot, or to moderately loud noises that continue for long periods of time.

- These noises can permanently damage the hair cells in the cochlea, and at least partial hearing loss occurs. Unfortunately, this gradual hearing loss usually isn't noticed until some hearing has been permanently destroyed.

- Any sound above 85 decibels (dB) can cause some hearing loss if the exposure is prolonged (Figure 11.14). Most portable music players can produce sounds up to 120 dB, which is louder than a lawn mower or a chain saw and is the equivalent to an ambulance siren.

- A **decibel** (**DES**-ih-bell) is commonly used as the measurement of the loudness of sound.

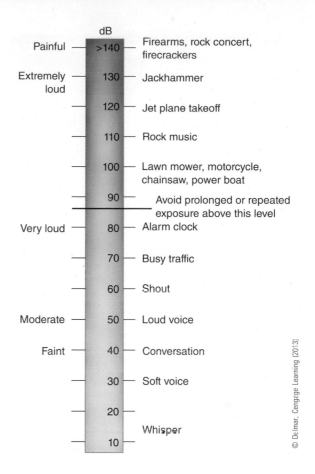

**FIGURE 11.14** A decibel scale of frequently heard sounds.

# DIAGNOSTIC PROCEDURES OF THE EARS AND HEARING

- An **audiological evaluation**, also known as *speech audiometry*, is the measurement of the ability to hear and understand speech sounds based on their pitch and loudness. This testing is best achieved in a sound-treated room with earphones. The resulting graph is an *audiogram* that represents the ability to hear a variety of sounds at various loudness levels.

- **Audiometry** (**aw**-dee-**OM**-eh-tree) is the use of an audiometer to measure hearing acuity (**audi/o** means hearing, and **-metry** means to measure). An *audiometer* is an electronic device that produces acoustic stimuli of a set frequency and intensity.

- Sound is measured in two different ways, in hertz and decibels. A **hertz** (Hz) (**HURTS**) is a measure of sound frequency that determines how high or low a pitch is. (Note: the singular and plural of *hertz* are the same.)

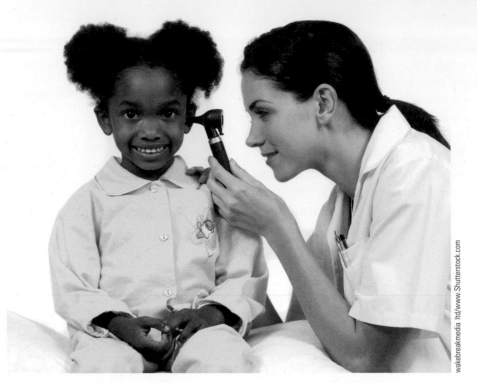

wakebreakmedia ltd/www.Shutterstock.com

**FIGURE 11.15** An otoscope is used to examine the external ear canal.

- An **otoscope**, which is an instrument used to examine the external ear canal, is discussed further in Chapter 15 (Figure 11.15).

- **Monaural testing** (mon-**AW**-rahl) involves one ear (**mon-** means one, **aur** means hearing, and **-al** means pertaining to). Compare with *binaural testing*.

- **Binaural testing** (bye-**NAW**-rul *or* bin-**AW**-rahl) involves both ears (**bin-** means two, **aur** means hearing, and **-al** means pertaining to). Compare with *monaural testing*.

- **Tympanometry** (**tim**-pah-**NOM**-eh-tree) is the use of air pressure in the ear canal to test for disorders of the middle ear (**tympan/o** means eardrum, and **-metry** means to measure). The resulting record is a *tympanogram*. This is used to test for middle ear fluid buildup or eustachian tube obstruction, or to evaluate a conductive hearing loss.

- **Weber and Rinne tests** use a tuning fork to distinguish between conductive and sensorineural hearing losses. The patient's perception of the tuning fork's vibrations helps evaluate his or her hearing ability by air conduction compared to that of bone conduction.

## ■ TREATMENT PROCEDURES OF THE EARS AND HEARING

### The Outer Ear

- **Otoplasty** (**OH**-toh-**plas**-tee) is the surgical repair, restoration, or alteration of the pinna of the ear (**ot/o** means ear, and **-plasty** means surgical repair). This is sometimes done as a cosmetic surgery called *ear pinning* to bring the ears closer to the head.

### The Middle Ear

- **Ear tubes,** formally known as *tympanostomy tubes*, are tiny ventilating tubes placed through the eardrum to provide ongoing drainage for fluids and to relieve pressure that can build up after childhood ear infections (Figure 11.16).

- A **mastoidectomy** (**mas**-toy-**DECK**-toh-mee) is the surgical removal of mastoid cells (**mastoid** means mastoid process, and **-ectomy** means surgical removal). This procedure is used to treat mastoiditis that cannot be controlled with antibiotics or in preparation for the placement of a cochlear implant.

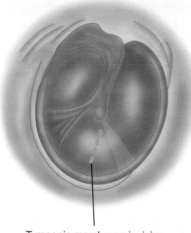 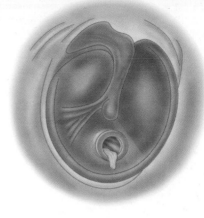

Tympanic membrane incision                    Tube placement to drain fluid

**FIGURE 11.16** Tympanoplasty and the placement of a pediatric ear tube.

- A **myringotomy** (**mir**-in-**GOT**-oh-mee) is a small surgical incision in the eardrum to relieve pressure from excess pus or fluid, or to create an opening for the placement of ear tubes (**myring** means eardrum, and **-otomy** means surgical incision).

- A **stapedectomy** (**stay**-peh-**DECK**-toh-mee) is the surgical removal of the top portion of the stapes bone and the insertion of a small prosthetic device known as a piston that conducts sound vibrations to the inner ear (**staped** means stapes, and **-ectomy** means surgical removal).

- **Tympanoplasty** (**tim**-pah-noh-**PLAS**-tee) is the surgical correction of a damaged middle ear, either to cure chronic inflammation or to restore function (**tympan/o** means eardrum, and **-plasty** means a surgical repair).

## The Inner Ear

- A **labyrinthectomy** (**lab**-ih-rin-**THECK**-toh-mee) is the surgical removal of all or a portion of the labyrinth (**labyrinth** means labyrinth, and **-ectomy** means surgical removal). This procedure is performed to relieve uncontrolled vertigo; however, it causes complete hearing loss in the affected ear.

- **Vestibular rehabilitation therapy** (VRT) (ves-**TIB**-you-lar) is a form of physical therapy designed to treat a wide variety of balance disorders, the majority of which are caused by problems in the inner ear and vestibular nerve.

## Treatments for Hearing Loss

- An **assistive listening device** (ALD) transmits, processes, or amplifies sound, and can be used with or without a hearing aid. An ALD can be helpful in eliminating distracting background noise. The Americans with Disabilities Act (ADA) requires that many public places provide assisted listening devices.

- A **cochlear implant** (**KOCK**-lee-ar) is an electronic device that bypasses the damaged portions of the ear and directly stimulates the auditory nerve (Figure 11.17). The external speech processor captures sounds and converts them into digital signals. Electrodes that are implanted into the cochlea receive the signals and stimulate the auditory nerve. The brain receives these signals and perceives them as sound; however, it may take several months to adjust to the difference in speech when it is received in this manner.

- **Fenestration** (**fen**-es-**TRAY**-shun) is a surgical procedure in which a new opening is created in the labyrinth to restore lost hearing (**fenestr/a** means window, and **-tion** means process).

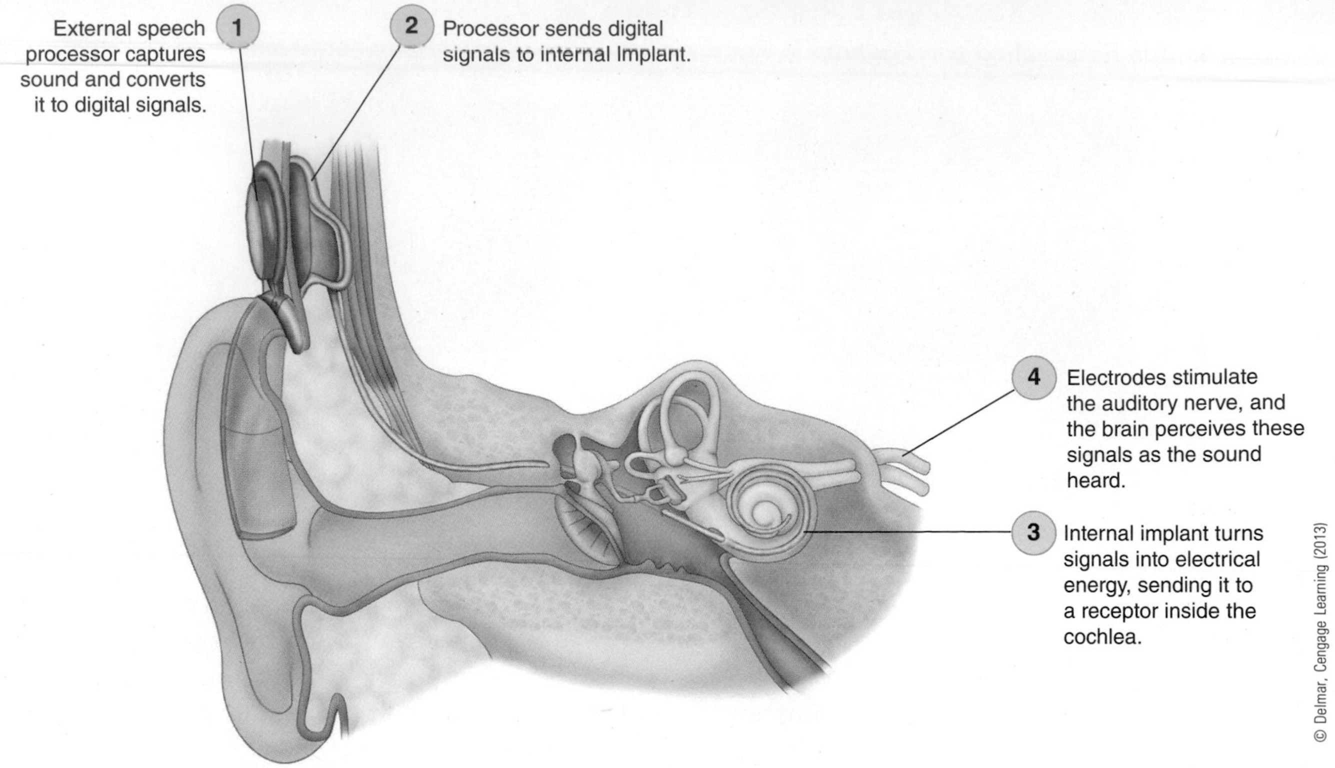

① External speech processor captures sound and converts it to digital signals.

② Processor sends digital signals to internal Implant.

④ Electrodes stimulate the auditory nerve, and the brain perceives these signals as the sound heard.

③ Internal implant turns signals into electrical energy, sending it to a receptor inside the cochlea.

© Delmar, Cengage Learning (2013)

**FIGURE 11.17** A cochlear implant transmits signals to electrodes that are implanted in the cochlea. This provides limited hearing for an individual who has been deaf since birth, or an adult who has a profound hearing loss.

## Hearing Aids

**Hearing aids** are electronic devices that are worn to correct a hearing loss. Sometimes a sensorineural hearing loss can be corrected with a hearing aid.

■ An *analog hearing aid* is an external electronic device that uses a microphone to detect and amplify sounds.

■ A *digital hearing aid* uses a computer chip to convert the incoming sound into a code that can be filtered before being amplified. This is designed to best compensate for a specific type of hearing loss.

## ■ ABBREVIATIONS RELATED TO THE SPECIAL SENSES

Table 11.3 presents an overview of the abbreviations related to the terms introduced in this chapter. Note: To avoid errors or confusion, always be cautious when using abbreviations.

## TABLE 11.3
## Abbreviations Related to the Special Senses

| | |
|---|---|
| **air conduction** = AC | **AC** = air conduction |
| **assistive listening device** = ALD | **ALD** = assistive listening device |
| **astigmatism** = AS | **AS** = astigmatism |
| **cataract** = CAT | **CAT** = cataract |
| **conjunctivitis** = CI | **CI** = conjunctivitis |
| **decibel** = dB | **dB** = decibel |
| **emmetropia** = EM, em | **EM, em** = emmetropia |
| **fluorescein angiography** = FA, FAG | **FA, FAG** = fluorescein angiography |
| **glaucoma** = G, glc | **G, glc** = glaucoma |
| **macular degeneration** = MD | **MD** = macular degeneration |
| **radial keratotomy** = RK | **RK** = radial keratotomy |
| **retinal detachment** = RD | **RD** = retinal detachment |
| **slit-lamp examination** = SLE | **SLE** = slit-lamp examination |
| **visual acuity** = VA | **VA** = visual acuity |
| **visual field** = VF | **VF** = visual field |

**StudyWARE CONNECTION**

For more practice and to test your mastery of this material, go to the StudyWARE™ to play interactive games and complete the quiz for this chapter.

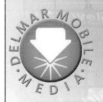

Downloadable audio is available for selected medical terms in this chapter to enhance your learning of medical terminology.

## ☐ Workbook Practice

Go to your workbook, and complete the exercises for this chapter.

## MATCHING WORD PARTS 1

Write the correct answer in the middle column.

| Definition | Correct Answer | Possible Answers |
|---|---|---|
| 11.1. cornea, hard | *kerat/o* | opt/o |
| 11.2. eyelid | *blepar/o* | -metry |
| 11.3. eye, vision | *opt/o* | kerat/o |
| 11.4. hearing | *-cusis* | -cusis |
| 11.5. to measure | *-metry* | blephar/o |

## MATCHING WORD PARTS 2

Write the correct answer in the middle column.

| Definition | Correct Answer | Possible Answers |
|---|---|---|
| 11.6. eardrum | *myring/o* | presby/o |
| 11.7. eye, vision | *ophthalm* | -opia |
| 11.8. iris of the eye | *irid/o* | ophthalm/o |
| 11.9. old age | *presby/o* | myring/o |
| 11.10. vision condition | *-opia* | irid/o |

## MATCHING WORD PARTS 3

Write the correct answer in the middle column.

| Definition | Correct Answer | Possible Answers |
|---|---|---|
| 11.11. ear | | tympan/o |
| 11.12. eardrum | | trop/o |

11.13.  hard, white of eye                    _____    **scler/o**

11.14.  retina                                _____    **retin/o**

11.15.  turn                                  _____    **ot/o**

## DEFINITIONS

Select the correct answer, and write it on the line provided.

11.16.  The _____ is the structure that maintains the shape of the eye and protects the

delicate inner layers of tissue.

  choroid               conjunctiva              cornea                   sclera

11.17.  The _____ is the snail-shaped structure of the inner ear.

  cochlea               incus                    tarsus                   stapes

11.18.  The _____ is also known as the blind spot of the eye.

  fovea centralis       macula                   optic disk               optic nerve

11.19.  The _____ lies between the outer ear and the middle ear.

  mastoid cells         oval window              posterior segment        tympanic membrane

11.20.  The _____ separates the middle ear from the inner ear.

  eustachian tube       inner canthus            oval window              tympanic membrane

11.21.  The auditory ossicle, which is also known as the anvil, is the _____.

  incus                 labyrinth                malleus                  stapes

11.22.  The term meaning common changes in the eyes that occur with aging is _____.

  ametropia             amblyopia                presbyopia               presbycusis

11.23.  In _____, a laser is used to repair a detached retina.

  keratoplasty          photocoagulation         retinopexy               trabeculoplasty

11.24.  The turning inward of the edge of the eyelid is known as _____.

  ectropion             emmetropia               entropion                esotropia

11.25.  An inflammation of the middle ear is also called _____.

  mastoiditis           otitis media             infectious myringitis    otalgia

## MATCHING CONDITIONS

Write the correct answer in the middle column.

| Definition | Correct Answer | Possible Answers |
|---|---|---|
| 11.26. cross-eyes | _____ | exotropia |
| 11.27. double vision | _____ | myopia |
| 11.28. farsightedness | _____ | hyperopia |
| 11.29. nearsightedness | _____ | esotropia |
| 11.30. walleye | _____ | diplopia |

## WHICH WORD?

Select the correct answer, and write it on the line provided.

11.31. A _____ is the unit of measurement of a lens's refractive power.

       decibel           diopter

11.32. The term meaning bleeding from the ears is _____.

       otorrhagia        otorrhea

11.33. A _____ is the surgical incision of the eardrum to create an opening for the placement of ear tubes.

       myringotomy       tympanoplasty

11.34. A visual field test to determine losses in peripheral vision is used to diagnose _____.

       cataracts        glaucoma

11.35. An inflammation of the uvea, causing swelling and irritation, is called _____.

       corneal abrasion       uveitis

## SPELLING COUNTS

Find the misspelled word in each sentence. Then write that word, spelled correctly, on the line provided.

11.36.  The eustashian tubes lead from the middle ear to the nasal cavity and the

throat. _____

11.37.  Cerunem, also known as earwax, is secreted by glands that line the external auditory

canal. _____

11.38.  Astegmatism is a condition in which the eye does not focus properly because of uneven curvatures of the

cornea. _____

11.39.  Laberinthitis is an inflammation of the labyrinth that can result in vertigo and

deafness. _____

11.40.  A Snellan chart is used to measure visual acuity. _____

## ABBREVIATION IDENTIFICATION

In the space provided, write the words that each abbreviation stands for.

11.41.  **CI**          _____

11.42.  **IOL**          _____

11.43.  **OD**          _____

11.44.  **IOP**          _____

11.45.  **MD**          _____

## TERM SELECTION

Select the correct answer, and write it on the line provided.

11.46.  A radial keratotomy is performed to treat _____.

cataracts          hyperopia          myopia          strabismus

11.47.  The condition in which the pupils are unequal in size is known as _____.

anisocoria          choked disk          macular degeneration          astigmatism

11.48.  A _____ is performed in preparation for the placement of a cochlear implant.

keratoplasty          labyrinthectomy          mastoidectomy          myringoplasty

11.49. The condition also known as a stye is _____.

blepharoptosis        chalazion        hordeolum        subconjunctival hemorrhage

11.50. The medical term for the condition commonly known as swimmer's ear is _____.

otalgia        otitis        otomycosis        otopyorrhea

## SENTENCE COMPLETION

Write the correct term or terms on the lines provided.

11.51. The ability of the lens to bend light rays so they focus on the retina is known

as _____.

11.52. A sense of whirling, dizziness, and the loss of balance is called _____.

11.53. A/An _____ is a specialist in measuring the accuracy of vision.

11.54. An inflammation of the cornea that can be due to many causes, including bacterial, viral, or fungal infec-

tions, is known as _____.

11.55. The medical term meaning color blindness is _____.

## WORD SURGERY

Divide each term into its component word parts. Write these word parts, in sequence, on the lines provided. When necessary, use a slash (/) to indicate a combining vowel. (You may not need all of the lines provided.)

11.56. **Anisocoria** is a condition in which the pupils are unequal in size.

_____    _____    _____    _____

11.57. **Emmetropia** is the normal relationship between the refractive power of the eye and the shape of the eye

that enables light rays to focus correctly on the retina.

_____    _____    _____    _____

11.58. **Otopyorrhea** is the flow of pus from the ear.

_____    _____    _____    _____

11.59. **Presbycusis** is a gradual loss of sensorineural hearing that occurs as the body ages.

_____    _____    _____    _____

11.60. **Xerophthalmia** is drying of eye surfaces, including the conjunctiva, that is often associated with aging.

_____    _____    _____    _____

## TRUE/FALSE

If the statement is true, write **True** on the line. If the statement is false, write **False** on the line.

11.61. _____ Rods in the retina are the receptors for color.

11.62. _____ Aqueous humor is drained through the canal of Schlemm.

11.63. _____ Visual field testing is performed to determine the presence of cataracts.

11.64. _____ Dacryoadenitis is an inflammation of the lacrimal gland caused by a bacterial, viral, or fungal infection.

11.65. _____ Tarsorrhaphy is the suturing together of the upper and lower eyelids.

## CLINICAL CONDITIONS

Write the correct answer on the line provided.

11.66. Following a boxing match, Jack Lawson required _____ to repair the injured pinna of his ear.

11.67. During his scuba diving expedition, Jose Ortega suffered from pressure-related ear discomfort. The medical term for this condition is _____.

11.68. Margo Spencer was diagnosed with closed-angle glaucoma affecting her left eye. She is scheduled to have a/an _____ performed to treat this condition.

11.69. Edward Cooke was diagnosed as having _____. This condition is characterized by blindness in one-half of the visual field.

11.70. While gathering branches after the storm, Vern Passman scratched the cornea of his eye. To diagnose the damage, his ophthalmologist performed _____ staining, which caused the corneal abrasions to appear bright green.

11.71. Ted Milligan was treated for an allergic reaction to being stung by a wasp. His reaction was swelling of the tissues around his eyes, and this is known as _____ edema.

11.72.  Adrienne Jacobus is unable to drive at night because she suffers from night blindness. The medical term

for this condition is _____.

11.73.  James Escobar complained of a ringing sound in his ears. His physician refers to this condition

as _____.

11.74.  The obstruction of a sebaceous gland caused the _____ to form on Ingrid Clareus

upper eyelid.

11.75.  Susie Harris was diagnosed as having _____. Her mother referred to this condition

as pinkeye.

## WHICH IS THE CORRECT MEDICAL TERM?

Select the correct answer, and write it on the line provided.

11.76.  Commonly known as choked disk, _____ is swelling and inflammation of the optic

nerve at the point of entrance into the eye through the optic disk.

         dilation              papilledema              tinnitus              xerophthalmia

11.77.  The presence of what appear to be flashes of light is known as _____.

         blind spot          retinal detachment           floaters              photopsia

11.78.  The term _____ describes any error of refraction in which images do not focus

properly on the retina.

         ametropia              diplopia              esotropia              hemianopia

11.79.  The _____ is the angle where the upper and lower eyelids meet.

         canthus          lacrimal glands          conjunctiva              tarsus

11.80.  The term _____ describes an accumulation of earwax that forms a solid mass by

adhering to the walls of the external auditory canal.

         canthus          impacted cerumen          otitis externa              mastoiditis

## CHALLENGE WORD BUILDING

These terms are *not* found in this chapter; however, they are made up of the following familiar word parts. If you need help in creating the term, refer to your medical dictionary.

| | |
|---|---|
| blephar/o | -algia |
| irid/o | -ectomy |
| lacrim/o | -edema |
| ophthalm/o | -itis |
| labyrinth/o | -ology |
| retin/o | -otomy |
| | -pathy |

11.81.  Pain felt in the iris is known as _____.

11.82.  Inflammation of the eyelid is known as _____.

11.83.  Inflammation of the lacrimal duct is _____.

11.84.  Based on word parts, the term _____ means any disease of the eyelid.

11.85.  The medical specialty concerned with the eye, its diseases, and refractive errors is known as _____.

11.86.  Swelling of the eyelid is known as _____.

11.87.  A surgical incision into the lacrimal duct is a/an _____.

11.88.  A surgical incision into the labyrinth of the inner ear is a/an _____.

11.89.  The term meaning any disease of the iris is _____.

11.90.  The surgical removal of the retina is known as a/an _____.

## LABELING EXERCISES

Identify the numbered items on the accompanying figures.

11.91. _____

11.92. anterior _____

11.93. crystalline _____

11.94. _____

11.95. _____ centralis

11.96. _____ or auricle

11.97. external _____ canal

11.98. _____ membrane

11.99. _____ tube

11.100. _____

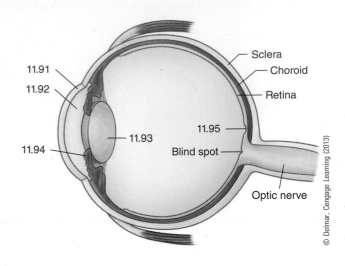

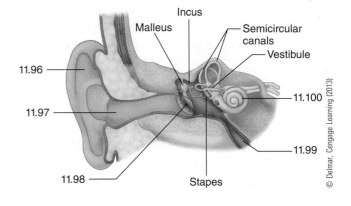

# THE HUMAN TOUCH
## Critical Thinking Exercise

The following story and questions are designed to stimulate critical thinking through class discussion or as a brief essay response. There are no right or wrong answers to these questions.

*William Davis is 62 years old. He was employed as a postal worker until his declining eyesight forced him into early retirement a few months ago. His wife, Mildred, died last year of complications from diabetes after a prolonged and expensive hospitalization. Mr. Davis does not trust the medical community, and because of this distrust, he has not been to a doctor since his wife's death.*

*Mr. Davis is not considered legally blind, but his presbyopia and an advancing cataract in his right eye are starting to interfere with his ability to take care of himself. He still drives to the market once a week, but other drivers get angry and honk at him. He pays for his groceries with a credit card because he is afraid the cashier will cheat him if he accidentally gives her the wrong bills. He complains that the cleaning lady hides things from him and deliberately leaves the furniture out of place. When she leaves, he can't find his slippers or an ashtray. Yesterday, he put his lit pipe down in a wooden bowl by accident.*

*His son insists on taking him to see the ophthalmologist who treated his wife's diabetic retinopathy. Dr. Hsing believes Mr. Davis's sight can be improved in the right eye by performing cataract surgery. Mr. Davis listens in fear as the doctor explains. "Without this procedure, your sight will only get worse."*

*Mr. Davis thinks about all the medical procedures that were tried on Mildred, and she died anyway. He doesn't want to go into the hospital, and he doesn't want any operations. But his son is talking about taking away his car if he doesn't do something about his failing sight. "What more can be taken away from me?" he thinks bitterly. "First my wife, then my job, and now my independence."*

## Suggested Discussion Topics

1. Discuss how Mr. Davis's loss of sight is affecting the way he treats others and is treated by them.

2. Mr. Davis is a patient at the clinic where you work. Discuss the ways you would adjust your usual routine to accommodate his needs.

3. Discuss why cataract surgery would be scary to Mr. Davis and what Dr. Hsing and his staff could do to ease his apprehension.

4. If Mr. Davis does not go ahead with the surgery, what help might he receive from an agency for the visually impaired? What other services might be available to help him deal with his grief and depression?

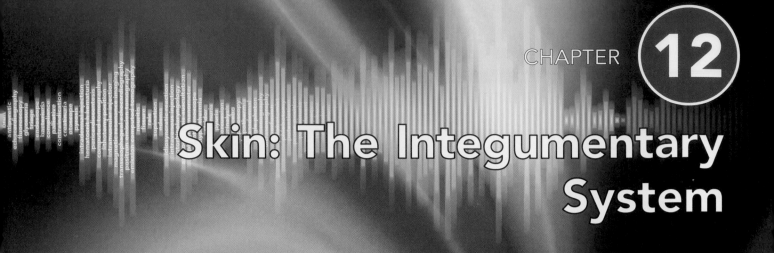

# Skin: The Integumentary System

## Overview of
## STRUCTURES, COMBINING FORMS, AND FUNCTIONS OF THE INTEGUMENTARY SYSTEM

| Major Structures | Related Combining Forms | Primary Functions |
|---|---|---|
| Skin | **cutane/o, dermat/o, derm/o** | Intact skin is the first line of defense for the immune system. Skin waterproofs the body and is the major receptor for the sense of touch. |
| Sebaceous Glands | **seb/o** | Secrete sebum (oil) to lubricate the skin and discourage the growth of bacteria on the skin. |
| Sweat Glands | **hidr/o** | Secrete sweat to regulate body temperature and water content, and these glands excrete some metabolic waste. |
| Hair | **pil/i, pil/o** | Aids in controlling the loss of body heat. |
| Nails | **onych/o, ungu/o** | Protect the dorsal surface of the last bone of each finger and toe. |

# Vocabulary Related to **THE INTEGUMENTARY SYSTEM**

This list contains essential word parts and medical terms for this chapter. These terms are pronounced in the student StudyWARE™ and Audio CDs that are available for use with this text. These and the other important **primary terms** are shown in boldface throughout the chapter. *Secondary terms*, which appear in *orange* italics, clarify the meaning of primary terms.

## Word Parts

- ☐ **cutane/o** skin
- ☐ **derm/o, dermat/o** skin
- ☐ **hidr/o** sweat
- ☐ **hirsut/o** hairy, rough
- ☐ **kerat/o** horny, hard
- ☐ **lip/o** fat, lipid
- ☐ **melan/o** black, dark
- ☐ **myc/o** fungus
- ☐ **onych/o** fingernail or toenail
- ☐ **pil/i, pil/o** hair
- ☐ **py/o** pus
- ☐ **rhytid/o** wrinkle
- ☐ **seb/o** sebum
- ☐ **urtic/o** rash, hives
- ☐ **xer/o** dry

## Medical Terms

- ☐ **actinic keratosis** (ack-**TIN**-ick **kerr**-ah-**TOH**-sis)
- ☐ **albinism** (**AL**-bih-niz-um)
- ☐ **alopecia** (**al**-oh-**PEE**-shee-ah)
- ☐ **blepharoplasty** (**BLEF**-ah-roh-**plas**-tee)
- ☐ **bulla** (**BULL**-ah)
- ☐ **capillary hemangioma** (**KAP**-uh-**ler**-ee hee-**man**-jee-**OH**-mah)
- ☐ **carbuncle** (**KAR**-bung-kul)
- ☐ **cellulitis** (**sell**-you-**LYE**-tis)
- ☐ **chloasma** (kloh-**AZ**-mah)
- ☐ **cicatrix** (sick-**AY**-tricks)
- ☐ **comedo** (**KOM**-eh-doh)
- ☐ **debridement** (dah-**BREED**-ment)
- ☐ **dermatitis** (**der**-mah-**TYE**-tis)
- ☐ **diaphoresis** (**dye**-ah-foh-**REE**-sis)
- ☐ **dysplastic nevi** (dis-**PLAS**-tick **NEE**-vye)
- ☐ **ecchymosis** (eck-ih-**MOH**-sis)
- ☐ **eczema** (**ECK**-zeh-mah)

- ☐ **erythema** (er-ih-**THEE**-mah)
- ☐ **erythroderma** (eh-**rith**-roh-**DER**-mah)
- ☐ **exanthem** (eck-**ZAN**-thum)
- ☐ **exfoliative dermatitis** (ecks-**FOH**-lee-**ay**-tiv **DER**-mah-**TYE**-tis)
- ☐ **folliculitis** (foh-**lick**-you-**LYE**-tis)
- ☐ **furuncles** (**FYOU**-rung-kulz)
- ☐ **granuloma** (**gran**-you-**LOH**-mah)
- ☐ **hematoma** (**hee**-mah-**TOH**-mah)
- ☐ **hirsutism** (**HER**-soot-izm)
- ☐ **ichthyosis** (ick-thee-**OH**-sis)
- ☐ **impetigo** (im-peh-**TYE**-goh)
- ☐ **keloid** (**KEE**-loid)
- ☐ **keratosis** (kerr-ah-**TOH**-sis)
- ☐ **koilonychia** (**koy**-loh-**NICK**-ee-ah)
- ☐ **lipedema** (lip-eh-**DEE**-mah)
- ☐ **lipoma** (lih-**POH**-mah)
- ☐ **macule** (**MACK**-youl)
- ☐ **malignant melanoma** (mel-ah-**NOH**-mah)
- ☐ **necrotizing fasciitis** (**NECK**-roh-**tiz**-ing **fas**-ee-**EYE**-tis)
- ☐ **onychocryptosis** (**on**-ih-koh-krip-**TOH**-sis)
- ☑ **onychomycosis** (**on**-ih-koh-my-**KOH**-sis)
- ☐ **papilloma** (**pap**-ih-**LOH**-mah)
- ☐ **papule** (**PAP**-youl)
- ☐ **paronychia** (**par**-oh-**NICK**-ee-ah)
- ☐ **pediculosis** (pee-**dick**-you-**LOH**-sis)
- ☐ **petechiae** (pee-**TEE**-kee-ee)
- ☐ **pruritus** (proo-**RYE**-tus)
- ☐ **psoriasis** (soh-**RYE**-uh-sis)
- ☐ **purpura** (**PUR**-pew-rah)
- ☐ **purulent** (**PYOU**-roo-lent)
- ☐ **rhytidectomy** (rit-ih-**DECK**-toh-mee)
- ☐ **rosacea** (roh-**ZAY**-shee-ah)
- ☐ **scabies** (**SKAY**-beez)
- ☐ **scleroderma** (**sklehr**-oh-**DER**-mah)
- ☐ **seborrhea** (**seb**-oh-**REE**-ah)
- ☐ **squamous cell carcinoma** (**SKWAY**-mus)
- ☐ **systemic lupus erythematosus** (sis-**TEH**-mik **LOO**-pus er-ih-**thee**-mah-**TOH**-sus)
- ☐ **tinea** (**TIN**-ee-ah)
- ☐ **urticaria** (**ur**-tih-**KARE**-ree-ah)
- ☐ **verrucae** (veh-**ROO**-kee)
- ☐ **vitiligo** (vit-ih-**LYE**-goh)
- ☐ **wheal** (**WHEEL**)
- ☐ **xeroderma** (zee-roh-**DER**-mah)

---

## LEARNING GOALS

On completion of this chapter, you should be able to:

1. Identify and describe the functions and structures of the integumentary system.

2. Identify the medical specialists associated with the integumentary system.

3. Recognize, define, spell, and pronounce the primary terms related to the structures and function, pathology, and the diagnostic and treatment procedures of the skin.

4. Recognize, define, spell, and pronounce the primary terms related to the structures and function, pathology, and the diagnostic and treatment procedures of hair, nails, and sebaceous glands.

---

## FUNCTIONS OF THE INTEGUMENTARY SYSTEM

The **integumentary system** (in-**teg**-you-**MEN**-tah-ree), which is made up of the skin and its related structures, performs important functions in maintaining the health of the body. The term *integument* comes from the Latin word meaning to cover or enclose.

### Functions of the Skin

The **skin** forms the protective outer covering the external surfaces of the entire body.

■ The skin waterproofs the body and prevents fluid loss.

■ Intact (unbroken) skin plays an important role in the immune system by blocking the entrance of pathogens into the body (see Chapter 6).

■ Skin is the major receptor for the sense of touch.

■ Skin helps the body synthesize vitamin D, an essential nutrient, from the sun's ultraviolet light, while screening out some harmful ultraviolet radiation.

■ The average adult has 2 square yards of skin, making it the largest bodily organ.

### Functions of Related Structures

The related structures of the integumentary system are the sebaceous glands, sweat glands, hair, and nails (Figure 12.1).

■ The **sebaceous glands** (seh-**BAY**-shus) secrete sebum (oil) that lubricates the skin and discourages the growth of bacteria on the skin.

■ The **sweat glands** help regulate body temperature and water content by secreting sweat. A small amount of metabolic waste is also excreted through the sweat glands.

■ **Hair** helps control the loss of body heat.

■ **Nails** protect the dorsal surface of the last bone of each toe and finger.

---

## THE STRUCTURES OF THE SKIN AND ITS RELATED STRUCTURES

### The Skin

The skin is a complex system of specialized tissues made up of three basic layers:

The skin is a complex system of specialized tissues made up of three basic layers: the *epidermis*, *dermis*, and *subcutaneous* layers (Figure 12.1). The term **cutaneous** (kyou-**TAY**-nee-us) means pertaining to the skin (**cutane** means skin, and **-ous** means pertaining to).

### *The Epidermis*

The **epidermis** (ep-ih-**DER**-mis), which is the outermost layer of the skin, is made up of several specialized epithelial tissues (**epi-** means above or upon, **derm** means skin, and **-is** is a noun ending).

The epidermis does not contain any blood vessels or connective tissue. It is therefore dependent on lower layers for nourishment.

■ **Epithelial tissues** (ep-ih-**THEE**-lee-al) form a protective covering for all of the internal *and* external surfaces of the body.

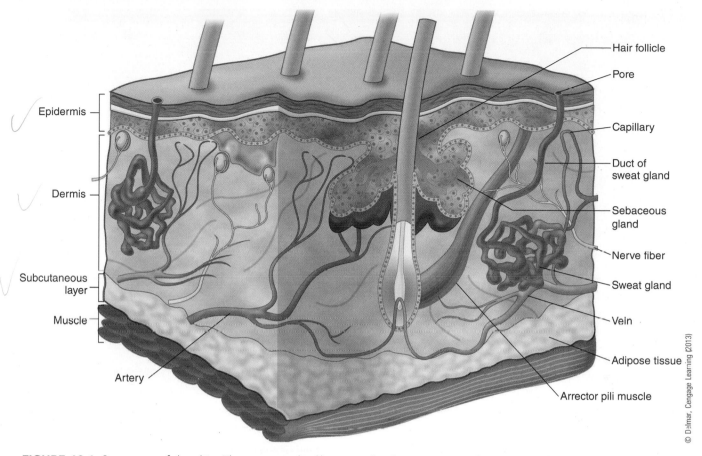

**FIGURE 12.1** Structures of the skin. The sweat and sebaceous glands are associated structures of the skin.

© Delmar, Cengage Learning (2013)

- **Squamous epithelial tissue** (**SKWAY**-mus) forms the upper layer of the epidermis. *Squamous* means scale-like. This layer consists of flat, scaly cells that are continuously shed.

- The **basal layer** (**BAY**-suhl) is the lowest layer of the epidermis. It is here that new cells are produced and then pushed upward. When these cells reach the surface, they die and become filled with keratin.

- **Keratin** (**KER**-ah-tin) is a fibrous, water-repellent protein. Soft keratin is a primary component of the epidermis. Hard keratin is found in the hair and nails.

- **Melanocytes** (**MEL**-ah-noh-sights) are special cells that are also found in the basal cell layer. These cells produce and contain a dark brown to black pigment known as melanin.

- **Melanin** (**MEL**-ah-nin) is the pigment that determines the color of the skin, which depends upon the type and amount of this pigment that is present (Figure 12.2). Melanin also produces spots of color such as freckles and age spots, which are discussed in later sections.

- Melanin has the important function of protecting the skin against some of the harmful ultraviolet rays of the sun. *Ultraviolet* (UV) refers to light that is beyond the visible spectrum at the violet end. Some UV rays help the skin produce vitamin D; however, other rays damage the skin.

## The Dermis

The **dermis** (**DER**-mis), also known as the *corium*, is the thick layer of living tissue directly below the epidermis. It contains connective tissue, blood and lymph vessels, and nerve fibers. Also found in the dermis are the *hair follicles*, *sebaceous glands*, and *sweat glands*, which are the related structures of the integumentary system (as well as the *nails*).

**Sensory nerve endings** in the dermis are the sensory receptors for stimuli such as touch, temperature, pain, and pressure.

## Tissues Within the Dermis

- **Collagen** (**KOL**-ah-jen), which means glue, is a tough, yet flexible, fibrous protein material found in the skin, and also in the bones, cartilage, tendons, and ligaments.

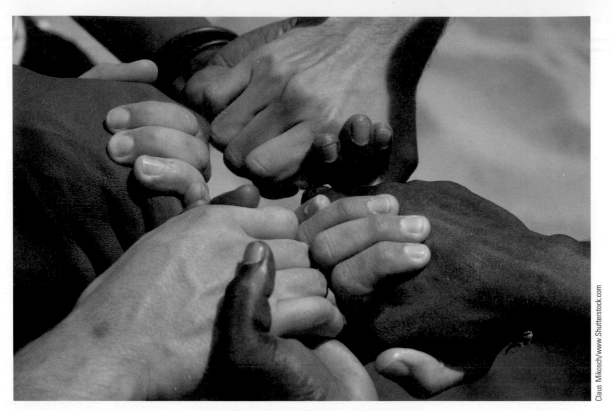

**FIGURE 12.2** The amount of melanin present in the skin determines its color.

- **Mast cells**, which are found in the connective tissue of the dermis, respond to injury, infection, or allergy by producing and releasing substances, including heparin and histamine.
- **Heparin** (**HEP**-ah-rin), which is released in response to an injury, is an anticoagulant. An *anticoagulant* prevents blood clotting.
- **Histamine** (**HISS**-tah-meen), which is released in response to allergens, causes the signs of an allergic response, including itching and increased mucus secretion.

### The Subcutaneous Layer

The **subcutaneous layer** (sub-kyou-**TAY**-nee-us) is located just below the layers of the skin and connects the skin to the surface muscles.

- This layer is made up of loose connective tissue and **adipose tissue** (**AD**-ih-pohs). *Adipose* means fat.
- *Cellulite* is a term used to describe deposits of dimpled fat around the buttocks and thighs. This is not a scientific term, and medical authorities agree that cellulite is simply ordinary fatty tissue. Note: Do not confuse cellulite with *cellulitis*, which is discussed later in this chapter.
- **Lipocytes** (**LIP**-oh-sights), also known as *fat cells*, are predominant in the subcutaneous layer where they manufacture and store large quantities of fat (**lip/o** means fat, and **-cytes** means cells).

### The Sebaceous Glands

**Sebaceous glands** (seh-**BAY**-shus) are located in the dermis layer of the skin and are closely associated with hair follicles (Figure 12.1).

- These glands secrete **sebum** (**SEE**-bum), which is an oily substance that is released through ducts opening into the hair follicles. From here, the sebum moves onto the surface and lubricates the skin.
- Because sebum is slightly acidic, it discourages the growth of bacteria on the skin.
- The milk-producing **mammary glands**, which are modified sebaceous glands, are sometimes classified with the integumentary system. However, they also are part of the reproductive system and are discussed in Chapter 14.

### The Sweat Glands

**Sweat glands**, also known as *sudoriferous glands*, are tiny, coiled glands found on almost all body surfaces. They are most numerous in the palms of the hands, the soles of the feet, the forehead, and in the armpits.

- **Pores** are the openings on the surface of the skin that act as the ducts of the sweat glands.

- **Perspiration**, commonly known as *sweat*, is secreted by sweat glands and is made up of 99% water plus some salt and metabolic waste products.

- Perspiring is one way in which the body excretes excess water.

- As the perspiration evaporates into the air, it also cools the body. Body odor associated with perspiration comes from the interaction of sweat with bacteria on the skin's surface.

- **Hidrosis** (high-**DROH**-sis) is the production and excretion of perspiration.

## The Hair

**Hair** fibers are rod-like structures composed of tightly fused, dead protein cells filled with hard keratin. The darkness and color of the hair is determined by the amount and type of melanin produced by the melanocytes that surround the core of the hair shaft.

- **Hair follicles** (**FOL**-lick-kulz) are the sacs that hold the root of the hair fibers. The shape of the follicle determines whether the hair is straight or curly.

- Although hair is dead tissue, it appears to grow because the cells at the base of the follicle divide rapidly and push the old cells upward. As these cells are pushed upward, they harden and undergo pigmentation.

- The **arrector pili** (ah-**RECK**-tor **PYE**-lye) are tiny muscle fibers attached to the hair follicles that cause the hair to stand erect. In response to cold or fright, these muscles contract, causing raised areas of skin known as goose bumps. This action reduces heat loss through the skin.

## The Nails

An **unguis** (**UNG**-gwis), which is commonly known as a fingernail or toenail, is the keratin plate that protects the dorsal surface of the last bone of each finger and toe (plural, *ungues*). Each nail consists of the following parts (Figure 12.3):

- The *nail body*, which is translucent, is closely molded to the surface of the underlying tissues. It is made up of hard, keratinized plates of epidermal cells.

- The *nail bed*, which joins the nail body to the underlying connective tissue, nourishes the nail. The blood vessels here give the nail its characteristic pink color.

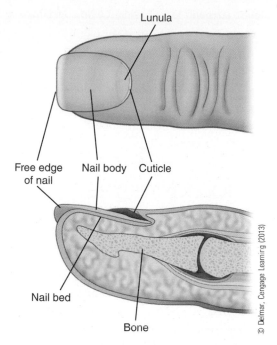

**FIGURE 12.3** Structures of the fingernails and toenails.

- The *free edge*, which is the portion of the nail not attached to the nail bed, extends beyond the tip of the finger or toe.

- The **lunula** (**LOO**-new-lah) is a pale half-moon-shaped region at every nail root, which is generally most easily seen in the thumbnail (plural, *lunulae*). This is the active area of the nail, where new keratin cells form. (**lun** means moon, and -**ula** means little).

- The **cuticle** is a narrow band of epidermis attached to the surface of the nail just in front of the root, protecting the new keratin cells as they form.

- The **nail root** fastens the nail to the finger or toe by fitting into a groove in the skin.

**StudyWARE** CONNECTION

To see the structures of the skin up close, view the **Skin** animation in the StudyWARE™.

## ■ MEDICAL SPECIALTIES RELATED TO THE INTEGUMENTARY SYSTEM

- A **dermatologist** (der-mah-**TOL**-oh-jist) is a physician who specializes in diagnosing and treating disorders of the skin (**dermat** means skin, and -**ologist** means specialist).

- A **plastic surgeon** is a physician who specializes in the surgical restoration and reconstruction of body structures. The term *plastic* is related to the suffix **-plasty**, meaning surgical repair.

- *Cosmetic surgeons* are plastic surgeons who perform operations such as breast augmentation, liposuction, and facelifts that are usually done for aesthetic rather than medical reasons.

# PATHOLOGY OF THE INTEGUMENTARY SYSTEM

## The Sebaceous Glands

- **Acne vulgaris** (**ACK**-nee vul-**GAY**-ris), commonly known as *acne*, is a chronic inflammatory disease characterized by pustular eruptions of the skin caused by an overproduction of sebum around the hair shaft. Although often triggered by hormones in puberty and adolescence, it also occurs in adults. *Vulgaris* is a Latin term meaning common.

- A **comedo** (**KOM**-eh-doh) is a noninfected lesion formed by the buildup of sebum and keratin in a hair follicle (plural, *comedones*) often associated with acne vulgaris. A comedo with an obstructed opening is called a *whitehead* (a closed comedo). A sebum plug that is exposed to air often oxidizes and becomes a *blackhead* (an open comedo).

- A **sebaceous cyst** (seh-**BAY**-shus **SIST**) is a closed sac associated with a sebaceous gland that is found just under the skin. These cysts contain yellow, fatty material and are usually found on the face, neck, or trunk.

- **Seborrhea** (seb-oh-**REE**-ah) is overactivity of the sebaceous glands that results in the production of an excessive amount of sebum (**seb/o** means sebum, and **-rrhea** means flow or discharge).

- **Seborrheic dermatitis** (seb-oh-**REE**-ick **der**-mah-**TYE**-tis) is an inflammation sometimes resulting from seborrhea that causes scaling and itching of the upper layers of the skin or scalp. Extensive *dandruff* is a form of seborrheic dermatitis, as is the scalp rash in infants known as *cradle cap*. In contrast, mild dandruff is usually caused by a yeast-like fungus on the scalp.

- A **seborrheic keratosis** (seb-oh-**REE**-ick **kerr**-ah-**TOH**-sis) is a benign skin growth that has a waxy or "pasted-on" look. These growths, which can vary in color from light tan to black, occur most commonly in the elderly.

## The Sweat Glands

- **Anhidrosis** (**an**-high-**DROH**-sis) is the abnormal condition of lacking sweat in response to heat (**an-** means without, **hidr** means sweat, and **-osis** means abnormal condition).

- **Diaphoresis** (**dye**-ah-foh-**REE**-sis) is profuse sweating (**dia-** means through or complete, **phor** means movement, and **-esis** means abnormal condition). This is a normal condition when brought on by heat or exertion, but can also be the body's response to emotional or physical distress.

- **Heat rash**, also known as *prickly heat*, is an intensely itchy rash caused by blockage of the sweat glands by bacteria and dead cells.

- **Hyperhidrosis** (**high**-per-high-**DROH**-sis) is a condition of excessive sweating in one area or over the whole body (**hyper-** means excessive, **hidr** means sweat, and **-osis** means abnormal condition).

- **Sleep hyperhidrosis**, commonly known as *night sweats*, is the occurrence of hyperhidrosis during sleep. There are many potential causes of this condition, including menopause, certain medications, and some infectious diseases.

## The Hair

- **Folliculitis** (foh-**lick**-you-**LYE**-tis) is an inflammation of the hair follicles (**follicul** means the hair follicle, and **-itis** means inflammation). This condition is especially common on arms, legs, and in the beard area of men.
  - One of the causes of folliculitis is a bacterium found in poorly chlorinated hot tubs or whirlpools. This leads to a condition called *hot tub folliculitis*.

- **Trichomycosis axillaris** (**try**-koh-my-**KOH**-sis ak-sih-**LAR**-is) is superficial bacterial infection of the hair shafts in areas with extensive sweat glands, such as the armpits (**trich/o** means hair, **myc** means fungus, and **-osis** means abnormal condition). *Axillaris* is Latin for axillary (**axill** means armpit, and **-ary** means pertaining to).

### Excessive Hairiness

- **Hirsutism** (**HER**-soot-izm) is the presence of excessive body and facial hair in women, usually occurring in a male pattern (**hirsut** means hairy, and **-ism** means condition). This condition can be hereditary or caused by a hormonal imbalance.

## Abnormal Hair Loss

- **Alopecia** (**al**-oh-**PEE**-shee-ah), also known as *baldness*, is the partial or complete loss of hair, most commonly on the scalp (**alopec** means baldness, and **-ia** means condition).

- **Alopecia areata** (ah-ree-**AY**-tuh) is an autoimmune disorder that attacks the hair follicles, causing well-defined bald areas on the scalp or elsewhere on the body (Figure 12.4). This condition often begins in childhood. *Areata* means occurring in patches.

- **Alopecia totalis** (toh-**TAL**-is), also known as *alopecia capitis totalis*, is an uncommon condition character-ized by the loss of all the hair on the scalp.

- **Alopecia universalis** (**yoo**-nih-vers-**AHL**-is) is the total loss of hair on all parts of the body. *Universalis* means total.

- **Female pattern baldness** is a condition in which the hair thins in the front and on the sides of the scalp and sometimes on the crown. This condition rarely leads to total hair loss.

- **Male pattern baldness** is a common hair-loss pattern in men, with the hairline receding from the front to the back until only a horseshoe-shaped area of hair remains in the back and at the temples.

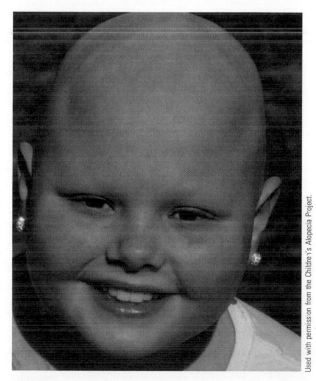

Used with permission from the Children's Alopecia Project.

**FIGURE 12.4** Alopecia areata is an autoimmune disorder that often begins in childhood.

## The Nails

- **Clubbing** is the abnormal curving of the nails that is often accompanied by enlargement of the fingertips. This condition can be hereditary, but usually is caused by changes associated with oxygen deficiencies related to coronary or pulmonary disease.

- **Koilonychia** (**koy**-loh-**NICK**-ee-ah), also known as *spoon nail*, is a malformation of the nails in which the outer surface is concave or scooped out like the bowl of a spoon (**koil** means hollow or concave, **onych** means fingernail or toenail, and **-ia** means condition). This condition is often an indication of iron-deficiency anemia (see Chapter 5).

- **Onychia** (oh-**NICK**-ee-ah), also known as *onychitis*, is an inflammation of the matrix of the nail that often results in the loss of the nail (**onych** means fingernail or toenail, and **-ia** means condition).

- **Onychocryptosis** (**on**-ih-koh-krip-**TOH**-sis) is com-monly known as an *ingrown toenail* (**onych/o** means fingernail or toenail, **crypt** means hidden, and **-osis** means abnormal condition). The edges of a toenail, usually on the big toe, curve inward and cut into the skin. The affected area is prone to inflammation or infection.

- **Onychomycosis** (**on**-ih-koh-my-**KOH**-sis) is a fungal infection of the nail (**onych/o** means fingernail or toenail, **myc** means fungus, and **-osis** means abnormal condition). Depending on the type of fungus involved, this condition can cause the nails to turn white, yellow, green, or black and to become thick or brittle.

- **Onychophagia** (**on**-ih-koh-**FAY**-jee-ah) means nail biting or nail eating (**onych/o** means fingernail or toenail, and **-phagia** means eating or swallowing).

- **Paronychia** (**par**-oh-**NICK**-ee-ah) is an acute or chronic infection of the skin fold around a nail (**par-** means near, **onych** means fingernail or toenail, and **-ia** means condition).

## Skin Pigmentation

- **Age spots,** also known as *solar lentigines* or *liver spots*, are discolorations caused by sun exposure. Although harmless, these spots sometimes resemble skin cancer growths.

- **Albinism** (**AL**-bih-niz-um) is a genetic condition characterized by a deficiency or the absence of pigment in the skin, hair, and irises of the eyes (**albin** means white, and **-ism** means condition).

This condition is the result of a missing enzyme that is necessary for the production of melanin. A person with this condition is known as an *albino*.

- **Chloasma** (kloh-**AZ**-mah), also known as *melasma* or the *mask of pregnancy*, is a pigmentation disorder characterized by brownish spots on the face. This can occur during pregnancy, especially among women with dark hair and fair skin, and usually disappears after delivery.

- **Vitiligo** (vit-ih-**LYE**-goh) is a skin condition resulting from the destruction of the melanocytes due to unknown causes. Vitiligo causes irregular patches of white skin, a process known as *depigmentation*. Hair growing in an affected area may also turn white.

## Bleeding into the Skin

- A **contusion** (kon-**TOO**-zhun) is an injury to underlying tissues without breaking the skin and is characterized by discoloration and pain (**contus** means bruise, and **-ion** means condition). This discoloration is caused by an accumulation of blood within the skin.

- An **ecchymosis** (eck-ih-**MOH**-sis), commonly known as a *bruise*, is a large, irregular area of purplish discoloration due to bleeding under the skin (**ecchym** means pouring out of juice, and **-osis** means abnormal condition) (Figure 12.5). The plural form is *ecchymoses*.

- **Purpura** (**PUR**-pew-rah) is the appearance of multiple purple discolorations on the skin caused by bleeding underneath the skin (**purpur** means purple, and **-a** is a noun ending). These areas of discoloration are smaller than an ecchymosis and larger than petechiae.

- **Petechiae** (pee-**TEE**-kee-ee) are very small, pinpoint hemorrhages that are less than 2 mm in diameter (singular, *petechia*). These hemorrhages sometimes result from high fevers.

- A **hematoma** (hee-mah-**TOH**-mah), which is usually caused by an injury, is a swelling of clotted blood trapped in the tissues (**hemat** means blood, and **-oma** means tumor). The body eventually reabsorbs this blood. A hematoma is often named for the area where it occurs. For example, a *subungual hematoma* is blood trapped under a finger or toenail.

## Surface Lesions

A **lesion** (**LEE**-zhun) is a pathologic change of the tissues due to disease or injury. Skin lesions are described by their appearance, location, color, and size as measured in centimeters (cm).

- A **crust**, also known as *scab*, is a collection of dried serum and cellular debris (Figure 12.6A).

- **Erosion** (eh-**ROH**-zhun) is the wearing away of a surface, such as the epidermis of the skin or the outer layer of a mucus membrane. This term can also describe the progressive loss of dental enamel.

- A **macule** (**MACK**-youl), also known as a *macula*, is a discolored flat spot that is less than 1 cm in diameter. Freckles, or flat moles, are examples of macules (Figure 12.6B).

- A **nodule** (**NOD**-youl) is a solid, raised skin lesion that is *larger than* 0.5 cm in diameter and deeper than a papule. In acne vulgaris, nodules can cause scarring.

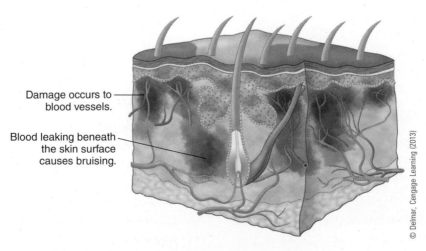

Damage occurs to blood vessels.

Blood leaking beneath the skin surface causes bruising.

© Delmar, Cengage Learning (2013)

**FIGURE 12.5** A cross-section of the skin showing the bleeding under the skin causing ecchymosis.

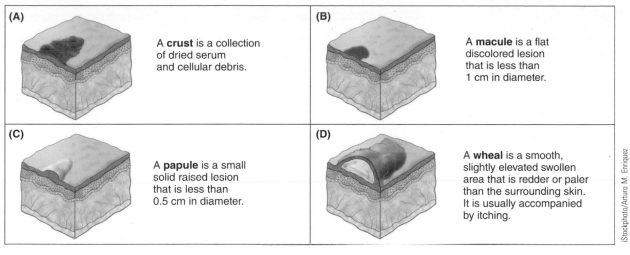

**(A)** A **crust** is a collection of dried serum and cellular debris.

**(B)** A **macule** is a flat discolored lesion that is less than 1 cm in diameter.

**(C)** A **papule** is a small solid raised lesion that is less than 0.5 cm in diameter.

**(D)** A **wheal** is a smooth, slightly elevated swollen area that is redder or paler than the surrounding skin. It is usually accompanied by itching.

iStockphoto/Arturo M. Enriquez

**FIGURE 12.6** Surface lesions of the skin. (A) Crust. (B) Macule. (C) Papule. (D) Wheal.

- A **papule** (**PAP**-youl) is a small, raised red lesion that is *less than* 0.5 cm in diameter and does not contain pus. Small pimples and insect bites are types of papules (Figure 12.6C).

- A **plaque** (**PLACK**) is a scaly, solid raised area of closely spaced papules. For example, the lesions of psoriasis are plaques (Figure 12.11). Note: The term *plaque* also means a fatty buildup in the arteries (see Chapter 5) and a soft substance that forms on the teeth (see Chapter 8)

- **Scales** are flakes or dry patches made up of excess dead epidermal cells. Some shedding of these scales is normal; however, excessive shedding is associated with skin disorders such as psoriasis.

- **Verrucae** (veh-**ROO**-kee), also known as *warts*, are small, hard skin lesions caused by the human papillomavirus (singular, *verruca*). *Plantar warts* are verrucae that develop on the sole of the foot. See Chapter 14 for more information on the human papillomavirus.

- A **wheal** (**WHEEL**), also known as a *welt*, is a small bump that itches. Wheals can appear as *urticaria*, or hives (which are discussed in a later section) as a symptom of an allergic reaction (Figure 12.6D).

### Fluid-Filled Lesions

- An **abscess** (**AB**-sess) is a closed pocket containing pus that is caused by a bacterial infection. An abscess can appear on the skin or within other structures of the body.

- **Purulent** (**PYOU**-roo-lent) means producing or containing pus.

- An **exudate** (**ECKS**-you-dayt) is a fluid, such as pus, that leaks out of an infected wound.

- A **cyst** (**SIST**) is an abnormal sac containing gas, fluid, or a semisolid material (Figure 12.7A). The term *cyst* can also refer to a sac or vesicle elsewhere in the body. The most common type of skin cyst is a sebaceous cyst.

- A **pustule** (**PUS**-tyoul), also known as a *pimple*, is a small, circumscribed lesion containing pus (Figure 12.7B). *Circumscribed* means contained within a limited area. Pustules can be cause by acne vulgaris, impetigo, or other skin infections.

- A **vesicle** (**VES**-ih-kul) is a small blister, *less than* 0.5 cm in diameter, containing watery fluid (Figure 12.7C). For example, the rash of poison ivy consists of vesicles (Figure 12.10).

- A **bulla** (**BULL**-ah) is a large blister that is usually *more than* 0.5 cm in diameter (plural, *bullae*) (Figure 12.7D).

### Lesions Through the Skin

- An **abrasion** (ah-**BRAY**-zhun) is an injury in which superficial layers of skin are scraped or rubbed away.

- A **fissure** (**FISH**-ur) is a groove or crack-like break in the skin. Fissures are, for example, the breaks in the skin between the toes caused by tinea pedis, or athlete's foot (Figure 12.8A). The term *fissure* also describes folds in the contours of the brain.

- A **laceration** (lass-er-**AY**-shun) is a torn or jagged wound, or an accidental cut wound.

- A **pressure sore**, previously known as a *decubitus ulcer* or *bedsore*, is an open ulcerated wound that is caused by prolonged pressure on an area of skin. Without proper care, these sores quickly become seriously infected and can result in tissue death.

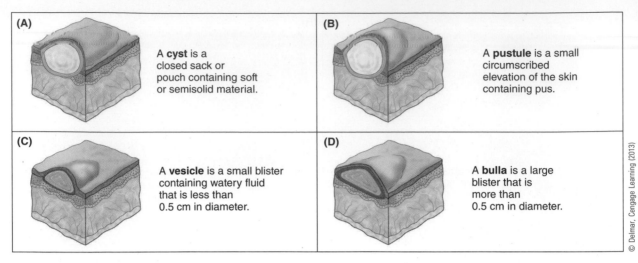

**FIGURE 12.7** Fluid-filled lesions in the skin. (A) Cyst. (B) Pustule. (C) Vesicle. (D) Bulla.

■ A **puncture wound** is a deep hole made by a sharp object such as a rusty nail or ice pick. This type of percutaneous wound carries a high risk of infection, particularly tetanus (see Chapter 6). *Percutaneous* means through the skin.

■ A *needlestick injury* is an accidental puncture wound caused by a used hypodermic needle, potentially transmitting an infection.

■ An **ulcer** (**UL**-ser) is an open lesion of the skin or mucous membrane resulting in tissue loss around the edges (Figure 12.8B). Note: Ulcers also occur inside the body. Those associated with the digestive system are discussed in Chapter 8.

## Birthmarks

A birthmark is a mole or blemish on the skin present at birth or shortly thereafter. Some birthmarks marks fade as a child gets older.

■ **Pigmented birthmarks** include **nevi**, also known as moles, as well as café-au-lait spots, stork bites, and other irregularities in skin color.

■ **Vascular birthmarks** are caused by blood vessels close to the skin's surface.

■ A **capillary hemangioma** (**KAP**-uh-**ler**-ee hee-**man**-jee-**OH**-mah), also known as a *strawberry birthmark*, is a soft, raised, pink or red vascular birthmark (**hem** means blood, **angi** means blood or lymph vessels, and **-oma** means tumor). A *hemangioma* is a benign tissue mass made up of newly formed small blood vessels that in birthmarks are visible through the skin (Figure 12.9). (Also see hemangioma in Chapter 5.)

■ A **port-wine stain** is a flat vascular birthmark made up of dilated blood capillaries, creating a large, reddish-purple discoloration on the face or neck. This type of birthmark will not resolve without treatment. See the later section "Laser and Light Source Treatments of Skin Conditions."

## Dermatitis

The term **dermatitis** (**der**-mah-**TYE**-tis) describes an inflammation of the skin (**dermat** means skin, and **-itis** means inflammation). This condition, which takes many forms, is usually characterized by redness, swelling, and itching.

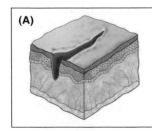

A **fissure** of the skin is a groove or crack-like sore.

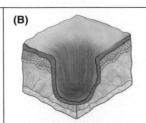

An **ulcer** is an open lesion of the skin or mucous membrane, resulting in tissue loss.

**FIGURE 12.8** Lesions extending through the skin. (A) Fissure. (B) Ulcer.

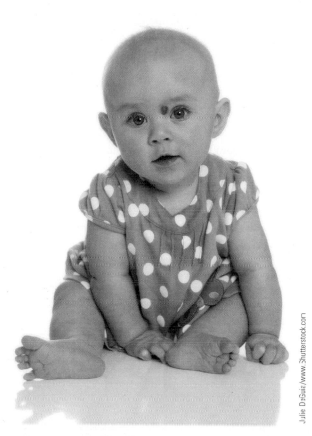

**FIGURE 12.9** A capillary hemangioma is a raised vascular birthmark made up of newly formed small blood vessels.

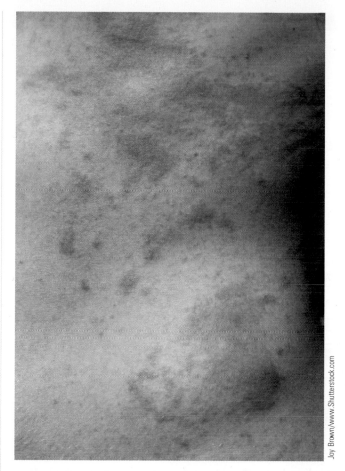

**FIGURE 12.10** Contact dermatitis on a young man's torso caused by poison ivy.

- **Contact dermatitis** (CD) is a localized allergic response caused by contact with an irritant, such as diaper rash. It can also be caused by exposure to an allergen, such as poison ivy, or an allergic reaction to latex gloves (Figure 12.10).

- **Eczema** (**ECK**-zeh-mah), also known as *atopic dermatitis*, is a form of persistent or recurring dermatitis usually characterized by redness, itching, and dryness, with possible blistering, cracking, oozing, or bleeding. This chronic condition, most often seen in infants and children, appears to be the result of a malfunction of the body's immune system.

- **Exfoliative dermatitis** (ecks-**FOH**-lee-**ay**-tiv **der**-mah-**TYE**-tis) is a condition in which there is widespread scaling of the skin. It is often accompanied by pruritus, erythroderma (redness), and hair loss. It may occur in severe cases of many common skin conditions, including eczema, psoriasis, and allergic reactions.

- **Pruritus** (proo-**RYE**-tus), also known as *itching*, is associated with most forms of dermatitis (**prurit** means itching, and **-us** is a singular noun ending). Note that this term ends in *-us*, not *-is*.

## Erythema

**Erythema** (er-ih-**THEE**-mah) is redness of the skin due to capillary dilation (**erythem** means flushed, and **-a** is a noun ending). *Dilation* describes the expansion of the capillary.

- *Erythema infectiosum*, also known as *fifth disease*, is a mildly contagious viral infection that is common in childhood. This infection produces a red, lace-like rash on the child's face that looks as if the child has been slapped. It is called "fifth disease" because its place on the list of six common childhood diseases that can cause an exanthem (which is discussed in a later bullet). Others include measles and rubella.

■ *Erythema multiforme* is a skin disorder resulting from a generalized allergic reaction to an illness, infection, or medication. This reaction, which affects the skin, the mucous membranes, or both, is characterized by a rash that may appear as nodules or papules (raised red bumps), macules (flat discolored areas), or vesicles or bullae (blisters).

■ *Erythema pernio*, also known as *chilblains*, is a purple-red inflammation that occurs when the small blood vessels below the skin are damaged, usually due to exposure to cold and damp weather. When warmth restores full circulation, the affected areas begin to itch; however, they usually heal without treatment.

■ *Sunburn* is a form of erythema in which skin cells are damaged by exposure to the ultraviolet rays in sunlight. This damage increases the chances of later developing skin cancer.

■ **Erythroderma** (eh-**rith**-roh-**DER**-mah) is abnormal redness of the entire skin surface (**erythr/o** means red, and -**derma** means skin).

■ **Exanthem** (eck-**ZAN**-thum) refers to a widespread rash, usually in children. A *rash* is a breaking out, or eruption, that changes the color or texture of the skin.

## General Skin Conditions

■ **Dermatosis** (**der**-mah-**TOH**-sis) is a general term used to denote skin lesions or eruptions of any type that are *not* associated with inflammation (**dermat** means skin, and -**osis** means abnormal condition).

■ **Ichthyosis** (**ick**-thee-**OH**-sis) is a group of hereditary disorders characterized by dry, thickened, and scaly skin (**ichthy** means dry or scaly, and -**osis** means abnormal condition). These conditions are caused either by the slowing of the skin's natural shedding process or by a rapid increase in the production of the skin's cells.

■ **Lipedema** (lip-eh-**DEE**-mah), also known as *painful fat syndrome*, is a chronic abnormal condition that is characterized by the accumulation of fat and fluid in the tissues just under the skin of the hips and legs (**lip** means fat, and -**edema** means swelling). This condition usually affects women and even with weight loss, this localized excess fat does not go away.

■ **Systemic lupus erythematosus** (sis-**TEH**-mik **LOO**-pus er-ih-**thee**-mah-**TOH**-sus) (SLE), also known as *lupus*, is an autoimmune disorder characterized by a

red, scaly rash on the face and upper trunk. In addition to the skin, this condition also attacks the connective tissue in other body systems, especially in the joints.

■ **Psoriasis** (soh-**RYE**-uh-sis) is a common skin disorder characterized by flare-ups in which red papules covered with silvery scales occur on the elbows, knees, scalp, back, or buttocks (Figure 12.11).

■ **Rosacea** (roh-**ZAY**-shee-ah), which is also known as *adult acne*, is characterized by tiny red pimples and broken blood vessels. This chronic condition of unknown cause usually develops in individuals with fair skin, between 30 and 60 years of ages.

■ **Rhinophyma** (**rye**-noh-**FIGH**-muh), also known as *bulbous nose*, usually occurs in older men (**rhin/o** means nose, and -**phyma** means growth). This condition is characterized by hyperplasia (overgrowth) of the tissues of the nose and is associated with advanced rosacea.

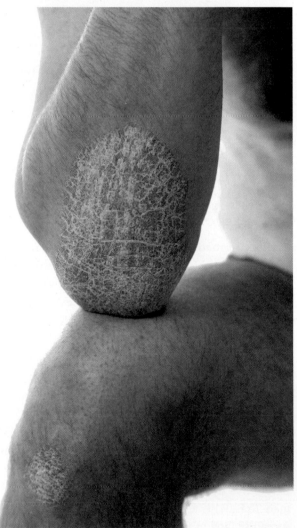

**FIGURE 12.11** Psoriasis is characterized by red papules covered with silvery scales.

Christine Langer-Pueschel/www.Shutterstock.com

- **Scleroderma** (**sklehr**-oh-**DER**-mah) is an autoimmune disorder in which the connective tissues become thickened and hardened, causing the skin to become hard and swollen (**scler/o** means hard, and **-derma** means skin). This condition can also affect the joints and internal organs.

- **Urticaria** (**ur**-tih-**KARE**-ree-ah), also known as *hives*, are itchy wheals caused by an allergic reaction (**urtic** means rash, and **-aria** means connected with).

- **Xeroderma** (zee-roh-**DER**-mah), also known as *xerosis*, is excessively dry skin (**xer/o** means dry, and **-derma** means skin).

## Bacterial Skin Infections

- A **carbuncle** (**KAR**-bung-kul) is a cluster of connected furuncles (boils).

- **Cellulitis** (**sell**-you-**LYE**-tis) is an acute, rapidly spreading bacterial infection within the connective tissues that is characterized by malaise, swelling, warmth, and red streaks. *Malaise* is a feeling of general discomfort or uneasiness that is often the first indication of an infection or other disease.

- **Furuncles** (**FYOU**-rung-kulz), also known as *boils*, are large, tender, swollen areas caused by a staphylococcal infection around hair follicles or sebaceous glands.

- **Gangrene** (**GANG**-green), which is tissue necrosis (death), is most commonly caused by a loss of circulation to the affected tissues. The tissue death is followed by bacterial invasion that causes putrefaction, and if this infection enters the bloodstream, it can be fatal. *Putrefaction* is decay that produces foul-smelling odors.

- **Impetigo** (**im**-peh-**TYE**-goh) is a highly contagious bacterial skin infection that commonly occurs in children. This condition is characterized by isolated pustules that become crusted and rupture.

- **Necrotizing fasciitis** (**NECK**-roh-**tiz**-ing **fas**-ee-**EYE**-tis) is a severe infection caused by Group A strep bacteria, which is also known as *flesh-eating bacteria*. *Necrotizing* means causing tissue death, and *fasciitis* is inflammation of fascia. These bacteria normally live harmlessly on the skin; however, if they enter the body through a skin wound, this serious infection can result. If untreated, the infected body tissue is destroyed, and the illness can be fatal.

- **Pyoderma** (**pye**-oh-**DER**-mah) is any acute, inflammatory, pus-forming bacterial skin infection such as impetigo (**py/o** means pus, and **-derma** means skin).

## Fungal Skin Infections

- **Mycosis** (my-**KOH**-sis) describes any abnormal condition or disease caused by a fungus (**myc** means fungus, and **-osis** means abnormal condition or disease).

- **Tinea** (**TIN**-ee-ah) is a fungal infection that can grow on the skin, hair, or nails. This condition is also known as *ringworm*, not because a worm is involved, but because as the fungus grows, it spreads out in a worm-like circle, leaving normal-looking skin in the middle (Figure 12.12).

  - *Tinea capitis* is found on the scalps of children. *Capitis* means head.

  - *Tinea corporis* is a fungal infection of the skin on the body. *Corporis* means body.

  - *Tinea cruris*, also known as *jock itch*, is found in the genital area.

  - *Tinea pedis*, also known as *athlete's foot*, is most commonly found between the toes. *Pedis* means feet.

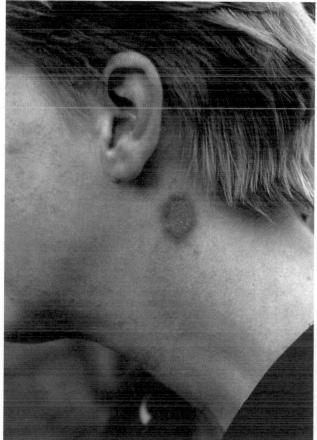

**FIGURE 12.12** Tinea is a fungal infection also known as ringworm.

*Tinea versicolor*, also known as *pityriasis versicolor*, is a fungal infection that causes painless, discolored areas on the skin. *Versicolor* means a variety of color.

## Parasitic Skin Infestations

An **infestation** is the dwelling of microscopic parasites on external surface tissue. Some parasites live temporarily on the skin. Others lay eggs and reproduce there.

- **Pediculosis** (pee-**dick**-you-**LOH**-sis) is an infestation with *lice* (**pedicul** means lice, and **-osis** means abnormal condition). In order to get rid of the infestation, the lice eggs, which are known as *nits*, must be destroyed. There are three types of lice, each attracted to a specific part of the body:
  - *Pediculosis capitis* is an infestation with head lice.
  - *Pediculosis corporis* is an infestation with body lice.
  - *Pediculosis pubis* is an infestation with lice in the pubic hair and pubic region.

- **Scabies** (**SKAY**-beez) is a skin infection caused by an infestation of *itch mites*. These tiny mites cause small, itchy bumps and blisters by burrowing into the top layer of human skin to lay their eggs. Medications applied to the skin kill the mites; however, itching may persist for several weeks.

## Skin Growths

- A **callus** (**KAL**-us) is a thickening of part of the skin on the hands or feet caused by repeated rubbing. Compare with *callus* in Chapter 3. A *clavus*, or *corn*, is a callus in the keratin layer of the skin covering the joints of the toes, usually caused by ill-fitting shoes.

- A **cicatrix** (sick-**AY**-tricks) is a normal scar resulting from the healing of a wound (plural, *cicatrices*).

- **Granulation tissue** is the tissue that normally forms during the healing of a wound. This tissue eventually forms the scar.

- **Granuloma** (**gran**-you-**LOH**-mah) is a general term used to describe a small, knot-like swelling of granulation tissue in the epidermis (**granul** meaning granular, and **-oma** means tumor). Granulomas can result from inflammation, injury, or infection.

- A **keloid** (**KEE**-loid) is an abnormally raised or thickened scar that expands beyond the boundaries of the original incision (**kel** means growth or tumor, and **-oid** means resembling). A tendency to form keloids is often inherited and is more common among people with dark-pigmented skin.

- A **keratosis** (**kerr**-ah-**TOH**-sis) is any skin growth, such as a wart or a callus, in which there is overgrowth and thickening of the skin (**kerat** means hard or horny, and **-osis** means abnormal condition) (plural, *keratoses*). Patches of keratosis in the mouth are known as *leukoplakia*. Note: **kerat/o** also refers to the cornea of the eye. (See Chapter 11.)

- A **lipoma** (lih-**POH**-mah) is a benign, slow-growing fatty tumor located between the skin and the muscle layer (**lip** means fatty, and **-oma** means tumor). This fatty tumor is usually harmless, and treatment is rarely necessary unless the tumor is in a bothersome location, is painful, or is growing rapidly.

- **Nevus** (**NEE**-vus), also known as a *mole*, is a small, dark, skin growth that develops from melanocytes in the skin (plural, *nevi*). Normally, these growths are benign.

- In contrast, **dysplastic nevi** (dis-**PLAS**-tick **NEE**-vye) are atypical moles that can develop into skin cancer.

- A **papilloma** (**pap**-ih-**LOH**-mah) is a benign, superficial wart-like growth on the epithelial tissue or elsewhere in the body, such as in the bladder (**papill** means resembling a nipple, and **-oma** means tumor).

- **Polyp** (**POL**-up) is a general term used most commonly to describe a mushroom-like growth from the surface of a mucous membrane, such as a polyp in the nose. These growths have many causes and are not necessarily malignant.

- **Skin tags** are small, flesh-colored or light-brown polyps that hang from the body by fine stalks. Skin tags are benign and tend to enlarge with age.

## Skin Cancer

**Skin cancer** is a harmful, malignant growth on the skin, which can have many causes, including repeated severe sunburns or long-term exposure to the sun. Skin cancer is becoming very common, affecting about one in five

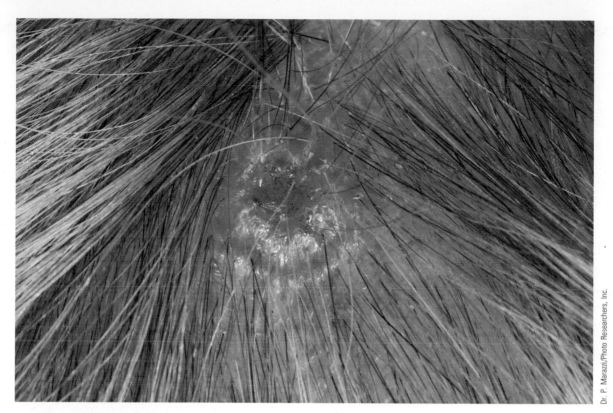

**FIGURE 12.13** Squamous cell carcinoma of the scalp.

Americans in his or her lifetime. There are three main types of skin cancer: basal cell carcinoma, squamous cell carcinoma, and melanoma.

■ An **actinic keratosis** (ack-**TIN**-ick **kerr**-ah-**TOH**-sis) is a precancerous skin growth that occurs on sun-damaged skin. It often looks like a red, tan, or pink scaly patch and feels like sandpaper. *Precancerous* describes a growth that is not yet malignant; however, if not treated, it is likely to become malignant.

■ A **basal cell carcinoma** is a malignant tumor of the basal cell layer of the epidermis. This is the most common and least harmful type of skin cancer because it is slow growing and rarely spreads to other parts of the body. The lesions, which occur mainly on the face or neck and tend to bleed easily, are usually pink, smooth, and are raised with a depression in the center (see carcinoma of the lip in Chapter 6, Figure 6.12).

■ **Squamous cell carcinoma** (**SKWAY**-mus) originates as a malignant tumor of the scaly squamous cells of the epithelium; however, it can quickly spread to other body systems. These cancers begin as skin lesions that appear to be sores that will not heal or that have a crusted look (Figure 12.13).

■ **Malignant melanoma** (mel ah **NOH** mah), also known as *melanoma*, is a type of skin cancer that occurs in the melanocytes (**melan** means black, and **-oma** means tumor). This is the most serious type of skin cancer and often the first signs are changes in the size, shape, or color of a mole (Figure 12.14).

## Burns

A **burn** is an injury to body tissues caused by heat, flame, electricity, sun, chemicals, or radiation. The severity of a burn is described according to the percentage of the total body skin surface affected (more than 15% is considered serious). It is also described according to the depth or layers of skin involved (Table 12.1 and Figure 12.15).

**StudyWARE** **CONNECTION**

Watch an animation on Burns in the StudyWARE™.

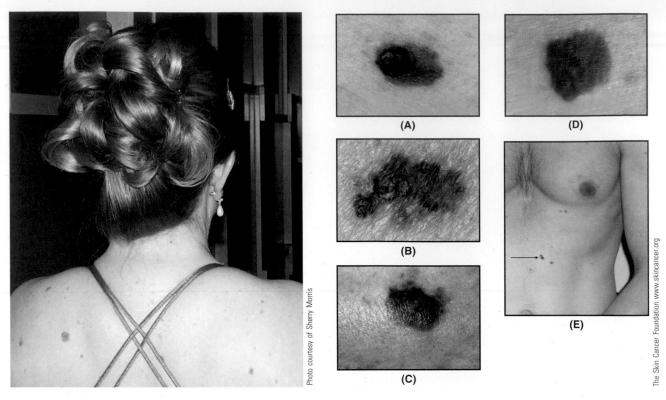

Photo courtesy of Sherry Morris

The Skin Cancer Foundation www.skincancer.org

**FIGURE 12.14**  Left: Melanoma visible on the left shoulder blade. Right: The A-B-C-D-E signs of melanoma are (A) asymmetry, (B) border irregularity, (C) color variation, and (D) diameter larger than a pencil eraser, (E) evolving, or changing in size, shape, or shade of color.

## TABLE 12.1
### Classification of Burn Severity

| Type of Burn | Also Known As | Layers of Skin Involved |
| --- | --- | --- |
| **First-degree burn** | *Superficial burn* | No blisters, superficial damage to the epidermis. |
| **Second-degree burn** | *Partial thickness burn* | Blisters, damage to the epidermis, and dermis. |
| **Third-degree burn** | *Full thickness burn* | Damage to the epidermis, dermis, and subcutaneous layers, and possibly also the muscle and bone below. |

## ■ DIAGNOSTIC PROCEDURES OF THE INTEGUMENTARY SYSTEM

A **biopsy** (**BYE**-op-see) is the removal of a small piece of living tissue for examination to confirm or establish a diagnosis (**bi** means pertaining to life, and **-opsy** means view of).

■ In an *incisional biopsy*, a piece, but not all, of the tumor or lesion is removed.

■ In an *excisional biopsy*, the entire tumor or lesion and a margin of surrounding tissue are removed. *Excision* means the complete removal of a lesion or organ.

■ In a *needle biopsy*, a hollow needle is used to remove a core of tissue for examination.

■ **Exfoliative cytology** (ecks-**FOH**-lee-**ay**-tiv sigh-**TOL**-oh-jee) is a technique in which cells are scraped from the tissue and examined under a microscope. *Exfoliation* is the removal of dead epidermal cells, often through sanding or chemabrasion (which is discussed in the next section), and is sometimes done for cosmetic purposes.

# ■ TREATMENT PROCEDURES OF THE INTEGUMENTARY SYSTEM

## Preventive Measures

**Sunscreen** that blocks out the harmful ultraviolet B (UVB) rays is sometimes measured in terms of the strength of the *sun protection factor*. Some sunscreens also give protection against ultraviolet A (UVA rays).

## Tissue Removal

- **Cauterization** (**kaw**-ter-eye-**ZAY**-zhun) is the destruction of tissue by burning.

- **Chemabrasion** (**kem**-ah-**BRAY**-zhun), also known as a *chemical peel*, is the use of chemicals to remove the outer layers of skin to treat acne scarring, fine wrinkling, and keratoses.

- **Cryosurgery** (**krye**-oh-**SIR**-jur-ee) is the destruction or elimination of abnormal tissue cells, such as warts or tumors, through the application of extreme cold by using liquid nitrogen (**cry/o** means cold, and **-surgery** means operative procedure).

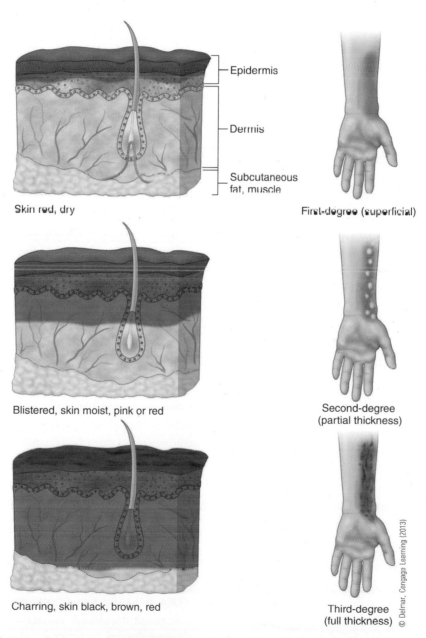

Epidermis

Dermis

Subcutaneous fat, muscle

Skin red, dry

First-degree (superficial)

Blistered, skin moist, pink or red

Second-degree (partial thickness)

Charring, skin black, brown, red

Third-degree (full thickness)

© Delmar, Cengage Learning (2013)

**FIGURE 12.15** The degree of a burn is determined by the layers of skin involved.

■ **Curettage** (**kyou**-reh-**TAHZH**) is the removal of material from the surface by scraping. One use of this technique is to remove basal cell tumors.

■ **Debridement** (dah-**BREED**-ment) is the removal of dirt, foreign objects, damaged tissue, and cellular debris from a wound to prevent infection and to promote healing.

■ In an **irrigation and debridement** procedure, pressurized fluid is used to clean out wound debris.

■ **Dermabrasion** (**der**-mah-**BRAY**-zhun) is a form of abrasion involving the use of a revolving wire brush or sandpaper. It is used to remove acne and chickenpox scars as well as for facial skin rejuvenation. *Microdermabrasion* removes only a fine layer of skin, so the results are temporary.

■ **Electrodesiccation** (ee-**leck**-troh-des-ih-**KAY**-shun) is a surgical technique in which tissue is destroyed using an electric spark. It is primarily used to eliminate small superficial growths and to seal off blood vessels.

■ An **incision** is a cut made with a surgical instrument. *Incision and drainage* (I & D) in an incision (cutting open) of a lesion, such as an abscess, and the draining of the contents.

■ **Mohs' surgery** is a technique used to treat various types of skin cancer. Individual layers of cancerous tissue are removed and examined under a microscope one at a time until a margin that is clear of all cancerous tissue has been achieved.

## Laser and Light Source Treatments of Skin Conditions

The term **laser** is an acronym in which the letters stand for **L**ight **A**mplification by **S**timulated **E**mission of **R**adiation. Lasers are used to treat skin conditions and other disorders of the body.

A laser tube can be filled with a solid, liquid, or gas substance that is stimulated to emit light at a specific wavelength. Some wavelengths are capable of destroying all skin tissue; others target tissue of a particular color.

■ *Port-wine stain* is treated using short pulses of laser light to remove the birthmark. Treatment can require many sessions, because only a small section is treated at a time.

■ *Rhinophyma* is treated by using a laser to reshape the nose by vaporizing the excess tissue.

■ Tattoos are removed by using lasers that target particular colors.

■ Some skin cancers, precancer of the lip, and warts that recur around nails and on the soles of feet are treated using lasers.

**Photodynamic therapy** (PDT) (**foh**-toh-dye-**NAH**-mik) is a technique used to treat damaged and precancerous skin, as well as various types of cancer.

■ A *photosensitizing drug* is administered topically or by injection. An incubation period is followed by exposure to a specific wavelength of light, administered either externally or endoscopically.

■ When the photosensitizers are thus activated, they produce a form of oxygen that kills nearby cells. PDT is used to treat tumors on or near the surface of the skin, or in the lining of internal organs such as the lungs and esophagus.

## Medications for Treatment of the Skin

**Retinoids** (**RET**-ih-noydz) are a class of chemical compounds derived from vitamin A that are used in skin care and treatment because of their effect on epithelial cell growth. The use of retinoids can, however, make the skin burn more easily.

■ *Isotretinoin*, known by its trade name of Accutane, is a powerful retinoid taken in pill form for the treatment of severe acne.

■ *Tretinoin* is the active ingredient in Retin-A and Renova, which are used to treat sun-damaged skin, acne, and wrinkles.

**Topical steroids** such as hydrocortisone and other more potent variations are used in the treatment of various skin disorders and diseases. These drugs, which are derivatives of the natural corticosteroid hormones produced by the adrenal glands, must be used cautiously to avoid potential side effects, which can include irreversible thinning of the skin.

## Cosmetic Procedures

■ **Blepharoplasty** (**BLEF**-ah-roh-**plas**-tee), also known as a *lid lift,* is the surgical reduction of the upper and lower eyelids by removing sagging skin (**blephar/o** means eyelid, and **-plasty** means surgical repair) (Figure 12.16). A small amount of fat from the patient's thighs or buttocks is sometimes injected in the hollow below the eye.

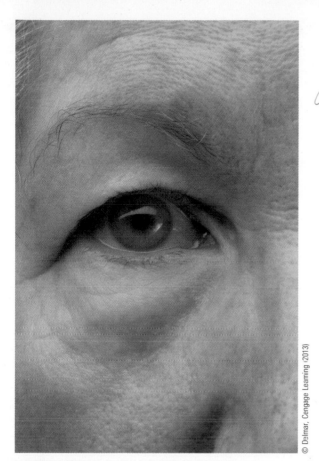

**FIGURE 12.16** Blepharoplasty is the surgical reduction of the eyelids by removing sagging skin that can interfere with the field of vision.

© Delmar, Cengage Learning (2013)

■ **Botox** is a formulation of *botulinum toxin*. This is the same neurotoxin responsible for the form of food poisoning known as botulism. When small sterile doses are injected into muscles on the forehead, it can temporarily block the nerve signals to the injected muscle for up to 3 to 4 months, reducing moderate to severe *frown lines* between the eyebrows. Botox is now also being used therapeutically to treat migraines and muscle spasms.

■ **Collagen replacement therapy** is a form of soft-tissue augmentation used to soften facial lines or scars, or to make lips appear fuller. Tiny quantities of collagen are injected under a line or scar to boost the skin's natural supply of collagen. The effect usually lasts for 3 to 12 months.

■ **Dermatoplasty** (**DER**-mah-toh-**plas**-tee), also known as a *skin graft*, is the replacement of damaged skin with healthy tissue taken from a donor site on the patient's body (**dermat/o** means skin, and **-plasty** means surgical repair).

■ **Electrolysis** (ee-leck-**TROL**-ih-sis) is the use of electric current to destroy hair follicles in order to produce the relatively permanent removal of undesired hair (**electr/o** means electric, and **-lysis** means destruction).

■ **Lipectomy** (lih-**PECK**-toh-mee) is the surgical removal of fat from beneath the skin to improve physical appearance (**lip** means fat, and **-ectomy** means surgical removal).

■ **Liposuction** (**LIP**-oh-**suck**-shun), also known as *suction-assisted lipectomy*, is the surgical removal of fat beneath the skin with the aid of suction.

■ **Rhytidectomy** (**rit**-ih-**DECK**-toh-mee), also known as a *facelift*, is the surgical removal of excess skin and fat from the face to eliminate wrinkles (**rhytid** means wrinkle, and **-ectomy** means surgical removal).

■ **Sclerotherapy** (**sklehr**-oh-**THER**-ah-pee) is the treatment of spider veins by injecting a saline *sclerosing solution* into the vein. This solution irritates the tissue, causing the veins to collapse and disappear. *Spider veins* are small, nonessential veins that can be seen through the skin.

## ABBREVIATIONS RELATED TO THE INTEGUMENTARY SYSTEM

Table 12.2 presents an overview of the abbreviations related to the terms introduced in this chapter. Note: To avoid errors or confusion, always be cautious when using abbreviations.

## TABLE 12.2
### Abbreviations Related to the Integumentary System

| | |
|---|---|
| basal cell carcinoma = BCC | BCC = basal cell carcinoma |
| cauterization = caut | caut = cauterization |
| eczema = Ecz, Ez | Ecz, Ez = eczema |
| irrigation and debridement = I & D | I & D = irrigation and debridement |
| malignant melanoma = MM | MM = malignant melanoma |
| necrotizing fasciitis = NF | NF = necrotizing fasciitis |
| photodynamic therapy = PDT | PDT = photodynamic therapy |
| psoriasis = Ps | Ps = psoriasis |
| scleroderma = SCD | SCD = scleroderma |
| squamous cell carcinoma = SCC | SCC = squamous cell carcinoma |
| subcutaneous = SC, subq | SC, subq = subcutaneous |
| systemic lupus erythematosus = SLE | SLE = systemic lupus erythematosus |

**StudyWARE CONNECTION**

For more practice and to test your mastery of this material, go to the StudyWARE™ to play interactive games and complete the quiz for this chapter.

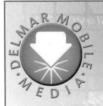

Downloadable audio is available for selected medical terms in this chapter to enhance your learning of medical terminology.

## ☐ Workbook Practice

Go to your workbook, and complete the exercises for this chapter.

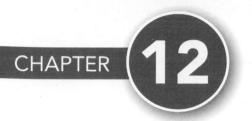
# LEARNING EXERCISES

## MATCHING WORD PARTS 1

Write the correct answer in the middle column.

| Definition | Correct Answer | Possible Answers |
|---|---|---|
| 12.1. skin | _____ | urtlc/o |
| 12.2. rash | _____ | rhytid/o |
| 12.3. red | _____ | hidr/o |
| 12.4. sweat | _____ | erythr/o |
| 12.5. wrinkle | _____ | cutane/o |

## MATCHING WORD PARTS 2

Write the correct answer in the middle column.

| Definition | Correct Answer | Possible Answers |
|---|---|---|
| 12.6. black, dark | _____ | pedicul/o |
| 12.7. fat, lipid | _____ | melan/o |
| 12.8. horny, hard | _____ | lip/o |
| 12.9. lice | _____ | kerat/o |
| 12.10. skin | _____ | dermat/o |

## MATCHING WORD PARTS 3

Write the correct answer in the middle column.

| Definition | Correct Answer | Possible Answers |
|---|---|---|
| 12.11. dry | _____ | xer/o |
| 12.12. fungus | _____ | seb/o |

12.13.  hairy, rough                   _____        **onych/o**

12.14.  nail                           _____        **myc/o**

12.15.  sebum                          _____        **hirsut/o**

## DEFINITIONS

Select the correct answer, and write it on the line provided.

12.16.  An acute, rapidly spreading bacterial infection within the connective tissues is known

as _____.

    abscess        cellulitis        fissure        ulcer

12.17.  Atypical moles that can develop into skin cancer are known as _____.

    dysplastic nevi        lipomas        malignant keratoses        papillomas

12.18.  The autoimmune disorder in which there are well-defined bald areas is known

as _____.

    alopecia areata        alopecia capitis        alopecia universalis        psoriasis

12.19.  A/An _____ is a swelling of clotted blood trapped in the tissues.

    abscess        contusion        hematoma        petechiae

12.20.  The term _____ means profuse sweating.

    anhidrosis        diaphoresis        hidrosis        ecchymosis

12.21.  A normal scar resulting from the healing of a wound is called a _____.

    cicatrix        keloid        keratosis        papilloma

12.22.  A large blister that is usually more than 0.5 cm in diameter is known as a/an _____.

    abscess        bulla        pustule        vesicle

12.23.  The removal of dirt, foreign objects, damaged tissue, and cellular debris from a wound is

called _____.

    cauterization        curettage        debridement        dermabrasion

12.24.  A _____ burn has blisters plus damage only to the epidermis and dermis.

    first-degree        fourth-degree        second-degree        third-degree

12.25.  Commonly known as warts, _____ are small, hard skin lesions caused by the

human papillomavirus.

nevi                    petechiae                    scabies                    verrucae

## MATCHING STRUCTURES

Write the correct answer in the middle column.

| Definition | Correct Answer | Possible Answers |
|---|---|---|
| 12.26.  fibrous protein found in hair, nails, and skin | _____ | unguis |
| 12.27.  fingernail or toenail | _____ | sebaceous glands |
| 12.28.  glands secreting sebum | _____ | mammary glands |
| 12.29.  milk-producing sebaceous glands | _____ | keratin |
| 12.30.  the layer of tissue below the epidermis | _____ | dermis |

## WHICH WORD?

Select the correct answer, and write it on the line provided.

12.31.  The medical term for the condition commonly known as an ingrown toenail

is _____.

onychomycosis          onychocryptosis

12.32.  The bacterial skin infection characterized by isolated pustules that become crusted and rupture is known

as _____. This highly contagious condition commonly occurs in children.

impetigo          xeroderma

12.33.  A torn or jagged wound or an accidental cut wound is known as a _____.

laceration          lesion

12.34.  The lesions of _____ carcinoma tend to bleed easily.

basal cell          squamous cell

12.35.   Group A strep, also known as flesh-eating bacteria, causes _____.

systematic lupus erythematosus                necrotizing fasciitis

## SPELLING COUNTS

Find the misspelled word in each sentence. Then write that word, spelled correctly, on the line provided.

12.36.   Soriasis is a disease of the skin characterized by itching and by red papules covered with

silvery scales. _____

12.37.   Exema is an inflammatory skin disease with possible blistering, cracking, oozing,

or bleeding. _____

12.38.   An absess is a localized collection of pus. _____

12.39.   Onichia is an inflammation of the nail bed that usually results in the loss of the

nail. _____

12.40.   Schleroderma is an autoimmune disorder in which the connective tissues become thickened and hard-

ened, causing the skin to become hard and swollen. _____

## ABBREVIATION IDENTIFICATION

In the space provided, write the words that each abbreviation stands for.

12.41.   **BCC**          _____

12.42.   **I & D**        _____

12.43.   **SLE**          _____

12.44.   **MM**           _____

12.45.   **SCC**          _____

## TERM SELECTION

Select the correct answer, and write it on the line provided.

12.46.   A _____ is a small, knot-like swelling of granulation tissue in the epidermis.

cicatrix            granuloma            keratosis            petechiae

12.47.   An infestation of lice is known as _____

pediculosis         itch mites           cicatrix             scabies

12.48. The term _____ is used to describe any redness of the skin due to dilated

capillaries.

    dermatitis          ecchymosis          erythema          urticaria

12.49. Flakes or dry patches made up of excess dead epidermal cells are known as _____.

    bullae          macules          plaques          scales

12.50. A cluster of connected boils is known as a/an _____.

    acne vulgaris          carbuncle          comedo          furuncle

## SENTENCE COMPLETION

Write the correct term or terms on the lines provided.

12.51. The term meaning producing or containing pus is _____.

12.52. The term meaning a fungal infection of the nail is _____.

12.53. Tissue death followed by bacterial invasion and putrefaction is known as _____.

12.54. A genetic condition characterized by a deficiency or absence of pigment in the skin, hair, and irises is

known as _____.

12.55. Commonly known as hives, _____ are itchy wheals caused by an allergic reaction.

## WORD SURGERY

Divide each term into its component word parts. Write these word parts, in sequence, on the lines provided. When necessary use a slash (/) to indicate a combining vowel. (You may not need all of the lines provided.)

12.56. A **rhytidectomy** is the surgical removal of excess skin for the elimination of wrinkles.

    _____          _____          _____          _____

12.57. **Onychomycosis** is a fungal infection of the nail.

    _____          _____          _____          _____

12.58. **Folliculitis** is an inflammation of the hair follicles that is especially common on the limbs and in the

beard area of men.

    _____          _____          _____          _____

12.59. **Pruritus**, which is commonly known as itching, is associated with most forms of dermatitis.

    _____          _____          _____          _____

12.60. **Ichthyosis** is a group of hereditary disorders that are characterized by dry, thickened, and scaly skin.

_____     _____     _____     _____

## TRUE/FALSE

If the statement is true, write **True** on the line. If the statement is false, write **False** on the line.

12.61. _____ An actinic keratosis is a precancerous skin growth that occurs on

sun-damaged skin.

12.62. _____ A skin tag is a malignant skin enlargement commonly found on older

clients.

12.63. _____ The arrector pili cause the raised areas of skin known as goose bumps.

12.64. _____ A keratosis is an abnormally raised scar.

12.65. _____ Lipedema, which is also known as painful fat syndrome, affects mostly

women.

## CLINICAL CONDITIONS

Write the correct answer on the line provided.

12.66. Carmella Espinoza underwent _____ for the treatment of spider veins.

12.67. Jordan Caswell is an albino. This disorder, which is known as _____, is due to a

missing enzyme necessary for the production of melanin.

12.68. Soon after Ying Li hit his thumb with a hammer, a collection of blood formed beneath the nail.

This condition is a subungual _____.

12.69. Trisha Bell fell off her bicycle and scraped off the superficial layers of skin on her knees. This type of

injury is known as a/an _____.

12.70. Molly Malone had a severe fever, and then she developed very small, pinpoint hemorrhages under her

skin. The doctor described these as being _____.

12.71. Many of the children in the Happy Hours Day Care Center required treatment

for _____, a skin infection caused by an infestation of itch mites.

12.72. Dr. Liu treated Jeanette Isenberg's skin cancer with _____ surgery. With this technique, individual layers of cancerous tissue are removed and examined under a microscope until all cancerous tissue has been removed.

12.73. Mrs. Garrison had cosmetic surgery that is commonly known as a lid lift. The medical term for this surgical treatment is a/an _____.

12.74. Manuel Fernandez developed a/an _____. This condition is a closed pocket containing pus that is caused by a bacterial infection.

12.75. Agnes Farrington calls them night sweats; however, the medical term for this condition is _____.

## WHICH IS THE CORRECT MEDICAL TERM?

Select the correct answer, and write it on the line provided.

12.76. The term that refers to an acute infection of the fold of skin around a nail is _____.

      onychia          onychocryptosis          paronychia          vitiligo

12.77. When the sebum plug of a _____ is exposed to air, it oxidizes and becomes a blackhead.

      chloasma          comedo          macule          pustule

12.78. The condition known as _____ is a skin disorder characterized by flare-ups of red papules covered with silvery scales.

      chloasma          psoriasis          rosacea

12.79. The medical term referring to a malformation of the nail is _____. This condition is also called spoon nail.

      clubbing          koilonychia          onychomycosis          paronychia

12.80. Commonly known as a mole, a/an _____ is a small, dark, skin growth that develops from melanocytes in the skin.

      keloid          nevus          papilloma          verrucae

## CHALLENGE WORD BUILDING

These terms are *not* found in this chapter; however, they are made up of the following familiar word parts. If you need help in creating the term, refer to your medical dictionary.

| | | |
|---|---|---|
| an- | dermat/o | -ia |
| hypo- | hidr/o | -ectomy |
| | melan/o | -itis |
| | myc/o | -malacia |
| | onych/o | -oma |
| | py/o | -derma |
| | | -osis |
| | | -pathy |
| | | -plasty |

12.81. Abnormal softening of the nails is known as ___onychomalacia___.

12.82. An abnormal condition resulting in the diminished flow of perspiration is known as ___hypohidrosis___.

12.83. The plastic surgery procedure to change the shape or size of the nose is a/an ___Rhinoplasty___.

12.84. A tumor arising from the nail bed is known as ___Onchyoma___.

12.85. The term meaning any disease marked by abnormal pigmentation of the skin is ___melanopathy___.

12.86. The surgical removal of a finger or toenail is a/an ___onychectomy___.

12.87. The term meaning pertaining to the absence of fingernails or toenails is ___Anonychia___.

12.88. The term meaning any disease of the skin is ___dermatology___.

12.89. Any disease caused by a fungus is ___Mycosis___. /Stomatomycosis ?

12.90. An excess of melanin present in an area of inflammation of the skin is known as ___dermatitis___? melano

## LABELING EXERCISES

Identify the numbered items on the accompanying figures.

12.91. _____

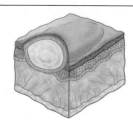

A **12.91** is a closed sack or pouch containing soft or semisolid material.

© Delmar, Cengage Learning (2013)

12.92. _____

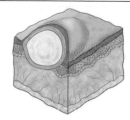

A **12.92** is a small circumscribed elevation of the skin containing pus.

© Delmar, Cengage Learning (2013)

12.93. _____

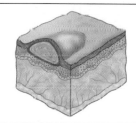

A **12.93** is a small blister containing watery fluid that is less than 0.5 cm in diameter.

© Delmar, Cengage Learning (2013)

12.94. _____

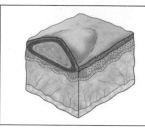

A **12.94** is a large blister that is more than 0.5 cm in diameter.

© Delmar, Cengage Learning (2013)

12.95. _____

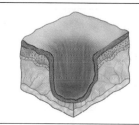

An **12.95** is an open lesion of the skin or mucous membrane, resulting in tissue loss.

© Delmar, Cengage Learning (2013)

12.96. _____ layer

12.97. _____ layer

12.98. _____ tissue

12.99. _____ gland

12.100. _____ gland

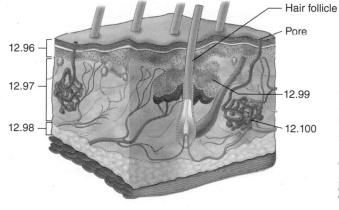

© Delmar, Cengage Learning (2013)

# THE HUMAN TOUCH
## Critical Thinking Exercise

The following story and questions are designed to stimulate critical thinking through class discussion or as a brief essay response. There are no right or wrong answers to these questions.

*"OK, guys, we're late again."* Shaylene Boulay calls out to her two oldest sons, Nathan Jr., 10, and Carl, 12. Grabbing the lunches Nate Sr. packed, she walks out the back door. *"Come on, Michael, school time!"* Shaylene peers under the porch for her 5-year-old. Their house is only a mile from the waterfront, and he loves to race cars between their dog Bubba's big paws in the cool sand underneath the porch. *"Look at you!"* As Shaylene dusts him off and heads to the truck, she notices that the rash of blisters on his leg is still bright red. *"Must be ant bites,"* she thinks.

*"Have a good day!"* Shaylene hands Nathan and Carl their lunches as they hop out of the truck at the middle school. Next stop, Oak Creek Elementary. As Michael starts to get out, clutching his brown lunch bag tightly, his kindergarten teacher comes rushing over. *"Michael, what are you doing here today? Didn't you give your mother the note from the nurse?"*

*"What note? Michael, honey, did you forget to give Mama something from school?"* Michael smiles sheepishly and reaches into his shorts pocket for a wadded up piece of paper. The note says: *"We believe Michael has impetigo. Since this condition is very contagious, please consult your doctor as soon as possible. We will need a note from the doctor before we can allow Michael to reenter class."*

*"Oh, no,"* Shaylene thinks. *"I'm due for my shift at the diner in 15 minutes. Nobody's home to watch Michael, and we don't have the money to see Dr. Gaines again. And what if this rash on my arm is that thing Michael has?"* She sits clutching the wheel of the old pickup, asking herself over and over, *"What am I gonna do?"*

## Suggested Discussion Topics

1. Discuss why the school wants Michael to have completed treatment before he returns to class.

2. You work in Dr. Gaines's office and you know that the Boulay's appointment today is about a potential contagious rash. What precautions should you take when the family arrives?

3. Discuss how you might explain to Shaylene what impetigo is, how it spreads, and what she can do to prevent her other children from getting it.

4. Shaylene is in a very difficult, and all too common, situation. Discuss possible answers to her question *"What am I gonna do?"*

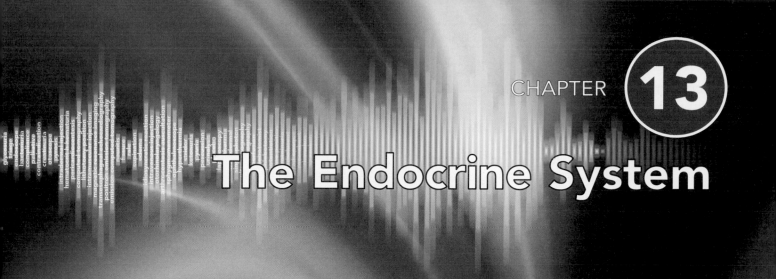

# The Endocrine System

## Overview of
## STRUCTURES, COMBINING FORMS, AND FUNCTIONS OF THE ENDOCRINE SYSTEM

| Major Structures | Related Combining Forms | Primary Functions |
| --- | --- | --- |
| Adrenal Glands | **adren/o** | Regulate electrolyte levels, influence metabolism, and respond to stress. |
| Gonads | **gonad/o** | Gamete (sex cell) producing glands |
| Male: Testicles | **testic/o** | Sperm-producing gland |
| Female: Ovaries | **ovari/o** | Ova (egg) producing gland |
| Pancreatic Islets | **pancreat/o** | Control blood sugar levels and glucose metabolism. |
| Parathyroid Glands | **parathyroid/o** | Regulate calcium levels throughout the body. |
| Pineal Gland | **pineal/o** | Influences the sleep-wakefulness cycle. |
| Pituitary Gland | **pituit/o, pituitar/o** | Secretes hormones that control the activity of the other endocrine glands. |
| Thymus | **thym/o** | Plays a major role in the immune reaction. |
| Thyroid Gland | **thyr/o, thyroid/o** | Stimulates metabolism, growth, and the activity of the nervous system. |

# Vocabulary Related to **THE ENDOCRINE SYSTEM**

This list contains essential word parts and medical terms for this chapter. These terms are pronounced in the student StudyWARE™ and Audio CDs that are available for use with this text. These and the other important **primary terms** are shown in boldface throughout the chapter. *Secondary terms*, which appear in *orange* italics, clarify the meaning of primary terms.

## Word Parts

- [ ] **acr/o** extremities (hands and feet), top, extreme point
- [ ] **adren/o** adrenal glands
- [ ] **crin/o** secrete
- [ ] **-dipsia** thirst
- [ ] **glyc/o** glucose, sugar
- [ ] **gonad/o** gonad, sex glands
- [ ] **-ism** condition, state of
- [ ] **pancreat/o** pancreas
- [ ] **parathyroid/o** parathyroid glands
- [ ] **pineal/o** pineal gland
- [ ] **pituitar/o** pituitary gland
- [ ] **poly-** many
- [ ] **somat/o** body
- [ ] **thym/o** thymus gland
- [ ] **thyr/o, thyroid/o** thyroid gland

## Medical Terms

- [ ] **acromegaly** (**ack**-roh-**MEG**-ah-lee)
- [ ] **Addison's disease** (**AD**-ih-sonz)
- [ ] **adrenalitis** (ah-**dree**-nal-**EYE**-tis)
- [ ] **aldosteronism** (al-**DOSS**-teh-roh-**niz**-em)
- [ ] **antidiuretic hormone** (**an**-tih-dye-you-**RET**-ick)
- [ ] **calcitonin** (**kal**-sih-**TOH**-nin)
- [ ] **Conn's syndrome** (**KONS**)
- [ ] **cortisol** (**KOR**-tih-sol)
- [ ] **cretinism** (**CREE**-tin-izm)
- [ ] **Cushing's syndrome** (**KUSH**-ingz)
- [ ] **diabetes insipidus** (**dye**-ah-**BEE**-teez in-**SIP**-ih-dus)
- [ ] **diabetes mellitus** (**dye**-ah-**BEE**-teez **MEL**-ih-tus)
- [ ] **diabetic retinopathy** (**ret**-ih-**NOP**-ah-thee)
- [ ] **electrolytes** (ee-**LECK**-troh-lytes)
- [ ] **epinephrine** (ep-ih-**NEF**-rin)
- [ ] **estrogen** (**ES**-troh-jen)
- [ ] **exophthalmos** (**eck**-sof-**THAL**-mos)

- [ ] **follicle-stimulating hormone** (**FOL**-lick-kul)
- [ ] **fructosamine test** (fruck-**TOHS**-ah-meen)
- [ ] **gestational diabetes mellitus** (jes-**TAY**-shun-al **dye**-ah-**BEE**-teez)
- [ ] **gigantism** (jigh-**GAN**-tiz-em)
- [ ] **glucagon** (**GLOO**-kah-gon)
- [ ] **glucose** (**GLOO**-kohs)
- [ ] **Graves' disease** (**GRAYVZ**)
- [ ] **growth hormone**
- [ ] **gynecomastia** (**guy**-neh-koh-**MAS**-tee-ah)
- [ ] **Hashimoto's disease** (hah-shee-**MOH**-tohz)
- [ ] **hypercalcemia** (**high**-per-kal-**SEE**-mee-ah)
- [ ] **hyperglycemia** (**high**-per-glye-**SEE**-mee-ah)
- [ ] **hyperinsulinism** (**high**-per-**IN**-suh-lin-izm)
- [ ] **hyperpituitarism** (**high**-per-pih-**TOO**-ih-tah-rizm)
- [ ] **hyperthyroidism** (**high**-per-**THIGH**-roid-izm)
- [ ] **hypoglycemia** (**high**-poh-gly-**SEE**-mee-ah)
- [ ] **hypothyroidism** (**high**-poh-**THIGH**-roid-izm)
- [ ] **insulin** (**IN**-suh-lin)
- [ ] **insulinoma** (in-suh-lin-**OH**-mah)
- [ ] **interstitial cell-stimulating hormone** (**in**-ter-**STISH**-al)
- [ ] **laparoscopic adrenalectomy** (ah-**dree**-nal-**ECK**-toh-mee)
- [ ] **leptin** (**LEP**-tin)
- [ ] **luteinizing hormone** (**LOO**-tee-in-eye-zing)
- [ ] **myxedema** (**mick**-seh-**DEE**-mah)
- [ ] **norepinephrine** (**nor**-ep-ih-**NEF**-rin)
- [ ] **oxytocin** (**ock**-see-**TOH**-sin)
- [ ] **pancreatitis** (**pan**-kree-ah-**TYE**-tis)
- [ ] **parathyroidectomy** (**par**-ah-**thigh**-roi-**DECK**-toh-mee)
- [ ] **pituitary adenoma** (pih-**TOO**-ih-**tair**-ee ad-eh-**NOH**-mah)
- [ ] **polydipsia** (pol-ee-**DIP**-see-ah)
- [ ] **polyphagia** (pol-ee-**FAY**-jee-ah)
- [ ] **polyuria** (pol-ee-**YOU**-ree-ah)
- [ ] **prediabetes**
- [ ] **progesterone** (proh-**JES**-ter-ohn)
- [ ] **prolactinoma** (proh-**lack**-tih-**NOH**-mah)
- [ ] **puberty** (**PYU**-ber-tee)
- [ ] **radioactive iodine treatment**
- [ ] **steroids** (**STEHR**-oidz)
- [ ] **testosterone** (tes-**TOS**-teh-rohn)
- [ ] **thymectomy** (thigh-**MECK**-toh-mee)
- [ ] **thymitis** (thigh-**MY**-tis)
- [ ] **thymosin** (**THIGH**-moh-sin)
- [ ] **thyroxine** (thigh-**ROCK**-sin)

## LEARNING GOALS

On completion of this chapter, you should be able to:

1. Describe the role of the endocrine glands in maintaining homeostasis.

2. Name and describe the functions of the primary hormones secreted by each of the endocrine glands.

3. Recognize, define, spell, and pronounce the primary terms relating to the pathology and the diagnostic and treatment procedures of the endocrine glands.

# FUNCTIONS OF THE ENDOCRINE SYSTEM

The primary function of the endocrine system is to produce hormones that work together to maintain homeostasis. **Homeostasis** (**hoh**-mee-oh-**STAY**-sis) is the processes through which the body maintains a constant internal environment (**home/o** means constant, and **-stasis** means control).

■ **Hormones** are chemical messengers that are secreted by endocrine glands directly into the bloodstream (see Chapter 2). This enables them to reach cells and organs throughout the body.

■ Each hormone has specialized functions in regulating the activities of specific cells, organs, or both.

■ Blood or urine tests are used to measure hormone levels. These tests are discussed in Chapter 15.

# STRUCTURES OF THE ENDOCRINE SYSTEM

**Endocrine glands** (**EN**-doh-krin), which produce hormones, do not have ducts (**endo-** means within, and **-crine** means to secrete).

There are 13 major glands that make up the endocrine system (Figure 13.1):

■ One **pituitary gland** (divided into two lobes)

■ One **pineal gland**

■ One **thyroid gland**

■ Four **parathyroid glands**

■ One **thymus**

■ One **pancreas** (**pancreatic islets**)

■ Two **adrenal glands**

■ Two **gonads** (either a pair of ovaries in females or a pair of testicles in males)

# THE PITUITARY GLAND

The **pituitary gland** (pih-**TOO**-ih-**tair**-ee), or *hypophysis*, is a pea-sized gland that is divided into two parts, the anterior and the posterior lobes. These lobes hang from a stalk-like structure located below the hypothalamus in the brain (Figure 13.2). The hypothalamus is part of the nervous system that produces hormones that controls many body functions (see Chapter 10).

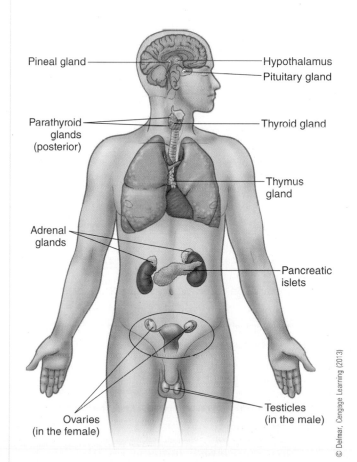

Pineal gland

Hypothalamus
Pituitary gland

Parathyroid glands (posterior)

Thyroid gland

Thymus gland

Adrenal glands

Pancreatic islets

Ovaries (in the female)

Testicles (in the male)

© Delmar, Cengage Learning (2013)

**FIGURE 13.1** Structures of the endocrine system.

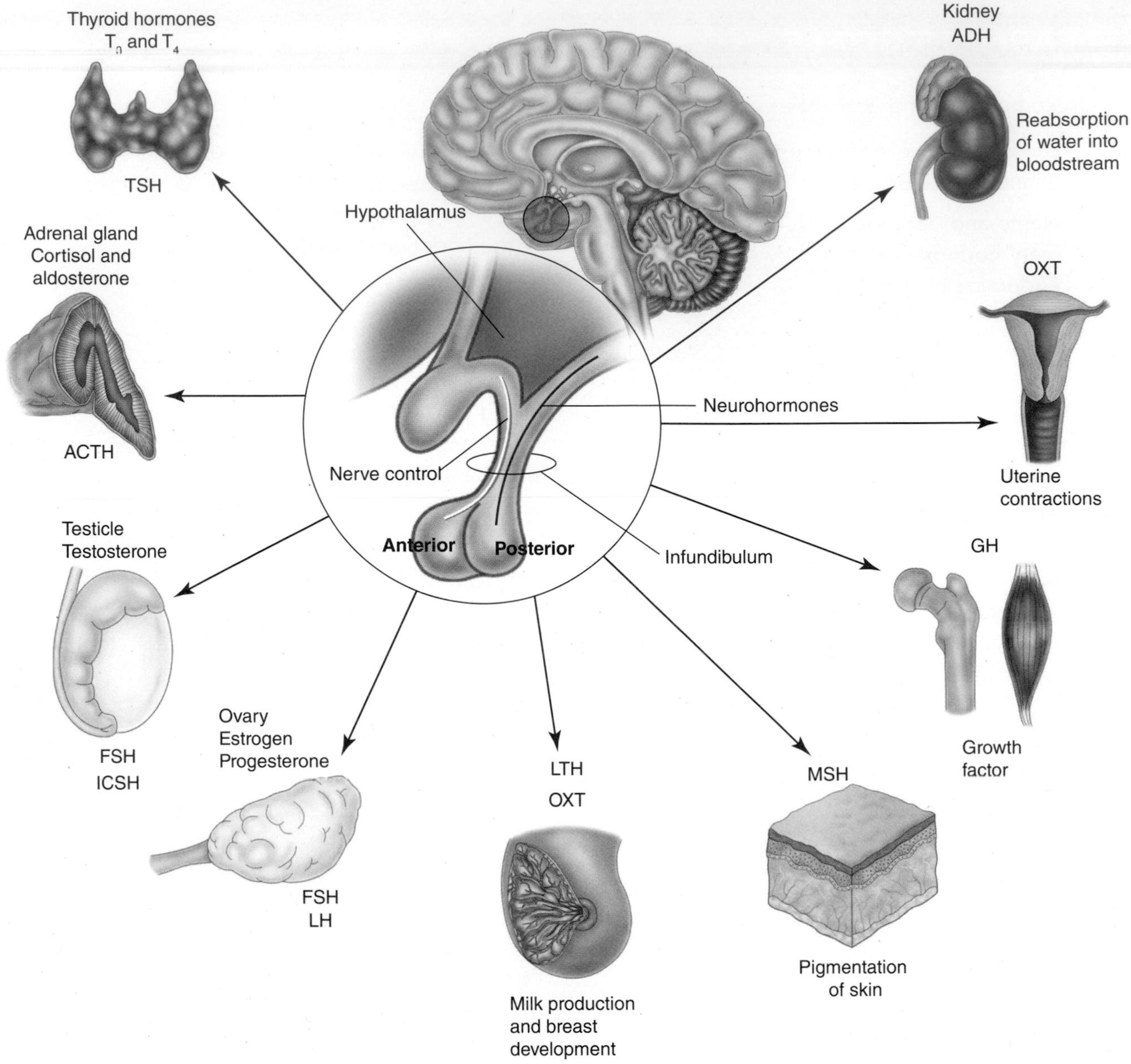

Thyroid hormones
T$_3$ and T$_4$
TSH

Adrenal gland
Cortisol and
aldosterone
ACTH

Testicle
Testosterone
FSH
ICSH

Ovary
Estrogen
Progesterone
FSH
LH

Hypothalamus

Nerve control

**Anterior** **Posterior**

Neurohormones

Infundibulum

LTH
OXT

Milk production
and breast
development

MSH

Pigmentation
of skin

Kidney
ADH

Reabsorption
of water into
bloodstream

OXT

Uterine
contractions

GH

Growth
factor

© Delmar, Cengage Learning (2013)

**FIGURE 13.2** The pituitary gland secretes hormones that control the activity of other endocrine glands. Hormones are often referred to by their abbreviations, all of which are explained below.

## Functions of the Pituitary Gland

The primary function of the pituitary gland is to secrete hormones that control the activity of other endocrine glands.

The pituitary gland acts in response to stimuli from neurohormones secreted by the hypothalamus. This creates a system of checks and balances to maintain an appropriate blood level of each hormone.

## Secretions of the Pituitary Gland: Anterior Lobe

■ The **adrenocorticotropic hormone** (ACTH) (ah-**DREE**-noh-**kor**-tih-coe-**TROP**-ik) stimulates the

growth and secretions of the adrenal cortex (**adren/o** means adrenal, **cortic/o** means cortex, **trop** means change, and **-ic** means pertaining to).

■ The **follicle-stimulating hormone** (FSH) stimulates the secretion of estrogen and the growth of ova (eggs) in the ovaries of the female. In the male, it stimulates the production of sperm in the testicles (testes).

■ The **growth hormone** (GII), also known as the *somatotropic hormone*, regulates the growth of bone, muscle, and other body tissues (**somat/o** means body, and **-tropic** means having an affinity for).

- The **interstitial cell-stimulating hormone** (ICSH) (**in**-ter-**STISH**-al) stimulates ovulation in the female. In the male, it stimulates the secretion of testosterone.

- The **lactogenic hormone** (LTH), also known as *prolactin*, stimulates and maintains the secretion of breast milk in the mother after childbirth (**lact/o** means milk, **gen** means producing, and **-ic** means pertaining to).

- The **luteinizing hormone** (LH) (**LOO**-tee-in-**eye**-zing) stimulates ovulation in the female. In the male, the luteinizing hormone stimulates the secretion of testosterone.

- The **melanocyte-stimulating hormone** (MSH) (mel-**LAN**-oh-sight) increases the production of melanin in melanocytes, thereby causing darkening of skin pigmentation (see Chapter 12). MSH production usually increases during pregnancy (see Chapter 14).

- The **thyroid-stimulating hormone** (TSH) stimulates the secretion of hormones by the thyroid gland.

## Secretions of the Pituitary Gland: Posterior Lobe

- The **antidiuretic hormone** (ADH) (**an**-tih-dye-you-**RET** ick), which is secreted by the hypothalamus and stored and released in the pituitary gland, helps control blood pressure by reducing the amount of water that is excreted through the kidneys (see Chapter 9). In contrast, a *diuretic* is administered to increase the amount of urine secretion.

- **Oxytocin** (OXT) (**ock**-see-**TOH**-sin) stimulates uterine contractions during childbirth (**oxy-** means swift, and **-tocin** means labor). After childbirth, oxytocin controls postnatal hemorrhage and stimulates the flow of milk from the mammary glands. *Pitocin* is a synthetic form of oxytocin that is administered to induce or speed up labor.

## THE PINEAL GLAND

The **pineal gland** (**PIN**-ee-al) is a very small endocrine gland, also known as the *pineal body*. It is located in the central portion of the brain.

### Functions and Secretions of the Pineal Gland

The secretions of the pineal gland influence the sleep-wakefulness cycle (Figure 13.3). These secretions include:

- The hormone **melatonin** (**mel**-ah-**TOH**-nin) influences the sleep-wakefulness portions of the circadian cycle. The term *circadian cycle* refers to the biological functions that occur within a 24-hour period.

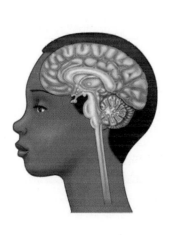

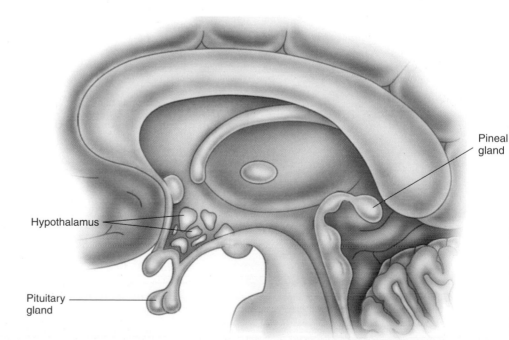

Pineal gland

Hypothalamus

Pituitary gland

**FIGURE 13.3** The pineal gland is located within the brain.

# THE THYROID GLAND

The butterfly-shaped **thyroid gland** lies on either side of the larynx, just below the thyroid cartilage (Figure 13.4).

## Functions and Secretions of the Thyroid Gland

One of the primary functions of the thyroid gland is to regulate the body's metabolism. The term *metabolism* describes all of the processes involved in the body's use of nutrients, including the rate at which they are used. Thyroid secretions also influence growth and the functioning of the nervous system.

- The two primary thyroid hormones regulate the rate of metabolism and affect the growth and rate of function of many other body systems. They are:
  - **thyroxine** ($T_4$) (thigh-**ROCK**-seen)
  - **triiodothyronine** ($T_3$) (try-**eye**-oh-doh-**THIGH**-roh-neen)
- The rate of secretion of these two hormones is controlled by the *thyroid-stimulating hormone* produced by the anterior lobe of the pituitary gland.
- **Calcitonin** (**kal**-sih-**TOH**-nin), which is produced by the thyroid gland, is a hormone that works with the parathyroid hormone to decrease calcium levels in the blood and tissues by moving calcium into storage in the bones and teeth.

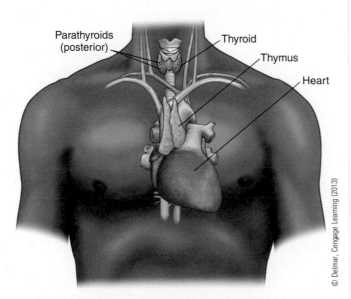

Parathyroids (posterior)
Thyroid
Thymus
Heart

© Delmar, Cengage Learning (2013)

**FIGURE 13.4** The thyroid, parathyroid, and thymus glands.

# THE PARATHYROID GLANDS

The four **parathyroid glands**, each of which is about the size of a grain of rice, are embedded in the posterior surface of the thyroid gland (Figure 13.4).

## Functions and Secretions of the Parathyroid Glands

The primary function of the parathyroid glands is to regulate calcium levels throughout the body. These calcium levels are important to the smooth functioning of the muscular and nervous systems. The secretions of the parathyroid glands include:

- The **parathyroid hormone** (PTH), which works with the hormone *calcitonin* that is secreted by the thyroid gland. Together, they regulate the calcium levels in the blood and tissues.
- Higher-than-normal levels of parathyroid hormone can increase calcium levels in the blood by mobilizing the release of calcium stored in bones and teeth.

# THE THYMUS

The **thymus** (**THIGH**-mus) is located near the midline in the anterior portion of the thoracic cavity. It is posterior to (behind) the sternum and slightly superior to (above) the heart (Figure 13.4).

## Functions and Secretions of the Thymus

The thymus functions as part of the endocrine system by secreting a hormone that functions as part of the immune system. The secretions of the thymus include:

- **Thymosin** (**THIGH**-moh-sin), which plays an important part in the immune system by stimulating the maturation of lymphocytes into T cells (see Chapter 6).

# THE PANCREAS (PANCREATIC ISLETS)

The **pancreas** (**PAN**-kree-as) is a feather-shaped organ located posterior to the stomach that functions as part of both the digestive and the endocrine systems (Figure 13.1).

The **pancreatic islets** (**pan**-kree-**AT**-ick **EYE**-lets) are those parts of the pancreas that have endocrine functions. An *islet* is a small isolated mass, or island, of one type of tissue within a larger mass of a different type.

## Functions and Secretions of the Pancreatic Islets

The endocrine functions of these islets are the control of blood sugar levels and glucose metabolism throughout the body. The secretions of the pancreatic islets include:

- **Glucose** (**GLOO**-kohs), also known as *blood sugar*, which is the basic form of energy used by the body.

- **Glucagon** (**GCG**) (**GLOO**-kah-gon) is the hormone secreted by the *alpha cells* of the pancreatic islets in response to low levels of glucose in the bloodstream. Glucagon increases the glucose level by stimulating the liver to convert glycogen into glucose for release into the bloodstream.

- **Insulin** (**IN**-suh-lin) is the hormone secreted by the *beta cells* of the pancreatic islets in response to high levels of glucose in the bloodstream. Insulin functions in two ways:

  1. When energy is needed, insulin allows glucose to enter the cells to be used as this energy.

  2. When additional glucose is *not* needed, insulin stimulates the liver to convert glucose into glycogen for storage.

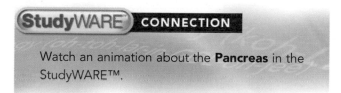

**StudyWARE CONNECTION**

Watch an animation about the **Pancreas** in the StudyWARE™.

## THE ADRENAL GLANDS

The **adrenal glands,** which are also known as the *suprarenals*, are so named because they are located with one on top of each kidney. Each of these glands consists of an outer portion, known as the *adrenal cortex*, and the middle portion, which is the *adrenal medulla*. Each of these parts has a specialized role (Figure 13.5).

## Functions of the Adrenal Glands

One of the primary functions of the adrenal glands is to control electrolyte levels within the body.

- **Electrolytes** (ee-**LECK**-troh-lytes) are mineral substances, such as sodium and potassium, that are normally found in the blood.

- Other important functions of the adrenal glands include helping regulate metabolism and interacting with the sympathetic nervous system in response to stress (see Chapter 10).

## Secretions of the Adrenal Cortex

- **Androgens** are sex hormones secreted by the gonads, the adrenal cortex, and fat cells (see later section on the gonads).

- **Corticosteroids** (**kor**-tih-koh-**STEHR**-oidz) are the steroid hormones produced by the adrenal cortex. The same term describes synthetically produced equivalents that are administered as medications.

  - **Aldosterone** (**ALD**) (al-**DOSS**-ter-ohn) is a corticosteroid that regulates the salt and water levels in the body by increasing sodium reabsorption and potassium excretion by the kidneys. *Reabsorption* means returning a substance to the bloodstream.

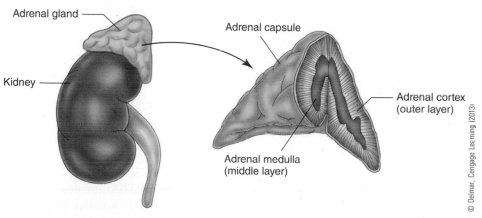

© Delmar, Cengage Learning (2013)

**FIGURE 13.5** One adrenal gland is located on top of each kidney. Each adrenal gland consists of the adrenal cortex and adrenal medulla.

- **Cortisol** (**KOR**-tih-sol), also known as *hydrocortisone*, is a corticosteroid that has an anti-inflammatory action. It also regulates the metabolism of carbohydrates, fats, and proteins in the body.

## Secretions of the Adrenal Medulla

- **Epinephrine** (Epi, EPI) (**ep**-ih-**NEF**-rin), also known as *adrenaline*, stimulates the sympathetic nervous system in response to physical injury or to mental stress such as fear. It makes the heart beat faster and can raise blood pressure. It also helps the liver release glucose (sugar) and limits the release of insulin.

- **Norepinephrine** (**nor**-ep-ih-**NEF**-rin) is both a hormone and a neurohormone. It is released as a hormone by the adrenal medulla and as a neurohormone by the sympathetic nervous system. It plays an important role in the "fight-or-flight response" by raising blood pressure, strengthening the heartbeat, and stimulating muscle contractions.

## ◼ THE GONADS

The **gonads** (**GOH**-nadz) are gamete-producing glands. These are ovaries in females and testicles in males.

## Functions of the Gonads

The gonads secrete the hormones that are responsible for the development and maintenance of the secondary sex characteristics that develop during puberty. *Secondary sex characteristics* refers to features that distinguish the two sexes, but are not directly related to reproduction. The additional functions of the gonads are discussed in Chapter 14.

- **Puberty** (**PYU**-ber-tee) is the process of physical changes by which a child's body becomes an adult body that is capable of reproducing (Figure 13.6). It is marked by maturing of the genital organs, development of secondary sex characteristics, and by the first occurrence of menstruation in the female. In the United States the average age is 12 for girls and 11 for boys.

- *Precocious puberty* is the early onset of the changes of puberty, usually before age 8 in girls and age 9 in boys. *Precocious* means exceptionally early in development or in occurrence.

**PUBERTY**

MALE

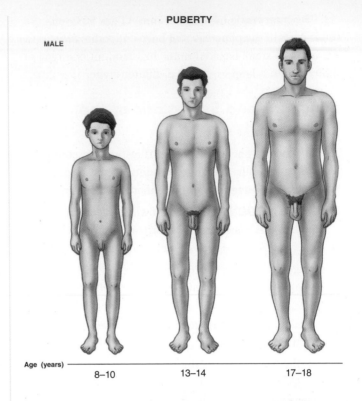

Age (years) ——————————————
8–10        13–14        17–18

FEMALE

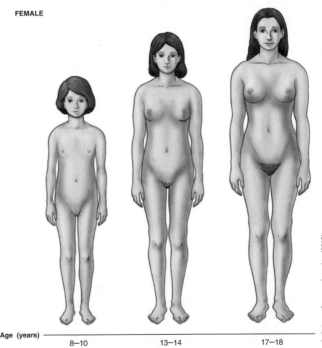

Age (years) ——————————————
8–10        13–14        17–18

© Delmar, Cengage Learning (2013)

**FIGURE 13.6** Puberty is the process through which secondary sex characteristics are gradually developed.

## Secretions of the Gonads

- **Estrogen** (E) (**ES**-troh-jen) is a hormone secreted by the ovaries that is important in the development and maintenance of the female secondary sex characteristics and in regulation of the menstrual cycle.

- **Progesterone** (proh-**JES**-ter-ohn) is the hormone released during the second half of the menstrual cycle by the corpus luteum in the ovary. Its function is to complete the preparation of the uterus for possible pregnancy (see Chapter 14).

- A **gamete** (**GAM**-eet) is a reproductive cell. These are *sperm* in the male and *ova* (*eggs*) in the female.

- **Gonadotropin** (**gon**-ah-doh-**TROH**-pin) is any hormone that stimulates the gonads (**gonad/o** means gonad, and **-tropin** means to simulate).

- **Androgens** (**AN**-droh-jenz) are sex hormones, primarily testosterone, secreted by the gonads, the adrenal cortex, and fat cells. Androgens promote the development and maintenance of the male sex characteristics, however, they are present in both men and women.

- **Testosterone** (tes-**TOS**-teh-rohn) is a steroid hormone secreted by the testicles and the adrenal cortex to stimulate the development of male secondary sex characteristics.

**StudyWARE CONNECTION**

Watch the **Endocrine System** animation in the StudyWARE™.

## Specialized Types of Hormones

Several specialized types of hormones do not fit the previous hormone definition, either because of their chemical structure or because they are not secreted by endocrine glands directly into the bloodstream.

### Steroids

**Steroids** (**STEHR**-oidz) are a large family of hormone-like substances that share the same fat-soluble chemical structure. Examples of steroids include cholesterol, testosterone, and some anti-inflammatory drugs.

- Steroids are secreted by endocrine glands or artificially produced as medications to relieve swelling and inflammation in conditions such as asthma.

- **Anabolic steroids** (**an**-ah-**BOL**-ick **STEHR**-oidz) are man-made substances that are chemically related to male sex hormones. They are used in the treatment of hormone problems in men and to help the body replace muscle mass lost due to disease. Athletes sometime use these steroids illegally to build muscle mass, a dangerous practice that can lead to lasting damage to the body.

### Hormones Secreted by Fat Cells

Adipose tissue is not commonly thought of as an endocrine gland; however, research has shown that fat cells do secrete at least one and possibly more hormones that play important roles in the balance and health of the body.

- **Leptin** (**LEP**-tin) is a protein hormone secreted by fat cells that is involved in the regulation of appetite.

- Leptin leaves the fat cells and travels in the bloodstream to the brain, where it acts on the hypothalamus to suppress appetite and burn fat stored in adipose tissue.

### Neurohormones

**Neurohormones** (**new**-roh-**HOR**-mohnz) are produced and released by neurons in the brain, rather than by the endocrine glands, and delivered to organs and tissues through the bloodstream. One example is neurohormones secreted by the hypothalamus that control the secretions of the pituitary gland (Figure 13.2).

## MEDICAL SPECIALTIES RELATED TO THE ENDOCRINE SYSTEM

- An **endocrinologist** (**en** doh krih **NOL** oh jist) is a physician who specializes in diagnosing and treating diseases and malfunctions of the endocrine glands (**endocrin** means to secrete within, and **-ologist** means specialist).

- A **certified diabetes educator** (CDE) is a health care professional qualified to teach people with diabetes how to manage their disease.

## PATHOLOGY OF THE ENDOCRINE SYSTEM

### The Pituitary Gland

- **Acromegaly** (**ack**-roh-**MEG**-ah-lee) is a rare chronic disease characterized by abnormal enlargement of the extremities (hands and feet) caused by the excessive secretion of growth hormone after puberty (**acr/o** means extremities, and **-megaly** means enlargement). Contrast with *gigantism*.

- **Gigantism** (jigh-**GAN**-tiz-em) is abnormal growth of the entire body that is caused by excessive secretion of growth hormone *before* puberty. Contrast with *acromegaly*.

- **Hyperpituitarism** (**high**-per-pih-**TOO**-ih-tah-rizm) is the excess secretion of growth hormone that causes acromegaly and gigantism (**hyper-** means excessive, **pituitar** means pituitary, and **-ism** means condition).

- **Short stature**, formerly known as *dwarfism*, is sometimes caused by deficient secretion of growth hormone (see Chapter 3).

- A **pituitary adenoma** (pih-**TOO**-ih-**tair**-ee ad-eh-**NOH**-mah) is also known as a *pituitary tumor*. There are two types of these slow-growing benign tumors of the pituitary gland.
  - *Functioning pituitary tumors* often produce hormones in large and unregulated amounts.
  - *Nonfunctioning pituitary tumors* do not produce any significant amounts of these hormones.

- **Galactorrhea** is a condition in which an excess of prolactin causes the breasts to produce milk spontaneously (see Chapter 14).

- A **prolactinoma** (proh-**lack**-tih-**NOH**-mah) is a benign tumor of the pituitary gland (**pro-** means on behalf of, **lactin** means milk, and **-oma** means tumor). This type of tumor, which causes the pituitary gland to produce too much of the lactogenic hormone known as prolactin, can cause infertility in women and erectile dysfunction in men, and can impair vision.

## Antidiuretic Hormone Conditions

- **Diabetes insipidus** (DI) (**dye**-ah-**BEE**-teez in-**SIP**-ih-dus), which is not related to *diabetes mellitus*, is caused by an insufficient production of the antidiuretic hormone ADH or by the inability of the kidneys to respond appropriately to this hormone.
  - When there is an insufficient quantity of ADH, which is secreted by the hypothalamus and stored and released in the pituitary gland, too much fluid is excreted by the kidneys. This causes *polydipsia* (excessive thirst) and *polyuria* (excessive urination). If this problem is not controlled, it can cause severe dehydration.
  - *Insipidus* comes from a Latin word meaning without taste, referring to the relatively low sodium (salt) content of the urine in patients with diabetes insipidus.

- **Syndrome of inappropriate antidiuretic hormone** (SIADH) is caused by the overproduction of the antidiuretic hormone ADH. This is often as a result of cancer or its treatment. High amounts of ADH keep the kidneys from excreting water, resulting in bloating and water retention that can dilute the blood, causing electrolyte imbalances, particularly hyponatremia.

## Pathology of the Pineal Gland

- A **pinealoma** (pin-ee-ah-**LOH**-mah) is a tumor of the pineal gland that can disrupt the production of melatonin (**pineal** means pineal gland, and **-oma** means tumor). This tumor can also cause insomnia by disrupting the circadian cycle.

## The Thyroid Gland

**Thyroid carcinoma**, or cancer, is the most common cancer of the endocrine system. This cancer affects more women than men and usually occurs between the ages of 25 and 65 years.

### Insufficient Thyroid Secretion

- **Hashimoto's disease** (hah-shee-**MOH**-tohz), also known as *chronic lymphocytic thyroiditis*, is an autoimmune disease in which the body's own antibodies attack and destroy the cells of the thyroid gland. This inflammation often leads to hypothyroidism.

- **Hypothyroidism** (**high**-poh-**THIGH**-roid-izm), also known as an *underactive thyroid*, is caused by a deficiency of thyroid secretion (**hypo-** means deficient, **thyroid** means thyroid, and **-ism** means condition). Symptoms include fatigue, depression, sensitivity to cold, and a decreased metabolic rate.

- **Cretinism** (**CREE**-tin-izm) is a congenital form of hypothyroidism. If treatment is not started soon after birth, cretinism causes arrested physical and mental development.

- **Myxedema** (**mick**-seh-**DEE**-mah), which is also known as *adult hypothyroidism*, is caused by an extreme deficiency of thyroid secretion. Symptoms include swelling, particularly around the eyes and cheeks, fatigue, and a subnormal temperature.

### Excessive Thyroid Secretion

- *Thyroid nodules* are lumps in the thyroid that can grow large enough to cause a goiter (see Graves' disease, below). Most nodules are benign; however some are malignant or produce too much thyroxine.

- A **thyroid storm**, also known as a *thyrotoxic crisis*, is a relatively rare, life-threatening condition caused by exaggerated hyperthyroidism. Patients experiencing a thyroid storm may complain of fever, chest pain, palpitations, shortness of breath, tremors, increased sweating, disorientation, and fatigue.

- **Hyperthyroidism** (**high**-per-**THIGH**-roid-izm), also known as *thyrotoxicosis*, is the overproduction of thyroid hormones (**hyper-** means excessive, **thyroid** means thyroid, and **-ism** means condition), which causes an imbalance of the metabolism. This causes symptoms including an increased metabolic rate, sweating, nervousness, and weight loss. The most common cause of hyperthyroidism is Graves' disease.

### Graves' Disease

**Graves' disease** (**GRAYVZ**) is a disorder of unknown cause in which the immune system attacks the thyroid gland and stimulates it to make excessive amounts of thyroid hormone (Figure 13.7). This results in hyperthyroidism and can also cause goiter, exophthalmos, or both. Note: A simple way to remember the difference between Hashimoto's disease (**hypo**thyroidism) and Graves' disease (**hyper**thyroidism) is that the Hashimoto's has an *o* in it and Graves' has an *e* in it.

- **Goiter** (**GOI**-ter), also known as *thyromegaly*, is an abnormal nonmalignant enlargement of the thyroid gland (**thyr/o** means thyroid, and **-megaly** means abnormal enlargement). This enlargement produces a swelling in the front of the neck. A goiter usually occurs when the thyroid gland is not able to produce enough thyroid hormone to meet the body's needs, either due to Graves' disease, other medical conditions, or an iodine deficiency.

- **Exophthalmos** (**eck**-sof-**THAL**-mos) is an abnormal protrusion of the eyeball out of the orbit (**ex-** means out, **ophthalm/o** means eye and **-s** is a noun ending).

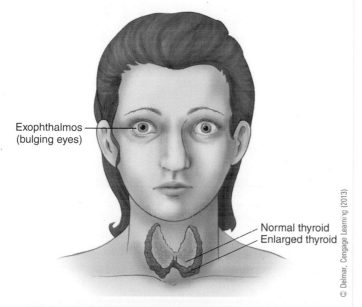

Exophthalmos (bulging eyes)

Normal thyroid
Enlarged thyroid

© Delmar, Cengage Learning (2013)

**FIGURE 13.7** Graves' disease can cause exophthalmos.

## The Parathyroid Glands

- **Hyperparathyroidism** (**high**-per-**par**-ah-**THIGH**-roid-izm), which is the overproduction of the parathyroid hormone, causes the condition known as hypercalcemia (**hyper-** means excessive, **parathyroid** means parathyroid, and **-ism** means condition). Hyperparathyroidism can result from a disorder of the parathyroid gland or from a disorder elsewhere in the body, such as kidney failure. Hyperparathyroidism is the opposite of *hypoparathyroidism*.

- **Hypercalcemia** (**high**-per-kal-**SEE**-mee-ah) is characterized by abnormally *high* concentrations of calcium circulating in the blood instead of being stored in the bones and teeth (**hyper-** means excessive, **calc** means calcium, and **-emia** means blood condition). This can lead to weakened bones and the formation of kidney stones. Hypercalcemia is the opposite of *hypocalcemia*.

- **Hypoparathyroidism** (**high**-poh-**par**-ah-**THIGH**-roid-izm) is caused by an insufficient or absent secretion of the parathyroid hormone (**hypo-** means deficient, **parathyroid** means parathyroid, and **-ism** means condition). This condition causes hypocalcemia, and in severe cases, it leads to tetany. *Tetany* is the condition of periodic, painful muscle spasms and tremors. Hypoparathyroidism is the opposite of *hyperparathyroidism*.

- **Hypocalcemia** (**high**-poh-kal-**SEE**-mee-ah) is characterized by abnormally *low* levels of calcium in the blood (**hypo-** means deficient, **calc** means calcium, and **-emia** means blood condition). Hypocalcemia is the opposite of *hypercalcemia*.

## The Thymus

- **Thymitis** (thigh-**MY**-tis) is an inflammation of the thymus gland (**thym** means thymus, and **-itis** means inflammation).

## The Pancreas

- An **insulinoma** (**in**-suh-lin-**OH**-mah) is a benign tumor of the pancreas that causes hypoglycemia by secreting additional insulin (**insulin** means insulin, and **-oma** means tumor).

- **Pancreatitis** (**pan**-kree-ah-**TYE**-tis) is an inflammation of the pancreas (**pancreat** means pancreas, and **-itis** means inflammation). A leading cause of pancreatitis is long-term alcohol abuse.

## Abnormal Blood Sugar Levels

■ **Hyperglycemia** (**high**-per-glye-**SEE**-mee-ah) is an abnormally high concentration of glucose in the blood (**hyper-** means excessive, **glyc** means sugar, and **-emia** means blood condition). Hyperglycemia is seen primarily in patients with diabetes mellitus. The symptoms include polydipsia, polyphagia, and polyuria. Hyperglycemia is the opposite of hypoglycemia.

■ **Polydipsia** (**pol**-ee-**DIP**-see-ah) is excessive thirst (**poly-** means many, and **-dipsia** means thirst).

■ **Polyphagia** (**pol**-ee-**FAY**-jee-ah) is excessive hunger (**poly-** means many, and **-phagia** means eating).

■ **Polyuria** (**pol**-ee-**YOU**-ree-ah) is excessive urination (**poly-** means many, and **-uria** means urination).

■ **Hyperinsulinism** (**high**-per-**IN**-suh-lin-izm) is the condition of excessive secretion of insulin in the bloodstream (**hyper-** means excessive, **insulin** means insulin, and **-ism** means condition). Hyperinsulinism can cause *hypoglycemia*.

■ **Hypoglycemia** (**high**-poh-glye-**SEE**-mee-ah) is an abnormally low concentration of glucose (sugar) in the blood (**hypo-** means deficient, **glyc** means sugar, and **-emia** means blood condition). Symptoms include nervousness and shakiness, confusion, perspiration, or feeling anxious or weak. Hypoglycemia is the opposite of *hyperglycemia*.

## Diabetes Mellitus

**Diabetes mellitus** (DM) (**dye**-ah-**BEE**-teez **MEL**-ih-tus) is a group of metabolic disorders characterized by hyperglycemia resulting from defects in insulin secretion, insulin action, or both. Diabetes mellitus is not related to diabetes insipidus.

■ This condition is described as type 1, type 2, and latent autoimmune diabetes in adults (type 1.5).

■ In the past, when a child developed diabetes, this condition was referred to as *juvenile diabetes*; however, the condition in children is now described as being either type 1 or type 2.

■ Many patients present with symptoms of both types of diabetes, and their treatment must be modified accordingly. The treatment goals for all types of diabetes are to most effectively control the blood sugar levels and to prevent complications.

■ *Metabolic syndrome* is a combination of medical conditions, including increased blood pressure, elevated insulin levels, excess body fat around the waist, or abnormal cholesterol levels. This syndrome increases the patient's risk of heart disease, stroke, and diabetes.

## Type 1 Diabetes

**Type 1 diabetes** is an autoimmune insulin deficiency disorder caused by the destruction of pancreatic islet beta cells. *Insulin deficiency* means that the pancreatic beta cells do not secrete enough insulin. (See Chapter 6 for more information about autoimmune disorders.)

■ Symptoms of type 1 diabetes include polydipsia, polyphagia, polyuria, weight loss, blurred vision, extreme fatigue, and slow healing.

■ Type 1 diabetes is treated with diet and exercise as well as carefully regulated insulin replacement therapy administered by injection or pump (Figure 13.8).

■ The onset of type 1 diabetes is often triggered by a viral infection.

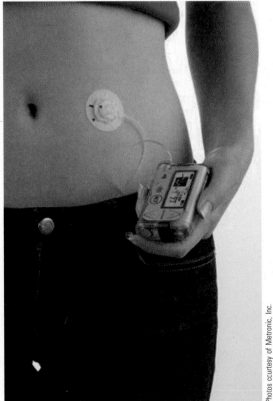

Photos ccurtesy of Metronic, Inc.

**FIGURE 13.8** An insulin pump can be worn on the patient's belt, administering controlled insulin replacement therapy.

## Type 2 Diabetes

**Type 2 diabetes** is an insulin resistance disorder. *Insulin resistance* means that insulin is being produced, but the body does not use it effectively. In an attempt to compensate for this lack of response, the body secretes more insulin. With the rise of childhood obesity, type 2 diabetes is increasingly common in children and young adults. Obese adults are also at high risk for this condition.

■ **Prediabetes** is a condition in which the blood sugar level is higher than normal, but not high enough to be classified as type 2 diabetes. However, this condition indicates an increased risk of developing type 2 diabetes, heart disease, and stroke.

■ Type 2 diabetics can have no symptoms for years. When symptoms do occur, they include those of type 1 diabetes plus recurring infections, irritability, and a tingling sensation in the hands or feet.

■ Type 2 diabetes is usually treated with diet, exercise, and oral medications, which include:

■ *Oral hypoglycemics*, which lower blood sugar by causing the pancreas to release more insulin or increasing the body's sensitivity to insulin.

■ *Glucophage* (*metformin hydrochloride*) and similar medications work within the cells to combat insulin resistance and to help insulin let blood sugar into the cells.

### Latent Autoimmune Diabetes in Adults

**Latent autoimmune diabetes in adults** (LADA), also known as *Type 1.5 diabetes*, is a condition in which type 1 diabetes develops in adults. It shares many of the characteristics of type 2 diabetes; however, autoimmune antibodies are present. *Latent* means present, but not visible.

■ LADA usually occurs in adults with a normal weight and family history of type 1 diabetes.

■ It is estimated that at least 10% of adults with diabetes have LADA. It is treated with diet, exercise, oral medications, and insulin.

### Gestational Diabetes Mellitus

**Gestational diabetes mellitus** (jes-**TAY**-shun-al **dye**-ah-**BEE**-teez) is a form of diabetes mellitus that occurs during some pregnancies. This condition usually disappears after delivery; however, many of these women have an increased risk to develop type 2 diabetes in later life.

## Diabetic Emergencies

Diabetic emergencies are due to either too much or too little blood sugar. Treatment depends on accurately diagnosing the cause of the emergency (Figure 13.9 A & B).

■ A **diabetic coma** is caused by very high blood sugar (hyperglycemia). Also known as *diabetic ketoacidosis*, this condition is treated by the prompt administration of insulin.

■ **Insulin shock** is caused by very low blood sugar (hypoglycemia). *Oral glucose*, which is a sugary substance that can quickly be absorbed into the bloodstream, is consumed to rapidly raise the blood sugar level.

## Diabetic Complications

Most diabetic complications result from the damage to capillaries and other blood vessels due to long-term exposure to excessive blood sugar.

■ **Diabetic retinopathy** (**ret**-ih-**NOP**-ah-thee) occurs when diabetes damages the tiny blood vessels in the retina. This causes blood to leak into the posterior segment of the eyeball and produce the damage of the loss of vision (see Chapter 11).

■ *Heart disease* occurs because excess blood sugar makes the walls of the blood vessels sticky and rigid. This encourages hypertension and atherosclerosis (see Chapter 5).

■ *Kidney disease* can lead to renal failure because damage to the blood vessels reduces blood flow through the kidneys (see Chapter 9).

■ *Peripheral neuropathy* is damage to the nerves affecting the hands and feet (see Chapter 10).

■ Poorly controlled blood sugar can also slow wound healing and increase the likelihood of wound infections. This can make minor injuries worse and lead to ulcers and gangrene, requiring amputation, particularly in the feet and legs.

## The Adrenal Glands

■ **Addison's disease** (**AD**-ih-sonz) occurs when the adrenal glands do not produce enough of the hormones cortisol or aldosterone. This condition is characterized by chronic, worsening fatigue and muscle weakness, loss of appetite, low blood pressure, and weight loss.

■ **Adrenalitis** (ah-**dree**-nal-**EYE**-tis) is inflammation of the adrenal glands (**adrenal** means adrenal glands, and **-itis** means inflammation).

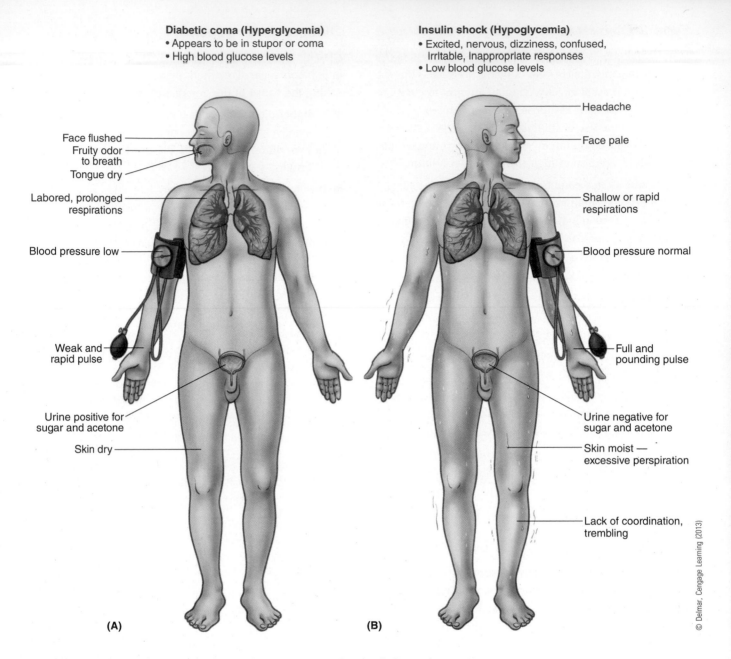

**Diabetic coma (Hyperglycemia)**
- Appears to be in stupor or coma
- High blood glucose levels

**Insulin shock (Hypoglycemia)**
- Excited, nervous, dizziness, confused, Irritable, Inappropriate responses
- Low blood glucose levels

Headache

Face flushed
Fruity odor to breath
Tongue dry

Face pale

Labored, prolonged respirations

Shallow or rapid respirations

Blood pressure low

Blood pressure normal

Weak and rapid pulse

Full and pounding pulse

Urine positive for sugar and acetone

Urine negative for sugar and acetone

Skin dry

Skin moist — excessive perspiration

Lack of coordination, trembling

(A)

(B)

© Delmar, Cengage Learning (2013)

**FIGURE 13.9** (A) Diabetic coma (hyperglycemia); (B) Insulin shock (hypoglycemia).

- **Aldosteronism** (al-**DOSS**-teh-roh-**niz**-em) is an abnormality of the electrolyte balance that is caused by the excessive secretion of aldosterone.

- **Conn's syndrome** (**KON**) is a disorder of the adrenal glands that is caused by the excessive production of aldosterone. This disease, which is a form of primary aldosteronism, can cause weakness, cramps, and convulsions.

- A **pheochromocytoma** (fee-oh-**kroh**-moh-sigh-**TOH**-mah) is a rare, benign tumor of the adrenal gland that causes too much release of epinephrine and norepinephrine, which are the hormones that regulate heart

rate and blood pressure (**phe/o** means dusky, **chrom/o** means color, **cyt** means cell, and **-oma** means tumor).

## Cushing's Syndrome

**Cushing's syndrome** (**KUSH**-ingz **SIN**-drohm), also known as *hypercortisolism*, is caused by prolonged exposure to high levels of cortisol. Cortisol has an anti-inflammatory action, and it regulates the metabolism of carbohydrates, fats, and proteins in the body. The symptoms include a rounded red "moon" face (Figure 13.10).

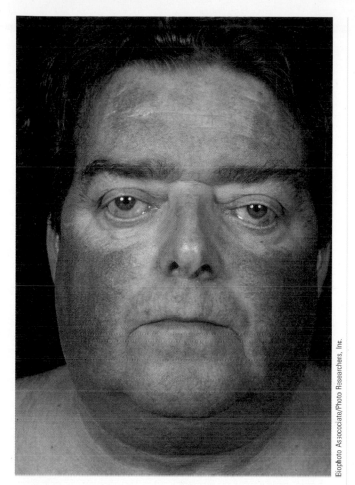

**FIGURE 13.10** Cushing's syndrome causes a characteristic rounded, red "moon" face.

This condition can be caused by overproduction of cortisol by the body or by prolonged use of corticosteroids. These steroid hormone medications are used to treat inflammatory diseases such as asthma, lupus, and rheumatoid arthritis and to keep the body from rejecting transplanted organs or tissue.

## The Gonads

- **Hypergonadism** (**high**-per-**GOH**-nad-izm) is the condition of excessive secretion of hormones by the sex glands (**hyper-** means excessive, **gonad** means sex gland, and **-ism** means condition). Compare with *hypogonadism*.

- **Hypogonadism** (**high**-poh-**GOH**-nad-izm) is the condition of deficient secretion of hormones by the sex glands (**hypo-** means deficient, **gonad** means sex gland, and **-ism** means condition). Compare with *hypergonadism*.

- **Gynecomastia** (**guy**-neh-koh-**MAS**-tee-ah) is the condition of excessive mammary development in the male (**gynec/o** means female, **mast** means breast, and **-ia** means abnormal condition). This is caused by a decrease in testosterone.

## DIAGNOSTIC PROCEDURES RELATED TO THE ENDOCRINE SYSTEM

### The Thyroid Gland

- A **radioactive iodine uptake test** (RAIU) uses radioactive iodine administered orally to measure thyroid function. The amount of radioactivity in the thyroid is measured 6 to 24 hours later using a handheld instrument called a gamma probe.

- A **thyroid-stimulating hormone assay** is a diagnostic test to measure the circulating blood level of thyroid-stimulating hormone. This test is used to detect abnormal thyroid activity resulting from excessive pituitary stimulation.

- A **thyroid scan**, which measures thyroid function, is a form of nuclear medicine that is discussed in Chapter 15.

### Diabetes Mellitus

- A **fasting blood sugar test**, also known as a *fasting plasma glucose (FPG) test*, measures the glucose (blood sugar) levels after the patient has not eaten for 8 to 12 hours. This test is used to screen for diabetes. It is also used to monitor treatment of this condition.

- An **oral glucose tolerance test** is performed to confirm a diagnosis of diabetes mellitus and to aid in diagnosing hypoglycemia.

- **Home blood glucose monitoring** measures the current blood sugar level. This test, which requires a drop of blood, is performed by the patient.

- **Hemoglobin A1c testing**, also known as *HbA1c*, and pronounced as "*H-B A-one-C*," is a blood test that measures the average blood glucose level over the previous 3 to 4 months.

- The **fructosamine test** (**fruck-TOHS**-ah-meen) measures average glucose levels over the previous 3 weeks. The fructosamine test is able to detect changes more rapidly than the HbA1c test.

## TREATMENT PROCEDURES RELATED TO THE ENDOCRINE SYSTEM

### The Pituitary Gland

- The **human growth hormone** (HGH) is a synthetic version of the growth hormone that is administered to stimulate growth when the natural supply of growth hormone is insufficient for normal development.

■ A **hypophysectomy** (high-**pof**-ih-**SECK**-toh-mee) is the removal of abnormal glandular tissue (**hypophys** refers to the pituitary gland, and **-ectomy** means removal). This surgery is performed through the nasal passages.

## The Pineal Gland

■ A **pinealectomy** (pin-ee-al-**ECK**-toh-mee) is the surgical removal of the pineal gland (**pineal** means pineal gland, and **-ectomy** means surgical removal).

## The Thyroid Gland

■ An **antithyroid drug** is a medication administered to slow the ability of the thyroid gland to produce thyroid hormones.

■ **Radioactive iodine treatment** (RAI) is the oral administration of radioactive iodine to destroy thyroid cells. This procedure, which disables at least part of the thyroid gland, is used to treat thyroid cancer and chronic hyperthyroid disorders such as Graves' disease.

■ A **lobectomy** (loh-**BECK**-toh-mee) is the surgical removal of one lobe of the thyroid gland. This term is also used to describe the removal of a lobe of the liver, brain, or lung.

■ **Synthetic thyroid hormones** are administered to replace lost thyroid function.

## The Parathyroid Glands

■ A **parathyroidectomy** (**par**-ah-**thigh**-roi-**DECK**-toh-mee), which is the surgical removal of one or more of the parathyroid glands, is performed to control hyperparathyroidism (**parathyroid** means parathyroid glands and **-ectomy** means surgical removal).

## The Thymus

■ A **thymectomy** (thigh-**MECK**-toh-mee) is the surgical removal of the thymus gland (**thym** means thymus, and **-ectomy** means surgical removal).

## The Pancreas

■ A **pancreatectomy** (pan-kree-ah-**TECK**-toh-mee) is the surgical removal of all or part of the pancreas (**pancreat** means pancreas, and **-ectomy** means surgical removal). A *total pancreatectomy* is performed to treat pancreatic cancer. This procedure also involves removing the spleen, gallbladder, common bile duct, and portions of the small intestine and stomach.

## The Adrenal Glands

■ A **laparoscopic adrenalectomy** (ah-**dree**-nal-**ECK**-toh-mee) is a minimally invasive surgical procedure to remove one or both adrenal glands (**adrenal** means adrenal gland, and **-ectomy** means surgical removal).

■ **Cortisone** (**KOR**-tih-sohn), also known as *hydrocortisone*, is the synthetic equivalent of corticosteroids produced by the body. Cortisone is administered to suppress inflammation and as an immunosuppressant (see Chapter 6).

■ A synthetic version of the hormone epinephrine is used as a vasoconstrictor to cause the blood vessels to contract. It is used to treat conditions such as allergic reactions, shock, and mild asthma. An *epinephrine autoinjector*, also known as an Epi pen, is a device used to inject a measured dose of epinephrine.

## ◼ ABBREVIATIONS RELATED TO THE ENDOCRINE SYSTEM

Table 13.1 presents an overview of the abbreviations related to the terms introduced in this chapter. Note: To avoid errors or confusion, always be cautious when using abbreviations.

**TABLE 13.1**

**Abbreviations Related to the Endocrine System**

| | |
|---|---|
| aldosterone = ALD | **ALD** = aldosterone |
| antidiuretic hormone = ADH | **ADH** = antidiuretic hormone |
| diabetes insipidus = DI | **DI** = diabetes insipidus |
| diabetes mellitus = DM | **DM** = diabetes mellitus |
| epinephrine = EPI, Epi | **Epi, EPI** = epinephrine |
| fasting blood sugar = FBS | **FBS** = fasting blood sugar |
| fructosamine test = FA | **FA** = fructosamine test |
| Graves' disease = GD | **GD** = Graves' disease |
| hypoglycemia = HG | **HG** = hypoglycemia |
| latent autoimmune diabetes = LADA | **LADA** = latent autoimmune diabetes |
| leptin = LEP, LPT | **LEP, LPT** = leptin |
| thyroid stimulating hormone = TSH | **TSH** = thyroid stimulating hormone |

**StudyWARE CONNECTION**

For more practice and to test your mastery of this material, go to the StudyWARE™ to play interactive games and complete the quiz for this chapter.

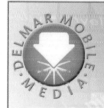

Downloadable audio is available for selected medical terms in this chapter to enhance your learning of medical terminology.

**☐ Workbook Practice**

Go to your workbook, and complete the exercises for this chapter.

## MATCHING WORD PARTS 1

Write the correct answer in the middle column.

| Definition | Correct Answer | Possible Answers |
|---|---|---|
| 13.1.  adrenal glands | _____ | acr/o |
| 13.2.  extremities | _____ | adren/o |
| 13.3.  ovaries or testicles | _____ | crin/o |
| 13.4.  thirst | _____ | -dipsia |
| 13.5.  to secrete | _____ | gonad/o |

## MATCHING WORD PARTS 2

Write the correct answer in the middle column.

| Definition | Correct Answer | Possible Answers |
|---|---|---|
| 13.6.  condition | _____ | pituitar/o |
| 13.7.  pancreas | _____ | pineal/o |
| 13.8.  parathyroid glands | _____ | parathyroid/o |
| 13.9.  pineal gland | _____ | pancreat/o |
| 13.10.  pituitary gland | _____ | -ism |

## MATCHING WORD PARTS 3

Write the correct answer in the middle column.

| Definition | Correct Answer | Possible Answers |
|---|---|---|
| 13.11.  body | _____ | thym/o |
| 13.12.  many | _____ | thyroid/o |

13.13.  sugar                _____        **somat/o**

13.14.  thyroid              _____        **poly-**

13.15.  thymus               _____        **glyc/o**

## DEFINITIONS

Select the correct answer, and write it on the line provided.

13.16.  The _____ hormone stimulates ovulation in the female.

    estrogen            follicle-stimulating            lactogenic            luteinizing

13.17.  The _____ gland secretes hormones that control the activity of the other endocrine glands.

    adrenal            hypothalamus            pituitary            thymus

13.18.  The _____ hormone stimulates the growth and secretions of the adrenal cortex.

    adrenocorticotropic            growth            melanocyte-stimulating            thyroid-stimulating

13.19.  _____ gland has functions as part of the endocrine system by secreting a hormone that functions as part of the endocrine and immune systems.

    adrenal            parathyroid            pineal            thymus

13.20.  The hormone _____ works with the parathyroid hormone to decrease calcium levels in the blood and tissues.

    aldosterone            calcitonin            glucagon            leptin

13.21.  Cortisol is secreted by the _____.

    adrenal cortex            adrenal medulla            pituitary gland            thyroid gland

13.22.  The amount of glucose in the bloodstream is increased by the hormone _____.

    adrenaline            glucagon            hydrocortisone            insulin

13.23.  Norepinephrine is secreted by the _____.

    adrenal cortex            adrenal medulla            pancreatic islets            pituitary gland

13.24.  The hormone _____ stimulates uterine contractions during childbirth.

    estrogen            oxytocin            progesterone            testosterone

13.25.  The development of the male secondary sex characteristics is stimulated by the hormone _____.

parathyroid              pitocin              progesterone              testosterone

## MATCHING STRUCTURES

Write the correct answer in the middle column.

| Definition | Correct Answer | Possible Answers |
|---|---|---|
| 13.26.  controls blood sugar levels | _____ | thyroid gland |
| 13.27.  controls the activity of other endocrine glands | _____ | pituitary gland |
| 13.28.  influences the sleep-wakefulness cycle | _____ | pineal gland |
| 13.29.  regulates electrolyte levels | _____ | pancreatic islets |
| 13.30.  stimulates metabolism | _____ | adrenal glands |

## WHICH WORD?

Select the correct answer, and write it on the line provided.

13.31.  The hormonal disorder that results from too much growth hormone in adults is known

as _____.

acromegaly              gigantism

13.32.  The growth hormone is secreted by the _____ lobe of the pituitary gland.

anterior lobe              posterior lobe

13.33.  Diabetes type 2 is an _____ disorder.

insulin deficiency        insulin resistance

13.34.  Insufficient production of ADH causes _____.

diabetes insipidus        Graves' disease

13.35.  _____ is caused by prolonged exposure to high levels of cortisol.

Addison's disease        Cushing's syndrome

## SPELLING COUNTS

Find the misspelled word in each sentence. Then write that word, spelled correctly, on the line provided.

13.36.   The lutinizing hormone stimulates ovulation in the female _____.

13.37.   Diabetes mellitas is a group of diseases characterized by defects in insulin production, use secretion,

insulin action, or both _____.

13.38.   Myxedemia is also known as adult hypothyroidism _____.

13.39.   The hormone progestarone is released during the second half of the menstrual

cycle _____.

13.40.   Thymoxin is secreted by the thymus gland _____.

## ABBREVIATION IDENTIFICATION

In the space provided, write the words that each abbreviation stands for.

13.41.   **ACTH**          _____

13.42.   **ADH**           _____    _____

13.43.   **DM**            _____

13.44.   **FBS**           _____

13.45.   **FSH**           _____

## TERM SELECTION

Select the correct answer, and write it on the line provided.

13.46.   A rare life-threatening condition caused by exaggerated hyperthyroidism is

called _____.

thyroid nodules             goiter              thyroid storm            Graves' disease

13.47.   The condition known as _____ is characterized by abnormally high concentrations

of calcium circulating in the blood instead of being stored in the bones.

hypercalcemia          hyperthyroidism          hypocalcemia          polyphagia

13.48. The four _____ glands, each of which is about the size of a grain of rice, are

embedded in the posterior surface of the thyroid gland.

        adrenal              pancreatic            parathyroid          pineal

13.49. A/An _____ is a benign tumor of the pituitary gland that causes it to produce too

much prolactin.

        insuloma           pheochromocytoma        pituitary adenoma       prolactinoma

13.50. The average blood glucose levels over the past 3 weeks is measured by the _____

test.

        blood sugar monitoring      fructosamine        glucose tolerance      hemoglobin A1c

## SENTENCE COMPLETION

Write the correct term on the line provided.

13.51. The mineral substances known as _____ are found in the blood and include

sodium and potassium.

13.52. The two primary hormones secreted by the thyroid gland are triiodothyronine ($T_3$)

and _____ ($T_4$).

13.53. Damage to the retina of the eye caused by diabetes mellitus is known as

diabetic _____.

13.54. The medical term meaning excessive hunger is _____.

13.55. Abnormal protrusion of the eye out of the orbit is known as _____.

## WORD SURGERY

Divide each term into its component word parts. Write these word parts, in sequence, on the lines provided. When necessary, use a slash (/) to indicate a combining vowel. (You may not need all of the lines provided.)

13.56. **Hyperpituitarism** is the excess secretion of growth hormone by the pituitary gland, causing acromegaly

and gigantism.

   _____      _____      _____      _____

13.57 **Hypoglycemia** is an abnormally low concentration of glucose in the blood.

   _____      _____      _____      _____

13.58. **Hyperinsulinism** is the condition of excessive secretion of insulin in the bloodstream.

_____     _____     _____     _____

13.59. **Gynecomastia** is the condition of excessive mammary development in the male.

_____     _____     _____     _____

13.60. **Hypocalcemia** is characterized by abnormally low levels of calcium in the blood.

_____     _____     _____     _____

## TRUE/FALSE

If the statement is true, write **True** on the line. If the statement is false, write **False** on the line.

13.61. _____ The beta cells of the pancreatic islets secrete glucagon in response to low

blood sugar levels.

13.62. _____ A pheochromocytoma is a rare, benign tumor of the adrenal gland that

causes too much release of epinephrine and norepinephrine.

13.63. _____ The hormone melatonin is secreted by the adrenal cortex.

13.64. _____ An insulinoma is a malignant tumor of the pancreas that causes hypoglyce-

mia by secreting insulin.

13.65. _____ Polyuria is excessive urination.

## CLINICAL CONDITIONS

Write the correct answer on the line provided.

13.66. During his nursing studies, Rodney Milne learned that the _____ hormone

helps control blood pressure by reducing the amount of water that is excreted through

the kidneys.

13.67. Eduardo Chavez complained of being thirsty all the time. His doctor noted this excessive thirst on his

chart as _____.

13.68. Mrs. Wei's symptoms included chronic, worsening fatigue, muscle weakness, loss of appetite, and weight

loss because her adrenal glands do not produce enough cortisol. Her doctor diagnosed this condition

as _____.

13.69. Linda Thomas was diagnosed as having a/an _____. This is a benign tumor of the

pancreas that causes hypoglycemia by secreting insulin.

13.70. Patrick Edward has the autoimmune disorder known as _____ in which the body's

own antibodies attack and destroy the cells of the thyroid gland.

13.71. Because Joe Dean's ultimate goal was to swim in the Olympics, he was tempted to make illegal use

of _____ steroids to increase his strength and muscle mass.

13.72. Holly Yates was surprised to learn that _____, which is a hormone secreted by fat

cells, travels to the brain and controls the balance of food intake and energy expenditure.

13.73. As a result of a congenital lack of thyroid secretion, the Vaugh-Eames child suffers

from _____, which is a condition of arrested physical and mental development.

13.74. Ray Grovenor is excessively tall and large. This condition, which was caused by excessive secretion of

growth hormone before puberty, is known as _____.

13.75. Rosita DeAngelis required the surgical removal of her pancreas. The medical term for this procedure is a/

an _____.

## WHICH IS THE CORRECT MEDICAL TERM?

Select the correct answer, and write it on the line provided.

13.76. Hormones called _____ are produced and released by neurons in the brain, rather

than by the endocrine glands, and delivered to organs and tissues through the bloodstream.

    hormones         neurohormones        neurotransmitters        steroids

13.77. A/An _____ is a slow-growing, benign tumor of the pituitary gland that is a func-

tioning tumor (secreting hormones) or a nonfunctioning tumor (not secreting hormones).

    hyperpituitarism        hypophysectomy        pituitary adenoma        prolactinoma

13.78. _____ disease, which is an autoimmune disorder caused by hyperthyroidism, is

often characterized by goiter, exophthalmos, or both.

    Addison's        Cushing's        Graves'        Hashimoto's

13.79. The diabetic emergency caused by very high blood sugar is a/an _____.

    diabetic coma        hypoglycemia        insulin shock        insuloma

13.80. The hormone _____, which is secreted by the pineal gland, influences the sleep-wakefulness cycles.

glucagon          melatonin          parathyroid          thymosin

## CHALLENGE WORD BUILDING

These terms are *not* found in this chapter; however, they are made up of the following familiar word parts. If you need help in creating the term, refer to your medical dictionary.

| | | |
|---|---|---|
| endo- | adren/o | -emia |
| | crin/o | -itis |
| | insulin/o | -megaly |
| | pancreat/o | -ology |
| | pineal/o | -oma |
| | thym/o | -otomy |
| | | -pathy |

13.81  The term meaning any disease of the adrenal glands is _____.

13.82. The study of endocrine glands and their secretions is known as _____.

13.83. Abnormal enlargement of the adrenal glands is known as _____.

13.84. The term meaning any disease of the thymus gland is _____.

13.85. Inflammation of the thyroid gland is known as _____.

13.86. A surgical incision into the pancreas is a/an _____.

13.87. A surgical incision into the thyroid gland is a/an _____.

13.88. The term meaning any disease of the pineal gland is _____.

13.89. Abnormally high levels of insulin in the blood are known as _____.

13.90. Inflammation of the adrenal glands is known as _____.

## LABELING EXERCISES

Identify the numbered items on the accompanying figure.

13.91. _____ gland

13.92. _____ glands

13.93. _____ gland

13.94. _____ of the

female

13.95. _____

13.96. _____ gland

13.97. _____ gland

13.98. _____ glands

13.99. _____ islets

13.100. _____ of the male

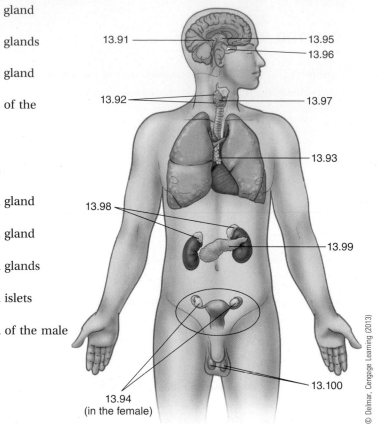

© Delmar, Cengage Learning (2013)

# THE HUMAN TOUCH
## Critical Thinking Exercise

The following story and questions are designed to stimulate critical thinking through class discussion or as a brief essay response. There are no right or wrong answers to these questions.

*By the time 14-year-old Jacob Tuls got home, he was sick enough for his mom to notice. He seemed shaky and confused, and was sweaty even though the fall weather was cool. "Jake, let's get you a glass of juice right away," his mother said as calmly as she could. She was all too familiar with the symptoms of hypoglycemia brought on by Jake's type 1 diabetes. Ever since he was diagnosed at age 6, she had carefully monitored his insulin, eating, and exercise. But now that he was in middle school, the ball was in his court, and it really worried her that he often seemed to mess up.*

*"Yeah, I know I shouldn't have gone so long without eating," Jake muttered once he was feeling better. "But you don't understand. I don't want to be different from the other kids." Before he could finish, his mom was on the telephone to the school nurse's office.*

*Jacob needed to inject himself with insulin three times a day. He knew what happened when his blood sugar got too high or if he didn't eat on schedule and it got too low. But when he was on a field trip with his friends, he hated to go to the chaperone and say that he needed to eat something right away. And he hated it when some kid walked in while he was injecting. His mom had made arrangements with the school nurse for him to go to her office to get some privacy, but whenever he didn't show up between fourth and fifth periods, she would come into the classroom to get him as if he was some kind of sick loser.*

*He was tired of having this disease, sick of shots, and angry that he could not sleep late and skip meals like other kids. He made a face at his mother as she talked on the telephone to the nurse, and slammed the back door on his way out to find his friend Joe.*

## Suggested Discussion Topics

1. Why is it more difficult for Jacob to maintain his injection routine in middle school than it was in elementary school?

2. Knowing that missing an insulin injection could cause a diabetic coma and possibly death, why do you think Jacob is not more conscientious in his self-care?

3. Do you think Jacob's schoolmates talk about him, or does he just think they do? Discuss both possibilities. What steps can Jacob take to help his classmates understand his condition?

4. Consider the cost of managing Jacob's diabetes for 1 year, for 10 years, for his lifetime. What if Jacob did not have insurance? What would happen if his mismanagement of his condition resulted in a hospital stay?

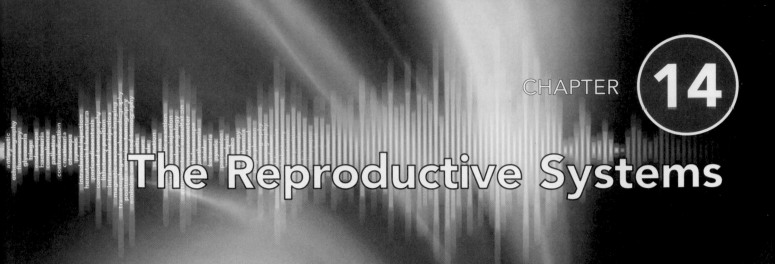

# The Reproductive Systems

## Overview of
## STRUCTURES, COMBINING FORMS, AND FUNCTIONS OF THE REPRODUCTIVE SYSTEMS

| Major Structures | Related Combining Forms | Primary Functions |
|---|---|---|
| **Male** | | |
| Penis | **pen/i, phall/i** | Used for sexual intercourse and urination. |
| Testicles | **orch/o, orchid/o, test/i, test/o** | Produce sperm and the hormone testosterone. |
| **Female** | | |
| Ovaries | **oophor/o, ovari/o** | Produce ova (eggs) and female hormones. |
| Fallopian Tubes | **salping/o** | Catch the mature ovum (egg) and transport it to the uterus. Also the site of fertilization. |
| Uterus | **hyster/o, metr/o, metri/o, uter/o** | Protects and supports the developing child. |
| Vagina | **vagin/o, colp/o** | Used for sexual intercourse, acts as channel for menstrual flow, and functions as the birth canal. |
| Placenta | **placent/o** | Exchanges nutrients and waste between the mother and fetus during pregnancy. |

# Vocabulary Related to THE REPRODUCTIVE SYSTEMS

This list contains essential word parts and medical terms for this chapter. These terms are pronounced in the student StudyWARE™ and Audio CDs that are available for use with this text. These and the other important **primary terms** are shown in boldface throughout the chapter. *Secondary terms*, which appear in *orange* italics, clarify the meaning of primary terms.

## Word Parts

- [ ] **cervic/o** cervix (neck of uterus)
- [ ] **colp/o** vagina
- [ ] **-gravida** pregnant
- [ ] **gynec/o** woman, female
- [ ] **hyster/o** uterus
- [ ] **mast/o** breast
- [ ] **men/o** menstruation, menses
- [ ] **orchid/o** testicles
- [ ] **ov/o** egg, ovum
- [ ] **ovari/o** ovary
- [ ] **-para** to give birth
- [ ] **-pexy** surgical fixation
- [ ] **salping/o** uterine (fallopian) tube
- [ ] **test/i** testicle, testis
- [ ] **vagin/o** vagina

## Medical Terms

- [ ] **amenorrhea** (ah-**men**-oh-**REE**-ah)
- [ ] **amniocentesis** (am-nee-oh-sen-**TEE**-sis)
- [ ] **andropause** (**AN**-droh-pawz)
- [ ] **Apgar score**
- [ ] **azoospermia** (ay-zoh-oh-**SPER**-mee-ah)
- [ ] **cervical dysplasia** (**SER**-vih-kal dis-**PLAY**-see-ah)
- [ ] **cervicitis** (ser-vih-**SIGH**-tis)
- [ ] **chlamydia** (klah-**MID**-ee-ah)
- [ ] **chorionic villus sampling** (kor-ee-**ON**-ick **VIL**-us)
- [ ] **colostrum** (kuh-**LOS**-trum)
- [ ] **colpopexy** (**KOL**-poh-**peck**-see)
- [ ] **colporrhaphy** (kol-**POR**-ah-fee)
- [ ] **colposcopy** (kol-**POS**-koh-pee)
- [ ] **dysmenorrhea** (dis-men-oh-**REE**-ah)
- [ ] **eclampsia** (eh-**KLAMP**-see-ah)
- [ ] **ectopic pregnancy** (eck-**TOP**-ick)
- [ ] **endocervicitis** (en-doh-ser-vih-**SIGH**-tis)

- [ ] **endometriosis** (en-doh-**mee**-tree-**OH**-sis)
- [ ] **epididymitis** (ep-ih-did-ih-**MY**-tis)
- [ ] **episiotomy** (eh-**piz**-ee-**OT**-oh-mee)
- [ ] **fibroadenoma** (**figh**-broh-**ad**-eh-**NOH**-mah)
- [ ] **fibrocystic breast disease** (**figh**-broh-**SIS**-tick)
- [ ] **galactorrhea** (gah-**lack**-toh-**REE**-ah)
- [ ] **gonorrhea** (**gon**-oh-**REE**-ah)
- [ ] **hematospermia** (**hee**-mah-toh-**SPER**-mee-ah)
- [ ] **hydrocele** (**HIGH**-droh-seel)
- [ ] **hypomenorrhea** (**high**-poh-men-oh-**REE**-ah)
- [ ] **hysterectomy** (**hiss**-teh-**RECK**-toh-mee)
- [ ] **hysterosalpingography** (**hiss**-ter-oh-**sal**-pin-**GOG**-rah-fee)
- [ ] **hysteroscopy** (**hiss**-ter-**OSS**-koh-pee)
- [ ] **leukorrhea** (**loo**-koh-**REE**-ah)
- [ ] **mastalgia** (mass-**TAL**-jee-ah)
- [ ] **mastopexy** (**MAS**-toh-**peck**-see)
- [ ] **menarche** (meh-**NAR**-kee)
- [ ] **menometrorrhagia** (**men**-oh-**met**-roh-**RAY**-jee-ah)
- [ ] **metrorrhea** (**mee**-troh-**REE**-ah)
- [ ] **neonate** (**NEE**-oh-nayt)
- [ ] **nulligravida** (**null**-ih-**GRAV**-ih-dah)
- [ ] **nullipara** (nuh-**LIP**-ah-rah)
- [ ] **obstetrician** (ob-steh-**TRISH**-un)
- [ ] **oligomenorrhea** (ol-ih-goh-**men**-oh-**REE**-ah)
- [ ] **oophorectomy** (oh-ahf-oh-**RECK**-toh-mee)
- [ ] **orchidectomy** (or-kih-**DECK**-toh-mee)
- [ ] **orchiopexy** (**or**-keeoh-**PECK**-see)
- [ ] **ovariorrhexis** (oh-**vay**-ree-oh-**RECK**-sis)
- [ ] **perimenopause** (pehr-ih-**MEN**-oh-pawz)
- [ ] **Peyronie's disease** (pay-roh-**NEEZ**)
- [ ] **placenta previa** (plah-**SEN**-tah **PREE**-vee-ah)
- [ ] **polycystic ovary syndrome** (pol-ee-**SIS**-tick)
- [ ] **preeclampsia** (pree-ee-**KLAMP**-see-ah)
- [ ] **priapism** (**PRYE**-ah-**piz**-em)
- [ ] **primigravida** (**prye**-mih-**GRAV**-ih-dah)
- [ ] **primipara** (prye-**MIP**-ah-rah)
- [ ] **pruritus vulvae** (proo-**RYE**-tus **VUL**-vee)
- [ ] **salpingo-oophorectomy** (sal-**ping**-goh oh-**ahf**-oh-**RECK**-toh-mee)
- [ ] **syphilis** (**SIF**-ih-lis)
- [ ] **trichomoniasis** (**trick**-oh-moh-**NYE**-ah-sis)
- [ ] **uterine prolapse** (proh-**LAPS**)
- [ ] **varicocele** (**VAR**-ih-koh-**seel**)
- [ ] **vasovasostomy** (vay-soh-vah-**ZOS**-toh-mee)

## LEARNING GOALS

On completion of this chapter, you should be able to:

1. Identify and describe the major functions and structures of the male reproductive system.

2. Recognize, define, spell, and pronounce the terms related to the pathology and the diagnostic and treatment procedures of the male reproductive system.

3. Name at least six sexually transmitted diseases.

4. Identify and describe the major functions and structures of the female reproductive system.

5. Recognize, define, spell, and pronounce the primary terms related to the pathology and the diagnostic and treatment procedures of the female reproductive system, and a woman during pregnancy, childbirth, and the postpartum period.

## ■ TERMS RELATED TO THE REPRODUCTIVE SYSTEMS OF BOTH SEXES

The **genitalia** (**jen**-ih-**TAY**-lee-ah) are the organs of reproduction and their associated structures.

■ *External genitalia* are reproductive organs located outside of the body cavity.

■ *Internal genitalia* are reproductive organs protected within the body.

The **perineum** (pehr-ih-**NEE**-um) is the external surface region in both males and females between the pubic symphysis and the coccyx.

■ The tissue of the *male perineum* extends from the scrotum to the area around the anus.

■ The tissue of the *female perineum* extends from the pubic symphysis to the area around the anus. (Figure 14.6).

## ■ FUNCTIONS OF THE MALE REPRODUCTIVE SYSTEM

The primary function of the male reproductive system is to produce sperm and deliver them into the female body so that one sperm can unite with a single ovum (egg) to create a new life. Some structures of the male reproductive system also function as part of the urinary system. These are discussed in Chapter 9.

## ■ STRUCTURES OF THE MALE REPRODUCTIVE SYSTEM

■ The *external male genitalia* are the penis and the scrotum, which contains two testicles.

■ The *internal male genitalia* include the remaining structures of the male reproductive system (Figures 14.1 and 14.2).

### The Scrotum and Testicles

The **scrotum** (**SKROH**-tum) is the sac-like structure that surrounds, protects, and supports the testicles. The scrotum is suspended from the pubic arch behind the penis and lies between the thighs.

The **testicles**, also known as *testes*, are the two small, egg-shaped glands that produce the sperm (singular, *testis*). These glands develop within the abdomen of the male fetus and normally descend into the scrotum before or soon after birth.

■ Sperm are formed within the **seminiferous tubules** (**see**-mih-**NIF**-er-us **TOO**-byouls) of each testicle (Figure 14.2).

■ The **epididymis** (**ep**-ih-**DID**-ih-mis) is a coiled tube at the upper part of each testicle. This tube runs down the length of the testicle, then turns upward toward the body. Here, it narrows to form the tube known as the *vas deferens*.

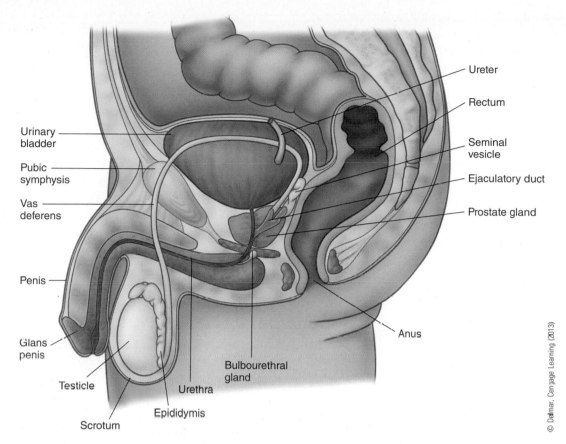

**FIGURE 14.1** Organs and ducts of the male reproductive system shown in a lateral cross-section.

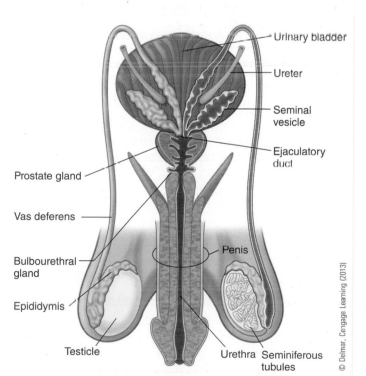

**FIGURE 14.2** Structures of the male reproductive system as shown in an anterior cross-section view.

■ The **spermatic cord** extends upward from the epididymis and is attached to each testicle. Each cord contains a vas deferens plus the arteries, veins, nerves, and lymphatic vessels required by each testicle.

## Semen Formation

**Sperm**, also known as *spermatozoa*, are the male gametes (reproductive cells). **Semen** (**SEE**-men) is the whitish fluid containing sperm that is ejaculated through the urethra at the peak of male sexual excitement. The term *ejaculate* means to expel suddenly.

■ **Spermatogenesis** (**sper**-mah-toh-**JEN**-eh-sis) is the process of sperm formation (**spermat/o** means sperm, and **-genesis** means creation).

■ The ideal temperature for sperm formation is 93.2°F. The scrotum aids in maintaining this temperature by adjusting how closely it holds the testicles to the body.

■ Sperm are formed in the seminiferous tubules of the testicles.

■ From here, the sperm move into the epididymis where they become motile and are temporarily stored. *Motile* means capable of spontaneous motion.

■ From the epididymis, the sperm travel upward into the body and enter the vas deferens. Here, the seminal vesicles and the prostate gland add their secretions to form semen.

## The Penis

The **penis** (**PEE**-nis) is the male sex organ that transports the sperm into the female vagina. The penis is composed of three columns of erectile tissue (Figures 14.1 and 14.2).

■ During sexual stimulation, the erectile tissue fills with blood under high pressure. This causes the swelling, hardness, and stiffness known as an *erection*.

■ The adjectives *penile* and *phallic* both mean relating to the penis (both **pen/i** and **phall/i** mean penis).

■ The **glans penis** (glanz **PEE**-nis), also known as the *head of the penis*, is the sensitive region located at the tip of the penis (Figure 14.1).

■ The **foreskin**, also known as the *prepuce*, is a retractable double-layered fold of skin and mucous membrane that covers and protects the glans penis.

## The Vas Deferens, Seminal Vesicles, and the Ejaculatory Duct

■ The **vas deferens** (vas **DEF**-er-enz), also known as the *ductus deferens*, are the long, narrow continuations of each epididymis. These structures lead upward and eventually join the urethra (Figures 14.1 and 14.2).

■ The **seminal vesicles** (**SEM**-ih-nal) are glands that secrete a thick, yellow substance to nourish the sperm cells. This secretion forms 60% of the volume of semen. These glands are located at the base of the urinary bladder and open into the vas deferens as it joins the urethra.

■ The **ejaculatory duct**, which begins at the vas deferens, passes through the prostate gland and empties into the urethra. During ejaculation, a reflex action caused by these ducts, semen passes into the urethra, which exits the body via the penis.

## The Prostate Gland

The **prostate gland** (**PROS**-tayt) lies under the bladder and surrounds the end of the urethra in the region where the vas deferens enters the urethra (Figures 14.1 and 14.2).

During ejaculation, the prostate gland secretes a thick, alkaline fluid into the semen that aids the motility of the sperm. *Motility* means ability to move. Disorders and treatment of the prostate gland are discussed in Chapter 9.

## The Bulbourethral Glands

The two **bulbourethral glands** (**bul**-boh-you-**REE**-thral), also known as *Cowper's glands*, are located just below the prostate gland. One of these glands is located on either side of the urethra, and they open into the urethra (Figures 14.1 and 14.2).

During sexual arousal, these glands secrete a fluid known as *pre-ejaculate*. This fluid helps flush out any residual urine or foreign matter in the urethra. It also lubricates the urethra for sperm to pass through. This fluid can contain sperm and is able to cause pregnancy even if ejaculation does not occur.

## The Urethra

The **urethra** passes through the penis to the outside of the body. In the male, the urethra serves both the reproductive and the urinary systems. Disorders of the urethra are discussed in Chapter 9.

## ■ MEDICAL SPECIALTIES RELATED TO THE MALE REPRODUCTIVE SYSTEM

A **urologist** (you-**ROL**-oh-jist) is a physician who specializes in diagnosing and treating diseases and disorders of the genitourinary system of males and the urinary system of females (**ur** means urine, and **-ologist** means specialist). The term *genitourinary* refers to both the genital and urinary organs.

# PATHOLOGY OF THE MALE REPRODUCTIVE SYSTEM

## The Penis

- **Balanitis** (**bal**-ah-**NIGH**-tis) is an inflammation of the glans penis that is usually caused by poor hygiene in men who have not had the foreskin removed by circumcision (**balan** means glans penis, and **-itis** means inflammation).

- **Phimosis** (figh-**MOH**-sis) is a narrowing of the opening of the foreskin so it cannot be retracted (pulled back) to expose the glans penis. This condition can be present at birth or become apparent during childhood.

- **Erectile dysfunction** (ED), also known as *impotence*, is the inability of the male to achieve or maintain a penile erection. A penis that is not erect is referred to as being *flaccid*, or limp.

- **Peyronie's disease** (pay-roh-**NEEZ**), also known as *penile curvature*, is a form of sexual dysfunction in which the penis is bent or curved during erection.

- **Priapism** (**PRYE**-ah-**piz**-em) is a painful erection that lasts 4 hours or more but is either not accompanied by sexual excitement or does not go away after sexual stimulation has ended. The condition can be caused by medications or by blood-related diseases such as sickle cell anemia or leukemia.

- **Premature ejaculation** is a condition in which the male reaches climax too soon, usually before or shortly after penetration of the female.

## The Testicles and Related Structures

- **Andropause** (**AN**-droh-pawz), which is referred to as *ADAM* (*Androgen Decline in the Aging Male*), is marked by the decrease of the male hormone testosterone (**andr/o** means male or masculine, and **-pause** means stopping). It usually begins in the late 40s and progresses very gradually over several decades. *Androgen* is a male sex hormone.

- **Cryptorchidism** (krip-**TOR**-kih-dizm), also known as an *undescended testicle*, is a developmental defect in which one or both of the testicles fail to descend into their normal position in the scrotum (**crypt** means hidden, **orchid** means testicle, and **-ism** means abnormal condition).

- **Epididymitis** (ep-ih-did-ih-**MY**-tis) is inflammation of the epididymis that is frequently caused by the spread of infection from the urethra or the bladder (**epididym** means epididymis, and **-itis** means inflammation) (Figure 14.3A).

- A **hydrocele** (**HIGH**-droh-seel) is a fluid-filled sac in the scrotum along the spermatic cord leading from the testicles (**hydr/o** means relating to water, and **-cele** means a hernia or swelling). Note: The term *hydrocele* is also used to describe the accumulation of fluid in any body cavity.

- A **spermatocele** (sper-**MAH**-toh-seel) is a cyst that develops in the epididymis and is filled with a milky fluid containing sperm (**spermat/o** means sperm, and **-cele** means hernia, tumor, or swelling).

- **Testicular cancer** is cancer that begins in the testicles. It is the most common cancer in American males between the ages of 15 and 34 years. This cancer is highly treatable when diagnosed early.

- **Testicular torsion** is a sharp pain in the scrotum caused by twisting of the vas deferens and blood vessels leading into the testicle. *Torsion* means twisting.

- **Testitis** (test-**TYE**-tis), also known as *orchitis*, is inflammation of one or both testicles (**test** means testicle, and **-itis** means inflammation) (Figure 14.3B).

- A **varicocele** (**VAR**-ih-koh-**seel**) is a knot of widening varicose veins in one side of the scrotum (**varic/o** means varicose veins, and **-cele** means a hernia or swelling). *Varicose veins* are abnormally swollen veins (Figure 14.3C).

### Sperm Count

A **normal sperm count** is 20 to 120 million or more sperm per milliliter (mL) of semen.

- **Azoospermia** (ay-**zoh**-oh-**SPER**-mee-ah) is the absence of sperm in the semen (**a-** means without, **zoo** means life, **sperm** means sperm, and **-ia** means abnormal condition).

- **Oligospermia** (**ol**-ih-goh-**SPER**-mee-ah) is a sperm count of below 20 million/mL (**olig/o** means few, **sperm** means sperm, and **-ia** means abnormal condition). This is also known as a *low sperm count* and is a common cause of *male infertility*.

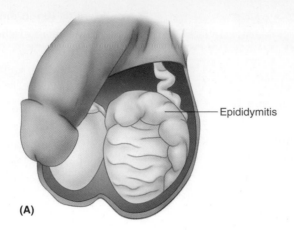

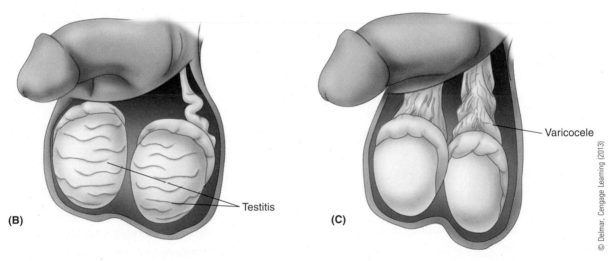

**FIGURE 14.3** Pathology of the testicles. (A) Epididymitis of the left testicle. (B) Testitis of both testicles. (C) A varicocele affecting the left testicle.

■ **Hematospermia** (**hee**-mah-toh-**SPER**-mee-ah) is the presence of blood in the seminal fluid (**hemat/o** means relating to blood, **sperm** means sperm, and **-ia** means abnormal condition). This condition can be caused by infections of the seminal vesicles, prostatitis, urethritis, or urethral strictures, which are discussed in Chapter 9.

## DIAGNOSTIC PROCEDURES OF THE MALE REPRODUCTIVE SYSTEM

■ **Sperm count**, also known as a *sperm analysis*, is the testing of freshly ejaculated semen to determine the volume plus the number, shape, size, and motility of the sperm.

■ **Testicular self-examination** is a self-help step in early detection of testicular cancer by detecting lumps, swelling, or changes in the skin of the scrotum.

**StudyWARE CONNECTION**

Watch the **Male Reproductive System** animation in the StudyWARE™ CD-ROM.

## TREATMENT PROCEDURES OF THE MALE REPRODUCTIVE SYSTEM

### General Treatment Procedures

■ **Circumcision** (**ser**-kum-**SIZH**-un) is the surgical removal of the foreskin of the penis. This optional procedure is usually performed within a few days of birth.

- An **orchidectomy** (**or**-kih-**DECK**-toh-mee), also spelled as *orchiectomy*, is the surgical removal of one or both testicles (**orchid** means testicle, and **-ectomy** means surgical removal).

- **Orchiopexy** (**or**-kee-oh-**PECK**-see) is the repair of an undescended testicle (**orchi/o** means testicle, and **-pexy** means surgical fixation). This is endoscopic surgery performed on infants before the age of 1 year to move the testicle into its normal position in the scrotum.

- A **varicocelectomy** (**var**-ih-koh-sih-**LECK**-toh-mee) is the removal of a portion of an enlarged vein to relieve a varicocele (**varic/o** means varicose vein, **cel** means swelling, and **-ectomy** means surgical removal).

## Male Sterilization

**Sterilization** is any procedure rendering an individual (male or female) incapable of reproduction.

- **Castration** (kas-**TRAY**-shun), also known as *bilateral orchidectomy*, is the surgical removal or destruction of both testicles.

- A **vasectomy** (vah-**SECK**-toh-mee) is the male sterilization procedure in which a small portion of the vas deferens is surgically removed (**vas** means vas deferens, and **-ectomy** means surgical removal). This prevents sperm from entering the ejaculate but does not change the volume of semen created by the body (Figure 14.4).

- A **vasovasostomy** (vay-soh-vah-**ZOS**-toh-mee), also known as a *vasectomy reversal*, is a procedure performed as an attempt to restore fertility to a vasectomized male (**vas/o** means blood vessel, **vas** means the vas deferens, and **-ostomy** means surgically creating an opening).

## ■ SEXUALLY TRANSMITTED DISEASES

**Sexually transmitted diseases** (STDs), which are also known as *venereal diseases* (VD) or sexually transmitted infections (STIs), are infections caused by either bacteria or a virus that affects both males and females. These conditions are commonly spread through sexual intercourse or other genital contact.

- A pregnant woman who is infected with one of these diseases can transmit it to her baby during birth. For this reason, all newborns receive an antibiotic ointment in each eye within an hour after birth to prevent *ophthalmia neonatorum*. This condition is a form of conjunctivitis that is caused by the bacteria responsible for chlamydia or gonorrhea.

  There are more than 20 types of STDs. The following are several of the more common diseases.

## Chlamydia

**Chlamydia** (klah-**MID**-ee-ah), which is caused by the bacterium *Chlamydia trachomatis*, is the most commonly reported STD in the United States. It is highly contagious and requires early treatment with antibiotics.

- In females, chlamydia can damage the reproductive organs. Even though symptoms are usually mild or absent, serious complications can cause irreversible damage, including infertility.

- In males, chlamydia is one of the causes of urethritis (see Chapter 9).

## Other Sexually Transmitted Diseases

- **Bacterial vaginosis** (BV) (**vaj**-ih-**NOH**-sis) is a condition in women in which there is an abnormal overgrowth of certain bacteria in the vagina (**vagin** means vagina, and **-osis** means abnormal condition or disease). This condition can cause complications during pregnancy and an increased risk of HIV infection if exposed to the virus. Symptoms sometimes include a discharge, odor, pain, itching, or burning.

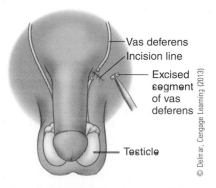

**FIGURE 14.4** In a vasectomy, a portion of the vas deferens is removed to prevent sperm from entering the semen.

- **Genital herpes** (**HER**-peez) is caused by the *herpes simplex virus type 1 or 2*. Symptoms include itching or burning before the appearance of lesions (sores) on the genitals or rectum. This condition is highly contagious, even when visible lesions are not present. Antiviral drugs ease symptoms and can suppress future outbreaks; however, currently there is no cure.

- **Genital warts**, which are caused by **human papillomaviruses** (HPV), are highly contagious. In the male, this virus infects the urethra. In the female, it infects the external genitalia, cervix, and vagina. It also increases the risk of cervical cancer. An HPV vaccine is available to prevent the spread of this disease. It is recommended that it be administered to girls between the ages of 11 and 12 or before they become sexually active.

- **Gonorrhea** (**gon**-oh-**REE**-ah) is a highly contagious condition caused by the bacterium *Neisseria gonorrhoeae*. In women, this condition affects the cervix, uterus, and fallopian tubes. In men, it affects the urethra by causing painful urination and an abnormal discharge. It can also affect the mouth, throat, and anus of both men and women.

- The **human immunodeficiency virus** (HIV) is transmitted through exposure to infected body fluids, particularly through sexual intercourse with an infected partner. HIV and AIDS are discussed in Chapter 6.

- **Syphilis** (**SIF**-ih-lis), which is caused by the bacterium *Treponema pallidum*, has many symptoms that are difficult to distinguish from other STDs. Syphilis is highly contagious and is passed from person to person through direct contact with a *chancre*, which is a sore caused by syphilis. This condition can be detected through the VDRL (**V**enereal **D**isease **R**esearch **L**aboratory) blood test before the lesions appear. The RPR test (**R**apid **P**lasma **R**eagin) is another blood test for syphilis.

- **Trichomoniasis** (**trick**-oh-moh-**NYE**-ah-sis), also known as *trich*, is an infection caused by the parasite *Trichomonas vaginalis*. One of the most common symptoms in infected women is a thin, frothy, yellow-green, foul-smelling vaginal discharge. Infected men often do not have symptoms; however, when symptoms are present, they include painful urination or a clear discharge from the penis.

## ◼ FUNCTIONS OF THE FEMALE REPRODUCTIVE SYSTEM

The primary function of the female reproductive system is the creation and support of new life.

- The ovaries produce mature eggs to be fertilized by the sperm.

- The uterus provides the environment and support for the developing child.

- After birth, the breasts produce milk to feed the child.

## ◼ STRUCTURES OF THE FEMALE REPRODUCTIVE SYSTEM

The structures of the female reproductive system are described as being the external female genitalia and the internal female reproductive organs (Figure 14.5).

### The External Female Genitalia

The *external female genitalia* are located posterior to the **mons pubis** (monz **PYOU**-bis), which is a rounded, fleshy prominence located over the pubic symphysis (Figure 14.6). These structures are known collectively as the **vulva** (**VUL**-vah) or the *pudendum*. The vulva consists of the labia, clitoris, Bartholin's glands, and vaginal orifice.

- The **labia majora** and **labia minora** (**LAY**-bee-ah mah-**JOR**-ah and **LAY**-bee-ah mih-**NOR**-ah) are the vaginal lips that protect the other external genitalia and the urethral meatus (singular, *labium*). The *urethral meatus*, which is the external opening of the urethra, is discussed in Chapter 9.

- The **clitoris** (**KLIT**-oh-ris) is an organ of sensitive, erectile tissue located anterior to the urethral meatus and the vaginal orifice.

- **Bartholin's glands** produce a mucus secretion to lubricate the vagina. These two small, round glands are located on either side of the vaginal orifice.

- The **vaginal orifice** is the exterior opening of the vagina. *Orifice* means opening. The **hymen** (**HIGH**-men) is a mucous membrane that partially covers this opening and can be torn either during the first instance of intercourse or other activity. This tissue can be absent in a woman who has not been sexually active.

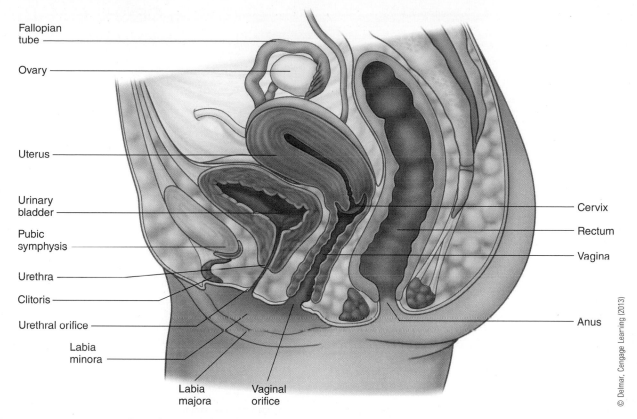

**FIGURE 14.5** Structures of the female reproductive system shown in a lateral cross-section.

## Breasts

**Breasts** are made up of fat, connective tissue, and the mammary glands (the word parts **mamm/o** and **mast/o** both mean breast). Each breast is fixed to the overlying skin and the underlying pectoral muscles by suspensory ligaments (Figure 14.7). Breast cancer, its diagnosis and treatment, are discussed in Chapter 6.

■ **Mammary glands**, also known as the *lactiferous glands*, are the milk-producing glands that develop during puberty.

■ The **lactiferous ducts** (lack-**TIF**-er-us), also known as *milk ducts*, carry milk from the mammary glands to the nipple (**lact** means milk, and **-iferous** means carrying or producing).

■ Breast milk flows through the **nipple**, which is surrounded by the dark-pigmented area known as the **areola** (ah-**REE**-oh-lah).

## The Internal Female Genitalia

The internal female genitalia are located within the pelvic cavity where they are protected by the bony pelvis. These structures include two ovaries, two fallopian tubes, the uterus, and the vagina (Figures 14.5 and 14.8).

## The Ovaries

The **ovaries** (**OH**-vah-rees) are a pair of small, almond-shaped organs located in the lower abdomen, one on either side of the uterus.

■ A **follicle** (**FOL**-lick-kul) is a fluid-filled sac containing a single ovum (egg). There are thousands of these sacs on the inside surface of the ovaries.

■ The **ova** (**OH**-vah), also known as *eggs*, are the female gametes (singular, *ovum*). These immature ova are present at birth. Normally, after puberty, one ovum matures and is released each month.

■ The ovaries also produce the sex hormones estrogen and progesterone, which are discussed in Chapter 13.

## The Fallopian Tubes

There are two **fallopian tubes** (fal-**LOH**-pee-an), which are also known as *uterine tubes*. These tubes extend from the upper end of the uterus to a point near but not attached to an ovary.

■ The **infundibulum** (in-fun-**DIB**-you-lum) is the funnel-shaped opening into the fallopian tube near the ovary.

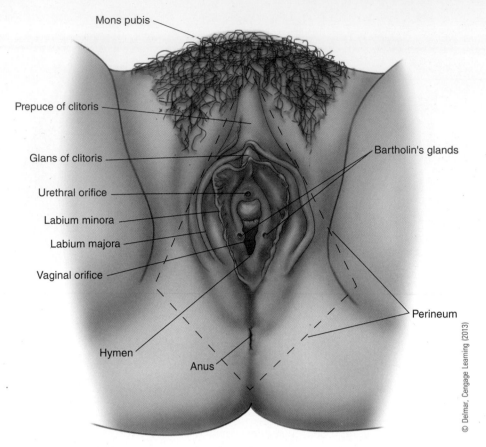

Mons pubis

Prepuce of clitoris

Glans of clitoris

Urethral orifice

Labium minora

Labium majora

Vaginal orifice

Hymen

Anus

Bartholin's glands

Perineum

© Delmar, Cengage Learning (2013)

**FIGURE 14.6** Female external genitalia.

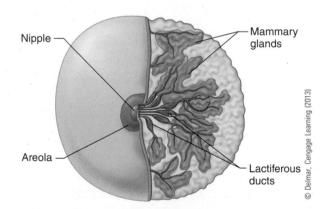

Nipple

Areola

Mammary glands

Lactiferous ducts

© Delmar, Cengage Learning (2013)

**FIGURE 14.7** Structures of the breast.

■ The **fimbriae** (**FIM**-bree-ee) are the fringed, finger-like extensions of this opening. Their role is to catch the mature ovum when it leaves the ovary (singular, *fimbria*).

■ Each month, one of these tubes carries a mature ovum from the ovary to the uterus (Figure 14.8). These tubes also carry sperm upward from the uterus toward the descending mature ovum so that fertilization can occur.

## The Uterus

The **uterus** (**YOU**-ter-us), formerly known as the *womb*, is a pear-shaped organ with muscular walls and a mucous membrane lining filled with a rich supply of blood vessels (Figure 14.8).

■ The uterus is located between the urinary bladder and the rectum and midway between the sacrum and the pubic bone.

■ In its normal position, which is known as **anteflexion** (**an**-tee-**FLECK**-shun), the body of the uterus is bent forward (**ante-** means forward, **flex** means bend, and **-ion** means condition) (Figure 14.5).

## The Parts of the Uterus

The body of the uterus consists of three major anatomic areas:

■ The **fundus** (**FUN**-dus) is the bulging, rounded part above the entrance of the fallopian tubes. Because the fundus rises during pregnancy, measuring the fundal height in relation to the pubic bone helps determine the baby's growth.

■ The **corpus** (**KOR**-pus), also known as the *body of the uterus*, is the middle portion.

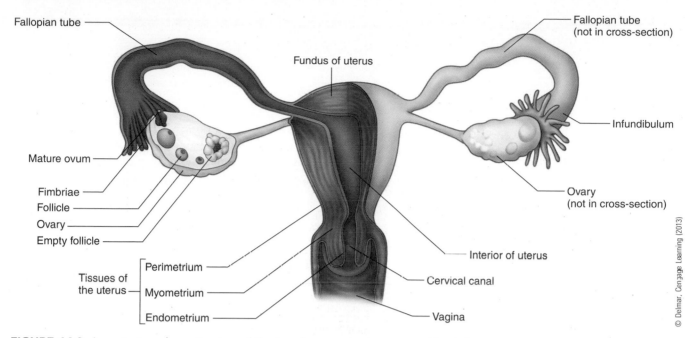

**FIGURE 14.8** An anterior schematic view of the female reproductive organs. The left ovary, shown here in cross-section, contains developing ova in different stages of maturation. Also shown on the left is a mature ovum that has just been released.

■ The **cervix** (**SER**-vicks), also known as the *cervix uteri*, is the lower, narrow portion that extends into the vagina. Within the cervix is the *cervical canal*, which ends at the *cervical os* at the vagina.

## The Tissues of the Uterus

The uterus is composed of three major layers of tissue:

■ The **perimetrium** (pehr-ih-**MEE**-tree-um), also known as the *uterine serosa*, is the tough, membranous outer layer (**peri-** means surrounding, **metri** means uterus, and **-um** is a singular noun ending). *Membranous* means pertaining to a thin layer of tissue.

■ The **myometrium** (my-oh-**MEE**-tree-um) is the muscular middle layer (**my/o** means muscle, **metri** means uterus, and **-um** is a singular noun ending).

■ The **endometrium** (en-doh-**MEE**-tree-um) is the inner layer, and it consists of specialized epithelial mucosa that is rich in blood vessels (**endo-** means within, **metri** means uterus, and **-um** is a singular noun ending). *Mucosa* means referring to mucous membrane.

## Vagina

The **vagina** (vah-**JIGH**-nah) is the muscular tube lined with mucosa that extends from the cervix to the outside of the body. The word parts **colp/o** and **vagin/o** both mean vagina (Figures 14.7 and 14.8).

## Menstruation

**Menstruation** (men-stroo-**AY**-shun), also known as *menses*, is the normal periodic discharge of the endometrial lining and unfertilized egg from uterus.

■ **Menarche** (**MEN**-ar-kee) is the beginning of the menstrual function (**men** means menstruation, and **-arche** means beginning). This function begins after the maturation that occurs during puberty. In the United States the average age is 12.

■ The average *menstrual cycle* consists of 28 days. These days are grouped into four phases and are summarized in Table 14.1.

■ **Menopause** (**MEN**-oh-pawz) is the normal termination of the menstrual function in a woman during middle age (**men/o** means menstruation and **-pause** means stopping). Menopause is considered to be confirmed when a woman has gone 1 year without having a period.

■ **Perimenopause** (pehr-ih-**MEN**-oh-pawz) is the term used to designate the transition phase between regular menstrual periods and no periods at all (**peri-** means surrounding, **men/o** means menstruation, and **-pause** means stopping). During this phase, which can last as long as 10 years, changes in hormone production can cause symptoms, including irregular menstrual cycles, hot flashes, mood swings, and disturbed sleep.

**TABLE 14.1**

**Phases of the Menstrual Cycle**

| | |
|---|---|
| Approximately Days 1–5 | *Menstrual phase.* These are the days when the endometrial lining of the uterus is sloughed off and discharged through the vagina as the menstrual flow. |
| Approximately Days 6–12 | *Postmenstrual phase.* After the menstrual period, the pituitary gland secretes follicle-stimulating hormone (FSH), causing an ovum to mature. Estrogen, which is secreted by the ovaries, stimulates the lining of the uterus to prepare itself to receive a zygote (fertilized egg). |
| Approximately Days 13–14 | *Ovulatory phase.* On approximately the 13th or 14th day of the cycle ovulation occurs. Ovulation is the release of a mature ovum. The mature egg leaves the ovary and travels slowly down the fallopian tube toward the uterus. During this time, the female is fertile and can become pregnant. |
| Approximately Days 15–28 | *Premenstrual phase.* If fertilization does not occur, hormone levels change to cause the breakdown of the uterine endometrium and the beginning of a new menstrual cycle. |

## ■ TERMS RELATED TO PREGNANCY AND CHILDBIRTH

### Ovulation

**Ovulation** (ov-you-**LAY**-shun) is the release of a mature egg from a follicle on the surface of one of the ovaries that happens on approximately the 13th or 14th day of a woman's menstrual cycle.

■ After the ovum (egg) is released, it is caught up by the fimbriae of the fallopian tube. Wave-like peristaltic actions move the ovum down the fallopian tube toward the uterus.

■ It usually takes an ovum about 5 days to pass through the fallopian tube. If sperm are present at that time, one will fertilize the ovum within the fallopian tube.

■ After the ovum has been released, the ruptured follicle enlarges, takes on a yellow fatty substance, and becomes the corpus luteum.

■ The **corpus luteum** (**KOR**-pus **LOO**-tee-um) secretes the hormone progesterone during the second half of the menstrual cycle. This maintains the growth of the uterine lining in preparation for the fertilized egg.

■ If the ovum is not fertilized, the corpus luteum dies, and the endometrium lining of the uterus sloughs off as the menstrual flow occurs.

■ If the ovum is fertilized, the corpus luteum continues to secrete the hormones required to maintain the pregnancy.

### Fertilization

■ During **coitus** (**KOH**-ih-tus), also known as *sexual intercourse* or *copulation*, the male ejaculates approximately 100 million sperm into the female's vagina. The sperm travel upward through the vagina, into the uterus, and on into the fallopian tubes.

■ **Conception** occurs when a sperm penetrates and fertilizes the descending ovum. This union, which is the beginning of a new life, forms a single cell known as a **zygote** (**ZYE**-goht).

■ After fertilization occurs in the fallopian tube, the zygote travels to the uterus where it is implanted. *Implantation* is the embedding of the zygote into the lining of the uterus.

■ From implantation through the 8th week of pregnancy, the developing child is known as an **embryo** (**EM**-bree-oh).

■ From the 9th week of pregnancy to the time of birth, the developing child in utero is known as a **fetus** (**fet** means unborn child, and **-us** is a singular noun ending). *In utero* means within the uterus (Figure 14.9).

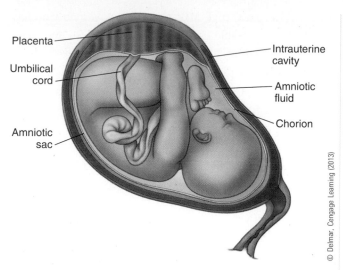

FIGURE 14.9 A normal pregnant uterus viewed in cross-section.

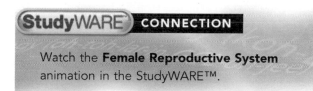

Watch the **Female Reproductive System** animation in the StudyWARE™.

## Multiple Births

If more than one egg is passing down the fallopian tube when sperm are present, the fertilization of more than one egg is possible.

- **Fraternal twins** result from the fertilization of separate ova by separate sperm cells. These develop into two separate embryos (Figure 14.10).

- **Identical twins** are formed by the fertilization of a single egg cell by a single sperm that divides to form two embryos. Each of these twins receives exactly the same genetic information from the parents.

- The term **multiples** is used to describe a birth involving more than two infants.

## The Chorion and Placenta

- The **chorion** (**KOR**-ee-on) is the thin outer membrane that encloses the embryo. It contributes to the formation of the placenta (Figure 14.9).

- The **placenta** (plah-**SEN**-tah) is a temporary organ that forms within the uterus to allow the exchange of nutrients, oxygen, and waste products between the mother and fetus without allowing maternal blood and fetal blood to mix. The placental barrier does not, however, keep chemicals and/or drugs from reaching the fetus.

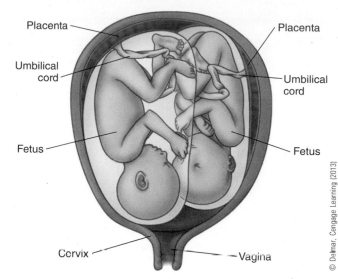

FIGURE 14.10 Fraternal twins in utero.

- The placenta also produces hormones necessary to maintain the pregnancy. These hormones are discussed in Chapter 13.

- After delivery of the newborn, the placenta and fetal membranes are expelled as the **afterbirth**.

## The Amniotic Sac

The **amniotic sac** (**am**-nee-**OT**-ick), which is also known as the *amnion*, is the innermost membrane that surrounds the embryo in the uterus (Figure 14.9). The common name for this structure is the *bag of waters*.

- The developing embryo is surrounded by the **amniotic cavity**. This is the fluid-filled space between the embryo and the amniotic sac.

- **Amnionic fluid** (**am**-nee-**ON**-ick), also known as *amniotic fluid*, is the liquid that protects the fetus and makes possible its floating movements.

## The Umbilical Cord

The **umbilical cord** (um-**BILL**-ih-kal) is the tube that carries blood, oxygen, and nutrients from the placenta to the developing child. It also transports waste from the fetus to be disposed of through the mother's excretory system. This cord is cut soon after the birth of the infant and before the delivery of the placenta.

- After birth, the **navel**, also known as the *belly button*, is formed where the umbilical cord was attached to the fetus.

## Gestation

**Gestation** (jes-**TAY**-shun), which lasts approximately 280 days (40 weeks), is the period of development of the child in the mother's uterus. Upon completion of this developmental time, the fetus is described as being *at term* and should be ready for birth (Figure 14.11).

- The term **pregnancy**, which is often used interchangeably with *gestation*, means the condition of having a developing child in the uterus.

- The length of pregnancy is described according to the number of weeks of gestation (usually 40 weeks total). For descriptive purposes, pregnancy can also be divided into three **trimesters** of about 13 weeks each.

- The **due date**, or *estimated date of confinement*, is calculated from the first day of the last menstrual period (LMP). *Confinement* is an old-fashioned term describing the period of rest for the mother that followed childbirth.

- **Quickening** is the first movement of the fetus in the uterus that can be felt by the mother. This usually occurs during the 16th to 20th week of pregnancy.

- **Braxton Hicks contractions** are intermittent painless uterine contractions that occur with increasing frequently as the pregnancy progresses. These contractions are not true labor pains and are usually infrequent, irregular, and essentially painless.

- The fetus is described as being **viable** when it is capable of living outside the uterus. Viability depends on the developmental age, birth weight, and developmental stage of the lungs of the fetus.

- The term **antepartum** (**an**-tee-**PAHR**-tum) refers to the final stage of pregnancy just before the onset of labor.

## The Mother

- A **nulligravida** (null-ih-**GRAV**-ih-dah) is a woman who has never been pregnant (**nulli-** means none, and **-gravida** means pregnant). Compare with *nullipara*.

- A **nullipara** (nuh-**LIP**-ah-rah) is a woman who has never borne a viable child (**nulli-** means none, and **-para** means to bring forth). Compare with *nulligravida*.

- A **primigravida** (**prye**-mih-**GRAV**-ih-dah) is a woman during her first pregnancy (**primi-** means first, and **-gravida** means pregnant). Compare with *primipara*.

- A **primipara** (prye-**MIP**-ah-rah) is a woman who has borne one viable child (**primi-** means first, and **-para** means to bring forth). Compare with *primigravida*.

- **Multiparous** (mul-**TIP**-ah-rus) means a woman who has given birth two or more times (**multi-** means many, and **-parous** means having borne one or more children).

## Childbirth

**Labor and delivery**, also known as *childbirth* or *parturition*, occurs in three stages, shown in Figure 14.11. The stages of labor and delivery are:

1. Dilation
2. Delivery of the baby
3. Expulsion of the afterbirth

### The First Stage

During the first (and longest) stage of labor, the changes that occur include the gradual **dilation** (dye-**LAY**-shun) and effacement of the cervix and the rupture of the amniotic sac. *Effacement* is the process by which the cervix prepares for delivery as it gradually softens, shortens, and becomes thinner (Figure 14.11B).

- **Fetal monitoring** is the use of an electronic device to record the fetal heart rate and the maternal uterine contractions during labor.

### The Second Stage

The second stage, which begins when the cervix is dilated to 10 centimeters, is the delivery of the infant. As the uterine contractions become stronger and more frequent, the mother pushes to help expel the child through the *birth canal* (vagina). Normally, the baby's head presents first. **Cephalic presentation** or *crowning* describes when the baby is coming head first. The head can be seen at the vaginal opening (Figure 14.11C).

### The Third Stage

The third stage is the expulsion of the placenta as the *afterbirth* (Figure 14.11D).

## Postpartum

The term **postpartum** (pohst-**PAR**-tum) means after childbirth.

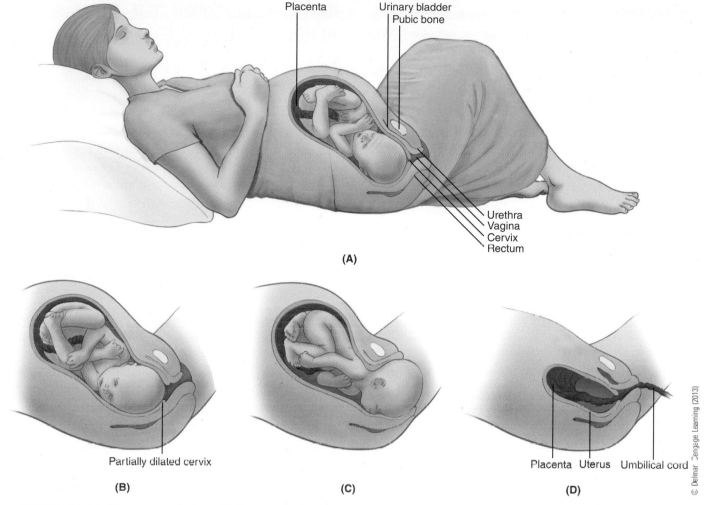

**FIGURE 14.11** The stages of labor. (A) Position of the fetus before labor. (B) First state of labor, cervical dilation. (C) Second stage of labor, fetal delivery. (D) Third stage of labor, delivery of the afterbirth (placenta and fetal membranes).

## The Mother

■ **Puerperium** (**pyou**-er-**PEE**-ree-um) is the time from the delivery of the placenta through approximately the first 6 weeks after the delivery. By the end of this period, most of the changes in the mother's body due to pregnancy have resolved, and the body has reverted to the nonpregnant state.

■ **Lochia** (**LOH**-kee-ah) is the postpartum vaginal discharge that typically continues for 4 to 6 weeks after childbirth (**loch** means childbirth, and **-ia** means pertaining to). It consists primarily of blood and mucus.

■ **Uterine involution** is the return of the uterus to its normal size and former condition after delivery. *Involution* means the return of an enlarged organ to its normal size.

■ **Colostrum** (kuh-**LOS**-trum) is a specialized form of milk that delivers essential nutrients and antibodies in a form that the newborn can digest. Colostrum is produced by the mammary glands in late pregnancy and during the first few days after giving birth.

■ **Lactation** (lack-**TAY**-shun) is the process of forming and secreting milk from the breasts as nourishment for the infant. The breast milk develops a few days after giving birth to replace the colostrum.

■ **Postpartum depression** is a mood disorder characterized by feelings of sadness and the loss of pleasure in normal activities that can occur shortly after giving birth. One cause of this depression is the rapid change in the hormone levels that occurs after giving birth. When the depression is severe, treatment is required.

## The Baby

The newborn infant is known as a **neonate** (NEE-oh-nayt) during the first 4 weeks after birth.

- **Vernix** (VER-nicks) is a greasy substance that protects the fetus in utero and can still be present at birth.

- **Meconium** (meh-KOH-nee-um) is the greenish material that collects in the intestine of a fetus and forms the first stools of a newborn.

## Apgar Scores

An **Apgar score** is a scale of 1 to 10 to evaluate a newborn infant's physical status at 1 and 5 minutes after birth.

- The newborn is evaluated by assigning numerical values (0 to 2) to each of five criteria: (1) heart rate, (2) respiratory effort, (3) muscle tone, (4) response stimulation, and (5) skin color.

- A total score of 8 to 10 indicates the best possible condition.

# ◼ MEDICAL SPECIALTIES RELATED TO THE FEMALE REPRODUCTIVE SYSTEM AND CHILDBIRTH

- A **gynecologist** (guy-neh-KOL-oh-jist), or GYN, is a physician who specializes in diagnosing and treating diseases and disorders of the female reproductive system (**gynec** means female, and **-ologist** means specialist).

- An **obstetrician** (ob-steh-TRISH-un), or OB, is a physician who specializes in providing medical care to women during pregnancy, childbirth, and immediately thereafter. This specialty is referred to as *obstetrics*.

- A *midwife* assists in labor and delivery. A certified nurse midwife (CNM) is an RN with specialized training in obstetrics and gynecology who provides primary care in normal pregnancies and deliveries.

- A **neonatologist** (nee-oh-nay-TOL-oh-jist) is a physician who specializes in diagnosing and treating disorders of the newborn (**neo-** means new, **nat** means born, and **-ologist** means specialist).

- An **infertility specialist**, also known as a *fertility specialist* helps infertile couples by diagnosing and treating problems associated with conception and maintaining pregnancy.

# ◼ PATHOLOGY OF THE FEMALE REPRODUCTIVE SYSTEM

## The Ovaries, Fallopian Tubes, and Ovulation

- **Anovulation** (an-ov-you-LAY-shun) is the absence of ovulation when it would be normally expected (**an-** means without, and **ovulation** means the release of a mature egg). This condition can be caused by stress, inadequate nutrition, or hormonal imbalances. Menstruation can continue, although ovulation does not occur.

- **Oophoritis** (oh-ahf-oh-RYE-tis) is inflammation of an ovary (**oophor** means ovary, and **-itis** means inflammation). This condition frequently occurs when salpingitis or pelvic inflammatory disease are present.

- **Ovarian cancer** originates within the cells of the ovaries. These cancer cells can break away from the ovary and spread (metastasize) to other tissues and organs within the abdomen or travel through the bloodstream to other parts of the body.

- **Ovariorrhexis** (oh-vay-ree-oh-RECK-sis) is the rupture of an ovary (**ovari/o** means ovary, and **-rrhexis** means to rupture).

- **Pelvic inflammatory disease** (PID) is any inflammation of the female reproductive organs that is not associated with surgery or pregnancy. This condition occurs most frequently as a complication of a sexually transmitted disease and can lead to infertility, ectopic pregnancy, and other serious disorders.

- **Polycystic ovary syndrome** (pol-ee-SIS-tick), also known as PCOS, is a condition caused by a hormonal imbalance in which the ovaries are enlarged by the presence of many cysts formed by incompletely developed follicles.

- **Pyosalpinx** (pye-oh-SAL-pinks) is an accumulation of pus in a fallopian tube (**py/o** means pus, and **-salpinx** means fallopian tube).

- **Salpingitis** (sal-pin-JIGH-tis) is an inflammation of a fallopian tube (**salping** means fallopian tube, and **-itis** means inflammation).

## The Uterus

- **Endometriosis** (en-doh-mee-tree-OH-sis) is a condition in which patches of endometrial tissue escape the uterus and become attached to other structures in the pelvic cavity (**endo-** means within, **metri** means uterus, and **-osis** means abnormal condition). It is a leading cause of infertility.

■ **Metrorrhea** (**mee**-troh-**REE**-ah) is an abnormal discharge, such as mucus or pus, from the uterus (**metr/o** means uterus, and **-rrhea** means flow or discharge).

■ **Endometrial cancer** (en-doh-**MEE**-tree-al) involves a cancerous growth that begins in the lining of the uterus. One of the earliest symptoms of this cancer that frequently occurs after menopause is abnormal bleeding from the uterus.

■ A **uterine fibroid**, also known as a *myoma*, is a benign tumor composed of muscle and fibrous tissue that occurs in the wall of the uterus (Figure 14.12).

■ A **uterine prolapse** (proh-**LAPS**), also known as a *pelvic floor hernia*, is the condition in which the uterus slides from its normal position in the pelvic cavity and sags into the vagina. *Prolapse* means the falling or dropping down of an organ or internal part.

## The Cervix

■ **Cervical cancer** is the second-most common cancer in women and usually affects women between the ages of 45 and 65 years. It is caused by human papillomaviruses (HPV), which can now be prevented through vaccination and can be detected early through routine Pap tests.

■ **Cervical dysplasia** (**SER**-vih-kal dis-**PLAY**-see-ah) is the presence of precancerous changes in the cells that make up the inner lining of the cervix. Without early detection and treatment, these cells can become malignant.

■ **Cervicitis** (**ser**-vih-**SIGH**-tis) is an inflammation of the cervix that is usually caused by an infection (**cervic** means cervix, and **-itis** means inflammation).

■ **Endocervicitis** (en-doh-**ser**-vih-**SIGH**-tis) is an inflammation of the mucous membrane lining of the cervix (**endo-** means within, **cervic** means cervix, and **-itis** means inflammation).

## The Vagina

■ **Colporrhexis** (**kol**-poh-**RECK**-sis) means tearing or laceration of the vaginal wall (**colp/o** means vagina, and **-rrhexis** means to rupture). A *laceration* is a torn, ragged wound or an accidental cut.

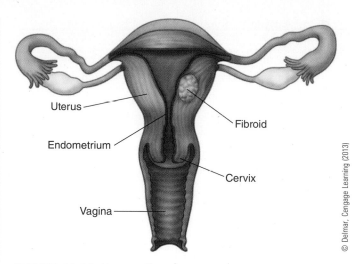

**FIGURE 14.12** Uterine fibroid.

*© Delmar, Cengage Learning (2013)*

■ **Dyspareunia** (**dis**-pah-**ROO**-nee-ah) is characterized by pain during sexual intercourse (**dys** means painful and **-pareunia** means sexual intercourse).

■ **Leukorrhea** (**loo**-koh-**REE**-ah) is a profuse, whitish mucus discharge from the uterus and vagina (**leuk/o** means white, and **-rrhea** means flow or discharge). Women normally may have some vaginal discharge; however, leukorrhea describes a change and increase in this discharge that can be due to an infection, malignancy, or hormonal changes.

■ **Vaginal candidiasis** (**kan**-dih-**DYE**-ah-sis), also known as a *yeast infection*, is a vaginal infection caused by the yeast-like fungus *Candida albicans*. The growth of this fungus is usually controlled by bacteria normally present in the vagina. When these bacteria are not able to control fungal growth, symptoms occur that include burning, itching, and a "cottage cheese-like" vaginal discharge.

■ **Vaginitis** (**vaj**-ih-**NIGH**-tis), also known as *colpitis*, is an inflammation of the lining of the vagina (**vagin** and **colp** both mean vagina, and **-itis** means inflammation). The most common causes of a vaginal inflammation are bacterial vaginosis, trichomoniasis, and vaginal candidiasis (discussed in the section "Sexually Transmitted Diseases").

## The External Genitalia

■ **Pruritus vulvae** (proo-**RYE**-tus **VUL**-vee) is a condition of severe itching of the external female genitalia. *Pruritus* means itching.

- **Vulvodynia** (vul-voh-**DIN**-ee-ah) is a painful syndrome of unknown cause (**vulv/o** means vulva, and **-dynia** means pain). It is characterized by chronic burning, pain during sexual intercourse, itching, or stinging irritation of the vulva.

- **Vulvitis** (vul-**VYE**-tis) is an inflammation of the vulva (**vulv** means vulva, and **-itis** means inflammation). Possible causes include fungal or bacterial infections, chafing, skin conditions, or allergies to products such as soaps and bubble bath.

## Breast Diseases

- **Breast cancer**, its diagnosis and treatment, are discussed in Chapter 6.

- A **fibroadenoma** (**figh**-broh-**ad**-eh-**NOH**-mah) is a round, firm, rubbery mass that arises from excess growth of glandular and connective tissue in the breast (Figure 14.13). These masses, which can grow to the size of a small plum, are benign and usually painless. Fibroadenomas often enlarge during pregnancy and shrink during menopause.

- **Fibrocystic breast disease** (**figh**-broh-**SIS**-tick) is the presence of single or multiple benign cysts in the breasts. This condition occurs more frequently in older women. A *cyst* is a closed sac containing fluid or semisolid material.

- **Galactorrhea** (gah-**lack**-toh-**REE**-ah) is the production of breast milk in a woman who is not breastfeeding (**galact/o** means milk, and **-rrhea** means flow or discharge). This condition is caused by a malfunction of the thyroid or pituitary gland.

- **Mastalgia** (mass-**TAL**-jee-ah), also known as *mastodynia*, is pain in the breast (**mast** means breast, and **-algia** means pain).

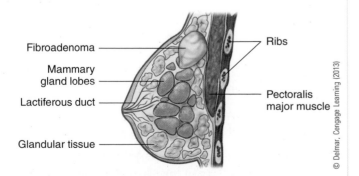

Fibroadenoma
Mammary gland lobes
Lactiferous duct
Glandular tissue
Ribs
Pectoralis major muscle

© Delmar, Cengage Learning (2013)

**FIGURE 14.13** A fibroadenoma of the breast.

- **Mastitis** (mas-**TYE**-tis) is a breast infection that is caused by bacteria that enter the breast tissue, most frequently during breastfeeding (**mast** means breast, and **-itis** means inflammation).

## Menstrual Disorders

- **Amenorrhea** (ah-**men**-oh-**REE**-ah) is an abnormal absence of menstrual periods for 90 days or more (**a-** means without, **men/o** means menstruation, and **-rrhea** means flow or discharge). This condition, which is normal only before puberty, during pregnancy, while breastfeeding, and after menopause, can be caused by stress, hormonal problems, poor nutrition, or excessive exercise.

- **Dysmenorrhea** (**dis**-men-oh-**REE**-ah) is pain caused by uterine cramps during a menstrual period (**dys-** means bad, **men/o** means menstruation, and **-rrhea** means flow or discharge). This pain, which occurs in the lower abdomen, can be sharp, intermittent, dull, or aching.

- **Dysfunctional uterine bleeding** (DUB) is a condition characterized by abnormal bleeding often due to an imbalance in hormone level changes.

- **Hypermenorrhea** (**high**-per-men-oh-**REE**-ah), also known as *menorrhagia*, is an excessive amount of menstrual flow over a period of more than 7 days (**hyper-** means excessive, **men/o** means menstruation, and **-rrhea** means flow or discharge). Hypermenorrhea is the opposite of *hypomenorrhea*.

- **Hypomenorrhea** (**high**-poh-men-oh-**REE**-ah) is an unusually small amount of menstrual flow during a shortened regular menstrual period (**hypo-** means deficient, **men/o** means menstruation, and **-rrhea** means flow or discharge). Hypomenorrhea is the opposite of *hypermenorrhea*.

- **Menometrorrhagia** (**men**-oh-**met**-roh-**RAY**-jee-ah), also known as *intermenstrual bleeding*, is excessive uterine bleeding at both the usual time of menstrual periods and at other irregular intervals (**men/o** means menstruation, **metr/o** means uterus, and **-rrhagia** means abnormal bleeding).

- **Oligomenorrhea** (**ol**-ih-goh-**men**-oh-**REE**-ah) is the term used to describe infrequent or very light menstruation in a woman with previously normal periods (**olig/o** means scanty, **men/o** means menstruation, and **-rrhea** means flow or discharge). Oligomenorrhea is the opposite of *polymenorrhea*.

- **Polymenorrhea** (**pol**-ee-**men**-oh-**REE**-ah) is the occurrence of menstrual cycles more frequently than is normal (**poly-** means many, **men/o** means menstruation, and **-rrhea** means flow or discharge). Polymenorrhea is the opposite of *oligomenorrhea*.

- **Premature menopause** is a condition in which the ovaries cease functioning before age 40 years due to disease, a hormonal disorder, or surgical removal. This causes infertility and often brings on menopausal symptoms.

- **Premenstrual syndrome** (PMS) is a group of symptoms experienced by some women within the 2-week period before menstruation. These symptoms can include bloating, swelling, headaches, mood swings, and breast discomfort.

- **Premenstrual dysphoric disorder** (PMDD) is a condition associated with severe emotional and physical problems that are closely linked to the menstrual cycle. Symptoms occur regularly in the second half of the cycle and end when menstruation begins or shortly thereafter.

## PATHOLOGY OF PREGNANCY AND CHILDBIRTH

### Pregnancy

- An **abortion** (ah-**BOR**-shun) is the interruption or termination of pregnancy before the fetus is viable. A *spontaneous abortion*, also known as a *miscarriage*, usually occurs early in the pregnancy and is due to an abnormality or genetic disorder.

- An *induced abortion*, caused by human intervention, is achieved through the use of drugs or suctioning. When done for medical purposes, it is known as a *therapeutic abortion*.

- An **ectopic pregnancy** (eck-**TOP**-ick), also known as an *extrauterine pregnancy*, is a potentially dangerous condition in which a fertilized egg is implanted and begins to develop outside of the uterus. *Ectopic* means out of place, and Figure 14.14 illustrates some of these potential locations.

- **Gestational diabetes mellitus** is discussed in Chapter 13.

- **Infertility** is the inability of a couple to achieve pregnancy after 1 year of regular, unprotected intercourse, or the inability of a woman to carry a pregnancy to a live birth.

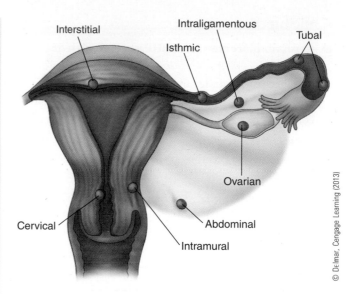

**FIGURE 14.14** Potential sites of an ectopic pregnancy.

- **Preeclampsia** (**pree**-ee-**KLAMP**-see-ah), also known as *pregnancy-induced hypertension* or *toxemia*, is a complication of pregnancy characterized by hypertension (high blood pressure), edema (swelling), and proteinuria (an abnormally high level of protein in the urine).

- **Eclampsia** (eh-**KLAMP**-see-ah), which is a more serious form of preeclampsia, is characterized by convulsions and sometimes coma. Treatment for this condition includes the delivery of the fetus.

### The Rh Factor

The **Rh factor** defines the presence or absence of the Rh antigen on red blood cells. (See Chapter 5.) The Rh factor can cause difficulties when an Rh negative (Rh−) mother is pregnant with an Rh positive (Rh+) baby. If a small amount of the baby's blood enters the mother's bloodstream, she can develop antibodies in an allergic response.

- A man who is Rh+ can father a baby that is either Rh+ or Rh−, potentially causing a reaction if the mother is Rh−. (If both parents are Rh−, there is no danger of incompatibility.)

- The antibodies that develop in the mother's body during pregnancy can cause anemia and other problems for the baby, and also be a factor in subsequent pregnancies if the mother is not treated.

- Blood tests of both parents can identify this potential problem. If it exists, the mother is vaccinated with a blood product called *Rh immunoglobulin* (RhIg).

## Childbirth

- **Abruptio placentae** (ah-**BRUP**-shee-oh plah-**SEN**-tee), or *placental abruption*, is a disorder in which the placenta separates from the uterine wall before the birth of the fetus. *Abruption* means breaking off. This condition is a leading cause of fetal death.

- **Breech presentation** occurs when the buttocks or feet of the fetus are positioned to enter the birth canal first instead of the head.

- **Placenta previa** (plah-**SEN**-tah **PREE**-vee-ah) is the abnormal implantation of the placenta in the lower portion of the uterus. *Previa* means appearing before or in front of. Symptoms include painless, sudden-onset bleeding during the third trimester.

- A **premature infant**, also known as a *preemie*, is a fetus born before the 37th week of gestation.

- A **stillbirth** is the birth of a fetus that died before, or during, delivery.

## ◼ DIAGNOSTIC PROCEDURES OF THE FEMALE REPRODUCTIVE SYSTEM

- **Colposcopy** (kol-**POS**-koh-pee) is the direct visual examination of the tissues of the cervix and vagina (**colp/o** means vagina, and **-scopy** means direct visual examination). This examination is performed using a binocular magnifier known as a *colposcope*.

- In an **endometrial biopsy**, a small amount of the tissue from the lining of the uterus is removed for microscopic examination. This test is most often used to determine the cause of abnormal vaginal bleeding.

- **Endovaginal ultrasound** (en-doh-**VAJ**-ih-nal) is performed to determine the cause of abnormal vaginal bleeding. This test is performed by placing an ultrasound transducer in the vagina so that the sound waves can create images of the uterus and ovaries.

- **Hysterosalpingography** (**hiss**-ter-oh-**sal**-pin-**GOG**-rah-fee) (HSG) is a radiographic examination of the uterus and fallopian tubes (**hyster/o** means uterus, **salping/o** means tube, and **-graphy** means the process of producing a picture or record). This test requires the instillation of radio-opaque contrast material into the uterine cavity and fallopian tubes to make them visible. *Instillation* means slowly pouring a liquid onto a body part or into a body cavity.

- **Hysteroscopy** (HYS) (**hiss**-ter-**OSS**-koh-pee) is the direct visual examination of the interior of the uterus and fallopian tubes (**hyster/o** means uterus, and **-scopy** means direct visual examination). This examination is performed by using the magnification of a *hysteroscope*.

- A **Pap smear** is an exfoliative biopsy of the cervix. It is performed to detect conditions that can be early indicators of cervical cancer (Figure 14.15). As used here, *exfoliative* means that cells are scraped from the tissue and examined under a microscope. A *speculum* is used to enlarge the opening of the vagina during the examination of the cervix and vagina.

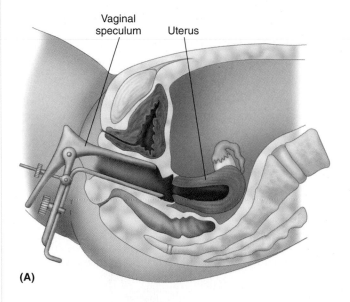

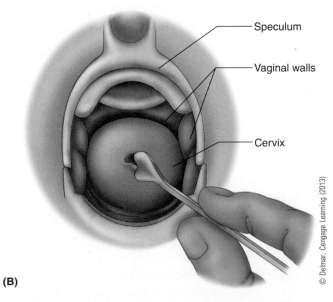

**FIGURE 14.15** For a pap smear, a speculum is used to enlarge the vaginal opening (A) and a few cervical cells are removed for study under a microscope (B).

■ *Ultrasound* and *laparoscopy*, which are also used to diagnose disorders of the reproductive system, are discussed further in Chapter 15.

## Diagnostic Procedures Related to Pregnancy and Childbirth

■ A **pregnancy test** is performed to detect an unusually high level of the *human chorionic gonadotropin* (HCG) hormone in either a blood or urine specimen, which is usually an indication of pregnancy. A home pregnancy test uses a urine specimen, whereas a pregnancy test based on a blood specimen at a doctor's office usually provides more reliable results.

■ **Fetal ultrasound** testing is discussed in Chapter 15.

■ **First trimester screening**, also known as *combined screening*, is performed between 11 and 13 weeks of pregnancy and involves an ultrasound and a finger-stick blood test. The combined results of these two measurements, plus the mother's age, detect if the fetus is at increased risk for Down syndrome, which is discussed in Chapter 2. Diagnostic tests, such as amniocentesis or chorionic villus sampling, are recommended for those at increased risk for this condition.

■ **Chorionic villus sampling** (CVS) (**kor**-ee-**ON**-ick **VIL**-us) is the examination of cells retrieved from the chorionic villi, which are minute, vascular projections on the chorion. This test is performed between the 8th and 10th weeks of pregnancy to search for genetic abnormalities in the developing fetus.

■ **Amniocentesis** (AMN) (**am**-nee-oh-sen-**TEE**-sis) is a surgical puncture with a needle to obtain a specimen of amniotic fluid (**amnio** means amnion and fetal membrane, and **-centesis** means a surgical puncture to remove fluid). This specimen, which is usually obtained after the 14th week of pregnancy, is used to evaluate fetal health and to diagnose certain congenital disorders.

■ **Pelvimetry** (pel-**VIM**-eh-tree) is a radiographic study to measure the dimensions of the pelvis to evaluate its capacity to allow passage of the fetus through the birth canal (**pelvi** means pelvis, and **-metry** means to measure).

## ■ TREATMENT PROCEDURES OF THE FEMALE REPRODUCTIVE SYSTEM

### Medications

■ A **contraceptive** is a measure taken to lessen the likelihood of pregnancy.

■ *Birth control pills* are a form of hormones that are administered as an oral contraceptive. Other forms of this type of contraceptive are available as an injection, a patch, and an inserted ring.

■ A **diaphragm** is a barrier contraceptive that prevents the sperm from reaching and fertilizing the egg.

■ An **intrauterine device** (IUD) is a molded plastic contraceptive inserted through the cervix into the uterus to prevent pregnancy (**intra-** means within, and **uterine** means uterus).

■ A **condom** will also prevent pregnancy when used correctly. It is the only contraceptive method mentioned here that will also prevent the transmission of sexually transmitted diseases (STDs).

■ **Hormone replacement therapy** (HRT) is the use of the female hormones estrogen and progestin to replace those the body no longer produces during and after perimenopause. *Progestin* is a synthetic form of the female hormone progesterone.

### The Ovaries and Fallopian Tubes

■ An **oophorectomy** (**oh**-ahf-oh-**RECK**-toh-mee), also known as an *ovariectomy*, is the surgical removal of one or both ovaries (**oophor** mean ovary, and **-ectomy** means surgical removal). If both ovaries are removed in a premenopausal woman, the patient experiences *surgical menopause*.

■ A **salpingectomy** (**sal**-pin-**JECK**-toh-mee) is the surgical removal of one or both fallopian tubes (**salping** means tube, and **-ectomy** means surgical removal).

■ A **salpingo-oophorectomy** (SO) (sal-**ping**-goh oh-**ahf**-oh-**RECK**-toh-mee) is the surgical removal of a fallopian tube and ovary (**salping/o** means tube, **oophor** means ovary, and **-ectomy** means surgical removal). A *bilateral salpingo-oophorectomy* is the removal of both of the fallopian tubes and ovaries.

- **Tubal ligation** is a surgical sterilization procedure in which the fallopian tubes are sealed or cut to prevent sperm from reaching a mature ovum.

## The Uterus, Cervix, and Vagina

- A **colpopexy** (**KOL**-poh-**peck**-see), also known as *vaginofixation*, is the surgical fixation of a prolapsed vagina to a surrounding structure such as the abdominal wall (**colp/o** means vagina, and **-pexy** means surgical fixation in place).

- **Conization** (**kon**-ih-**ZAY**-shun), also known as a *cone biopsy*, is the surgical removal of a cone-shaped specimen of tissue from the cervix. This is performed as a diagnostic procedure or to remove abnormal tissue.

- **Colporrhaphy** (kol-**POR**-ah-fee) is the surgical suturing of a tear in the vagina (**colp/o** means vagina, and **-rrhaphy** means surgical suturing).

- **Dilation and curettage** (dye-**LAY**-shun and **kyou**-reh-**TAHZH**), commonly known as a *D & C*, is a surgical procedure in which the cervix is dilated and the endometrium of the uterus is scraped away. This can be performed as a diagnostic or a treatment procedure. *Dilation* means the expansion of an opening. *Curettage* is the removal of material from the surface by scraping with an instrument known as a curette.

- A **myomectomy** (**my**-oh-**MECK**-toh-mee) is the surgical removal of uterine fibroids (**myom** means muscle tumor, and **-ectomy** means surgical removal).

## Hysterectomies

A **hysterectomy** (**hiss**-teh-**RECK**-toh-mee) is the surgical removal of the uterus (**hyster** means uterus, and **-ectomy** means surgical removal). The procedure is further described depending upon the structures that are removed (Figure 14.16).

- In a **total hysterectomy**, also known as a *complete hysterectomy*, the uterus and cervix are removed. This procedure can be performed through the vagina or laparoscopically through the abdomen.

- In a *partial* or *subtotal hysterectomy*, the uterus is removed and the cervix is left in place.

- A **radical hysterectomy**, also known as a *bilateral hysterosalpingo-oophorectomy*, is most commonly performed to treat uterine cancer (Figure 14.16B). This procedure includes the surgical removal of the ovaries and fallopian tubes, the uterus and cervix, plus nearby

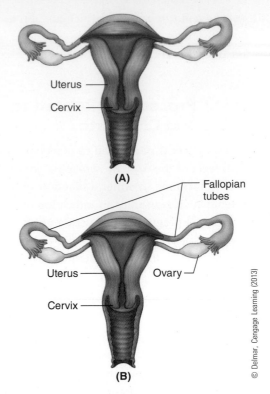

**FIGURE 14.16** Types of hysterectomies, with the areas removed shown in blue. (A) In a total hysterectomy, the uterus and cervix are removed. (B) In a radical hysterectomy, the ovaries, fallopian tubes, uterus, and cervix are removed.

© Delmar, Cengage Learning (2013)

lymph nodes. If this surgery is performed before natural menopause, the patient immediately experiences *surgical menopause*.

## Mammoplasty

**Mammoplasty** (**MAM**-oh-**plas**-tee), also spelled *mammaplasty*, is a general term for a cosmetic operation on the breasts (**mamm/o** means breast, and **-plasty** means surgical repair).

- **Breast augmentation** is mammoplasty performed to increase breast size. *Augmentation* means the process of adding to make larger. Breast augmentation is the opposite of breast reduction.

- **Breast reduction** is mammoplasty performed to decrease and reshape excessively large, heavy breasts. Breast reduction is the opposite of breast augmentation.

- **Mastopexy** (**MAS**-toh-**peck**-see), also called a breast lift, is a mammoplasty to affix sagging breasts in a more elevated position (**mast/o** means breast, and **-pexy** means surgical fixation).

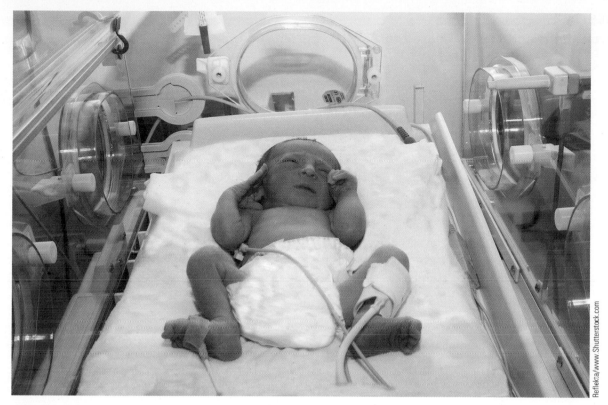

**FIGURE 14.17** An incubator provides a newborn infant with an environment of the controlled temperature, humidity, and oxygen.

■ *Breast reconstruction* following a mastectomy is discussed in Chapter 6.

## Treatment Procedures Related to Pregnancy and Childbirth

■ A **cesarean section** (seh-**ZEHR**-ee-un **SECK**-shun), also known as a *C-section*, is the delivery of the child through an incision in the maternal abdominal and uterine walls. This is usually performed when a vaginal birth would be unsafe for either the mother or baby.

■ *VBAC* is the acronym used to describe **v**aginal **b**irth **a**fter a **c**esarean.

■ An **episiotomy** (eh-**piz**-ee-**OT**-oh-mee) is a surgical incision made into the perineum to enlarge the vaginal orifice to prevent tearing of the tissues as the infant moves out of the birth canal (**episi** means vulva, and **-otomy** means a surgical incision).

■ An **episiorrhaphy** (eh-**piz**-ee-**OR**-ah-fee) is the surgical suturing to repair an episiotomy (**episi/o** means vulva, and **-rrhaphy** means surgical suturing).

■ An **incubator** (**IN**-kyou-**bate**-or) is an apparatus for maintaining an environment of controlled

temperature, humidity, and oxygen concentration for a premature or ill newborn (Figure 14.17).

## Assisted Reproduction

The term **assisted reproductive technology** describes techniques used to aid an infertile couple in achieving a viable pregnancy.

■ **Artificial insemination**, also called intrauterine insemination (IUI), is a technique in which sperm from a woman's partner or from a donor are introduced into the vagina or uterus during the ovulatory phase of her menstrual cycle.

■ **In vitro fertilization** is a procedure in which mature ova are removed from the mother to be fertilized. The resulting embryos are transferred into the uterus with the hope that they will implant and continue to develop as in a normal pregnancy. *In vitro* means in an artificial environment such as a test tube.

■ A *gestational carrier* is an option for a woman with ovaries but no uterus. Her egg is fertilized by her partner's sperm and placed inside another woman's uterus (the carrier).

**TABLE 14.2**

**Abbreviations and Terms Related to Assisted Fertilization**

| | |
|---|---|
| **AMA** | **Advanced maternal age** is the term applied to women in their late 30s to late 40s. As one of these women age, the possibility of her becoming pregnant decreases. |
| **AI** | **Artificial insemination** is a technique in which sperm from a woman's partner or from a donor are introduced into the vagina or uterus during the ovulatory phase of her menstrual cycle. |
| **ART** | The term **assisted reproductive technology** describes techniques used to aid an infertile couple in achieving a viable pregnancy. |
| **IVF** | **In vitro fertilization** is a procedure in which mature ova are removed from the mother to be fertilized. The resulting embryos are transferred into the uterus with the hope that they will implant and continue to develop as a normal pregnancy. *In vitro* means in an artificial environment such as a test tube. |

■ A woman who volunteers to be inseminated with the sperm of a man who is not her partner in order to conceive and carry a child for the man and his partner is referred to as a *surrogate*.

## ■ ABBREVIATIONS RELATED TO THE REPRODUCTIVE SYSTEMS

Table 14.3 presents an overview of the abbreviations related to the terms introduced in this chapter. Note: To avoid errors or confusion, always be cautious when using abbreviations.

**StudyWARE CONNECTION**

For more practice and to test your mastery of this material, go to the StudyWARE™ to play interactive games and complete the quiz for this chapter.

**☐ Workbook Practice**

Go to your workbook, and complete the exercises for this chapter.

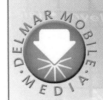

*Downloadable audio is available for selected medical terms in this chapter to enhance your learning of medical terminology.*

## TABLE 14.3
### Abbreviations Related to the Reproductive Systems

| | |
|---|---|
| amniocentesis = AMN | AMN = amniocentesis |
| bacterial vaginosis = BV | BV = bacterial vaginosis |
| cesarean section = CS | CS = cesarean section |
| hormone replacement therapy = HRT | HRT = hormone replacement therapy |
| human papillomaviruses = HPV | HPV = human papillomaviruses |
| hysterosalpingography = HSG | HSG = hysterosalpingography |
| hysteroscopy = HYS | HYS = hysteroscopy |
| intrauterine device = IUD | IUD = intrauterine device |
| labor and delivery = L & D | L & D = labor and delivery |
| neonatal intensive care unit = NICU | NICU = neonatal intensive care unit |
| pelvic inflammatory disease = PID | PID = pelvic inflammatory disease |
| premenstrual syndrome = PMS | PMS = premenstrual syndrome |

# LEARNING EXERCISES

## MATCHING WORD PARTS 1

Write the correct answer in the middle column.

| Definition | Correct Answer | Possible Answers |
|---|---|---|
| 14.1. cervix | _____ | **men/o** |
| 14.2. female | _____ | **gynec/o** |
| 14.3. menstruation | _____ | **-gravida** |
| 14.4. pregnant | _____ | **colp/o** |
| 14.5. vagina | _____ | **cervic/o** |

## MATCHING WORD PARTS 2

Write the correct answer in the middle column.

| Definition | Correct Answer | Possible Answers |
|---|---|---|
| 14.6. egg | _____ | **vagin/o** |
| 14.7. ovary | _____ | **test/i** |
| 14.8. testicle | _____ | **ov/o** |
| 14.9. uterus | _____ | **ovari/o** |
| 14.10. vagina | _____ | **hyster/o** |

## MATCHING WORD PARTS 3

Write the correct answer in the middle column.

| Definition | Correct Answer | Possible Answers |
|---|---|---|
| 14.11. breast | _____ | **salping/o** |
| 14.12. none | _____ | **-pexy** |

14.13. surgical fixation _____ -para

14.14. to give birth _____ nulli-

14.15. tube _____ mast/o

## DEFINITIONS

Select the correct answer, and write it on the line provided.

14.16. The term that describes the inner layer of the uterus is _____.

corpus　　　endometrium　　　myometrium　　　perimetrium

14.17. The term describing the single cells formed immediately after conception is _____.

embryo　　　fetus　　　gamete　　　zygote

14.18. The mucus that lubricates the vagina is produced by the _____.

Bartholin's glands　　　bulbourethral glands　　　Cowper's glands　　　hymen glands

14.19. The finger-like structures of the fallopian tube that catch the ovum are the _____.

fimbriae　　　fundus　　　infundibulum　　　oviducts

14.20. The term _____ is used to designate the transition phase between regular menstrual periods and no periods at all.

menarche　　　menopause　　　perimenopause　　　puberty

14.21. The medical term for the condition also known as a yeast infection is _____.

colporrhea　　　leukorrhea　　　pruritus vulvae　　　vaginal candidiasis

14.22. Sperm are formed within the _____ of each testicle.

ejaculatory ducts　　　epididymis　　　seminiferous tubules　　　urethra

14.23. During puberty, the term _____ describes the beginning of the menstrual function.

menarche　　　menopause　　　menses　　　menstruation

14.24. In the female, the region between the vaginal orifice and the anus is known as the _____.

clitoris　　　mons pubis　　　perineum　　　vulva

14.25. The release of a mature egg by the ovary is known as _____.

coitus            fertilization            menstruation            ovulation

## MATCHING STRUCTURES

Write the correct answer in the middle column.

| Definition | Correct Answer | Possible Answers |
|---|---|---|
| 14.26. carry milk from the mammary glands | _____ | vulva |
| 14.27. surrounds the testicles | _____ | scrotum |
| 14.28. external female genitalia | _____ | lactiferous ducts |
| 14.29. protects the tip of the penis | _____ | foreskin |
| 14.30. sensitive tissue near the vaginal opening | _____ | clitoris |

## WHICH WORD?

Select the correct answer, and write it on the line provided.

14.31. The term used to describe a woman during her first pregnancy is a _____.

       primigravida            primipara

14.32. The fluid produced by the mammary glands during the first few days after giving birth

is _____.

       colostrum            meconium

14.33. The term _____ describes an inflammation of the cervix that is usually caused by

an infection.

       cervicitis            vulvitis

14.34. From implantation through the 8th week of pregnancy, the developing child is known as

a/an _____.

       embryo            fetus

14.35. A _____ is a woman who has never borne a viable child.

       nulligravida            nullipara

## SPELLING COUNTS

Find the misspelled word in each sentence. Then write that word, spelled correctly, on the line provided.

14.36.   The prostrate gland secretes a thick fluid that aids the motility of the sperm. _____

14.37.   The normal periodic discharge from the uterus is known as menstration. _____

14.38.   The third stage of labor and delivery is the expulsion of the plasenta as the

afterbirth. _____

14.39.   The term hemataspermia is the presence of blood in the seminal fluid. _____

14.40.   The surgical removal of the foreskin of the penis is known as cercumsion. _____

## ABBREVIATION IDENTIFICATION

In the space provided, write the words that each abbreviation stands for.

14.41.   **AMA**         _____

14.42.   **PID**         _____

14.43.   **PMDD**       _____

14.44.   **IUD**         _____

14.45.   **VD**          _____

## TERM SELECTION

Select the correct answer, and write it on the line provided.

14.46.   An accumulation of pus in the fallopian tube is known as _____.

oophoritis          pelvic inflammatory disease          pyosalpinx          salpingitis

14.47.   A _____ is a knot of widening varicose veins in one side of the scrotum.

hydrocele          phimosis          priapism          varicocele

14.48.   The direct visual examination of the tissues of the cervix and vagina using a binocular magnifier is known

as _____.

colposcopy          endovaginal ultrasound          hysteroscopy          laparoscopy

14.49. The term used to describe infrequent or very light menstruation in a woman with previously normal

periods is _____.

        amenorrhea        hypomenorrhea        oligomenorrhea        polymenorrhea

14.50. The examination of cells retrieved from the edge of the placenta between the 8th and 10th weeks of

pregnancy is known as _____.

        amniocentesis        chorionic villus sampling        fetal monitoring        pelvimetry

## SENTENCE COMPLETION

Write the correct term or terms on the lines provided.

14.51. The dark-pigmented area surrounding the nipple is known as the _____.

14.52. A fluid-filled sac in the scrotum along the spermatic cord leading from the testicles is known as

a/an _____.

14.53. The serious complication of pregnancy that is characterized by convulsions and sometimes coma is

known as _____. The treatment for this condition is delivery of the fetus.

14.54. Surgical suturing of a tear in the vagina is known as _____.

14.55. The _____ is the tube that carries blood, oxygen, and nutrients from the placenta

to the developing child.

## WORD SURGERY

Divide each term into its component word parts. Write these word parts, in sequence, on the lines provided. When necessary use a slash (/) to indicate a combining vowel. (You may not need all of the lines provided.)

14.56. **Endocervicitis** is an inflammation of the mucous membrane lining of the cervix.

    _____        _____        _____        _____

14.57. **Menometrorrhagia** is excessive uterine bleeding at both the usual time of menstrual periods and at other

irregular intervals.

    _____        _____        _____        _____

14.58. **Hysterosalpingography** is a radiographic examination of the uterus and fallopian tubes.

    _____        _____        _____        _____

14.59. **Galactorrhea** is the production of breast milk in a woman who is not breastfeeding.

_____        _____        _____        _____

14.60. **Azoospermia** is the absence of sperm in the semen.

_____        _____        _____        _____

## TRUE/FALSE

If the statement is true, write **True** on the line. If the statement is false, write **False** on the line.

14.61. _____ Peyronie's disease causes a sexual dysfunction in which the penis is bent or

curved during erection.

14.62. _____ Braxton Hicks contractions are the first true labor pains.

14.63. _____ An Apgar score is an evaluation of a newborn infant's physical status

at 1 and 5 minutes after birth.

14.64. _____ Breast augmentation is mammoplasty that is performed to reduce breast

size.

14.65. _____ An ectopic pregnancy is a potentially dangerous condition in which a

fertilized egg is implanted and begins to develop outside of the uterus.

## CLINICAL CONDITIONS

Write the correct answer on the line provided.

14.66. Baby Ortega was born with cryptorchidism. When this testicle had not descended by the time he was 9

months old, a/an _____ was performed.

14.67. When she went into labor with her first child, Mrs. Hoshi's baby was in a breech presentation.

Because of risks associated with this, her obstetrician delivered the baby surgically by performing

a/an _____.

14.68. Dawn Grossman was diagnosed as having uterine fibroids that required surgical removal. Her gynecolo-

gist scheduled Dawn for a/an _____.

14.69. Rita Chen, who is 25 years old and knows that she is not pregnant, is concerned because she has not had

a menstrual period for 3 months. Her doctor described this condition as _____.

14.70. Enrico Flores' physician removed a portion of each vas deferens. The medical term for this sterilization

procedure is a/an _____.

14.71. Tiffany Thomas developed a thin, frothy, yellow-green, foul-smelling vaginal discharge. She was diag-

nosed as having _____, which is caused by the parasite *Trichomonas vaginalis*.

14.72. Mr. Wolford, who is age 65, has been reading a lot about the decrease of testosterone in older men.

His physician told him that the medical term for this condition is _____.

14.73. Just before the delivery of her baby, Barbara Klein's obstetrician performed a/

an _____ to prevent tearing of the tissues.

14.74. Jane Marsall's pregnancy was complicated by the abnormal implantation of the placenta in the lower

portion of the uterus. The medical term for this condition is _____.

14.75. Immediately after birth, the Reicher baby was described as being a newborn or

a/an _____.

## WHICH IS THE CORRECT MEDICAL TERM?

Select the correct answer, and write it on the line provided.

14.76. The postpartum vaginal discharge during the first several weeks after childbirth is known

as _____.

colostrum          involution          lochia          meconium

14.77. Abdominal pain caused by uterine cramps during a menstrual period is known

as _____.

dysmenorrhea       hypermenorrhea     menometrorrhagia     polymenorrhea

14.78. The term that describes an inflammation of the glans penis is _____.

phimosis          balanitis          epididymitis          testitis

14.79. An inflammation of the lining of the vagina is known as _____. The most common

causes of this condition are bacterial vaginosis, trichomoniasis, and vaginal candidiasis.

cervical dysplasia       cervicitis       colporrhexis       vaginitis

14.80.  The term that describes a profuse whitish mucus discharge from the uterus and vagina

is _____. This type of discharge can be due to an infection, malignancy, or

hormonal changes.

        endocervicitis        leukorrhea        pruritus vulvae        vaginitis

## CHALLENGE WORD BUILDING

These terms are *not* found in this chapter; however, they are made up of the following familiar word parts. If you need help in creating the term, refer to your medical dictionary.

| endo- | hyster/o | -cele |
|---|---|---|
|  | mast/o | -dynia |
|  | metr/i | -itis |
|  | oophor/o | -pexy |
|  | orchid/o | -plasty |
|  | vagin/o | -rrhaphy |
|  | vulv/o | -rrhexis |

14.81.  The term meaning a hernia protruding into the vagina is _____.

14.82.  The term meaning the surgical repair of one or both testicles is _____.

14.83.  The term meaning an inflammation of the endometrium is _____.

14.84.  The term meaning the surgical repair of an ovary is a/an _____.

14.85.  The term meaning pain in the vagina is _____.

14.86.  The term meaning surgical suturing of the uterus is _____.

14.87.  The term meaning a hernia of the uterus, particularly during pregnancy, is

a/an _____.

14.88.  The term meaning the surgical fixation of a displaced ovary is _____.

14.89.  The term meaning the rupture of the uterus, particularly during pregnancy,

is _____.

14.90.  The term meaning an inflammation of the vulva and the vagina is _____.

## LABELING EXERCISES

Identify the numbered items on these accompanying figures.

14.91. _____ bladder

14.92. _____ gland

14.93. _____

14.94. _____

14.95. _____

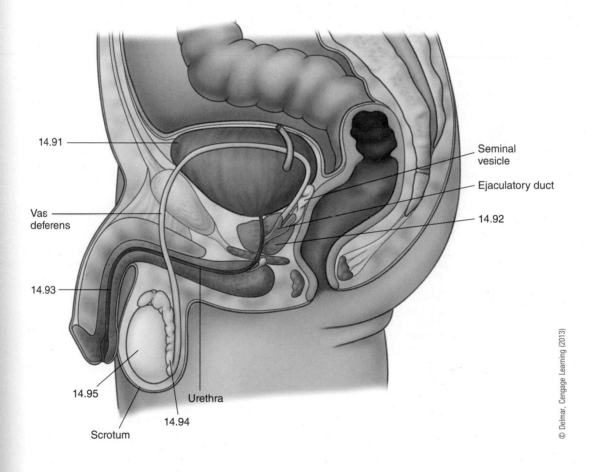

14.91
Vas deferens
14.93
14.95
Scrotum
14.94
Urethra
Seminal vesicle
Ejaculatory duct
14.92

© Delmar, Cengage Learning (2013)

14.96.  _____ or uterine tube

14.97.  body of the _____

14.98  _____ bladder

14.99.  _____

14.100.  _____

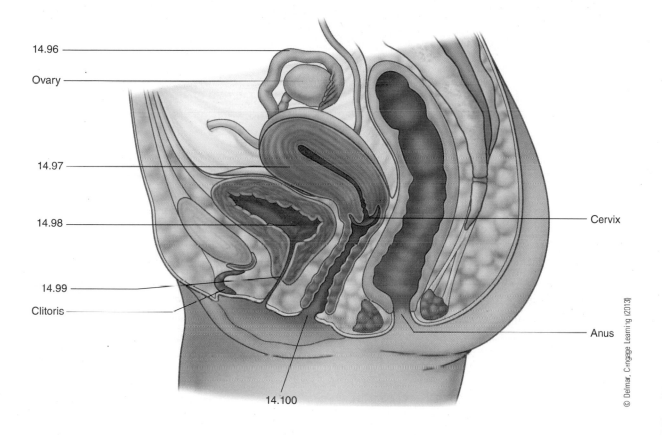

14.96 ————

Ovary ————

14.97 ————

14.98 ————

14.99 ————

Clitoris ————

Cervix

Anus

14.100

© Delmar, Cengage Learning (2013)

# THE HUMAN TOUCH
## Critical Thinking Exercise

The following story and questions are designed to stimulate critical thinking through class discussion or as a brief essay response. There are no right or wrong answers to these questions.

*"But Sam, you promised!" Jamie Chu began.*

*"Please do not get so upset," her husband interrupted. "I know I agreed to a vasectomy, but Grandmother may have a point. I do not have a son. Our family name has to be considered. I just feel that we should think about this."*

*"But Sam, we already discussed it. You're scheduled for the procedure." It seemed to Jamie that they had already spent plenty of time considering the number of children they wanted and talking about various contraceptive methods. Jamie had problems taking the pill, and Sam didn't like using a condom. A tubal ligation could have been the answer, but Jamie had a fear of not waking up from the anesthesia. Besides, she had been the one to go through two pregnancies and childbirths. Sam had reluctantly agreed that it was his turn to take responsibility for family planning.*

*Their two daughters, 2-year-old Nanyn and her big sister, Nadya, made the perfect size family, Jamie thought. She had grown up in a large family. A lot of her childhood was spent taking care of her brothers and sisters, and she rarely had her mother's undivided attention. She didn't want that for her children.*

*Sam's story was different. Before his parents immigrated to America, they had had four daughters. His father was so proud when Sam was born, a son to carry on the family tradition.*

*It had taken quite a long time to convince Sam that a family of only daughters could be considered complete. And now Grandmother was questioning that decision.*

## Suggested Discussion Topics

1. In a sexual relationship, which partner is responsible for birth control and why?
2. If a couple cannot agree about family size or birth control methods, what options are available to them?
3. Discuss how cultural differences and religious beliefs influence choices like family size and birth control.
4. Some cultures value male children over female children. Discuss why you think this is so and how the changing cultural role of women may affect these values.

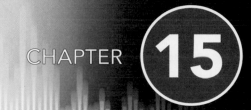

# Diagnostic Procedures, Nuclear Medicine, and Pharmacology

## Overview of
## DIAGNOSTIC PROCEDURES, NUCLEAR MEDICINE, AND PHARMACOLOGY

| Major Headings | Including |
|---|---|
| Basic Diagnostic Procedures | Vital signs <br> Auscultation <br> Palpation and percussion <br> Basic examination instruments |
| Examination Positions | Recumbent positions <br> Sims' position <br> Knee-chest position <br> Lithotomy position |
| Laboratory Tests | Blood tests <br> Urinalysis |
| Endoscopy | Endoscopes |
| Centesis | Diagnostic procedures involving the removal of body fluids |
| Imaging Techniques | Radiography <br> Computed tomography <br> Magnetic resonance imaging <br> Fluoroscopy <br> Ultrasonography |
| Nuclear Medicine | Nuclear medicine |
| Pharmacology | Prescription and over-the-counter drugs <br> Generic and brand-name drugs <br> Terminology related to pharmacology <br> Medications for pain management <br> Methods of drug administration |
| Complementary and Alternative Therapies | Alternative medicine <br> Complementary medicine |

# Vocabulary Related to DIAGNOSTIC PROCEDURES, NUCLEAR MEDICINE, AND PHARMACOLOGY

This list contains essential word parts and medical terms for this chapter. These terms are pronounced in the student StudyWARE™ and Audio CDs that are available for use with this text. These and the other important **primary terms** are shown in boldface throughout the chapter. *Secondary terms*, which appear in *orange* italics, clarify the meaning of primary terms.

## Word Parts

- ☐ **albumin/o** albumin, protein
- ☐ **calc/i** calcium, lime, the heel
- ☐ **-centesis** surgical puncture to remove fluid
- ☐ **creatin/o** creatinine
- ☐ **glycos/o** glucose, sugar
- ☐ **-graphy** the process of producing a picture or record
- ☐ **hemat/o** blood, relating to the blood
- ☐ **lapar/o** abdomen, abdominal wall
- ☐ **-otomy** cutting, surgical incision.
- ☐ **phleb/o** vein
- ☐ **radi/o** radiation, x-rays
- ☐ **-scope** instrument for visual examination
- ☐ **-scopy** visual examination
- ☐ **son/o** sound
- ☐ **-uria** urination, urine

## Medical Terms

- ☐ **acetaminophen** (ah-**seet**-ah-**MIN**-oh-fen)
- ☐ **acupuncture** (**AK**-que-**punk**-tyour)
- ☐ **albuminuria** (**al**-byou-mih-**NEW**-ree-ah)
- ☐ **analgesic** (an-al-**JEE**-zick)
- ☐ **antipyretic** (**an**-tih-pye-**RET**-ick)
- ☐ **arthrocentesis** (**ar**-throh-sen-**TEE**-sis)
- ☐ **auscultation** (aws-kul-**TAY**-shun)
- ☐ **bacteriuria** (back-**tee**-ree-**YOU**-ree-ah)
- ☐ **bruit** (**BREW**-ee)
- ☐ **calciuria** (**kal**-sih-**YOU**-ree-ah)
- ☐ **compliance**
- ☐ **computed tomography** (toh-**MOG**-rah-fee)
- ☐ **contraindication**
- ☐ **creatinuria** (kree-**at**-ih-**NEW**-ree-ah)
- ☐ **echocardiography** (**eck**-oh-**kar**-dee-**OG**-rah-fee)
- ☐ **endoscope** (**EN**-doh-**skope**)
- ☐ **fluoroscopy** (**floo**-or-**OS**-koh-pee)

- ☐ **glycosuria** (**glye**-koh-**SOO**-ree-ah)
- ☐ **hematocrit** (hee-**MAT**-oh-krit)
- ☐ **hematuria** (**hee**-mah-**TOO**-ree-ah)
- ☐ **hyperthermia** (**high**-per-**THER**-mee-ah)
- ☐ **hypothermia** (**high**-poh-**THER**-mee-ah)
- ☐ **idiosyncratic reaction** (**id**-ee-oh-sin-**KRAT**-ick)
- ☐ **interventional radiology**
- ☐ **intradermal injection**
- ☐ **intramuscular injection**
- ☐ **intravenous injection**
- ☐ **ketonuria** (**kee**-toh-**NEW**-ree-ah)
- ☐ **laparoscopy** (**lap**-ah-**ROS**-koh-pee)
- ☐ **lithotomy position** (lih-**THOT**-oh-mee)
- ☐ **magnetic resonance imaging**
- ☐ **ophthalmoscope** (ahf-**THAL**-moh-skope)
- ☐ **otoscope** (**OH**-toh-skope)
- ☐ **palliative** (**PAL**-ee-**ay**-tiv)
- ☐ **parenteral** (pah-**REN**-ter-al)
- ☐ **percussion** (per-**KUSH**-un)
- ☐ **perfusion** (per-**FYOU**-zuhn)
- ☐ **pericardiocentesis** (**pehr**-ih-**kar**-dee-oh-sen-**TEE**-sis)
- ☐ **phlebotomy** (fleh-**BOT**-oh-mee)
- ☐ **placebo** (plah-**SEE**-boh)
- ☐ **positron emission tomography**
- ☐ **prone position**
- ☐ **proteinuria** (**proh**-tee-in-**YOU**-ree-ah)
- ☐ **pyuria** (pye-**YOU**-ree-ah)
- ☐ **radiolucent** (**ray**-dee-oh-**LOO**-sent)
- ☐ **radiopaque** (**ray**-dee-oh-**PAYK**)
- ☐ **rale** (**RAHL**)
- ☐ **recumbent** (ree-**KUM**-bent)
- ☐ **rhonchi** (**RONG**-kye)
- ☐ **Sims' position**
- ☐ **single photon emission computed tomography**
- ☐ **speculum** (**SPECK**-you-lum)
- ☐ **sphygmomanometer** (**sfig**-moh-mah-**NOM**-eh-ter)
- ☐ **stethoscope** (**STETH**-oh-skope)
- ☐ **stridor** (**STRYE**-dor)
- ☐ **subcutaneous injection** (**sub**-kyou-**TAY**-nee-us)
- ☐ **transdermal**
- ☐ **transesophageal echocardiography** (**trans**-eh-sof-ah-**JEE**-al-**eck**-oh-**kar**-dee-**OG**-rah-fee)
- ☐ **ultrasonography** (**ul**-trah-son-**OG**-rah-fee)
- ☐ **urinalysis** (**you**-rih-**NAL**-ih-sis)

## LEARNING GOALS

On completion of this chapter, you should be able to:

1. Describe the vital signs recorded for most patients.

2. Recognize, define, spell, and pronounce the primary terms associated with basic examination procedures and positions.

3. Recognize, define, spell, and pronounce the primary terms associated with frequently performed blood and urinalysis laboratory tests.

4. Recognize, define, spell, and pronounce the primary terms associated with radiography and other imaging techniques.

5. Describe the uses of nuclear medicine in diagnosis and treatment.

6. Recognize, define, spell, and pronounce the primary pharmacology terms introduced in this chapter.

7. Describe the most common types of complementary and alternative therapies and their uses.

# ■ DIAGNOSTIC PROCEDURES

A wide range of diagnostic tools are used to determine the patient's general state of health and to look for specific medical conditions.

## Basic Examination Procedures

Basic examination procedures are performed during the assessment of the patient's condition. As used in medicine, the term **assessment** means the evaluation or appraisal of the patient's condition. This information is used in reaching a diagnosis and in formulating a patient care plan.

## Observation

The first step in a physical assessment is to observe the patient's overall appearance, emotional affect, and ambulation.

■ *Overall appearance* includes a number of factors: how appropriately the patient is dressed, whether there is any body odor, or if there are signs of possible difficulties with self-care.

■ *Emotional affect* refers to the patient's expression, tone of voice, mood, and emotions. *Affect* means the outward expression of emotion.

■ *Ambulation* means the way the patient walks, including gait, any unsteadiness, or possible difficulty.

## Vital Signs

**Vital signs** are the four key indications that the body systems are functioning. These signs, which are recorded for most patient visits, are *temperature*, *pulse*, *respiration*, and *blood pressure*. The abbreviation *VSS* stands for vital signs stable.

### Temperature

An average normal body **temperature** is 98.6°F (Fahrenheit) or 37.0°C (Celsius).

■ An oral body temperature of 100°F or higher is a **fever**. A fever is most commonly caused by an infection, an injury, or medications.

■ Temperature readings are named for the location in which they are taken: *oral* (in the mouth), *aural* (in the ear), *axillary* (in the armpit), and *rectal* (in the rectum). Caution: *oral* and *aural* sound alike; however, they require different styles of thermometers and are taken in different locations.

■ Temperature readings vary slightly depending upon the location in which they are taken.

■ **Hyperthermia** (**high**-per-**THER**-mee-ah) is an extremely high fever (**hyper-** means excessive, **therm** means heat, and **-ia** means pertaining to).

■ **Hypothermia** (**high**-poh-**THER**-mee-ah) is an abnormally low body temperature (**hypo-** means deficient, **therm** means heat, and **-ia** means pertaining to).

## Pulse

The **pulse** is the rhythmic pressure against the walls of an artery that is caused by the beating of the heart. The pulse rate reflects the number of times the heart beats each minute and is recorded as *bpm* (beats per minute). As shown in Figure 15.1, the pulse can be measured at different points on the body.

■ The *normal resting heart rate* differs by age group. In adults, a normal resting heart rate is from 60–100 bpm. Generally heart rates are higher in children, and for a newborn the resting heart rate ranges from 100–160 bpm. Athletes, however, can have a normal resting heart rate of 40–60 bpm.

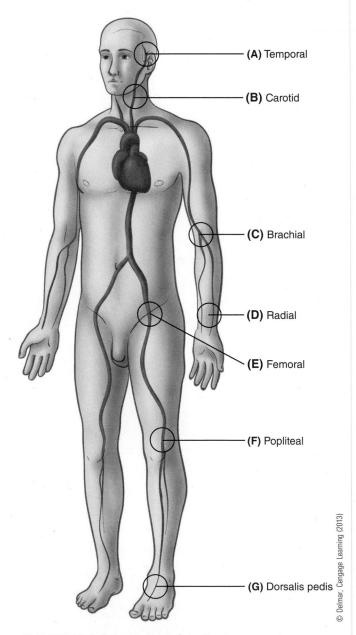

**(A)** Temporal

**(B)** Carotid

**(C)** Brachial

**(D)** Radial

**(E)** Femoral

**(F)** Popliteal

**(G)** Dorsalis pedis

© Delmar, Cengage Learning (2013)

**FIGURE 15.1** Pulse points of the body.

## Respiration

**Respiration**, which is also known as the **respiratory rate** (RR), is the number of complete breaths per minute. A single respiration consists of one inhalation and one exhalation (see Chapter 7). The normal respiratory rate for adults ranges from 12 to 20 respirations per minute.

## Blood Pressure

**Blood pressure** is the force of the blood against the walls of the arteries. This force is measured using a **sphygmomanometer** (**sfig**-moh-mah-**NOM**-eh-ter). When using manual style, as shown in Figure 15.2, a stethoscope is required to listen to the blood sounds. A digital sphygmomanometer is automated and does not require the use of a stethoscope.

Blood pressure is recorded as a ratio with the **systolic** (sis-**TOL**-ick) over the **diastolic** (dye-ah-**STOL**-ick) reading. The systolic is the first beat heard. The diastolic is the last beat heard. Memory aid: *SSSS-systolic* is like steam going up. *DDDD-diastolic* is as in going down (Figure 15.3).

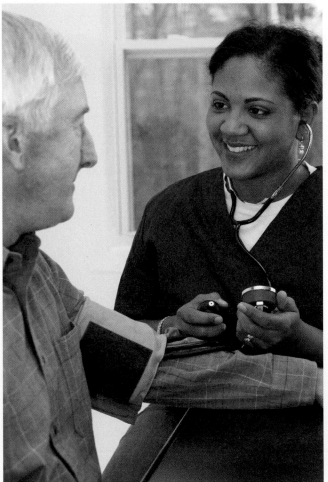

Rob Marmion/www.Shutterstock.com

**FIGURE 15.2** A manual sphygmomanometer being used with a stethoscope to measure blood pressure.

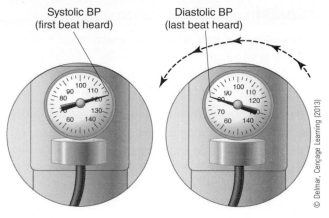

FIGURE 15.3 Using a stethoscope, the systolic pressure is the first sound heard and the diastolic pressure is the last beat heard.

Blood pressure ranges are explained in Table 5.3 of Chapter 5.

## Pain

In certain settings, such as a hospital, **pain** is considered to be the fifth vital sign. Since this is a subjective symptom that cannot be measured objectively, it must be determined as reported by the patient.

- Using a *pain rating scale*, the patient is asked to describe his or her level of pain from 0 (no pain) to 10 (severe pain). Facial expressions are used to ask children to rate their pain (Figure 15.4).

- *Acute pain*, which comes on quickly, can be severe and lasts only a relatively short time. It can be caused by disease, inflammation, or injury to the tissues. When the cause of the pain is diagnosed and treated, the pain goes away.

- *Chronic pain*, which can be mild or severe, persists over a longer period of time than acute pain and is resistant to most medical treatments. It often causes severe problems for the patient.

## Auscultation

The term **auscultation** (**aws**-kul-**TAY**-shun) means listening for sounds within the body and is usually performed through a stethoscope (**auscult/a** means to listen, and **-tion** means the process of) (Figure 15.5).

## Respiratory Sounds

Respiratory sounds heard through a stethoscope provide information about the condition of the lungs and pleura as the patient breathes (see Chapter 7).

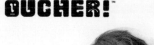

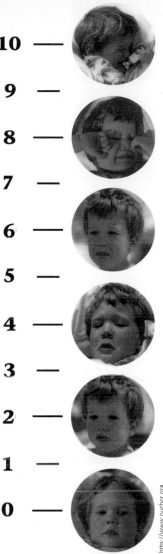

FIGURE 15.4 A pediatric pain scale such as the Oucher Pain Assessment Tool uses facial expressions instead of numbers. (The Caucasion version of the Oucher, developed and copyrighted by Judith E. Beyer, RN, Ph.D., 1983. Used with permission.)

- A **rale** (**RAHL**), also known as a *crackle*, is an abnormal crackle-like lung sound heard through a stethoscope during inspiration (breathing in).

- **Rhonchi** (**RONG**-kye) are coarse rattling sounds that are somewhat like snoring. These sounds are usually caused by secretions in the bronchial airways (singular *rhonchus*).

- **Stridor** (**STRYE**-dor) is an abnormal, high-pitched, musical breathing sound caused by a blockage in the throat or in the larynx (voice box).

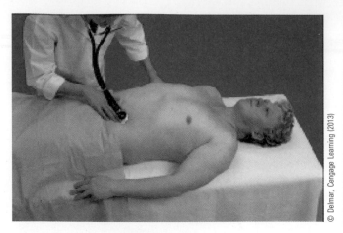

© Delmar, Cengage Learning (2013)

**FIGURE 15.5** Auscultation is listening through a stethoscope to sounds within the body.

## Heart Sounds

The heartbeat heard through a stethoscope has two distinct sounds. These are known as the "lubb dupp" or "lub dub" sounds.

- The *lubb sound* is heard first. It is caused by the tricuspid and mitral valves closing between the atria and the ventricles.

- The *dupp sound*, which is shorter and higher pitched, is heard next. It is caused by the closing of the semilunar valves in the aorta and pulmonary arteries as blood is pumped out of the heart.

- A **bruit** (**BREW**-ee) is an abnormal sound or murmur heard during auscultation of an artery. These sounds are usually due to a partially blocked, narrowed, or diseased artery. A *thrill* is an abnormal rhythmic vibration felt when palpating an artery. (Note: the term *bruit* is also sometimes pronounced **BROOT**.)

- A **heart murmur** is an abnormal heart sound that is most commonly a sign of defective heart valves. Heart murmurs are described by volume and the stage of the heartbeat when the murmur is heard.

## Abdominal Sounds

**Abdominal sounds**, also known as *bowel sounds*, are normal noises made by the intestines. Auscultation of the abdomen is performed to evaluate these sounds and to detect abnormalities. For example, increased bowel sounds can indicate a bowel obstruction. The absence of these sounds can indicate ileus, which is the stopping of intestinal peristalsis (see Chapter 8).

## Palpation and Percussion

- **Palpation** (pal-**PAY**-shun) is an examination technique in which the examiner's hands are used to feel the texture, size, consistency, and location of certain body parts (Figure 15.6).

- **Percussion** (per-**KUSH**-un) is a diagnostic procedure designed to determine the density of a body part by the sound produced by tapping the surface with the fingers. As shown in Figure 15.7, this is performed on the back to determine the presence of normal air content in the lungs.

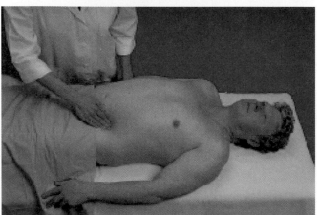

© Delmar, Cengage Learning (2013)

**FIGURE 15.6** Palpation is an examination technique in which the examiner's hands are used to feel the texture, size, consistency, and location of certain body parts.

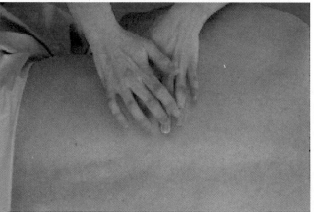

© Delmar, Cengage Learning (2013)

**FIGURE 15.7** Percussion is a diagnostic procedure in which the examiner's hands are used to determine the density of a body area.

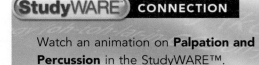

**StudyWARE CONNECTION**

Watch an animation on **Palpation and Percussion** in the StudyWARE™.

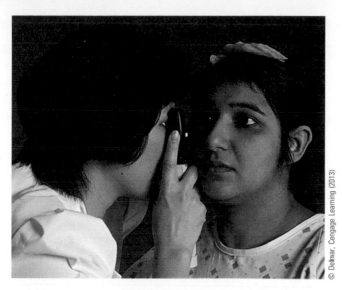

**FIGURE 15.8** An ophthalmoscope is used to examine the interior of the eye.

## Basic Examination Instruments

- An **ophthalmoscope** (ahf-**THAL**-moh-skope) is an instrument used to examine the interior of the eye (**ophthalm/o** means eye, and **-scope** means instrument for visual examination) (Figure 15.8).

- An **otoscope** (**OH**-toh-skope) is an instrument used to visually examine the external ear canal and tympanic membrane (**ot/o** means ear, and **-scope** means instrument for visual examination) (see Chapter 11, Figure 11.15).

- A **speculum** (**SPECK**-you-lum) is an instrument used to enlarge the opening of any canal or cavity to facilitate inspection of its interior (see Chapter 14, Figure 14.15 A).

- A **stethoscope** (**STETH**-oh-skope) is an instrument used to listen to sounds within the body (**steth/o** means chest and **-scope** means instrument for examination) (Figures 15.2 and 15.5).

## RECUMBENT EXAMINATION POSITIONS

Specific basic examination positions are used to examine different areas of the body. The term **recumbent** (ree-**KUM**-bent) describes any position in which the patient is lying down. This can be on the back, front, or side. In radiography, the term *decubitus* describes the patient lying in a recumbent position.

These are positions in which the patient is *face up*:

- In the **horizontal recumbent position**, also known as the *supine position*, the patient is lying on the back, face up. This position is used for examination and treatment of the anterior surface of the body and for x-rays.

- In the **dorsal recumbent position**, the patient is lying on the back, face up, with the knees bent. This position is used for the examination and treatment of the abdominal area and for vaginal or rectal examinations.

- In the **lithotomy position** (lih-**THOT**-oh-mee) the patient is lying on the back, face up, with the feet and legs raised and supported in stirrups. This position is used for vaginal and rectal examinations and during childbirth.

These are positions in which the patient is *face down* or *on his/her side*:

- In a **prone position**, the patient is lying on the abdomen face down. The arms may be placed under the head for comfort. This position is used for the examination and treatment of the back and buttocks.

- In the **Sims' position**, the patient is lying on the left side with the right knee and thigh drawn up with the left arm placed along the back. This position is used in the examination and treatment of the rectal area.

- In the **knee-chest position**, the patient is lying face down with the hips bent so that the knees and chest rest on the table. This position is also used for rectal examinations.

## LABORATORY TESTS

When a laboratory test is ordered **stat**, the results are needed immediately, and the tests have top priority in the laboratory. *Stat* comes from the Latin word meaning immediately.

### Blood Tests

When used in regard to laboratory tests, the term **profile** means tests that are frequently performed as a group on automated multi-channel laboratory testing equipment.

### Obtaining Specimens

- A **phlebotomist** (fleh-**BOT**-oh-mist) is a medical professional who is trained to draw blood from patients for various laboratory tests and other procedures (Figure 15.9).

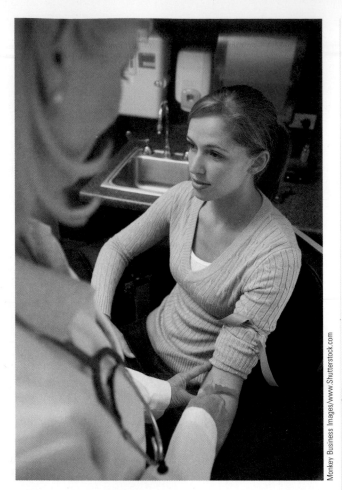

Monkey Business Images/www.Shutterstock.com

**FIGURE 15.9** A phlebotomist draws a blood sample from a patient for testing.

- **Phlebotomy** (fleh-**BOT**-oh-mee), also known as *venipuncture*, is the puncture of a vein for the purpose of drawing blood (**phleb** means vein, and **-otomy** means a surgical incision).

- An **arterial stick** is the puncture of an artery, usually on the inside of the wrist, to obtain arterial blood. Arterial blood differs from venous blood mostly in the concentration of dissolved gases it contains.

- A **capillary puncture** is the technique used when only a small amount of blood is needed as a specimen for a blood test. Named for where it is performed, a capillary puncture is usually known as a *finger, heel*, or an *earlobe stick*.

## Complete Blood Cell Counts

A **complete blood cell count** (CBC) is a series of tests performed as a group to evaluate several blood conditions. Blood disorders are discussed in Chapter 5.

- **Erythrocyte sedimentation rate** (ESR) (eh-**RITH**-roh site), also known as a *sed rate*, is a test based on the speed with which the red blood cells separate from the plasma and fall to the bottom of a specialized test tube. An elevated sed rate indicates the presence of inflammation in the body. Normal range is <15–20 mm/hr (millimeters per hour) for adults under 50, and <20–30 mm/hr for adults over 50.

- The term **hematocrit** (hee-**MAT**-oh-krit) describes the percentage, by volume, of a blood sample occupied by red cells (**hemat/o** means blood, and **-crit** means to separate). This test is used to diagnose abnormal states of *hydration* (fluid levels in the body), *polycythemia* (excess red blood cells), and *anemia* (deficient red blood cells).

- A **platelet count** measures the number of platelets in a specified amount of blood and is a screening test to evaluate platelet function. It is also used to monitor changes in the blood associated with chemotherapy and radiation therapy. These changes include *thrombocytosis* (an abnormal increase in the number of platelets) and *thrombocytopenia* (an abnormal decrease in the number of platelets).

- A **red blood cell count** (RBC) is a determination of the number of erythrocytes in the blood. A depressed count can indicate anemia or a hemorrhage lasting more than 24 hours.

- A **total hemoglobin test** (Hb) is usually part of a complete blood count (**hem/o** means blood, and **-globin** means protein). Elevated Hb levels indicate a higher than normal hemoglobin concentration in the plasma due to polycythemia or dehydration. Low Hb indicates lower than normal hemoglobin concentration due to anemia, recent hemorrhage, or fluid retention.

- A **white blood cell count** (WBC) is a determination of the number of leukocytes in the blood. An elevated count can be an indication of infection or inflammation.

- A **white blood cell** (WBC) **differential count** tests to see what percentage of the total white blood cell count is composed of each of the five types of leukocytes. This provides information about the patient's immune system, detects certain types of leukemia, and determines the severity of infection.

## Additional Blood Tests

- A **basic metabolic panel** (BMP, or Profile 8) is a group of eight specific blood tests that provide important information about the current status of the patient's *kidneys, electrolyte balance, blood sugar,* and *calcium levels.* Significant changes in these test results can indicate acute problems such as kidney failure, insulin shock or diabetic coma, respiratory distress, or heart rhythm changes.

- A **blood urea nitrogen test** (BUN test) measures the amount of nitrogen in the blood due to the waste product urea. This test is performed to obtain an indication of kidney function. **Urea** (you-**REE**-ah) is the major end product of protein metabolism found in urine and blood.

- **Crossmatch tests** are performed to determine the compatibility of blood donor and the recipient before a blood transfusion. Agglutination is a positive reaction that indicates the donor unit is not a suitable match. *Agglutination* is the clumping together of red blood cells.

- A **C-reactive protein test** (CRP) is performed to identify high levels of inflammation within the body. The information provided by this test is obtained by the presence of the C-reactive protein, which is produced by the liver only during episodes of acute inflammation. Although this test does not identify the specific cause of the inflammation, an elevated level can indicate a heart attack, a coronary artery disease, or an autoimmune disorder.

- A **lipid panel** measures the amounts of total cholesterol, high-density lipoprotein (HDL), low-density lipoprotein (LDL), and triglycerides in a blood sample.

- **Prothrombin time** (proh-**THROM**-bin), also known as *pro time,* is a test used to diagnose conditions associated with abnormalities of clotting time and to monitor anticoagulant therapy. A longer prothrombin time can be caused by serious liver disease, bleeding disorders, blood-thinning medicines, or a lack of vitamin K.

- A **serum bilirubin test** measures the ability of the liver ability to take up, process, and secrete bilirubin into the bile. This test is useful in determining whether a patient has liver disease or a blocked bile duct.

- A **thyroid-stimulating hormone assay** measures circulating blood levels of thyroid-stimulating hormone (TSH) that can indicate abnormal thyroid activity (see Chapter 13).

- An **arterial blood gas analysis** (ABG) measures the pH, oxygen, and carbon dioxide levels of arterial blood. This test is used to evaluate lung and kidney function and overall metabolism.

## Urinalysis

**Urinalysis** (**you**-rih-**NAL**-ih-sis) is the examination of the physical and chemical properties of urine to determine the presence of abnormal elements.

- *Routine urinalysis* is performed to screen for urinary and systemic disorders. This test utilizes a dipstick. This is a plastic strip impregnated with chemicals that react with substances in the urine and change color when abnormalities are present (Figure 15.10).

- *Microscopic examination* of the specimen is performed when more-detailed testing of the specimen is necessary, for example, to identify casts. **Casts** are fibrous or protein materials, such as pus and fats, that are thrown off into the urine in kidney disease. (Note: The term *cast* is also used to describe a rigid dressing, traditionally made of gauze and plaster, used to immobilize a bone that has been fractured.)

## pH Values of Urine

The average normal **pH** range of urine is from 4.5 to 8.0. The abbreviation *pH* describes the degree of acidity or alkalinity of a substance.

- A pH value *below* 7 indicates acid urine and is an indication of acidosis. *Acidosis* is excessive acid in the body fluids.

- A pH value *above* 7 indicates alkaline urine and can indicate conditions such as a urinary tract infection.

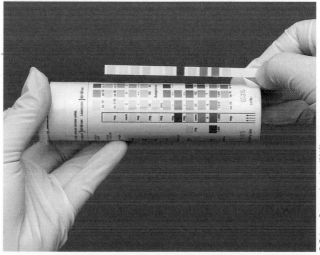

© Delmar, Cengage Learning (2013)

**FIGURE 15.10** A dipstick is used for routine urinalysis.

## Specific Gravity

The **specific gravity** of urine reflects the amount of wastes, minerals, and solids that are present.

■ *Low specific gravity* (dilute urine) is characteristic of diabetes insipidus, which is discussed in Chapter 13.

■ *High specific gravity* (concentrated urine) occurs in conditions such as dehydration, liver failure, or shock.

## Conditions and Drug Use Identified Through Urinalysis

■ **Albuminuria** (**al**-byou-mih-**NEW**-ree-ah) is the presence of the protein albumin in the urine. High test levels are a sign of impaired kidney function (**albumin** means albumin or protein, and **-uria** means urine). *Albumin* is a form of protein found in most body tissues.

■ **Bacteriuria** (back-**tee**-ree-**YOU**-ree-ah) is the presence of bacteria in the urine (**bacteri** means bacteria, and **-uria** means urine).

■ **Calciuria** (**kal**-sih-**YOU**-ree-ah) is the presence of calcium in the urine (**calci** means calcium, and **-uria** means urine). Abnormally high levels can be diagnostic for hyperparathyroidism as described in Chapter 13. Lower-than-normal levels can indicate osteomalacia, which is discussed in Chapter 3.

■ **Creatinuria** (kree-**at**-ih-**NEW**-ree-ah) is an increased concentration of creatinine in the urine (**creatin** means creatinine, and **-uria** means urine). *Creatinine* is a waste product of muscle metabolism that is normally removed by the kidneys. The presence of excess creatinine is an indication of increased muscle breakdown or a disruption of kidney function.

■ A **drug-screening urine test** is a rapid method of identifying the presence in the body of one or more drugs of abuse such as cocaine, heroin, and marijuana. These tests are also used to detect the use of performance-enhancing drugs by athletes.

■ **Glycosuria** (**glye**-koh-**SOO**-ree-ah) is the presence of glucose in the urine (**glycos** means glucose, and **-uria** means urine). This condition is most commonly caused by diabetes.

■ **Hematuria** (**hee**-mah-**TOO**-ree-ah) is the presence of blood in the urine (**hemat** means blood, and **-uria** means urine). This condition can be caused by kidney stones, infection, kidney damage, or bladder cancer.

■ **Ketonuria** (**kee**-toh-**NEW**-ree-ah) is the presence of ketones in the urine (**keton** means ketones, and **-uria** means urine). *Ketones* are formed when the body breaks down fat and their presence in urine can indicate starvation or uncontrolled diabetes.

■ **Proteinuria** (**proh**-tee-in-**YOU**-ree-ah) is the presence of an abnormal amount of protein in the urine (**protein** means protein, and **-uria** means urine). This condition is usually a sign of kidney disease.

■ **Pyuria** (pye-**YOU**-ree-ah) is the presence of pus in the urine (**py** means pus, and **-uria** means urine). When pus is present, the urine is turbid in appearance. *Turbid* means has a cloudy or smoky appearance.

■ A **urine culture and sensitivity tests**, also known as a *urine C and S*, is a laboratory test that is used to identify the cause of a urinary tract infection and to determine which antibiotic would be the most effective treatment.

## ■ ENDOSCOPY

**Endoscopy** (en-**DOS**-koh-pee) is the visual examination of the interior of a body cavity (**endo** means within, and **-scopy** means visual examination). These procedures are usually named for the organs involved.

**Endoscopic surgery** is a surgical procedure that is performed through very small incisions with the use of an endoscope and specialized instruments. These procedures are named for the body parts involved, for example, arthroscopic surgery, which is discussed in Chapter 3.

### Endoscopes

An **endoscope** (**EN**-doh-**skope**) is a small flexible tube with a light and a lens on the end (**endo** means within and **–scope** is an instrument for visual examination). These fiber-optic instruments are named for the body parts they are designed to examine. For example, a hysteroscope is used to examine the interior of the uterus, while a laparoscope is used to examine the interior of the abdomen (Figure 15.11).

### Laparoscopic Procedures

**Laparoscopy** (lap-ah-**ROS**-koh-pee) is the visual examination of the interior of the abdomen with the use of a laparoscope that is passed through a small incision in the abdominal wall (**lapar/o** means abdomen, and **-scopy** means visual examination).

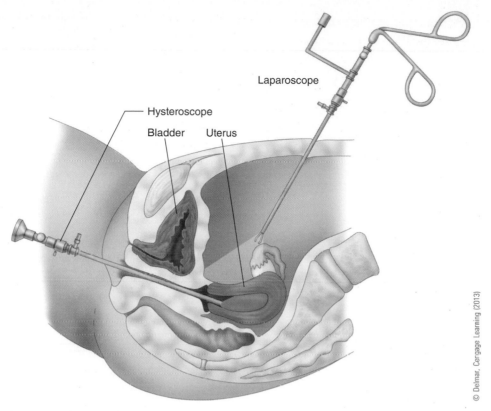

Laparoscope

Hysteroscope

Bladder     Uterus

© Delmar, Cengage Learning (2013)

**FIGURE 15.11** A laparoscope is used to examine the interior of the abdomen. A hysteroscope is used to examine the interior of the uterus.

Laparoscopic surgery involves the use of a laparoscope plus specialized instruments inserted into the abdomen through small incisions (Figure 15.11). A laparoscope is used for several purposes:

■ Explore and examine the interior of the abdomen.

■ Take specimens to be biopsied.

■ Perform surgical procedures such as the endoscopic removal of a diseased gallbladder (see Chapter 8).

## CENTESIS

**Centesis** (sen-TEE-sis) is a surgical puncture to remove excess fluid or to remove fluid for diagnostic purposes. Note: Centesis is used alone as a noun or as a suffix in conjunction with the combining form describing the body part being treated.

■ **Abdominocentesis** (ab-**dom**-ih-noh-sen-**TEE**-sis) is the surgical puncture of the abdominal cavity to remove fluid (**abdomin/o** means abdomen, and -**centesis** means a surgical puncture to remove fluid).

■ *Amniocentesis*, which is a diagnostic test performed during pregnancy, is discussed in Chapter 14.

■ **Arthrocentesis** (**ar**-throh-sen-**TEE** sis) is a surgical puncture of the joint space to remove synovial fluid for analysis to determine the cause of pain or swelling in a joint (**arthr/o** means joint, and -**centesis** means a surgical puncture to remove fluid).

■ **Cardiocentesis** (**kar**-dee-oh-sen-**TEE**-sis), also known as *cardiopuncture*, is the puncture of a chamber of the heart for diagnosis or therapy (**cardi/o** means heart, and -**centesis** means a surgical puncture to remove fluid).

■ **Pericardiocentesis** (**pehr**-ih-**kar**-dee-oh-sen-**TEE** sis) is the puncture of the pericardial sac for the purpose of removing fluid (**peri-** means surrounding, **cardi/o** means heart, and -**centesis** means a surgical puncture to remove fluid). This procedure is performed to treat pericarditis (see Chapter 5).

## IMAGING TECHNIQUES

Imaging techniques are used to visualize and examine internal body structures. The three most commonly used techniques are compared in Table 15.1.

## TABLE 15.1

### Imaging Systems Compared

| Method | How It Works |
|---|---|
| **Radiography** (x-ray) | Uses x-radiation (x-rays) passing through the patient to expose a film or create a digital image that shows the body in profile. In the resulting film, hard tissues are light, soft tissues are shades of gray, and air is black. |
| **Computed tomography** (CT) | Uses x-radiation (x-rays) with computer assistance to produce multiple cross-sectional views of the body. Hard tissues are light, and soft tissues appear as shades of gray. |
| **Magnetic resonance imaging** (MRI) | Uses a combination of radio waves and a strong magnetic field to produce images. Hard tissues are dark, and soft tissues appear as shades of gray. |

## Contrast Medium

A **contrast medium** is administered by swallowing, via an enema, or intravenously to make specific body structures visible. Specialized substances are used depending on the imaging systems and the body parts to be enhanced. These media are either radiopaque or radiolucent.

- **Radiopaque** (**ray**-dee-oh-**PAYK**) means that the substance *does not allow x-rays to pass through* and appears white or light gray on the resulting film. Radiopaque is the opposite of radiolucent.

- **Radiolucent** (**ray**-dee-oh-**LOO**-sent) means that the substance, such as air or nitrogen gas, *does allow x-rays to pass through* and appears black or dark gray on the resulting film. Radiolucent is the opposite of radiopaque.

- An **intravenous contrast medium** is injected into a vein to make the flow of blood through blood vessels and organs visible (**intra-** means within, **ven** means vein, and **-ous** means pertaining to). This technique, which is usually named for the vessels or organs involved, is illustrated in.

### Barium

**Barium** (chemical symbol Ba) is a radiopaque contrast medium used primarily to visualize the gastrointestinal tract (Figure 15.12). It is administered orally as a *barium swallow* for an upper GI study. It is administered rectally as a *barium enema* for a lower GI study. Radiography and fluoroscopy are used to trace the flow of the barium.

## Radiology

Conventional **radiology** creates an image of hard-tissue internal structures by the exposure of sensitized film to x-radiation (**radi** means radiation, and **-ology** means study of). The resulting film is known as a **radiograph** or *radiogram*; however, it is commonly referred to as an *x-ray*.

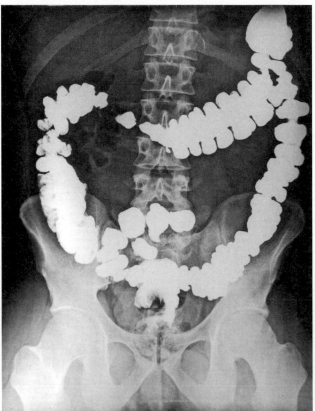

©Danilo Ascione/Shutterstock.com

**FIGURE 15.12** A radiograph (x-ray) of the abdomen using a contrast medium.

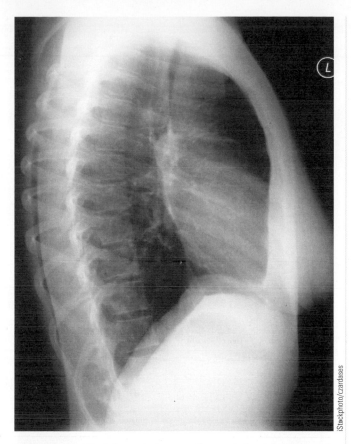

**FIGURE 15.13** A lateral chest radiograph (x-ray). Bones of the spine are white, and the soft tissues are shades of gray. The surrounding air is black.

- X-radiation, which is also referred to as *ionizing radiation,* is beneficial in producing diagnostic images and in treating cancer; however, excess exposure to this radiation is dangerous, and the effects are cumulative. Because x-radiation is invisible, has no odor, and cannot be felt, appropriate precautions must always be taken to protect the technician and the patient.

- *Radiopaque hard tissues,* such as bone and tooth enamel, appear white or light gray on the radiograph.

- *Radiolucent soft tissues,* such as muscles, and skin, appear as shades of gray to black on the radiograph (Figure 15.13).

- A **radiologist** (ray-dee-**OL**-oh-jist) is a physician who specializes in diagnosing and treating diseases and disorders with x-rays and other forms of radiant energy (**radi** means radiation, and -**ologist** means specialist).

- **Interventional radiology** is the use of radiographic imaging to guide a procedure such as a biopsy. It is also used to confirm the placement of an inserted object such as a stent or feeding tube.

## Radiographic Positioning

The term **radiographic positioning** describes the placement of the patient's body and the part of the body that is closest to the x-ray film. For example, in a *left lateral position,* the left side of the patient's body is placed nearest the film.

## Radiographic Projections

The term **radiographic projection** describes the path that the x-ray beam follows through the patient's body from the entrance to the exit.

- When the name of the projection combines two terms into a single word, the term listed first is the one that the x-ray penetrates first.

- The basic projections described in the next section can be used for most body parts. These projections can be exposed with the patient in a standing or recumbent position.

## Dental Radiography

Specialized techniques and equipment are used in obtaining dental radiographs.

- The term **extraoral radiography** means that the film is placed and exposed outside of the mouth. A **panoramic radiograph**, commonly known as a *Panorex,* shows all of the structures in both dental arches in a single film.

- **Intraoral radiography** means that the film is placed within the mouth and exposed by a camera positioned next to the exterior of the cheek (Figure 15.14).

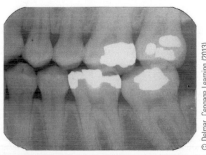

**FIGURE 15.14** Intraoral dental radiographs. The white areas are fillings that restore decayed teeth.

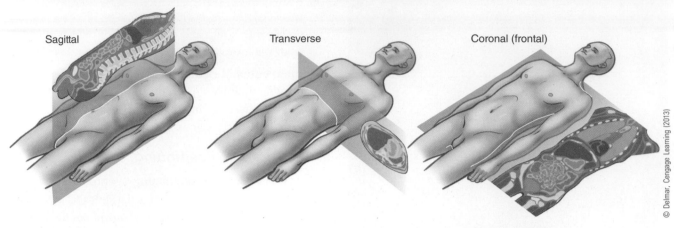

Sagittal    Transverse    Coronal (frontal)

© Delmar, Cengage Learning (2013)

**FIGURE 15.15** Computed tomography (CT scan) provides cross-sectional views of different body planes.

## Computed Tomography

**Computed tomography** (CT) (toh-**MOG**-rah-fee) uses a thin, fan-shaped x-ray beam that rotates around the patient to produce multiple cross-sectional views of the body (**tom/o** means to cut, section, or slice, and **-graphy** means the process of recording a picture or record) (Figure 15.15).

- Information gathered by radiation detectors is downloaded to a computer, analyzed, and converted into gray-scale images corresponding to anatomic slices of the body (Figure 15.16). These images are viewed on a monitor, stored as digital files, or printed as films.

- Computed tomography is more effective than MRI at imaging compact bone and is frequently preferred for patients with head injuries or strokes.

- **Tomotherapy** is the combination of *tomography* with *radiation therapy* to precisely target the tumor being treated (**tom/o** means slice and **-therapy** means treatment). In this type of therapy, radiation is delivered slice-by-slice to the tumor and is able to avoid healthy tissue.

- Computed tomography scans can be performed with or without contrast dye. The contrast dye contains iodine, which can trigger allergic reactions in patients who have iodine or seafood allergies.

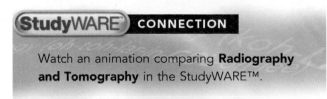

## Magnetic Resonance Imaging

**Magnetic resonance imaging**, or **MRI**, uses a combination of radio waves and a strong magnetic field to create

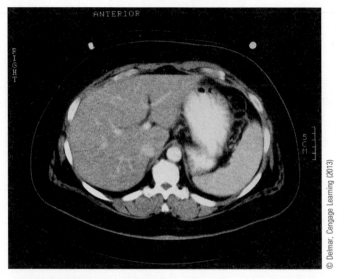

ANTERIOR

RIGHT

© Delmar, Cengage Learning (2013)

**FIGURE 15.16** An abdominal computed tomography scan in which the liver is predominant in the upper left and the stomach is visible in the upper right.

signals that are sent to a computer and converted into images of any plane through the body. These images are used to construct images of internal organs and tissues that often do not show up well in radiographs. An MRI is a noninvasive means of examining soft tissues such as those of the heart, blood vessels, brain, spinal cord, joints, muscles, and internal organs (Figure 15.17).

- MRI images can be produced in *coronal*, *sagittal*, or *oblique* planes and are created without the use of x-radiation.

- Because of the use of powerful magnets, the presence of metal implants such as a knee replacement, an artificial pacemaker, or metal stents can be contraindications for using an MRI on a patient.

- *Closed architecture MRI*, which is the most commonly used type of equipment, produces the most

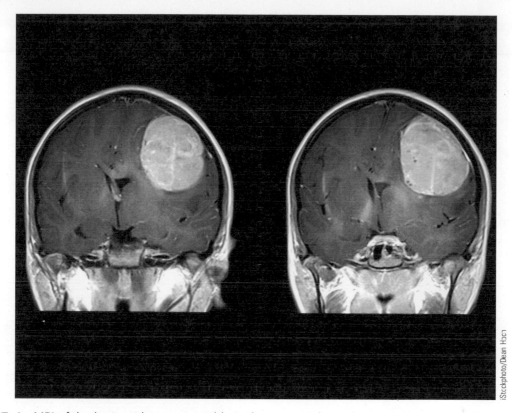

**FIGURE 15.17** An MRI of the brain with a tumor visible in the upper right.

accurate images; however, patients can be uncomfortable because of the noise generated by the machine and the feeling of being closed in.

■ As an alternative *open architecture MRI* is designed to be less confining and is more comfortable for some patients.

■ Some MRI exams use gadolinium contrast. Unlike computed tomography scan contrast dye, this does not use iodine, which is an allergy risk for those who have iodine or seafood allergies.

■ **Magnetic resonance angiography** (MRA), also known as *magnetic resonance angio*, helps locate problems within blood vessels throughout the body. This diagnostic imaging, which sometimes includes the use of a contrast dye, is frequently used as an alternative to the conventional angiography discussed in Chapter 5.

## Fluoroscopy

**Fluoroscopy** (floo-or-**OS**-koh-pee) is the visualization of body parts in motion by projecting x-ray images on a luminous fluorescent screen (**fluor/o** means glowing, and **-scopy** means visual examination). *Luminous* means glowing.

■ **Cineradiography** (sin-eh-**ray**-dee-**OG**-rah-fee) is the recording of the fluoroscopy images (**cine-** means relationship to movement, **radi/o** means radiation,

and **-graphy** means process of recording a picture or record).

■ Fluoroscopy can also be used in conjunction with conventional x-ray techniques to capture x-ray images of specific parts of the examination.

## Ultrasonography

**Ultrasonography** (**ul**-trah-son-**OG**-rah-fee), commonly referred to as *ultrasound* or *diagnostic ultrasound*, is imaging of deep body structures by recording the echoes of sound wave pulses that are above the range of human hearing ( **ultra-** means beyond, **son/o** means sound, and **-graphy** means the process of recording a picture or record).

■ A **sonogram** (**SOH**-noh-gram) is the image created by ultrasonography (**son/o** means sound, and **-gram** means a picture or record). These images are created by a *sonographer*, who is a technician specifically trained in this technique.

■ This technique is most effective for viewing solid organs of the abdomen and soft tissues where the signal is not stopped by intervening bone or air. Common uses of ultrasound include evaluating fetal development, detecting the presence of gallstones, or confirming the presence of a mass found on a mammogram.

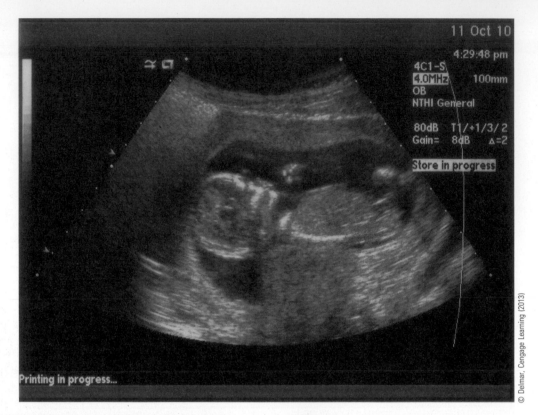

© Delmar, Cengage Learning (2013)

**FIGURE 15.18** Fetal ultrasound at about 15 weeks.

- *Carotid ultrasonography* is the use of sound waves to image the carotid artery to detect an obstruction that could cause an ischemic stroke (see Chapter 10).

- **Echocardiography** (**eck**-oh-**kar**-dee-**OG**-rah-fee) is an ultrasonic diagnostic procedure used to evaluate the structures and motion of the heart (**ech/o** means sound, **cardi/o** means heart, and **-graphy** means the process of recording a picture or record). The resulting record is an *echocardiogram*.

- A **Doppler echocardiogram** is performed in the same way as an echocardiogram; however, this procedure measures the speed and direction of the blood flow within the heart.

- **Fetal ultrasound** is a noninvasive procedure used to image and evaluate fetal development during pregnancy (Figures 15.18 and 15.19). *3D/4D ultrasound* is a technique that uses specialized equipment to create photograph-like images of the developing child.

- **Transesophageal echocardiography** (TEE) (**trans**-eh-**sof**-ah-**JEE**-al **eck**-oh-**kar**-dee-**OG**-rah-fee) is an ultrasonic imaging technique used to evaluate heart structures. This diagnostic test is performed from inside the esophagus, and because the esophagus is so close to the heart, this technique produces clearer images than those obtained with echocardiography.

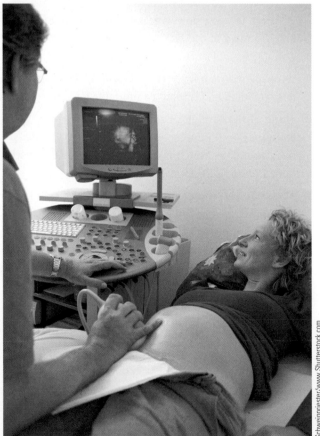

Schweinpriester/www.Shutterstock.com

**FIGURE 15.19** Fetal ultrasound is a noninvasive procedure used to image and evaluate fetal development before birth.

# NUCLEAR MEDICINE

In **nuclear medicine**, radioactive substances known as **radiopharmaceuticals** are administered for either diagnostic or treatment purposes. When used for diagnostic purposes, this is referred to as **nuclear imaging**, and these images document the structure and function of the organ or organs being examined.

- Each radiopharmaceutical contains a *radionuclide tracer*, also known as a *radioactive tracer*, which is specific to the body system being examined.

- Radiopharmaceuticals emit gamma rays that are detected by a gamma-ray camera attached to a computer. The data is used to generate an image showing the pattern of absorption that can be indicative of pathology.

## Nuclear Scans

A **nuclear scan**, also known as a *scintigram*, is a diagnostic procedure that uses nuclear medicine technology to gather information about the structure and function of organs or body systems that cannot be seen on conventional x-rays.

### Bone Scans

A **bone scan** is a nuclear scanning test that identifies new areas of bone growth or breakdown. The results are obtained after a radionuclide tracer is injected into the bloodstream, and the patient then waits while the material travels through the body tissues.

This testing can be done to evaluate damage to the bones, detect cancer that has metastasized (spread) to the bones, and monitor conditions that can affect the bones. A bone scan can often detect a problem days to months earlier than a regular x-ray. Only pathology in the bones absorbs the radionuclide, and these are visible as dark areas.

### Thyroid Scans

For a **thyroid scan**, a radiopharmaceutical containing radioactive iodine is administered. This scan makes use of the thyroid gland's ability to concentrate certain radioactive isotopes to generate images of it. A thyroid scan provides information about the size, shape, location, and relative activity of different parts of the thyroid gland.

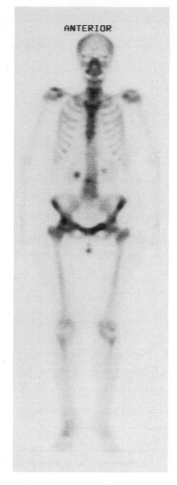
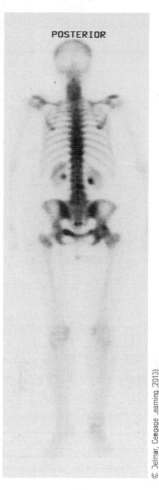

ANTERIOR　　　POSTERIOR

© Delmar, Cengage Learning (2013)

**FIGURE 15.20** A bone scan of the whole body showing the anterior and posterior view.

## Single Photon Emission Computed Tomography

**Single photon emission computed tomography**, also known as *SPECT*, is a type of nuclear imaging test that produces 3D computer-reconstructed images showing perfusion through tissues and organs. **Perfusion** (per-**FYOU**-zhun) means the flow of blood through an organ.

- SPECT scanning is used primarily to view the flow of blood through arteries and veins in the brain.

- It is also useful in diagnosing blood-deprived areas of brain following a stroke and tumors.

## Positron Emission Tomography

**Positron emission tomography**, also known as *PET imaging*, combines tomography with radionuclide tracers to produce enhanced images of selected body organs or areas.

- PET scans of the whole body are often used to detect cancer and to examine the effects of cancer therapy.

- PET scans of the heart are used to determine blood flow to the heart muscle. This procedure helps evaluate signs of coronary artery disease or to differentiate nonfunctional heart muscle from tissue that would benefit from a procedure such as angioplasty or coronary artery bypass surgery.

- PET scans of the brain are used to evaluate patients who have memory disorders of an undetermined cause, suspected or proven brain tumors, or seizure disorders that are not responsive to medical therapy and are therefore candidates for surgery.

## ■ PHARMACOLOGY

**Pharmacology** is the study of the nature, uses, and effects of drugs for medical purposes (**pharmac** means drug, and **-ology** means study of).

- A **pharmacist** is a licensed specialist who formulates and dispenses prescribed medications.

## Frequently Used Drug Administration Abbreviations and Symbols

Many abbreviations used in prescriptions and drug administration come from Latin terms. It may be helpful to look at the original words to remember their meanings and common abbreviations. See Table 15.2.

The Joint Commission has released a list of "do not use" abbreviations designed to cut back on medication errors by eliminating some commonly confused abbreviations (see Chapter 1 for more information about this). When in doubt, write it out!

Many of the symbols used in prescriptions are similar to those used in mathematics (see Table 15.3).

## Prescription and Over-the-Counter Drugs

- A **prescription** drug is a medication that can legally be dispensed only by a pharmacist with an order from a licensed professional such as a physician or dentist.

**TABLE 15.2**

**Frequently Used Drug Administration Abbreviations**

| Abbreviation | Meaning | Latin Origin |
|---|---|---|
| **ac** | before meals | *ante cibum* |
| **ad lib** | as desired | *ad libitum* |
| **amt** | amount | |
| **bid** | twice a day | *bis in die* |
| **NPO** | nothing by mouth | *nil per os* |
| **pc** | after meals | *post cibum* |
| **po** | by mouth | *per os* |
| **prn** | as needed | *pro re nata* |
| **qh** | every hour | *quaque* plus *h* for *hour* |
| **qid** | four times a day | *quater in die* |
| **Rx** | prescription | *recipe (to take)* |
| **sig** | to be labeled accordingly | *signa (to write)* |
| **tid** | three times a day | *ter in die* |

**TABLE 15.3**

**Frequently Used Drug Administration Symbols**

| Symbol | Meaning |
|---|---|
| @ | at |
| c̄ | with |
| ↑ | increase |
| ↓ | decrease |
| > | greater than |
| ≥ | greater than or equal to |
| < | less than |
| ≤ | less than or equal to |
| ♀ | female |
| ♂ | male |

■ An **over-the-counter** drug, also known as an *OTC*, is a medication that can be purchased without a prescription.

## Generic and Brand-Name Drugs

■ A **generic** drug is usually named for its chemical structure and is not protected by a brand name or trademark. For example, *diazepam* is the generic name of a drug frequently used as skeletal muscle relaxant, sedative, and anti-anxiety agent.

■ A **brand-name** drug is sold under the name given the drug by the manufacturer. A brand name is always spelled with a capital letter. For example, *Valium* is a brand name for diazepam.

## Terminology Related to Pharmacology

■ An **addiction** is compulsive, uncontrollable dependence on a drug, alcohol, or other substance. It can also be a habit or practice that cannot be stopped without causing severe emotional, mental, or physiologic reactions.

■ Drug **tolerance** is when the body has become accustomed to a medication after being on it for a length of time, and higher doses are required to achieve the desired effect.

■ An **adverse drug reaction** (ADR), also known as a *side effect*, is an undesirable reaction that accompanies the principal response for which the drug was taken.

■ **Compliance** is the patient's consistency and accuracy in following the regimen prescribed by a physician or other health care professional. As used here, *regimen* means directions or rules.

■ A **contraindication** is a factor in the patient's condition that makes the use of a medication or specific treatment dangerous or ill advised.

■ A **drug interaction** is the result of drugs reacting with each other, often in ways that are unexpected or potentially harmful. Such interactions can occur when medications are taken along with herbal remedies or when more than one prescription drug is taken at the same time.

■ An **idiosyncratic reaction** (**id**-ee-oh-sin-**KRAT**-ick) is an unexpected reaction to a drug that is peculiar to the individual.

■ A **palliative** (**PAL**-ee-**ay**-tiv) is a substance that eases the pain or severity of the symptoms of a disease, but does not cure it. *Palliative care* is treatment that focuses on alleviating pain and relieving symptoms rather than curing the disease.

■ A **paradoxical reaction** is the result of medical treatment that yields the exact opposite of normally expected results. *Paradoxical* means not being normal or the usual kind.

■ A **placebo** (plah-**SEE**-boh) is an inactive substance, such as a sugar pill or liquid, that is administered only for its suggestive effects. In medical research, a placebo is administered to one group and the drug being studied is administered to another group.

■ An **antipyretic** (**an**-tih-pye-**RET**-ick) is medication administered to prevent or reduce fever (**anti-** means against, **pyret** means fever, and **-ic** means pertaining to). These medications, such as aspirin and acetaminophen, act by lowering a raised body temperature; however, they do not affect a normal body temperature when a fever is not present.

■ An **anti-inflammatory** relieves inflammation and pain without affecting consciousness.

## Medications for Pain Management
### Analgesics

The term **analgesic** (an-al-**JEE**-zick) refers to the class of drugs that relieves pain without affecting consciousness. These include such drugs as aspirin, acetaminophen, and ibuprofen.

*Non-narcotic analgesics*, such as aspirin, are sold over the counter for mild to moderate pain. Prescription pain relievers, sold through a pharmacy under the direction of a physician, are used for more moderate to severe pain.

*Narcotic analgesics*, such as morphine, Demerol, and codeine, are available by prescription only to relieve severe pain. These medications also have a sedative (calming) effect and can cause physical dependence or addiction. Sedatives are discussed in Chapter 10.

- **Acetaminophen** (ah-**seet**-ah-**MIN**-oh-fen) is an analgesic that reduces pain and fever, but does not relieve inflammation; however, it does not have the negative side effects of NSAIDS. This substance is basic ingredient found in Tylenol and its generic equivalents.

- **Nonsteroidal anti-inflammatory drugs**, commonly known as *NSAIDs*, are non-narcotic analgesics administered to control pain by reducing inflammation and swelling. NSAIDS, such as aspirin and ibuprofen, are available over the counter. Stronger NSAIDs are available by prescription. Medications in this group can cause side effects, including attacking the stomach lining and thinning the blood.

- **Ibuprofen** (eye-byoo-**pro**-fen) is a non-steroidal anti-inflammatory medicine that is sold over the counter under the brand names of Advil and Motrin. This medication acts an analgesic and an antipyretic.

- Although pain management is not their primary role, **anticonvulsants** and **antidepressants** have been found to be effective as part of some chronic pain management programs. *Anticonvulsants* are traditionally administered to prevent seizures such as those associated with epilepsy. *Antidepressants* are primarily administered to prevent or relieve depression.

## Additional Pain Control Methods

- **Pain-relieving creams** are applied topically to relieve pain due to conditions such as osteoarthritis and rheumatoid arthritis. The primary active ingredient in these ointments is *capsaicin*, a chemical found in chili peppers.

- **Transcutaneous electronic nerve stimulation**, also known as *TENS*, is a method of pain control by wearing a device that delivers small electrical impulses, as needed, to the nerve endings through the skin (**trans-** means across, **cutane** means skin, and **-ous** means pertaining to). These electrical impulses cause changes in muscles, such as numbness or contractions, which produce temporary pain relief. The term *transcutaneous* means performed through the unbroken skin.

## Methods of Drug Administration

- **Inhalation administration** describes vapors and gases taken in through the nose or mouth and absorbed into the bloodstream through the lungs. One example is the use of a metered-dose inhaler to treat asthma (see Chapter 7) or the gases used for general anesthesia (see Chapter 10).

- **Oral administration** refers to medications taken by mouth to be absorbed through the walls of the stomach or small intestine. These drugs can be in the form of liquids, tablets (pills), or capsules. Medications to be released in the small intestine are covered with an *enteric coating* to prevent them from being absorbed in the stomach.

- **Rectal administration** is the insertion of medication in the rectum either in the form of a suppository or a liquid. A *suppository* is medication in a semi-solid form that is introduced into the rectum. The suppository melts at body temperature, and the medication is absorbed through the surrounding tissues.

- **Sublingual administration** is the placement of medication under the tongue where it is allowed to dissolve slowly (**sub-** means under, **lingu** means tongue, and **-al** means pertaining to). Because the sublingual tissues are highly vascular, the medication is quickly absorbed directly into the bloodstream. *Highly vascular* means containing many blood vessels.

- A **topical application** is a liquid or ointment that is rubbed into the skin on the area to be treated, for example, *cortisone ointment* is applied topically to relieve itching and to speed healing; *antibiotic ointments* are applied over minor wounds to prevent infection.

- A **transdermal** medication is administered from a patch that is applied to unbroken skin (**trans-** means through or across, **derm** means skin, and **-al** means pertaining to). The medication, which is continuously released by the patch, is absorbed through the skin and transmitted to the bloodstream so that it can produce a systemic effect. These multilayered patches are used to convey medications, such as nitroglycerin for angina, hormones for hormone replacement therapy, or nicotine patches for smoking cessation.

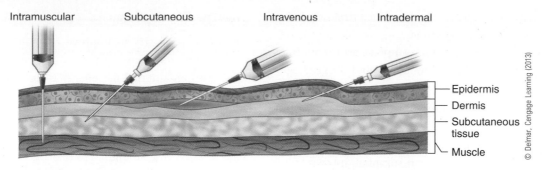

**FIGURE 15.21** Types of injections.

## Parenteral Administration

The term **parenteral** (pah-**REN**-ter-al) means taken into the body or administered in a manner other than through the digestive tract. The most common use of parenteral administration is by injection through a *hypodermic syringe* (Figure 15.21).

■ A **subcutaneous injection** (SC) is made into the fatty layer just below the skin.

■ An **intradermal injection** is made into the middle layers of the skin.

■ An **intramuscular injection** (IM) is made directly into muscle tissue (**intra-** means within, **muscul** means muscle, and **-ar** means pertaining to).

■ An **intravenous injection** (IV) is made directly into a vein (**intra-** means within, **ven** means vein, and **-ous** means pertaining to).

■ A **PICC line,** which is the abbreviation for *peripherally inserted central catheter*, is frequently used for a patient who will need IV therapy for more than 7 days.

■ A **bolus** (**BOH**-lus), which is also known as a *bolus infusion*, is a single, concentrated dose of drug usually injected into a blood vessel over a short period of time. The term *bolus* is also used in relation to the digestive system (see Chapter 8).

## ■ COMPLEMENTARY AND ALTERNATIVE MEDICINE

There is a wide range of **complementary and alternative medicine** (CAM) available to patients today. Some have been researched and proven effective, but others have little research to support their claims. These therapies can be used to supplement or replace allopathic medicine.

■ **Allopathic medicine** (ah-low-**PAH**-thick) is another term for conventional, or Western, medical practices and systems of health care.

■ **Alternative medicine** is a general term for practices and systems of health care other than allopathic approaches used *in place of* these treatments.

■ **Complementary medicine** is a general term for practices and systems of health care other than allopathic approaches used to *supplement* these treatments.

■ **Integrative medicine** is a model of health care based on both allopathic and alternative medicine.

■ The term **holistic** (hoe-**LISS**-tick) refers to a treatment approach that takes into consideration the whole body and its environment, including the mind, body, and spirit.

## Alternative Medicine

Some forms of alternative medicine are rooted in traditional systems, such as Ayurvedic medicine and traditional Chinese medicine, while others have been developed more recently, such as homeopathy. It is important to be aware of any herbal supplements or remedies that patients may be taking, as some can interact negatively with other medications or have potentially dangerous side effects.

■ **Ayurvedic medicine** (ay-uhr-**VEH**-dick) is the traditional Hindu system of medicine, emphasizing a holistic approach to preventive treatment through hygiene, exercise, herbal preparations, and yoga, and the treatment of illnesses with herbal medicines, physiotherapy, and diet.

■ **Traditional Chinese medicine** is a system of ancient Chinese medicinal treatments including acupuncture, diet, herbal therapy, meditation, physical exercise, and massage, to prevent, diagnose, and treat disease. Parts of traditional Chinese medicine, such as acupuncture, are also used as complementary medicine.

■ **Naturopathy** (nay-cher-**AH**-pah-thee), also known as *naturopathic medicine*, is a combination of nutrition, medicinal supplements and herbs, water therapy, homeopathy, and lifestyle modifications used to identify and treat the root causes of symptoms and disease instead of surgery and drugs. It emphasizes supporting the body's own innate healing ability and the healing power of nature.

- **Homeopathy** (**hoh**-mee-**OP**-ah-thee) involves the use of substances created from plant or mineral products diluted a thousand-fold in water or alcohol. Homeopaths believe that the body can stimulate its own healing responses when the right trigger is given in minute doses, producing symptoms similar to the disease being treated.

## Complementary Medicine

Types of complementary medicine can be broken down into three categories: mind-body therapies, hands-on therapies, and energy therapies.

### Mind-Body Therapies

*Mind-body therapies* try to reduce stress and prevent its negative effects on the body. They can be used for stress reduction, pain management, lifestyle changes, and depression. These therapies are based on the belief that emotions, such as stress, trigger physiological responses. By becoming aware of and reducing stressful emotions and thoughts, it is possible to decrease physical stress and its negative effects.

- **Biofeedback** is a patient-guided treatment that teaches individuals to control muscle tension, pain, body temperature, brain waves, and other bodily functions through relaxation, visualization, and other cognitive control techniques.

- **Guided imagery** is a type of treatment in which a patient follows verbal prompts to envision a specific, peaceful location in detail, distancing him- or herself from any pain or stress the patient is currently experiencing.

- **Hypnosis** is a type of therapy in which a patient is placed in a state of focused concentration and narrowed attention that makes him or her more susceptible to suggestions, and then given suggestions directed toward the patient's treatment goal.

- **Mindfulness meditation** focuses on becoming aware of thoughts and emotions and their physiological responses, as well as accepting them and maintaining a calm, constant awareness.

### Energy Therapies

*Energy therapies* try to improve or maintain health by manipulating the body's energy flow, or qi. *Qi* is believed to be the fundamental life energy responsible for health and vitality. These therapies are based on the belief that illness is linked to blocked or insufficient energy levels.

- **Acupressure** (**AK**-que-**presh**-ur) is a traditional Chinese touch therapy involving finger pressure applied to specific areas of the body to restore the flow of qi.

- **Acupuncture** (**AK**-que-**punk**-tyour) is a traditional Chinese medical practice using very thin acupuncture needles inserted into specific points of the body to restore the flow of qi (Figure 15.22)

- **Qi Gong** (**CHEE**-gong) is a Chinese system of movement, breathing techniques, and meditation designed to improve and enhance the flow of qi.

### Hands-on Therapies

*Hands-on therapies* try to improve body function by physically manipulating or massaging the body. They can be used for neck or back pain, relaxation, and increased range of motion. This therapy is based on the belief that the body functions more efficiently when it is in proper alignment, and that it is possible to identify and correct poor movement and posture habits.

- **Chiropractic manipulative therapy** is a system of mechanical spinal adjustments made by a chiropractor to correct biomechanical problems in the skeletal framework of the body. See Chapter 3 for the definition of *chiropractor*.

- **Osteopathic manipulative therapy** is mechanical spinal adjustment used in conjunction with conventional medical therapies by an osteopath. See Chapter 3 for the definition of *osteopath*.

- **Craniosacral therapy** (**kray**-nee-oh-**SAK**-ral) is the use of gentle touch to help the body release tension, stress, and trauma to correct restrictions resulting from stress on the central nervous system (**crani/o** means skull, and **sacral** means referring to the sacrum).

- **Myofascial release** (**my**-oh-**FASH**-ee-ahl) is a specialized soft-tissue manipulation technique used to ease the pain of conditions such as fibromyalgia, myofascial pain syndrome, movement restrictions, temporomandibular joint disorders (TMJ), and carpal tunnel syndrome (**my/o** means muscle, and **fascial** refers to the fascia) (See Chapter 4).

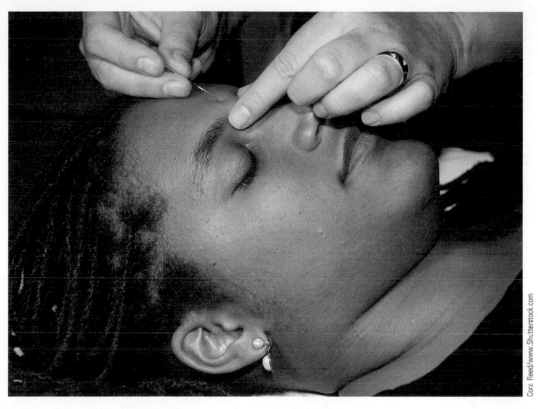

Core Reed/www.Shutterstock.com

**FIGURE 15.22** Acupuncture uses thin needles inserted into specific body points.

■ **Neuromuscular therapy** (NMT) is a form of massage that uses soft-tissue manipulation focusing on applying pressure to trigger points to treat injuries and alleviate pain. A *trigger point* is a particularly taut band of muscle that is tender to the touch.

## ■ ABBREVIATIONS RELATED TO DIAGNOSTIC PROCEDURES, NUCLEAR MEDICINE, AND PHARMACOLOGY

Table 15.4 presents an overview of the abbreviations related to the terms introduced in this chapter. Note: To avoid errors or confusion, always be cautious when using abbreviations.

### StudyWARE CONNECTION

For more practice and to test your mastery of this material, go to the StudyWARE™ to play interactive games and complete the quiz for this chapter.

### ☐ Workbook Practice

Go to your workbook and complete the exercises for this chapter.

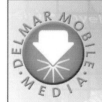

*Downloadable audio is available for selected medical terms in this chapter to enhance your learning of medical terminology.*

## TABLE 15.4
## Abbreviations Related to the Diagnostic Procedures, Nuclear Medicine, and Pharmacology

| | |
|---|---|
| **adverse drug reaction** = ADR | **ADR** = adverse drug reaction |
| **beats per minute** = bpm | **bpm** = beats per minute |
| **blood pressure** = BP | **BP** = blood pressure |
| **blood urea nitrogen** = BUN | **BUN** = blood urea nitrogen |
| **complete blood count** = CBC | **CBC** = complete blood count |
| **computed tomography scan** = CT scan | **CT scan** = computed tomography scan |
| **endoscopy** = endo | **endo** = endoscopy |
| **erythrocyte sedimentation rate** = ESR | **ESR** = erythrocyte sedimentation rate |
| **hematocrit** = Hct | **Hct** = hematocrit |
| **magnetic resonance imaging** = MRI | **MRI** = magnetic resonance imaging |
| **red blood count** = RBC | **RBC** = red blood count |
| **respiratory rate** = RR | **RR** = respiratory rate |
| **temperature, pulse, respiration** = TPR | **TPR** = temperature, pulse, respiration |
| **white blood count** = WBC | **WBC** = white blood count |

# LEARNING EXERCISES

## MATCHING WORD PARTS 1

Write the correct answer in the middle column.

| Definition | Correct Answer | Possible Answers |
|---|---|---|
| 15.1.   abdomen | _____ | **lapar/o** |
| 15.2.   albumin, protein | _____ | **glycos/o** |
| 15.3.   calcium | _____ | **creatin/o** |
| 15.4.   creatinine | _____ | **calc/i** |
| 15.5.   sugar | _____ | **albumin/o** |

## MATCHING WORD PARTS 2

Write the correct answer in the middle column.

| Definition | Correct Answer | Possible Answers |
|---|---|---|
| 15.6.   surgical puncture to remove fluid | _____ | **son/o** |
| 15.7.   blood | _____ | **-otomy** |
| 15.8.   surgical incision | _____ | **hemat/o** |
| 15.9.   process of producing a picture or record | _____ | **-graphy** |
| 15.10.  sound | _____ | **-centesis** |

## MATCHING WORD PARTS 3

Write the correct answer in the middle column.

| Definition | Correct Answer | Possible Answers |
|---|---|---|
| 15.11.  direct visual examination | _____ | -uria |
| 15.12.  radiation | _____ | -scopy |
| 15.13.  urine | _____ | -scope |
| 15.14.  vein | _____ | radi/o |
| 15.15.  visual examination instrument | _____ | phleb/o |

## DEFINITIONS

Select the correct answer, and write it on the line provided.

15.16.  The type of therapy in which a patient is placed in a state of focused concentration and narrowed atten-

tion that makes him or her more susceptible to suggestions, and then given suggestions directed toward

the treatment goal is called _____.

    mindfulness meditation          hypnosis          biofeedback          guided imagery

15.17.  A/An _____ is used to enlarge the opening of any body canal or cavity to facilitate

inspection of its interior.

        endoscope          otoscope          speculum          sphygmomanometer

15.18.  The imaging technique that produces multiple cross-sectional images using x-radiation

is _____.

        computed tomography          fluoroscopy          magnetic resonance imaging          radiography

15.19.  Drug _____ is when the body has become accustomed to a medication after being

on it for a length of time, and higher doses are required to achieve the desired effect.

        tolerance          compliance          side effect          paradoxical reaction

15.20.  The diagnostic technique _____ creates images of deep body structures by record-

ing the echoes of pulses of sound waves that are above the range of human hearing.

        cineradiography          extraoral radiography          fluoroscopy          ultrasonography

15.21.  The presence of calcium in the urine is known as _____.

        albuminuria               calciuria              creatinuria           glycosuria

15.22.  A/An _____ test is used to identify high levels of inflammation within the body.

       blood urea nitrogen        C-reactive protein        erythrocyte sedimentation      serum bilirubin

15.23.  In the _____ position, the patient is lying on the back with the knees bent.

       dorsal recumbent        horizontal recumbent        knee-chest        supine

15.24.  A _____ is an abnormal sound heard during auscultation of an artery.

          bruit              rale             rhonchi          stridor

15.25.  The presence of pus in the urine, which causes the urine to be cloudy or smoky in appearance, is

      called _____.

        glycosuria              ketonuria            hematuria           pyuria

## MATCHING TECHNIQUES

Write the correct answer in the middle column.

| Definition | Correct Answer | Possible Answers |
| --- | --- | --- |
| 15.26.  produces cross-sectional views | _____ | x-rays |
| 15.27.  produces views in only one direction | _____ | MRI |
| 15.28.  the removal of fluid for diagnostic purposes | _____ | fluoroscopy |
| 15.29.  uses a luminous fluorescent screen | _____ | centesis |
| 15.30.  uses radio waves and a magnetic field | _____ | CT |

## WHICH WORD?

Select the correct answer, and write it on the line provided.

15.31.  A/An _____ reaction is an unexpected reaction to a drug that is peculiar to the

      individual.

       idiosyncratic             palliative

15.32. _____ tomography combines tomography with radionuclide tracers to produce

enhanced images of selected body organs or areas.

Positron emission                Single photon emission computed

15.33.  A substance that does not allow x-rays to pass through is described as being _____.

radiolucent                radiopaque

15.34.  When film is placed within the mouth and exposed by a camera positioned next to the cheek, this is

called _____ radiography.

extraoral                intraoral

15.35.  A _____ drug is sold under the name given the drug by the manufacturer. These

drug names are always spelled with a capital letter.

brand-name                generic

## SPELLING COUNTS

Find the misspelled word in each sentence. Then write that word, spelled correctly, on the line provided.

15.36.  Listening through a stethoscope for sounds within the body to determine the condition of the lungs,

pleura, heart, and abdomen is known as asultation. _____

15.37.  A sphygnomanometer is used to measure blood pressure. _____

15.38.  Fluroscopy is the visualization of body parts in motion by projecting x-ray images on a luminous fluores-

cent screen. _____

15.39.  A conterindication is a factor in the patient's condition that makes the use of a medication or specific

treatment dangerous or ill advised.

15.40.  An opthalmoscope is used to examine the interior of the eye. _____

## ABBREVIATION IDENTIFICATION

In the space provided, write the words in English that each abbreviation stands for.

10.41.  **ESR**                _____

10.42.  **NPO**                _____

10.43.  **prn**                _____

10.44.  **TPR**    _____

10.45.  **WBC**    _____

## TERM SELECTION

Select the correct answer, and write it on the line provided.

15.46.  Drawing fluid from the sac surrounding the heart is known as _____.

      abdominocentesis        cardiocentesis        pericardiocentesis        arthrocentesis

15.47.  The presence of blood in the urine is known as _____.

      albuminuria        creatinuria        hematuria        ketonuria

15.48.  _____ is a combination of nutrition, medicinal supplements and herbs, water therapy, homeopathy, and lifestyle modifications used to identify and treat the root causes of symptoms and disease.

      naturopathy        homeopathy        Qi Gong        biofeedback

15.49.  A/An _____ relieves inflammation and pain without affecting consciousness.

      acetaminophen        analgesic        anti-inflammatory        palliative

15.50.  The term _____ means the administration of a medication by a manner other than through the digestive tract (more commonly through injection).

      hypodermic        parenteral        transcutaneous        transdermal

## SENTENCE COMPLETION

Write the correct term on the line provided.

15.51.  The term *radiographic* _____ describes the path that the x-ray beam follows through the body from entrance to exit.

15.52.  The term _____ describes an abnormal, high-pitched, musical breathing sound that is heard during inspiration.

15.53.  A/An _____ is a medical professional trained to draw blood from patients for laboratory tests and other procedures.

15.54.  A/An _____ is an instrument used to visually examine the external ear and tympanic membrane.

15.55. _____ is a traditional Chinese touch therapy involving finger pressure applied to specific areas of the body to restore the flow of qi.

## WORD SURGERY

Divide each term into its component word parts. Write these word parts, in sequence, on the lines provided. When necessary use a slash (/) to indicate a combining vowel. (You may not need all of the lines provided.)

15.56. **Abdominocentesis** is a surgical puncture of the joint space to remove synovial fluid for analysis to determine the cause of pain or swelling in a joint.

_____   _____   _____   _____

15.57. **Cineradiography** is the recording of fluoroscopy images.

_____   _____   _____   _____

15.58. **Echocardiography** is an ultrasonic diagnostic procedure used to evaluate the structures and motion of the heart.

_____   _____   _____   _____

15.59. **Bacteriuria** is the presence of bacteria in the urine.

_____   _____   _____   _____

15.60. **Pharmacology** is the study of the nature, uses, and effects of drugs for medical purposes.

_____   _____   _____   _____

## TRUE/FALSE

If the statement is true, write **True** on the line. If the statement is false, write **False** on the line.

15.61. _____ Neuromuscular therapy is a form of massage that uses soft-tissue manipulation focusing on applying pressure to trigger points.

15.62. _____ Casts are fibrous or protein materials, such as pus and fats, that are thrown off into the urine in kidney disease.

15.63. _____ A placebo contains medication and has the potential to cure a disease.

15.64. _____ An MRI creates images by combining sound wave pulses and strong magnets.

15.65. _____ Compliance means that the patient has accurately followed instructions.

## CLINICAL CONDITIONS

Write the correct answer on the line provided.

15.66.  The urinalysis for Sophia O'Keefe showed the presence of ketones. The medical term for this condition

is _____.

15.67.  Dr. Jamison suspected her patient had an infection. An elevated count in the

patient's _____ cell count test would confirm her diagnosis.

15.68.  Kelly Harrison was extremely cold after being stranded in a snowstorm. When rescued, the paramedics

said she was suffering from _____.

15.69.  During his examination of the patient, Dr. Wong used _____ to feel the texture,

size, consistency, and location of certain body parts.

15.70.  Dr. McDowell ordered a blood transfusion. Before the transfusion, _____ tests were

required to determine the compatibility of donor's and recipient's blood.

15.71.  In preparation for his upper GI series, Dwight Oshone swallowed a liquid containing the contrast

medium _____.

15.72.  Maria Martinez required _____ echocardiography to evaluate the structures of her

heart.

15.73.  Another term for conventional, or Western, medical practices is _____.

15.74.  The urinalysis for Kathleen McCaffee showed _____. This is the presence of glu-

cose in the urine.

15.75.  Dr. Roberts used _____ during the examination. This technique involves tapping

the surface of the body with a finger or instrument.

## WHICH IS THE CORRECT MEDICAL TERM?

Select the correct answer, and write it on the line provided.

15.76. A/An _____ drug reaction is an undesirable reaction that accompanies the principal response for which the drug was taken.

      adverse           idiosyncratic           placebo           synergism

15.77. The urinalysis indicated _____. This is an increased concentration of creatinine in the urine.

      creatinuria           glycosuria           ketonuria           proteinuria

15.78. The energy therapy where finger pressure is applied to specific areas of the body is called _____.

      Qi Gong           acupuncture           acupressure           hypnosis

15.79. During a/an _____ examination, some patients feel uncomfortable because of the noise generated by the machine and the feeling of being closed in.

      CT           MRI           PET           x-ray

15.80. The examination position that has the patient lying on the back with the feet and legs raised and supported in stirrups is the _____ position.

      dorsal recumbent           lithotomy           prone           Sims'

## CHALLENGE WORD BUILDING

These terms are *not* found in this chapter; however, they are made up of the following familiar word parts. If you need help in creating the term, refer to your medical dictionary.

| | | |
|---|---|---|
| **hyper-** | **albumin/o** | **-centesis** |
| **hypo-** | **calc/i** | **-emia** |
| | **cyst/o** | **-gram** |
| | **glycos/o** | **-scope** |
| | **protein/o** | **-uria** |
| | **pleur/o** | |
| | **py/o** | |

15.81. The term meaning the presence of abnormally low concentrations of protein in the blood

is _____.

15.82. The term meaning abnormally high levels of albumin in the blood is _____.

15.83. The term meaning unusually large amounts of sugar in the urine is _____.

15.84. The instrument used to visually examine the interior of the urinary bladder is

a/an _____.

15.85. The term meaning a surgical puncture of the chest wall with a needle to obtain fluid from the pleural

cavity is _____. This procedure is also known as thoracentesis.

15.86. An x-ray examination of the bladder is called a _____

15.87. The term meaning an abnormally low level of calcium in the circulating blood

is _____.

15.88. The term meaning abnormally large amounts of calcium in the urine is _____.

15.89. The term meaning the presence of pus-forming organisms in the blood is _____.

15.90. The term meaning the presence of excess protein in the urine is _____.

## LABELING EXERCISES

Identify the numbered items on the accompanying figures.

15.91.   This is the _____ position.

15.92.   This is the _____ recumbent position.

15.93.   This is the _____ position.

15.94.   This is the _____ recumbent position.

15.95.   This is the _____ position.

15.96.   This is the _____ position.

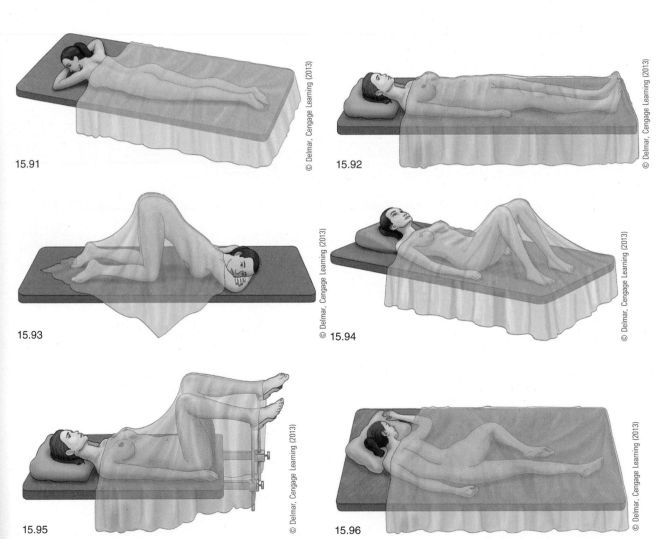

15.91

15.92

15.93

15.94

15.95

15.96

© Delmar, Cengage Learning (2013)

15.97.   This is a/an _____ injection.

15.98.   This is a/an _____ injection.

15.99.   This is a/an _____ injection.

15.100  This is a/an _____ injection.

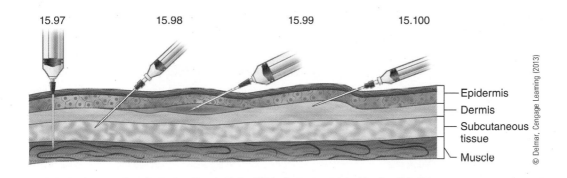

© Delmar, Cengage Learning (2013)

# THE HUMAN TOUCH
## Critical Thinking Exercise

The following story and questions are designed to stimulate critical thinking through class discussion or as a brief essay response. There are no right or wrong answers to these questions.

*Terrance Ortega had finally made it. Standing behind the counter of the pharmacy at SuperDrug, he thought back on his years at pharmacology school. He had studied hard, and it paid off when he landed this job.*

*A young man approached the counter and said, "I'm James Tirendale, and I'm here to pick up my mom Ginny's prescription for MS Contin." He flashed a handwritten scrawled note from his mother. "Sure thing, James, let me just find that for you."*

*Terrance headed to the counter where filled prescriptions were kept and grabbed the one marked "Ginny Tirendale." Sure enough, there was a prescription for MS Contin; a palliative usually prescribed for pain.*

*He explained to James the adverse affects that this drug could have, that it was to be administered orally, and that it was not to be crushed or cut. James paid cash and headed out of the store in a hurry.*

*Later that day, a woman on crutches came up to the pharmacy counter. She explained that her name was Ginny Tirendale and that she needed to pick up some pain medication because she had just had knee surgery. A confused look came over Terrance's face. "Your son already picked that up, Ms. Tirendale," he explained. "Oh no!" Ginny replied, "I knew I should not have told him I was coming here this afternoon. He must have realized which drug I was prescribed and got here before me."*

*Suddenly Terrance realized that he should have looked at the note more closely or called Ms. Tirendale before giving out a prescription for a drug with such a high "street value." It occurred to him that an adverse drug reaction could occur if MS Contin was taken with alcohol, and it could easily lead to psychological and physical dependence if abused. What if her son didn't know that and died, or sold it to someone else who abused it?*

## Suggested Discussion Topics

1. What precaution had James taken in case the pharmacist asked questions?
2. Suppose Terrance was suspicious about allowing James pick up the prescription. Discuss the steps Terrance might have taken, including involving his supervisor.
3. Terrance appears to blame himself for what happened with the MS Contin prescription. What might the pharmacy have done to ensure that medicine is always given to the right person, no matter who is on duty?
4. Ms. Tirendale is obviously suspicious of her son's actions regarding the prescription. Discuss the steps she might take to help him if she thinks he is abusing drugs.

# Comprehensive Medical Terminology Review

## Overview of
## COMPREHENSIVE MEDICAL TERMINOLOGY REVIEW

**Study Tips**

Hints to help you review more effectively.

**Answer Sheets**

Write the *letter* of the correct answer for the questions in the review tests. Although only one set of answer sheets are included, you can take these tests as often as you want.

**Review Session**

A 100-multiple-choice-question review session to help you determine where you need more study emphasis. However, be aware that none of these questions are from the actual final test.

**Simulated Medical Terminology Final Test**

A 100-multiple-choice-question "mock" final test to help you evaluate your progress. However, be aware that none of these questions are from the actual final test.

**Answer Keys**

The answer keys for self-grading these practice tests are at the end of the respective review sections.

# ■ STUDY TIPS

## Use Your Vocabulary Lists

■ Photocopy the vocabulary list for each chapter from your textbook, and add any terms suggested by your instructor. This creates a study aid that is easy to carry with you for additional review whenever you have a free minute.

■ Review the terms on each list. When you have mastered a term, put a check in the box next to it. If you cannot spell and define a term, highlight it for further study.

■ Look up the meanings of the highlighted terms in the textbook, and work on mastering them.

■ When using a list is not convenient, consider listening to the **Audio CDs** that accompany this text. The 60 words in the vocabulary list at the beginning of each chapter are pronounced and defined on these CDs.

■ Caution: Do not limit your studying to these lists. Although they contain important terms, there are many additional important words in each chapter that you need to know.

## Use Your Flash Cards

■ Use the flash cards from the back of this book.

■ As you go through them, remove from the stack all the word parts you can define.

■ Keep working until you have mastered all of the word parts.

## Make Your Own Study List

■ By now you should have greatly reduced the number of terms still to be mastered. Make a list of these terms and word parts, and concentrate on them.

## Review Your Learning Exercises

As your corrected Learning Exercises are returned, save them. At review time go through these sheets and note where you made mistakes. Ask yourself, *"Do I know the correct answer now?"* If not, add the term or word part to your study list.

For the True/False questions in the Learning Exercises, you can challenge yourself to change all the "false" answers into true ones. For example, "Cholangiography is an endoscopic diagnostic procedure," is false. Ask yourself: "What is the correct definition of cholangiography?"

## Help Someone Else

One of the greatest ways to really learn something is to teach it! If a classmate is having trouble, tutoring that person will help both of you learn the material.

## Use the Practice Sessions

The next two pages are answer sheets to be used with the Review Session and Simulated Medical Terminology Final Test that follow. The answer keys for self-grading these tests are at the end of the respective sections.

# REVIEW SESSION ANSWER SHEET

Write the **letter** of the correct answer on the line next to the question number.

Name _____

RS.1. _____

RS.2. _____

RS.3. _____

RS.4. _____

RS.5. _____

RS.6. _____

RS.7. _____

RS.8. _____

RS.9. _____

RS.10. _____

RS.11. _____

RS.12. _____

RS.13. _____

RS.14. _____

RS.15. _____

RS.16. _____

RS.17. _____

RS.18. _____

RS.19. _____

RS.20. _____

RS.21. _____

RS.22. _____

RS.23. _____

RS.24. _____

RS.25. _____

RS.26. _____

RS.27. _____

RS.28. _____

RS.29. _____

RS.30. _____

RS.31. _____

RS.32. _____

RS.33. _____

RS.34. _____

RS.35. _____

RS.36. _____

RS.37. _____

RS.38. _____

RS.39. _____

RS.40. _____

RS.41. _____

RS.42. _____

RS.43. _____

RS.44. _____

RS.45. _____

RS.46. _____

RS.47. _____

RS.48. _____

RS.49. _____

RS.50. _____

RS.51. _____

RS.52. _____

RS.53. _____

RS.54. _____

RS.55. _____

RS.56. _____

RS.57. _____

RS.58. _____

RS.59. _____

RS.60. _____

RS.61. _____

RS.62. _____

RS.63. _____

RS.64. _____

RS.65. _____

RS.66. _____

RS.67. _____

RS.68. _____

RS.69. _____

RS.70. _____

RS.71. _____

RS.72. _____

RS.73. _____

RS.74. _____

RS.75. _____

RS.76. _____

RS.77. _____

RS.78. _____

RS.79. _____

RS.80. _____

RS.81. _____

RS.82. _____

RS.83. _____

RS.84. _____

RS.85. _____

RS.86. _____

RS.87. _____

RS.88. _____

RS.89. _____

RS.90. _____

RS.91. _____

RS.92. _____

RS.93. _____

RS.94. _____

RS.95. _____

RS.96. _____

RS.97. _____

RS.98. _____

RS.99. _____

RS.100. _____

# ■ SIMULATED MEDICAL TERMINOLOGY FINAL TEST ANSWER SHEET

Write the **letter** of the correct answer on the line next to the question number.

**Name** _____

| | | | |
|---|---|---|---|
| FT.1. _____ | FT.26. _____ | FT.51. _____ | FT.76. _____ |
| FT.2. _____ | FT.27. _____ | FT.52. _____ | FT.77. _____ |
| FT.3. _____ | FT.28. _____ | FT.53. _____ | FT.78. _____ |
| FT.4. _____ | FT.29. _____ | FT.54. _____ | FT.79. _____ |
| FT.5. _____ | FT.30. _____ | FT.55. _____ | FT.80. _____ |
| FT.6. _____ | FT.31. _____ | FT.56. _____ | FT.81. _____ |
| FT.7. _____ | FT.32. _____ | FT.57. _____ | FT.82. _____ |
| FT.8. _____ | FT.33. _____ | FT.58. _____ | FT.83. _____ |
| FT.9. _____ | FT.34. _____ | FT.59. _____ | FT.84. _____ |
| FT.10. _____ | FT.35. _____ | FT.60. _____ | FT.85. _____ |
| FT.11. _____ | FT.36. _____ | FT.61. _____ | FT.86. _____ |
| FT.12. _____ | FT.37. _____ | FT.62. _____ | FT.87. _____ |
| FT.13. _____ | FT.38. _____ | FT.63. _____ | FT.88. _____ |
| FT.14. _____ | FT.39. _____ | FT.64. _____ | FT.89. _____ |
| FT.15. _____ | FT.40. _____ | FT.65. _____ | FT.90. _____ |
| FT.16. _____ | FT.41. _____ | FT.66. _____ | FT.91. _____ |
| FT.17. _____ | FT.42. _____ | FT.67. _____ | FT.92. _____ |
| FT.18. _____ | FT.43. _____ | FT.68. _____ | FT.93. _____ |
| FT.19. _____ | FT.44. _____ | FT.69. _____ | FT.94. _____ |
| FT.20. _____ | FT.45. _____ | FT.70. _____ | FT.95. _____ |
| FT.21. _____ | FT.46. _____ | FT.71. _____ | FT.96. _____ |
| FT.22. _____ | FT.47. _____ | FT.72. _____ | FT.97. _____ |
| FT.23. _____ | FT.48. _____ | FT.73. _____ | FT.98. _____ |
| FT.24. _____ | FT.49. _____ | FT.74. _____ | FT.99. _____ |
| FT.25. _____ | FT.50. _____ | FT.75. _____ | FT.100. _____ |

# REVIEW SESSION

RS.1. An abnormally rapid rate of respiration usually of more than 20 breaths per minute is known as _____.

a. bradypnea

b. eupnea

c. hyperventilation

d. tachypnea

RS.2. An abnormally slow heart rate of less than 60 beats per minute is known as _____.

a. atrial fibrillation

b. bradycardia

c. palpitation

d. tachycardia

RS.3. The suffix _____ means surgical fixation.

a. **-desis**

b. **-lysis**

c. **-pexy**

d. **-ptosis**

RS.4. The presence of glucose in the urine is known as _____.

a. albuminuria

b. calciuria

c. glycosuria

d. hematuria

RS.5. A collection of pus within a body cavity is known as a/an _____.

a. cyst

b. empyema

c. hernia

d. tumor

RS.6. The grating sound heard when the ends of a broken bone move together is known as _____.

a. closed reduction

b. osteoclasis

c. callus

d. crepitation

RS.7. The abnormal development or growth of cells is known as _____.

a. anaplasia

b. dysplasia

c. hyperplasia

d. hypertrophy

RS.8. Which form of anemia is a genetic disorder?

a. aplastic

b. hemolytic

c. megaloblastic

d. sickle cell

RS.9. The processes through which the body maintains a constant internal environment are known as _____.

a. hemothorax

b. homeostasis

c. hypophysis

d. metabolism

RS.10. _____ is an inflammation of the myelin sheath of peripheral nerves, characterized by rapidly worsening muscle weakness that can lead to temporary paralysis.

a. Bell's palsy

b. Guillain-Barré syndrome

c. Lou Gehrig's disease

d. Raynaud's phenomenon

RS.11. The term _____ describes weakness or wearing away of body tissues and structures caused by pathology or by disuse of the muscle over a long period of time.

a. adhesion

b. ankylosis

c. atrophy

d. contracture

RS.12. The suffix _____ means blood or blood condition.

a. -emia

b. -oma

c. -pnea

d. -uria

RS.13. The procedure in which an anastomosis is created between the upper portion of the stomach and the duodenum is a/an _____.

a. esophagogastrectomy

b. esophagoplasty

c. gastroduodenostomy

d. gastrostomy

RS.14. Another term for conventional, or Western, medical practices and systems of health care is _____ medicine.

a. alternative

b. complementary

c. allopathic

d. integrative

RS.15. The term _____ means abnormal enlargement of the liver.

a. hepatitis

b. hepatomalacia

c. hepatomegaly

d. hepatorrhexis

RS.16. The term describing the prolapse of a kidney is _____.

a. hydronephrosis

b. nephroptosis

c. nephropyosis

d. nephropexy

RS.17. Which of these conditions is commonly known as a bruise?

a. ecchymosis

b. epistaxis

c. hematoma

d. lesion

RS.18. The acute respiratory infection known as _____ is characterized in children and infants by obstruction of the larynx, hoarseness, and a barking cough.

a. asthma

b. croup

c. diphtheria

d. pneumonia

RS.19. _____ is an autoimmune disease in which the body's own antibodies attack and destroy the cells of the thyroid gland.

a. Conn's disease

b. Hashimoto's disease

c. Lou Gehrig's disease

d. Graves' disease

RS.20. Which sexually transmitted disease can be detected through the VDRL blood test before the lesions appear?

a. chlamydia

b. gonorrhea

c. syphilis

d. trichomoniasis

RS.21. A blood clot attached to the interior wall of a vein or artery is known as a/an _____.

a. embolism

b. embolus

c. thrombosis

d. thrombus

RS.22. The term _____ describes the removal of a body part or the destruction of its function through the use of surgery, hormones, drugs, heat, chemicals, electrocautery, or other methods.

a. ablation

b. abrasion

c. cryosurgery

d. exfoliative cytology

RS.23. The term _____ describes any restriction to the opening of the mouth caused by trauma, surgery, or radiation associated with the treatment of oral cancer.

   a. atresia

   b. cachexia

   c. mastication

   d. trismus

RS.24. A woman who has borne one viable child is referred to as a _____.

   a. nulligravida

   b. nullipara

   c. primigravida

   d. primipara

RS.25. The term _____ means inflammation of the pancreas.

   a. insulinoma

   b. pancreatectomy

   c. pancreatitis

   d. pancreatotomy

RS.26. The condition in which excess cerebrospinal fluid accumulates in the ventricles of the brain is known as _____.

   a. encephalocele

   b. hydrocephalus

   c. hydronephrosis

   d. hydroureter

RS.27. A _____ is the surgical fixation of a prolapsed vagina to a surrounding structure.

   a. colpopexy

   b. colporrhaphy

   c. cystopexy

   d. cystorrhaphy

RS.28. The combining form **metr/o** means _____.

   a. breast

   b. cervix

   c. menstruation

   d. uterus

RS.29. Which statement is accurate regarding cystic fibrosis (CF)?

   a. CF is a congenital disorder in which red blood cells take on a sickle shape.

   b. CF is also known as iron overload disease.

   c. CF is a genetic disorder that affects the lungs and digestive system.

   d. CF is characterized by short-lived red blood cells.

RS.30. The condition _____, which is thinner than average bone density, causes the patient to be at an increased risk of developing osteoporosis.

   a. osteochondroma

   b. osteopenia

   c. osteosclerosis

   d. rickets

RS.31. A/An _____ is a specialist who provides medical care to women during pregnancy, childbirth, and immediately thereafter.

   a. geriatrician

   b. gynecologist

   c. neonatologist

   d. obstetrician

RS.32. _____ is characterized by exophthalmos.

   a. Conn's syndrome

   b. Graves' disease

   c. Hashimoto's disease

   d. Huntington's disease

RS.33. The hormone _____ stimulates uterine contractions during childbirth.

   a. estrogen

   b. oxytocin

   c. progesterone

   d. testosterone

RS.34. A/An _____ is an unfavorable response due to prescribed medical treatment.

a. idiopathic disorder

b. nosocomial infection

c. infectious disease

d. iatrogenic illness

RS.35. The surgical freeing of a kidney from adhesions is known as _____.

a. nephrolithiasis

b. nephrolysis

c. nephropyosis

d. pyelitis

RS.36. _____ is the tissue death of an artery or arteries.

a. arterionecrosis

b. arteriostenosis

c. atherosclerosis

d. arthrosclerosis

RS.37. The _____ plane divides the body vertically into unequal left and right portions.

a. frontal

b. midsagittal

c. sagittal

d. transverse

RS.38. The term _____ means toward or nearer the midline.

a. distal

b. dorsal

c. medial

d. ventral

RS.39. A _____ was performed as a definitive test to determine if Alice Wilkinson has osteoporosis.

a. bone marrow biopsy

b. dual x-ray absorptiometry

c. MRI

d. nuclear bone scan

RS.40. The term _____ means movement of a limb away from the midline of the body.

a. abduction

b. adduction

c. extension

d. flexion

RS.41. When he fell, Manuel tore the posterior femoral muscles in his left leg. This is known as a/an _____ injury.

a. Achilles tendon

b. hamstring

c. myofascial

d. shin splint

RS.42. Mrs. Valladares has a bacterial infection of the lining of her heart. This condition is known as bacterial _____.

a. endocarditis

b. myocarditis

c. pericarditis

d. valvulitis

RS.43. The condition of _____ is commonly known as tooth decay.

a. dental caries

b. dental plaque

c. gingivitis

d. periodontal disease

RS.44. Henry was diagnosed as having an inflammation of the bone marrow and adjacent bone. Which term describes this condition?

a. encephalitis

b. meningitis

c. osteomyelitis

d. myelosis

RS.45. The term for an inflammation of the sheath surrounding a tendon is _____.

a. bursitis

b. tendinitis

c. fascitis

d. tenosynovitis

RS.46. The term _____ describes drooping of the upper eyelid that is usually due to paralysis.

a. ptosis

b. dacryocystitis

c. scleritis

d. dacryoadenitis

RS.47. The combining form _____ means old age.

a. **percuss/o**

b. **presby/o**

c. **prurit/o**

d. **pseud/o**

RS.48. Mr. Ramirez had a heart attack. His physician recorded this as _____.

a. angina

b. a myocardial infarction

c. congestive heart failure

d. ischemic heart disease

RS.49. _____ is an abnormal increase in the number of red cells in the blood due to excess production of these cells by the bone marrow.

a. anemia

b. polycythemia

c. thrombocytosis

d. thrombocytopenia

RS.50. The common skin disorder _____ is characterized by flare-ups in which red papules covered with silvery scales occur on the elbows, knees, scalp, back, or buttocks.

a. ichthyosis

b. systemic lupus erythematosus

c. psoriasis

d. rosacea

RS.51. _____ is a group of disorders involving the parts of the brain that control thought, memory, and language.

a. Alzheimer's disease

b. catatonic behavior

c. persistent vegetative state

d. Reye's syndrome

RS.52. A/An _____ is a physician who specializes in physical medicine and rehabilitation with the focus on restoring function.

a. exercise physiologist

b. orthopedist

c. physiatrist

d. rheumatologist

RS.53. The term _____ describes a bone disorder of unknown cause that destroys normal bone structure and replaces it with fibrous tissue.

a. costochondritis

b. fibrous dysplasia

c. osteomyelitis

d. periostitis

RS.54. Slight paralysis of one side of the body is known as _____.

a. hemiparesis

b. hemiplegia

c. myoparesis

d. quadriplegia

RS.55. The _____ are the specialized cells that play an important role in blood clotting.

a. basophils

b. erythrocytes

c. leukocytes

d. thrombocytes

RS.56. The term _____ describes blood in the urine.

 a. hemangioma

 b. hematemesis

 c. hematoma

 d. hematuria

RS.57. The _____ receives the sound vibrations and relays them to the auditory nerve fibers.

 a. cochlea

 b. eustachian tube

 c. organ of Corti

 d. semicircular canal

RS.58. The _____ patrol the body, searching for antigens that produce infections. When such a cell is found, these cells grab, swallow, and internally break apart the captured antigen.

 a. B cells

 b. dendritic cells

 c. interleukins

 d. T cells

RS.59. The medical term for the congenital condition commonly known as clubfoot is _____.

 a. hallux valgus

 b. rickets

 c. spasmodic torticollis

 d. talipes

RS.60. A _____ is a normal scar resulting from the healing of a wound.

 a. callus

 b. cicatrix

 c. crepitus

 d. keloid

RS.61. The _____ is commonly known as the collar bone.

 a. clavicle

 b. olecranon

 c. patella

 d. sternum

RS.62. _____ are long, slender spiral-shaped bacteria that have flexible walls and are capable of movement.

 a. bacilli

 b. spirochetes

 c. staphylococcus

 d. streptococcus

RS.63. A/An _____ is a malignant tumor usually involving the upper shaft of long bones, the pelvis, or knee.

 a. adenocarcinoma

 b. Hodgkin's lymphoma

 c. osteochondroma

 d. osteosarcoma

RS.64. Which of these diseases is transmitted to humans by the bite of an infected blacklegged tick?

 a. cytomegalovirus

 b. human immunodeficiency virus

 c. Lyme disease

 d. West Nile virus

RS.65. _____ involves compression of nerves and blood vessels due to swelling within the enclosed space created by the fascia that separates groups of muscles.

 a. chronic fatigue syndrome

 b. compartment syndrome

 c. fibromyalgia syndrome

 d. myofascial pain syndrome

RS.66. A/An _____, also known as a *boil*, is a large, tender, swollen area caused by a staphylococcal infection around a hair follicle or sebaceous gland.

a. abscess

b. carbuncle

c. furuncle

d. pustule

RS.67. Which term refers to a class of drugs that relieves pain without affecting consciousness?

a. analgesic

b. barbiturate

c. hypnotic

d. sedative

RS.68. Fine muscle tremors, rigidity, and a slow or shuffling gait are all symptoms of the progressive condition known as _____.

a. multiple sclerosis

b. muscular dystrophy

c. myasthenia gravis

d. Parkinson's disease

RS.69. A form of vasculitis that affects the arms, upper body, neck, and head with symptoms including headache and touch sensitivity is known as _____.

a. temporal arteritis

b. hemangioma

c. migraine

d. peripheral vascular disease

RS.70. During her pregnancy, Ruth had a skin condition commonly known as the mask of pregnancy. The medical term for this condition is _____.

a. chloasma

b. albinism

c. exanthem

d. vitiligo

RS.71. _____ is caused by the failure of the bones of the limbs to grow to an appropriate length.

a. acromegaly

b. gigantism

c. hyperpituitarism

d. short stature

RS.72. In a _____ fracture, a bone is splintered or crushed.

a. comminuted

b. compound

c. compression

d. spiral

RS.73. The combining form _____ means vertebra or vertebral column.

a. **synovi/o**

b. **spondyl/o**

c. **scoli/o**

d. **splen/o**

RS.74. Which heart chamber receives oxygen-poor blood from all tissues, except the lungs?

a. left atrium

b. left ventricle

c. right atrium

d. right ventricle

RS.75. Which substance is commonly known as good cholesterol?

a. high-density lipoprotein cholesterol

b. homocysteine

c. low-density lipoprotein cholesterol

d. triglycerides

RS.76. Which symbol means less than?

a. $>$

b. $\geq$

c. $<$

d. $\downarrow$

RS.77. When medication is placed under the tongue and allowed to dissolve slowly, this is known as _____ administration.

a. oral

b. parenteral

c. sublingual

d. topical

RS.78. A sonogram is the image created by _____.

a. computerized tomography

b. fluoroscopy

c. magnetic resonance imaging (MRI)

d. ultrasonography

RS.79. Which combining form means red?

a. **melan/o**

b. **leuk/o**

c. **erythr/o**

d. **cyan/o**

RS.80. An autoimmune disorder characterized by a severe reaction to foods containing gluten is known as _____.

a. irritable bowel syndrome

b. diverticulosis

c. dyspepsia

d. celiac disease

RS.81. The term _____ describes inflammation of the gallbladder.

a. cholecystectomy

b. cholecystitis

c. cholecystotomy

d. cholelithiasis

RS.82. The term _____ means vomiting.

a. emesis

b. epistaxis

c. reflux

d. singultus

RS.83. The bluish discoloration of the skin caused by a lack of adequate oxygen is known as _____.

a. cyanosis

b. erythema

c. jaundice

d. pallor

RS.84. _____ is a disorder of the adrenal glands due to excessive production of aldosterone.

a. Conn's syndrome

b. Crohn's disease

c. Cushing's syndrome

d. Raynaud's phenomenon

RS.85. A/An _____ is any substance that the body regards as being foreign.

a. allergen

b. antibody

c. antigen

d. immunoglobulin

RS.86. Which condition has purple discolorations on the skin due to bleeding underneath the skin?

a. dermatosis

b. pruritus

c. purpura

d. suppuration

RS.87. A brief disturbance in brain function in which there is a loss of awareness often described as a staring episode is known as a/an _____ seizure.

a. petit mal

b. tonic-clonic

c. absence

d. grand mal

RS.88. A band of fibrous tissue that holds structures together abnormally is a/an _____.

a. adhesion

b. ankylosis

c. contracture

d. ligation

RS.89. Which procedure is performed to treat spider veins?

a. blepharoplasty

b. Botox

c. liposuction

d. sclerotherapy

RS.90. The instrument used to examine the external ear canal is known as a/an _____.

a. anoscope

b. ophthalmoscope

c. otoscope

d. speculum

RS.91. Which condition is breast cancer at its earliest stage before the cancer has broken through the wall of the milk duct?

a. ductal carcinoma in situ

b. infiltrating lobular carcinoma

c. inflammatory breast cancer

d. invasive lobular carcinoma

RS.92. Enlarged and swollen veins at the lower end of the esophagus are known as _____.

a. esophageal aneurysms

b. esophageal varices

c. hemorrhoids

d. varicose veins

RS.93. _____ is a progressive autoimmune disorder characterized by inflammation that causes demyelination of the myelin sheath.

a. systemic lupus erythematosus

b. multiple sclerosis

c. muscular dystrophy

d. spina bifida

RS.94. The abdominal region located below the stomach is known as the _____ region.

a. epigastric

b. hypogastric

c. left hypochondriac

d. umbilical

RS.95. Which of these sexually transmitted disease is a bacterial infection?

a. acquired immunodeficiency syndrome

b. gonorrhea

c. genital herpes

d. trichomoniasis

RS.96. Narrowing of the opening of the foreskin so that it cannot be retracted to expose the glans penis is known as _____.

a. balanitis

b. Peyronie's disease

c. phimosis

d. priapism

RS.97. A/An _____ is an exfoliative screening biopsy for the detection and diagnosis of conditions of the cervix and surrounding tissues.

a. endometrial biopsy

b. lymph node dissection

c. Pap smear

d. sentinel node biopsy

RS.98. The term _____ is used to describe practices and systems of health care used to supplement traditional Western medicine.

a. allopathic medicine

b. complementary medicine

c. alternative medicine

d. homeopathy

RS.99. The term _____ describes turning the palm upward or forward.

a. circumduction

b. pronation

c. rotation

d. supination

RS.100. The term _____ describes the inflammation of a vein.

a. vasculitis

b. arteritis

c. phlebitis

d. phlebostenosis

# ■ REVIEW SESSION ANSWER KEY

| | | | |
|---|---|---|---|
| RS.1. D | RS.26. B | RS.51. A | RS.76. C |
| RS.2. B | RS.27. A | RS.52. C | RS.77. C |
| RS.3. C | RS.28. D | RS.53. B | RS.78. D |
| RS.4. C | RS.29. C | RS.54. A | RS.79. C |
| RS.5. B | RS.30. B | RS.55. D | RS.80. D |
| RS.6. D | RS.31. D | RS.56. D | RS.81. B |
| RS.7. B | RS.32. B | RS.57. C | RS.82. A |
| RS.8. D | RS.33. B | RS.58. B | RS.83. A |
| RS.9. B | RS.34. D | RS.59. D | RS.84. A |
| RS.10. B | RS.35. B | RS.60. B | RS.85. C |
| RS.11. C | RS.36. A | RS.61. A | RS.86. C |
| RS.12. A | RS.37. C | RS.62. B | RS.87. C |
| RS.13. C | RS.38. C | RS.63. D | RS.88. A |
| RS.14. C | RS.39. B | RS.64. C | RS.89. D |
| RS.15. C | RS.40. A | RS.65. B | RS.90. C |
| RS.16. B | RS.41. B | RS.66. C | RS.91. A |
| RS.17. A | RS.42. A | RS.67. A | RS.92. B |
| RS.18. B | RS.43. A | RS.68. D | RS.93. B |
| RS.19. B | RS.44. C | RS.69. A | RS.94. B |
| RS.20. C | RS.45. D | RS.70. A | RS.95. B |
| RS.21. D | RS.46. A | RS.71. D | RS.96. C |
| RS.22. A | RS.47. B | RS.72. A | RS.97. C |
| RS.23. D | RS.48. B | RS.73. B | RS.98. B |
| RS.24. D | RS.49. B | RS.74. C | RS.99. D |
| RS.25. C | RS.50. C | RS.75. A | RS.100. C |

# ■ SIMULATED FINAL TEST

FT.1. The term _____ describes a torn or jagged wound.

a. fissure

b. fistula

c. laceration

d. lesion

FT.2. The bone and soft tissues that surround and support the teeth are known as the _____.

a. dentition

b. rugae

c. gingiva

d. periodontium

FT.3. A chronic condition in which the heart is unable to pump out all of the blood that it receives is known as _____.

a. atrial fibrillation

b. heart failure

c. tachycardia

d. ventricular fibrillation

FT.4. Inflammation of the connective tissues that encloses the spinal cord and brain is known as _____.

a. encephalitis

b. encephalopathy

c. meningitis

d. myelopathy

FT.5. _____ is the partial or complete blockage of the small and/or large intestine that is caused by the stopping of normal intestinal peristalsis.

a. Crohn's disease

b. ileus

c. intussusception

d. intestinal obstruction

FT.6. The term _____ describes a condition in which the eye does not focus properly because of uneven curvatures of the cornea.

a. ametropia

b. astigmatism

c. ectropion

d. entropion

FT.7. A procedure in which pressurized fluid is used to clean out wound debris is known as _____.

a. irrigation and debridement

b. dilation and curettage

c. incision and drainage

d. dermabrasion

FT.8. The term _____ describes persistent severe burning pain that usually follows an injury to a sensory nerve.

a. causalgia

b. hyperesthesia

c. paresthesia

d. peripheral neuropathy

FT.9. A/An _____ is performed to reduce the risk of a stroke caused by a disruption of the blood flow to the brain.

a. aneurysmectomy

b. arteriectomy

c. carotid endarterectomy

d. coronary artery bypass graft

FT.10. The term _____ means bleeding from the ear.

a. barotrauma

b. otomycosis

c. otopyorrhea

d. otorrhagia

FT.11. The medical term meaning itching is _____.

a. perfusion

b. pruritus

c. purpura

d. suppuration

FT.12. _____ is a condition characterized by episodes of severe chest pain due to inadequate blood flow to the myocardium.

a. angina

b. claudication

c. cyanosis

d. myocardial infarction

FT.13. The greenish material that forms the first stools of a newborn is known as _____.

a. colostrum

b. lochia

c. meconium

d. vernix

FT.14. A/An _____ is the result of medical treatment that yields the exact opposite of normally expected results.

a. drug interaction

b. paradoxical reaction

c. placebo

d. idiosyncratic reaction

FT.15. A _____ is a prediction of the probable course and outcome of a disease or disorder.

a. differential diagnosis

b. diagnosis

c. prognosis

d. syndrome

FT.16. _____ is a yellow discoloration of the skin, mucous membranes, and the eyes.

a. vitiligo

b. jaundice

c. erythema

d. albinism

FT.17. A/An _____ occurs at the lower end of the radius when a person tries to break a fall by landing on his or her hands.

a. Colles' fracture

b. comminuted fracture

c. osteoporotic hip fracture

d. spiral fracture

FT.18. The term _____ describes excessive urination during the night.

a. nocturia

b. polydipsia

c. polyuria

d. urinary retention

FT.19. A closed sac associated with a sebaceous gland that contains yellow, fatty material is known as a _____.

a. comedo

b. sebaceous cyst

c. seborrheic dermatitis

d. seborrheic keratosis

FT.20. The term _____ describes the condition commonly known as swollen glands.

a. adenoiditis

b. vasculitis

c. lymphadenitis

d. lymphangioma

FT.21. A/An _____ is a sudden, involuntary contraction of one or more muscles.

a. adhesion

b. contracture

c. spasm

d. sprain

FT.22. _____ is the respiratory disease commonly known as whooping cough.

a. coup

b. diphtheria

c. emphysema

d. pertussis

FT.23. The lymphocytes that play an important role in the killing of cancer cells and cells infected by viruses are known as _____.

a. cytokines

b. natural killer cells

c. B cells

d. T cells

FT.24. _____ is an abnormal lateral curvature of the spine.

a. kyphosis

b. lordosis

c. lumbago

d. scoliosis

FT.25. The surgical creation of an artificial excretory opening between the ileum and the outside of the abdominal wall is a/an _____.

a. colostomy

b. enteropexy

c. gastroptosis

d. ileostomy

FT.26. Which examination technique is the visualization of body parts in motion by projecting x-ray images on a luminous fluorescent screen?

a. computed tomography

b. fluoroscopy

c. magnetic resonance imaging

d. radiography

FT.27. As the condition known as _____ progresses, the chest sometimes assumes an enlarged barrel shape.

a. asthma

b. diphtheria

c. emphysema

d. epistaxis

FT.28. The term _____ means to stop or control bleeding.

a. hemorrhage

b. hemostasis

c. homeostasis

d. thrombocytopenia

FT.29. An accumulation of pus in the fallopian tube is known as _____.

a. leukorrhea

b. otopyorrhea

c. pyosalpinx

d. salpingitis

FT.30. A _____ is the bruising of brain tissue as a result of a head injury.

a. cerebral contusion

b. concussion

c. hydrocele

d. meningocele

FT.31. The term _____ means vomiting blood.

a. epistaxis

b. hemarthrosis

c. hematemesis

d. hyperemesis

FT.32. _____ is a diagnostic procedure designed to determine the density of a body part by the sound produced by tapping the surface with the fingers.

a. auscultation

b. palpation

c. percussion

d. range of motion

FT.33. Abnormally rapid, deep breathing resulting in decreased levels of carbon dioxide in the blood is known as _____.

a. apnea

b. dyspnea

c. hyperventilation

d. hypoventilation

FT.34. The term _____ describes difficult or painful urination.

a. dyspepsia

b. dysphagia

c. dystrophy

d. dysuria

FT.35. A _____ is a false personal belief that is maintained despite obvious proof or evidence to the contrary.

a. delusion

b. dementia

c. mania

d. phobia

FT.36. In _____, the normal rhythmic contractions of the atria are replaced by rapid irregular twitching of the muscular heart wall.

a. atrial fibrillation

b. bradycardia

c. tachycardia

d. ventricular fibrillation

FT.37. The eye condition known as _____ is characterized by increased intraocular pressure.

a. cataracts

b. glaucoma

c. macular degeneration

d. monochromatism

FT.38. _____ is the presence of blood in the seminal fluid.

a. azoospermia

b. hematuria

c. hematospermia

d. prostatorrhea

FT.39. The condition of common changes in the eyes that occur with aging is known as _____.

a. hyperopia

b. presbycusis

c. presbyopia

d. strabismus

FT.40. Which body cavity protects the brain?

a. anterior

b. cranial

c. caudal

d. ventral

FT.41. A hernia of the bladder through the vaginal wall is known as a _____.

a. cystocele

b. cystopexy

c. vaginocele

d. vesicovaginal fistula

FT.42. Which condition of a young child is characterized by the inability to develop normal social relationships?

a. autism

b. attention deficit disorder

c. dyslexia

d. mental retardation

FT.43. A ringing, buzzing, or roaring sound in one or both ears is known as _____.

a. labyrinthitis

b. syncope

c. tinnitus

d. vertigo

FT.44. A/An _____ is an outbreak of a disease occurring over a large geographic area that is possibly worldwide.

a. endemic

b. epidemic

c. pandemic

d. syndrome

FT.45. _____ is an abnormal accumulation of serous fluid in the peritoneal cavity.

a. ascites

b. aerophagia

c. melena

d. bolus

FT.46. A _____ is a discolored flat spot that is less than 1 cm in diameter, such as a freckle.

a. macule

b. papule

c. plaque

d. vesicle

FT.47. The Western blot test is used to _____.

a. confirm an HIV infection

b. detect hepatitis C

c. diagnose Kaposi's sarcoma

d. test for tuberculosis

FT.48. The term _____ describes excessive uterine bleeding at both the usual time of menstrual periods and at other irregular intervals.

a. dysmenorrhea

b. hypermenorrhea

c. menometrorrhagia

d. oligomenorrhea

FT.49. _____ is a form of sexual dysfunction in which the penis is bent or curved during erection.

a. erectile dysfunction

b. Peyronie's disease

c. phimosis

d. priapism

FT.50. A/An _____ is an abnormal sound or murmur heard during auscultation of an artery.

a. auscultation

b. bruit

c. rhonchi

d. stridor

FT.51. The condition commonly known as wear-and-tear arthritis is _____.

a. gouty arthritis

b. osteoarthritis

c. rheumatoid arthritis

d. spondylosis

FT.52. The term _____ means to free a tendon from adhesions.

a. tenodesis

b. tenolysis

c. tenorrhaphy

d. insertion

FT.53. The malignant condition known as _____ is distinguished by the presence of Reed-Sternberg cells.

a. Hodgkin's lymphoma

b. leukemia

c. non-Hodgkin's lymphoma

d. osteosarcoma

FT.54. The chronic, degenerative disease characterized by scarring that causes disturbance of the structure and function of the liver is _____.

a. cirrhosis

b. hepatitis

c. hepatomegaly

d. jaundice

FT.55. _____ removes waste products directly from the bloodstream of patients whose kidneys no longer function.

a. diuresis

b. epispadias

c. hemodialysis

d. peritoneal dialysis

FT.56. The medical term for the condition commonly known as fainting is _____.

a. comatose

b. singultus

c. stupor

d. syncope

FT.57. _____ is a condition in which there is an insufficient supply of oxygen in the tissues due to a restricted blood flow to a part of the body.

a. angina

b. infarction

c. ischemia

d. perfusion

FT.58. A collection of blood in the pleural cavity is known as a _____.

a. hemophilia

b. hemoptysis

c. hemostasis

d. hemothorax

FT.59. The return of swallowed food into the mouth is known as _____.

a. dysphagia

b. emesis

c. pyrosis

d. regurgitation

FT.60. An inflammation of the lacrimal gland that can be a bacterial, viral, or fungal infection is known as _____.

a. anisocoria

b. dacryoadenitis

c. exophthalmos

d. hordeolum

FT.61. The contraction of the pupil, normally in response to exposure to light, but also possibly due to the use of prescription or illegal drugs, is known as _____.

a. nystagmus

b. mydriasis

c. miosis

d. mycosis

FT.62. The term _____ means excessive urination.

a. enuresis

b. oliguria

c. overactive bladder

d. polyuria

FT.63. The surgical removal of the gallbladder is known as a _____.

a. cholecystectomy

b. cholecystostomy

c. cholecystotomy

d. choledocholithotomy

FT.64. An elevated _____ indicates the presence of inflammation in the body.

a. complete blood cell count

b. erythrocyte sedimentation rate

c. platelet count

d. total hemoglobin test

FT.65. A/An _____ is a groove or crack-like break in the skin.

a. abrasion

b. fissure

c. laceration

d. ulcer

FT.66. A/An _____ injection is made into the fatty layer just below the skin.

a. intradermal

b. intramuscular

c. intravenous

d. subcutaneous

FT.67. The _____ has roles in both the immune and endocrine systems.

a. pancreas

b. pituitary

c. spleen

d. thymus

FT.68. The medical term _____ describes an inflammation of the brain.

a. encephalitis

b. mastitis

c. meningitis

d. myelitis

FT.69. The hormone secreted by fat cells is known as _____.

a. interstitial cell-stimulating hormone

b. growth hormone

c. leptin

d. neurohormone

FT.70. A type of catheter made of a flexible tube with a balloon filled with sterile water at the end to hold it in place in the bladder is known as a _____ catheter.

   a. Foley

   b. indwelling

   c. suprapubic

   d. intermittent

FT.71. A/An _____ is acquired in a hospital or clinic setting.

   a. functional disorder

   b. iatrogenic illness

   c. idiopathic disorder

   d. nosocomial infection

FT.72. A type of pneumonia contracted during a stay in the hospital when the patient's defenses are impaired is known as _____ pneumonia.

   a. hospital-acquired

   b. aspiration

   c. community-acquired

   d. walking

FT.73. The term _____ describes an eye disorder that can develop as a complication of diabetes.

   a. diabetic neuropathy

   b. diabetic retinopathy

   c. papilledema

   d. retinal detachment

FT.74. The physical wasting with the loss of weight and muscle mass due to diseases such as advanced cancer is known as _____.

   a. cachexia

   b. anorexia nervosa

   c. bulimia nervosa

   d. malnutrition

FT.75. The term _____ means difficulty in swallowing.

   a. aerophagia

   b. dyspepsia

   c. dysphagia

   d. eructation

FT.76. A/An _____ occurs when a blood vessel in the brain leaks or ruptures.

   a. cerebral hematoma

   b. embolism

   c. hemorrhagic stroke

   d. ischemic stroke

FT.77. The hormonal disorder known as _____ results from the pituitary gland producing too much growth hormone in adults.

   a. acromegaly

   b. cretinism

   c. gigantism

   d. pituitarism

FT.78. The term _____ describes the condition commonly known an ingrown toenail.

   a. cryptorchidism

   b. onychocryptosis

   c. onychomycosis

   d. priapism

FT.79. An _____ is the instrument used to examine the interior of the eye.

   a. ophtalmoscope

   b. ophthalmoscope

   c. opthalmoscope

   d. opthlmoscope

FT.80. A/An _____ is a protrusion of part of the stomach upward into the chest through an opening in the diaphragm.

   a. esophageal hernia

   b. esophageal varices

   c. hiatal hernia

   d. hiatal varices

FT.81. An _____ is a surgical incision made to enlarge the vaginal orifice to facilitate childbirth.

    a. episiorrhaphy

    b. episiotomy

    c. epispadias

    d. epistaxis

FT.82. Severe itching of the external female genitalia is known as _____.

    a. colpitis

    b. leukorrhea

    c. pruritus vulvae

    d. vaginal candidiasis

FT.83. _____ is a urinary problem caused by interference with the normal nerve pathways associated with urination.

    a. neurogenic bladder

    b. overactive bladder

    c. polyuria

    d. overflow incontinence

FT.84. A/An _____ is an instrument used to enlarge the opening of any canal or cavity to facilitate inspection of its interior.

    a. endoscope

    b. speculum

    c. sphygmomanometer

    d. stethoscope

FT.85. A _____, also known as *scab*, is a collection of dried serum and cellular debris.

    a. crust

    b. nodule

    c. plaque

    d. scale

FT.86. A _____ is a type of cancer that occurs in blood-making cells found in the red bone marrow.

    a. carcinoma

    b. myeloma

    c. osteochondroma

    d. sarcoma

FT.87. _____ can occur when a foreign substance, such as vomit, is inhaled into the lungs.

    a. aspiration pneumonia

    b. bacterial pneumonia

    c. walking pneumonia

    d. Pneumocystis pneumonia

FT.88. The condition known as _____ is ankylosis of the bones of the middle ear that causes a conductive hearing loss.

    a. labyrinthitis

    b. mastoiditis

    c. osteosclerosis

    d. otosclerosis

FT.89. The procedure known as _____ is the surgical fusion of two bones to stiffen a joint.

    a. arthrodesis

    b. arthrolysis

    c. synovectomy

    d. tenodesis

FT.90. The suffix _____ means rupture.

    a. **-rrhage**

    b. **-rrhaphy**

    c. **-rrhea**

    d. **-rrhexis**

FT.91. An abnormal fear of being in small or enclosed spaces is known as _____.

    a. acrophobia

    b. agoraphobia

    c. social phobia

    d. claustrophobia

FT.92. _____ is the distortion or impairment of voluntary movement such as in a tic or spasm.

a. bradykinesia

b. dyskinesia

c. hyperkinesia

d. myoclonus

FT.93. Which structure secretes bile?

a. gallbladder

b. liver

c. pancreas

d. spleen

FT.94. _____ is the process of recording the electrical activity of the brain.

a. echoencephalograph

b. electroencephalography

c. electromyography

d. magnetic resonance imaging

FT.95. The suffix _____ means surgical fixation.

a. **-lysis**

b. **-rrhaphy**

c. **-desis**

d. **-pexy**

FT.96. The eye condition that causes the loss of central vision, but not total blindness, is known as _____.

a. cataracts

b. glaucoma

c. macular degeneration

d. presbyopia

FT.97. A/An _____ is performed to remove excess skin and fat for the elimination of wrinkles.

a. ablation

b. blepharoplasty

c. rhytidectomy

d. sclerotherapy

FT.98. The condition known as _____ describes total paralysis affecting only one side of the body.

a. hemiparesis

b. hemiplegia

c. paraplegia

d. quadriplegia

FT.99. _____ is a new cancer site that results from the spreading process.

a. in situ

b. metabolism

c. metastasis

d. metastasize

FT.100. Which of these hormones is produced by the pituitary gland?

a. adrenocorticotropic hormone

b. calcitonin

c. cortisol

d. epinephrine

# ■ SIMULATED MEDICAL TERMINOLOGY FINAL TEST ANSWER KEY

| | | | |
|---|---|---|---|
| FT.1. C | FT.26. B | FT.51. B | FT.76. C |
| FT.2. D | FT.27. C | FT.52. B | FT.77. A |
| FT.3. B | FT.28. B | FT.53. A | FT.78. B |
| FT.4. C | FT.29. C | FT.54. A | FT.79. B |
| FT.5. B | FT.30. A | FT.55. C | FT.80. C |
| FT.6. B | FT.31. C | FT.56. D | FT.81. B |
| FT.7. A | FT.32. C | FT.57. C | FT.82. C |
| FT.8. A | FT.33. C | FT.58. D | FT.83. A |
| FT.9. C | FT.34. D | FT.59. D | FT.84. B |
| FT.10. D | FT.35. A | FT.60. B | FT.85. A |
| FT.11. B | FT.36. A | FT.61. C | FT.86. B |
| FT.12. A | FT.37. B | FT.62. D | FT.87. A |
| FT.13. C | FT.38. C | FT.63. A | FT.88. D |
| FT.14. B | FT.39. C | FT.64. B | FT.89. A |
| FT.15. C | FT.40. B | FT.65. B | FT.90. D |
| FT.16. B | FT.41. A | FT.66. D | FT.91. D |
| FT.17. A | FT.42. A | FT.67. D | FT.92. B |
| FT.18. A | FT.43. C | FT.68. A | FT.93. B |
| FT.19. B | FT.44. C | FT.69. C | FT.94. B |
| FT.20. C | FT.45. A | FT.70. A | FT.95. D |
| FT.21. C | FT.46. A | FT.71. D | FT.96. C |
| FT.22. D | FT.47. A | FT.72. A | FT.97. C |
| FT.23. B | FT.48. C | FT.73. B | FT.98. B |
| FT.24. D | FT.49. B | FT.74. A | FT.99. C |
| FT.25. D | FT.50. B | FT.75. C | FT.100. A |

# PREFIXES, COMBINING FORMS, AND SUFFIXES

## Pertaining to

| | |
|---|---|
| **-ac** | pertaining to |
| **-al** | pertaining to |
| **-ar** | pertaining to |
| **-ary** | pertaining to |
| **-eal** | pertaining to |
| **-ial** | pertaining to |
| **-ical** | pertaining to |
| **-ic** | pertaining to |
| **-ine** | pertaining to |
| **-ior** | pertaining to |
| **-ory** | pertaining to |
| **-ous** | pertaining to |
| **-tic** | pertaining to |

## Abnormal Conditions

| | |
|---|---|
| **-ago** | abnormal condition, disease |
| **-esis** | abnormal condition, disease |

| | |
|---|---|
| **-ia** | abnormal condition, disease |
| **-iasis** | abnormal condition, disease |
| **-ion** | condition |
| **-ism** | condition, state of |
| **-osis** | abnormal condition, disease |

## Noun Endings

| | |
|---|---|
| **-a** | noun ending |
| **-ae** | plural noun ending |
| **-e** | noun ending |
| **-i** | plural noun ending |
| **-um** | singular noun ending |
| **-us** | singular noun ending |
| **-y** | noun ending |

# A

| | |
|---|---|
| a- | no, not, without, away from, negative |
| -a | noun ending |
| ab- | away from, negative, absent |
| abdomin/o | abdomen |
| -able | capable of, able to |
| abort/o | premature expulsion of a nonviable fetus |
| abrad/o, abras/o | rub or scrape off |
| abrupt/o | broken away from |
| abs- | away from |
| abscess/o | collection of pus, going away |
| absorpt/o | suck up, suck in |
| -ac | pertaining to |
| acanth/o | spiny, thorny |
| acetabul/o | acetabulum (hip socket) |
| -acious | characterized by |
| acne/o | point or peak |
| acous/o, acoust/o | hearing, sound |
| acquir/o | get, obtain |
| acr/o | extremities (hands and feet), top, extreme point |
| acromi/o | acromion, point of shoulder blade |
| actin/o | light |
| acu/o | sharp, severe, sudden |
| acuit/o, acut/o | sharp, sharpness |
| acust/o, -acusia, -acusis | hearing, sense of hearing |
| ad- | toward, to, in the direction of |
| aden/o | gland |
| adenoid/o | adenoids |
| adhes/o | stick to, cling to |
| adip/o | fat |
| adnex/o | bound to |
| adren/o, adrenal/o | adrenal glands |
| aer/o | air, gas |
| aesthet/o | sensation, sense of perception |
| af- | toward, to |
| affect/o | exert influence on |
| agglutin/o | clumping, stick together |
| aggress/o | attack, step forward |
| -ago | abnormal condition, disease |
| agor/a | marketplace |
| -agra | excessive pain, seizure, attack of severe pain |
| -aise | comfort, ease |
| -al | pertaining to |

| | |
|---|---|
| alb/i, alb/o, albin/o | white |
| albumin/o | albumin, protein |
| alg/e, algi/o, alg/o, algesi/o | relationship to pain |
| -algesia, -algesic | painful, pain sense |
| -algia | pain, suffering, painful condition |
| align/o | bring into line or correct position |
| aliment/o | to nourish |
| all/o, all- | other, different from normal, reversal |
| alopec/o | baldness, mangy |
| alveol/o | alveolus, air sac, small sac |
| ambi- | both sides, around or about, double |
| ambly/o | dull, dim |
| ambul/o, ambulat/o | walk |
| ametr/o | out of proportion |
| -amine | nitrogen compound |
| amni/o | amnion, fetal membrane |
| amph- | around, on both sides, doubly |
| amput/o, amputat/o | cut away, cut off a part of the body |
| amyl/o | starch |
| an- | no, not, without |
| an-, ana- | up, apart, backward, excessive |
| an/o | anus, ring |
| -an | characteristic of, pertaining to |
| -ancy | state of |
| andr/o | male, masculine |
| aneurysm/o | aneurysm |
| angi/o | blood or lymph vessel |
| angin/o | angina, choking, strangling |
| anis/o | unequal |
| ankyl/o | crooked, bent, stiff |
| anomal/o | irregularity |
| ante- | before, in front of, forward |
| anter/o | before, front |
| anthrac/o | coal, coal dust |
| anti- | against |
| anxi/o, anxiet/o | anxiety, anxious, uneasy |
| aort/o | aorta |
| ap- | toward, to |
| -apheresis | removal |
| aphth/o | ulcer |
| apic/o | apex |
| ap-, apo- | separation, away from, opposed, detached |
| aplast/o | defective development, lack of development |

| | |
|---|---|
| **aponeur/o** | aponeurosis (type of tendon) |
| **apoplect/o** | a stroke |
| **append/o,** | appendix |
| **appendic/o** | |
| **aqu/i, aqu/o,** | water |
| **aque/o** | |
| **-ar** | pertaining to |
| **arachn/o** | spiderweb, spider |
| **arc/o** | bow, arc, or arch |
| **-arche** | beginning |
| **areat/o** | occurring in patches or circumscribed areas |
| **areol/o** | little open space |
| **-aria** | connected with |
| **arrect/o** | upright, lifted up, raised |
| **arter/o, arteri/o** | artery |
| **arthr/o** | joint |
| **articul/o** | joint |
| **-ary** | pertaining to |
| **as-** | toward, to |
| **asbest/o** | asbestos |
| **-ase** | enzyme |
| **aspir/o, aspirat/o** | to breathe in |
| **asthen-, -asthenia** | weakness, lack of strength |
| **asthmat/o** | gasping, choking |
| **astr/o** | star, star-shaped |
| **at-** | toward, to |
| **atel/o** | incomplete, imperfect |
| **ather/o** | plaque, fatty substance |
| **athet/o** | uncontrolled |
| **-ation** | state or action |
| **atop/o** | strange, out of place |
| **atres/i** | without an opening |
| **atri/o** | atrium |
| **attenuat/o** | diluted, weakened |
| **aud-, audi/o,** | ear, hearing, the sense of hearing |
| **audit/o** | |
| **aur/i, aur/o** | ear, hearing |
| **auscult/a, auscult/o** | listen |
| **aut/o** | self |
| **-ax** | noun ending |
| **ax/o** | axis, main stem |
| **axill/o** | armpit |

## B

| | |
|---|---|
| **bacill/o** | rod-shaped bacterium (plural, *bacteria*) |
| **bacteri/o** | bacteria (singular, *bacterium*) |
| **balan/o** | glans penis |

| | |
|---|---|
| **bar/o** | pressure, weight |
| **bartholin/o** | Bartholin's gland |
| **bas/o** | base, opposite of acid |
| **bi-** | twice, double, two |
| **bi/o** | life |
| **bifid/o** | split, divided into two parts |
| **bifurcat/o** | divide or fork into two branches |
| **bil/i** | bile, gall |
| **bilirubin/o** | bilirubin |
| **bin-** | two |
| **-blast** | embryonic, immature, formative element |
| **blephar/o** | eyelid |
| **borborygm/o** | rumbling sound |
| **brachi/o** | arm |
| **brachy-** | short |
| **brady-** | slow |
| **brev/i, brev/o** | short |
| **bronch/i, bronchi/o,** | bronchial tube, bronchus |
| **bronch/o** | |
| **bronchiol/o** | bronchiole, bronchiolus |
| **brux/o** | grind |
| **bucc/o** | cheek |
| **burs/o** | bursa, sac of fluid near joint |

## C

| | |
|---|---|
| **cadaver/o** | dead body, corpse |
| **calcane/o** | calcaneus, heel bone |
| **calc/i** | calcium, lime, the heel |
| **calci-, calc/o** | calcium |
| **calcul/o** | stone, little stone |
| **cali/o, calic/o** | cup, calyx |
| **call/i, callos/o** | hard, hardened and thickened |
| **calor/i** | heat |
| **canalicul/o** | little canal or duct |
| **canth/o** | corner of the eye |
| **capill/o** | hair |
| **capit/o** | head |
| **capn/o** | carbon dioxide, sooty or smoky appearance |
| **capsul/o** | little box |
| **carb/o** | carbon |
| **carbuncl/o** | carbuncle |
| **carcin/o** | cancerous |
| **cardi/o, card/o** | heart |
| **cari/o** | rottenness, decay |
| **carot/o** | stupor, sleep |
| **carp/o** | wrist bones |
| **cartilag/o** | cartilage, gristle |

| | |
|---|---|
| caruncul/o | bit of flesh |
| cat-, cata-, cath- | down, lower, under |
| catabol/o | a breaking down |
| cathart/o | cleansing, purging |
| cathet/o | insert, send down |
| caud/o | lower part of body, tail |
| caus/o, caust/o | burning, burn |
| cauter/o, caut/o | heat, burn |
| cav/i, cav/o | hollow, cave |
| cavern/o | containing hollow spaces |
| cec/o | cecum |
| -cele | hernia, tumor, swelling |
| celi/o, cel/o | abdomen, belly |
| cement/o | cementum, a rough stone |
| cent- | hundred |
| -centesis | surgical puncture to remove fluid |
| cephal/o | head |
| cera- | wax |
| cerebell/o | cerebellum |
| cerebr/o | cerebrum, brain |
| cerumin/o | cerumen, earwax |
| cervic/o | neck, cervix (neck of uterus) |
| cheil/o | lip or lips |
| cheir/o | hand |
| chem/i, chem/o, chemic/o | drug, chemical |
| chir/o | hand |
| chlor/o | green |
| chlorhydr/o | hydrochloric acid |
| chol/e | bile, gall |
| cholangi/o | bile duct |
| cholecyst/o | gallbladder |
| choledoch/o | common bile duct |
| cholesterol/o | cholesterol |
| chondr/i, chondr/o | cartilage |
| chord/o | spinal cord, cord |
| chori/o, chorion/o | chorion, membrane |
| choroid/o | choroid layer of eye |
| chrom/o, chromat/o | color |
| chron/o | time |
| chym/o | to pour, juice |
| cib/o | meal |
| cicatric/o | scar |
| -cidal | pertaining to killing |
| -cide | causing death |
| cili/o | eyelashes, microscopic hair-like projections |
| cine- | relationship to movement |
| circ/i | ring or circle |

| | |
|---|---|
| circulat/o | circulate, go around in a circle |
| circum- | around, about |
| circumcis/o | cutting around |
| circumscrib/o | confined, limited in space |
| cirrh/o | orange-yellow, tawny |
| cis/o | cut |
| -clasis, -clast | break down |
| claudicat/o | limping |
| claustr/o | barrier |
| clav/i | key |
| clavicul/o, cleid/o | clavicle, collar bone |
| clitor/o | clitoris |
| -clonus | violent action |
| clus/o | shut or close |
| -clysis | irrigation, washing |
| co- | together, with |
| coagul/o, coagulat/o | clotting, coagulation |
| coarct/o, coarctat/o | press together, narrow |
| cocc/i, cocc/o, -coccus | spherical bacteria |
| coccyg/o | coccyx, tailbone |
| cochle/o | spiral, snail, snail shell |
| coher/o, cohes/o | cling, stick together |
| coit/o | a coming together |
| col/o | colon, large intestine |
| coll/a | glue |
| colon/o | colon, large intestine |
| colp/o | vagina |
| column/o | pillar |
| com- | together, with |
| comat/o | deep sleep |
| comminut/o | break into pieces |
| communic/o | share, to make common |
| compatibil/o | sympathize with |
| con- | together, with |
| concav/o | hollow |
| concentr/o | condense, intensify, remove excess water |
| concept/o | become pregnant |
| conch/o | shell |
| concuss/o | shaken together, violently agitated |
| condyl/o | knuckle, knob |
| confus/o | confusion, disorder |
| coni/o | dust |
| conjunctiv/o | conjunctiva, joined together, connected |
| consci/o | aware, awareness |
| consolid/o | become firm or solid |

| | |
|---|---|
| constipat/o | pressed together, crowded together |
| constrict/o | draw tightly together |
| contact/o | touched, infected |
| contagi/o | infection, unclean, touching of something |
| contaminat/o | render unclean by contact, pollute |
| contine/o, continent/o | keep in, contain, hold back, restrain |
| contra- | against, counter, opposite |
| contracept/o | prevention of conception |
| contus/o | bruise |
| convalesc/o | recover, become strong |
| convex/o | arched, vaulted |
| convolut/o | coiled, twisted |
| convuls/o | pull together |
| copi/o | plentiful |
| copulat/o | joining together, linking |
| cor/o | pupil |
| cord/o | cord, spinal cord |
| cordi/o | heart |
| core/o | pupil |
| cori/o | skin, leather |
| corne/o | cornea |
| coron/o | coronary, crown |
| corp/u, corpor/o | body |
| corpuscul/o | little body |
| cort- | covering |
| cortic/o | cortex, outer region |
| cost/o | rib |
| cox/o | hip, hip joint |
| crani/o | skull |
| -crasia | a mixture or blending |
| creatin/o | creatinine |
| crepit/o, crepitat/o | crackling, rattling |
| crin/o, -crine | secrete |
| cris/o, critic/o | turning point |
| -crit | to separate |
| cry/o | cold |
| crypt/o | hidden |
| cubit/o | elbow |
| culd/o | cul-de-sac, blind pouch |
| cult/o | cultivate |
| -cusis | hearing |
| cusp/i | point, pointed flap |
| cutane/o | skin |
| cyan/o | blue |
| cycl/o | ciliary body of eye, cycle |
| -cyesis | pregnancy |
| cyst-, -cyst | bladder, bag |
| cyst/o | urinary bladder, cyst, sac of fluid |

| | |
|---|---|
| cyt/o, -cyte | cell |
| -cytic | pertaining to a cell |
| -cytosis | condition of cells |

# D

| | |
|---|---|
| dacry/o | tear, lacrimal duct (tear duct) |
| dacryocyst/o | lacrimal sac (tear sac) |
| dactyl/o | fingers, toes |
| de- | down, lack of, from, not, removal |
| debrid/e | open a wound |
| deca-, deci- | ten, tenth |
| decidu/o | shedding, falling off |
| decubit/o | lying down |
| defec/o, defecat/o | to free from waste, clear |
| defer/o | carrying down or out |
| degenerat/o | gradual impairment, breakdown, diminished function |
| deglutit/o | swallow |
| deliri/o | wandering in the mind |
| delt/o | Greek letter delta, triangular shape |
| delus/o | delude, mock, cheat |
| -dema | swelling (fluid) |
| dem/i, dem/o | people, population |
| demi- | half |
| dendr/o | branching, resembling a tree |
| dent/i, dent/o | tooth, teeth |
| depilate/o | hair removal |
| depress/o | press down, lower, pressed or sunk down |
| dermat/o, derm/o | skin |
| desic/o | drying |
| -desis | to bind, tie together |
| deteriorat/o | worsening or gradual impairment |
| dextr/o | right side |
| di- | twice, twofold, double |
| dia- | through, between, apart, complete |
| diaphor/o | sweat |
| diaphragmat/o | diaphragm, wall across |
| diastole/o | standing apart, expansion |
| didym/o | testes, twins, double |
| diffus/o | pour out, spread apart |
| digest/o | divide, distribute |
| digit/o | finger or toe |
| dilat/o, dilatat/o | spread out, expand |
| -dilation | widening, stretching, expanding |
| dilut/o | dissolve, separate |
| diphther/o | membrane |
| dipl/o | double |

| | |
|---|---|
| **dips/o, -dipsia** | thirst |
| **dis-** | negative, apart, absence of |
| **dislocat/o** | displacement |
| **dissect/o** | cutting apart |
| **disseminat/o** | widely scattered |
| **dist/o** | far |
| **distend/o, distent/o** | stretch apart, expand |
| **diur/o, diuret/o** | tending to increase urine output |
| **divert/i** | turning aside |
| **domin/o** | controlling, ruling |
| **don/o** | give |
| **dors/i, dors/o** | back of body |
| **-dote** | what is given |
| **-drome** | to run, running |
| **-duct** | opening |
| **duct/o** | to lead, carry |
| **duoden/i, duoden/o** | duodenum, first part of small intestine |
| **-dural** | pertaining to dura mater |
| **-dynia** | pain |
| **dys-** | bad, difficult, painful |

# E

| | |
|---|---|
| **e-** | out of, from |
| **-e** | noun ending |
| **-eal** | pertaining to |
| **ec-** | out, outside |
| **ecchym/o** | pouring out of juice |
| **ech/o** | sound |
| **eclamps/o, eclampt/o** | flashing or shining forth |
| **ectasia, -ectasis** | stretching, dilation, enlargement |
| **ecto-** | out, outside |
| **-ectomy** | surgical removal, cutting out, excision |
| **-ectopy** | displacement |
| **eczemat/o** | eruption |
| **-edema** | swelling |
| **edem-, edemat/o** | swelling, fluid, tumor |
| **edentul/o** | without teeth |
| **ef-** | out |
| **effect/o** | bring about a response, activate |
| **effus/o** | pouring out |
| **ejaculat/o** | throw or hurl out |
| **electr/o** | electricity, electric |
| **eliminat/o** | expel from the body |
| **em-** | in |

| | |
|---|---|
| **emaciat/o** | wasted by disease |
| **embol/o** | something inserted or thrown in |
| **embry/o** | fertilized ovum, embryo |
| **-emesis** | vomiting |
| **emet/o** | vomit |
| **-emia** | blood, blood condition |
| **emmetr/o** | in proper measure |
| **emolli/o** | make soft, soften |
| **en-** | in, within, into |
| **encephal/o** | brain |
| **end-, endo-** | in, within, inside |
| **endocrin/o** | secrete within |
| **enem/o** | end in, inject |
| **enter/o** | small intestine |
| **ento-** | within |
| **epi-** | above, upon, on |
| **epidemi/o** | among the people, an epidemic |
| **epididym/o** | epididymis |
| **epiglott/o** | epiglottis |
| **episi/o** | vulva |
| **epithel/i, epitheli/o** | epithelium |
| **equin/o** | pertaining to a horse |
| **-er** | one who |
| **erect/o** | upright |
| **erg/o, -ergy** | work |
| **erot/o** | sexual love |
| **eruct/o, eructat/o** | belch forth |
| **erupt/o** | break out, burst forth |
| **erythem/o, erythemat/o** | flushed, redness |
| **erythr/o** | red |
| **es-** | out of, outside, away from |
| **-esis** | abnormal condition, disease |
| **eso-** | inward |
| **esophag/o** | esophagus |
| **-esthesia, esthesi/o** | sensation, feeling |
| **esthet/o** | feeling, nervous sensation, sense of perception |
| **estr/o** | female |
| **ethm/o** | sieve |
| **eti/o** | cause |
| **eu-** | good, normal, well, easy |
| **-eurysm** | widening |
| **evacu/o, evacuat/o** | empty out |
| **ex-** | out of, outside, away from |
| **exacerbat/o** | aggravate, irritate |
| **exanthemat/o** | rash |
| **excis/o** | cutting out |

| | |
|---|---|
| excori/o, excoriat/o | abrade or scratch |
| excret/o | separate, discharge |
| excruciat/o | intense pain, agony |
| exhal/o, exhalat/o | breathe out |
| exo- | out of, outside, away from |
| exocrin/o | secrete out of |
| expector/o | cough up |
| expir/o, expirat/o | breathe out |
| exstroph/o | turned or twisted out |
| extern/o | outside, outer |
| extra- | on the outside, beyond, outside |
| extreme/o, extremit/o | extremity, outermost |
| extrins/o | from the outside, contained outside |
| exud/o, exudat/o | to sweat out |

## F

| | |
|---|---|
| faci/o | face, form |
| -facient | making, producing |
| fasci/o | fascia, fibrous band |
| fascicul/o | little bundle |
| fatal/o | pertaining to fate, death |
| fauc/i | narrow pass, throat |
| febr/l | fever |
| fec/i, fec/o | dregs, sediment, waste |
| femor/o | femur, thigh bone |
| fenestr/a | window |
| fer/o | bear, carry |
| -ferent | carrying |
| -ferous | bearing, carrying, producing |
| fertil/o | fertile, fruitful, productive |
| fet/i, fet/o | fetus, unborn child |
| flbr/o | fibrous tissue, fiber |
| fibrill/o | muscular twitching |
| fibrin/o | fibrin, fibers, threads of a clot |
| fibros/o | fibrous connective tissue |
| fibul/o | fibula |
| -fic, fic/o | making, producing, forming |
| -fication | process of making |
| -fida | split |
| filtr/o, filtrat/o | filter, to strain through |
| fimbri/o | fringe |
| fiss/o, fissur/o | crack, split, cleft |
| fistul/o | tube or pipe |
| flat/o | flatus, breaking wind, rectal gas |
| flex/o | bend |
| flu/o | flow |
| fluor/o | glowing, luminous |

| | |
|---|---|
| foc/o | focus, point |
| foll/i | bag, sac |
| follicul/o | follicle, small sac |
| foramin/o | opening, foramen |
| fore- | before, in front of |
| -form, form/o | resembling, in the shape of |
| fove/o | pit |
| fract/o | break, broken |
| frigid/o | cold |
| front/o | forehead, brow |
| -fuge | to drive away |
| funct/o, function/o | perform, function |
| fund/o | bottom, base, ground |
| fung/i | fungus |
| furc/o | forking, branching |
| furuncul/o | furunculus, a boil, an infection |
| -fusion | pour |

## G

| | |
|---|---|
| galact/o | milk |
| gamet/o | wife or husband, egg or sperm |
| gangli/o, ganglion/o | ganglion |
| gangren/o | eating sore, gangrene |
| gastr/o | stomach, belly |
| gastrocnemi/o | gastrocnemius, calf muscle |
| gemin/o | twin, double |
| gen-, gen/o, -gen | producing, forming |
| -gene | production, origin, formation |
| -genic, -genesis | creation, reproduction |
| genit/o | produced by, birth, reproductive organs |
| -genous | producing |
| ger/i | old age |
| germin/o | bud, sprout, germ |
| geront/o | old age |
| gest/o, gestat/o | bear, carry young or offspring |
| gigant/o | giant, very large |
| gingiv/o | gingival tissue, gums |
| glauc/o | gray |
| glen/o | socket or pit |
| gli/o | neurologic tissue, supportive tissue of nervous system |
| globin/o, -globulin | protein |
| globul/o | little ball |
| glomerul/o | glomerulus |
| glott/i, glott/o | back of the tongue |
| gluc/o | glucose, sugar |

| | |
|---|---|
| glute/o | buttocks |
| glyc/o, glycos/o | glucose, sugar |
| glycer/o | sweet |
| glycogen/o | glycogen, animal starch |
| -gnosia | knowledge, to know |
| -gog, -gogue | make flow |
| goitr/o | goiter, enlargement of the thyroid gland |
| gon/e, gon/o | seed |
| gonad/o | gonad, sex glands |
| goni/o | angle |
| grad/i | move, go, step, walk |
| -gram | a picture or record |
| granul/o | granule(s) |
| -graph | a picture or record, machine for recording record |
| -graphy | the process of producing a picture or record |
| gravid/o | pregnancy |
| -gravida | pregnant |
| gynec/o | woman, female |
| gyr/o | turning, folding |

## H

| | |
|---|---|
| hal/o, halit/o | breath |
| hallucin/o | hallucination, to wander in the mind |
| hem/e | deep red iron-containing pigment |
| hem/o, hemat/o | blood, relating to the blood |
| hemi- | half |
| hemoglobin/o | hemoglobin |
| hepat/o | liver |
| hered/o, heredit/o | inherited, inheritance |
| herni/o | hernia |
| herpet/o | creeping |
| -hexia | habit |
| hiat/o | opening |
| hidr/o | sweat |
| hirsut/o | hairy, rough |
| hist/o, histi/o | tissue |
| holo- | all |
| hom/o | same, like, alike |
| home/o | sameness, unchanging, constant |
| hormon/o | hormone |
| humer/o | humerus (upper arm bone) |
| hydr/o, hydra- | relating to water |
| hygien/o | healthy |
| hymen/o | a membrane, hymen |
| hyper- | excessive, increased |

| | |
|---|---|
| hyp- | deficient, decreased |
| hypn/o | sleep |
| hypo- | deficient, decreased |
| hyster/o | uterus |

## I

| | |
|---|---|
| -ia | abnormal condition, disease, plural of -ium |
| -ial | pertaining to |
| -ian | specialist |
| -iasis | abnormal condition, disease |
| iatr/o | physician, treatment |
| -iatrics | field of medicine, healing |
| -iatrist | specialist |
| -iatry | field of medicine |
| -ible | capable of, able to |
| -ic | pertaining to |
| ichthy/o | dry, scaly |
| -ician | specialist |
| icter/o | jaundice |
| idi/o | peculiar to the individual or organ, one, distinct |
| -iferous | bearing, carrying, producing |
| -ific | making, producing |
| -iform | shaped or formed like, resembling |
| -igo | attack, diseased condition |
| -ile | capable of |
| ile/o | ileum, small intestine |
| ili/o | ilium, hip bone |
| illusi/o | deception |
| im- | not |
| immun/o | immune, protection, safe |
| impact/o | pushed against, wedged against, packed |
| impress/o | pressing into |
| impuls/o | pressure or pushing force, drive, urging on |
| in- | in, into, not, without |
| incis/o | cutting into |
| incubat/o | incubation, hatching |
| indurat/o | hardened |
| -ine | pertaining to |
| infarct/o | filled in, stuffed |
| infect/o | infected, tainted |
| infer/o | below, beneath |
| infest/o | attack, assail, molest |
| inflammat/o | flame within, set on fire |
| infra- | below, beneath, inferior to |
| infundibul/o | funnel |

| | |
|---|---|
| ingest/o | carry or pour in |
| inguin/o | groin |
| inhal/o, inhalat/o | breathe in |
| inject/o | to force or throw in |
| innominat/o | unnamed, nameless |
| inocul/o | implant, introduce |
| insipid/o | tasteless |
| inspir/o, inspirat/o | breathe in |
| insul/o | island |
| insulin/o | insulin |
| intact/o | untouched, whole |
| inter- | between, among |
| intermitt/o | not continuous |
| intern/o | within, inner |
| interstiti/o | the space between things |
| intestin/o | intestine |
| intim/o | innermost |
| intoxic/o | put poison in |
| intra- | within, inside |
| intrins/o | contained within |
| intro- | within, into, inside |
| introit/o | entrance or passage |
| intussuscept/o | take up or receive within |
| involut/o | rolled up, curled inward |
| iod/o | iodine |
| -ion | action, process, state or condition |
| ion/o | ion, to wander |
| -ior | pertaining to |
| ipsi- | same |
| ir- | in |
| -is | noun ending |
| ir/i, ir/o, irid/o, irit/o | iris, colored part of eye |
| is/o | same, equal |
| isch/o | to hold back |
| ischi/o | ischium |
| -ism | condition, state of |
| iso- | equal |
| -ist | a person who practices, specialist |
| -isy | noun ending |
| -itis | inflammation |
| -ium | structure, tissue |
| -ive | performs, tends toward |
| -ize | to make, to treat |

## J

| | |
|---|---|
| jejun/o | jejunum |
| jugul/o | throat |
| juxta- | beside, near, nearby |

## K

| | |
|---|---|
| kary/o | nucleus, nut |
| kata-, kath- | down |
| kel/o | growth, tumor |
| kerat/o | horny, hard, cornea |
| ket/o, keton/o | ketones, acetones |
| kines/o, kinesi/o, -kinesia | movement |
| -kinesis | motion |
| klept/o | to steal |
| koil/o | hollow or concave |
| kraur/o | dry |
| kyph/o | bent, hump |

## L

| | |
|---|---|
| labi/o | lip |
| labyrinth/o | maze, labyrinth, the inner ear |
| lacer/o, lacerat/o | torn, mangled |
| lacrim/o | tear, tear duct, lacrimal duct |
| lact/i, lact/o | milk |
| lactat/o | secrete milk |
| lamin/o | lamina |
| lapar/o | abdomen, abdominal wall |
| laps/o | slip, fall, slide |
| -lapse | to slide, fall, sag |
| laryng/o | larynx, throat |
| lat/i, lat/o | broad |
| later/o | side |
| lav/o, lavat/o | wash, bathe |
| lax/o, laxat/o | loosen, relax |
| leiomy/o | smooth (visceral) muscle |
| lent/i | the lens of the eye |
| lenticul/o | shaped like a lens, pertaining to a lens |
| -lepsy | seizure |
| lept/o | thin, slender |
| -leptic | to seize, take hold of |
| lepto- | small, soft |
| letharg/o | drowsiness, oblivion |
| leuk/o | white |
| lev/o, levat/o | raise, lift up |
| lex/o, -lexia | word, phrase |
| libid/o, libidin/o | sexual drive, desire, passion |
| ligament/o | ligament |
| ligat/o | binding or tying off |
| lingu/o | tongue |
| lipid/o, lip/o | fat, lipid |
| -listhesis | slipping |

| | |
|---|---|
| **lith/o, -lith** | stone, calculus |
| **-lithiasis** | presence of stones |
| **lob/i, lob/o** | lobe, well-defined part of an organ |
| **loc/o** | place |
| **loch/i** | childbirth, confinement |
| **-logy** | study of |
| **longev/o** | long-lived, long life |
| **lord/o** | curve, swayback, bent |
| **lumb/o** | lower back, loin |
| **lumin/o** | light |
| **lun/o, lunat/o** | moon |
| **lunul/o** | crescent |
| **lup/i, lup/o** | wolf |
| **lute/o** | yellow |
| **lux/o** | to slide |
| **lymph/o** | lymph, lymphatic tissue |
| **lymphaden/o** | lymph node or gland |
| **lymphangi/o** | lymph vessel |
| **-lysis** | breakdown, separation, setting free, destruction, loosening |
| **-lyst** | agent that causes lysis or loosening |
| **-lytic** | to reduce, destroy |

# M

| | |
|---|---|
| **macro-** | large, abnormal size or length, long |
| **macul/o** | spot |
| **magn/o** | great, large |
| **major/o** | larger |
| **mal-** | bad, poor, evil |
| **-malacia** | abnormal softening |
| **malign/o** | bad, evil |
| **malle/o** | malleus, hammer |
| **malleol/o** | malleolus, little hammer |
| **mamm/o** | breast |
| **man/i** | madness, rage |
| **man/i, man/o** | hand |
| **mandibul/o** | mandible, lower jaw |
| **-mania** | obsessive preoccupation |
| **manipul/o** | use of hands |
| **manubri/o** | handle |
| **masset/o** | chew |
| **mast/o** | breast |
| **mastic/o, masticat/o** | chew |
| **mastoid/o** | mastoid process |
| **matern/o** | maternal, of a mother |
| **matur/o** | ripe |
| **maxill/o** | maxilla (upper jaw) |
| **maxim/o** | largest, greatest |

| | |
|---|---|
| **meat/o** | opening or passageway |
| **medi/o** | middle |
| **mediastin/o** | mediastinum, middle |
| **medic/o** | medicine, physician, healing |
| **medicat/o** | medication, healing |
| **medull/o** | medulla (inner section), middle, soft, marrow |
| **mega-, megal/o** | large, great |
| **-megaly** | enlargement |
| **mei/o** | less, meiosis |
| **melan/o** | black, dark |
| **mellit/o** | honey, honeyed |
| **membran/o** | membrane, thin skin |
| **men/o** | menstruation, menses |
| **mening/o, meningi/o** | membranes, meninges |
| **menisc/o** | meniscus, crescent |
| **mens/o** | menstruate, menstruation, menses |
| **menstru/o, menstruat/o** | occurring monthly |
| **ment/o** | mind, chin |
| **mes-** | middle |
| **mesenter/o** | mesentery |
| **mesi/o** | middle, median plane |
| **meso-** | middle |
| **meta-** | change, beyond, subsequent to, behind, after or next |
| **metabol/o** | change |
| **metacarp/o** | metacarpals, bones of the hand |
| **metatars/o** | bones of the foot between the tarsus and toes |
| **-meter** | measure, instrument used to measure |
| **metr/i, metr/o, metri/o** | uterus |
| **-metrist** | one who measures |
| **-metry** | to measure |
| **micr/o, micro-** | small |
| **mictur/o, micturit/o** | urinate |
| **mid-** | middle |
| **midsagitt/o** | from front to back, at the middle |
| **milli-** | one-thousandth |
| **-mimetic** | mimic, copy |
| **mineral/o** | mineral |
| **minim/o** | smallest, least |
| **minor/o** | smaller |
| **mio-** | smaller, less |
| **-mission** | to send |
| **mit/o** | a thread |
| **mitr/o** | a miter, having two points on top |

| | |
|---|---|
| **mobil/o** | capable of moving |
| **monil/i** | string of beads, genus of parasitic mold or fungus |
| **mono-** | one, single |
| **morbid/o** | disease, sickness |
| **moribund/o** | dying |
| **morph/o** | shape, form |
| **mort/i, mort/o, mort/u** | death, dead |
| **mortal/i** | pertaining to death, subject to death |
| **mot/o, motil/o** | motion, movement |
| **mu/o** | close, shut |
| **muc/o, mucos/o** | mucus |
| **multi-** | many, much |
| **muscul/o** | muscle |
| **mut/a** | genetic change |
| **mut/o** | unable to speak, inarticulate |
| **mutagen/o** | causing genetic change |
| **my/o** | muscle |
| **myc/e, myc/o** | fungus |
| **mydri/o** | wide |
| **mydrias/i** | dilation of the pupil |
| **myel/o** | spinal cord, bone marrow |
| **myocardi/o** | myocardium, heart muscle |
| **myom/o** | muscle tumor |
| **myos/o** | muscle |
| **myring/o** | tympanic membrane, eardrum |
| **myx/o, myxa-** | mucus |

## N

| | |
|---|---|
| **nar/i** | nostril |
| **narc/o** | numbness, stupor |
| **nas/i, nas/o** | nose |
| **nat/i** | birth |
| **natr/o** | sodium |
| **nause/o** | nausea, seasickness |
| **necr/o** | death |
| **-necrosis** | tissue death |
| **neo-, ne/o** | new, strange |
| **nephr/o** | kidney |
| **nerv/o, neur/i, neur/o** | nerve, nerve tissue |
| **neutr/o** | neither, neutral |
| **nev/o** | birthmark, mole |
| **nid/o** | next |
| **niter-, nitro-** | nitrogen |
| **noct/i** | night |
| **nod/o** | knot, swelling |

| | |
|---|---|
| **nodul/o** | little knot |
| **nom/o** | law, control |
| **non-** | no |
| **nor-** | chemical compound |
| **norm/o** | normal or usual |
| **nuch/o** | the nape |
| **nucle/o** | nucleus |
| **nucleol/o** | little nucleus, nucleolus |
| **nulli-** | none |
| **numer/o** | number, count |
| **nunci/o** | messenger |
| **nutri/o, nutrit/o** | nourishment, food, nourish, feed |
| **nyct/o, nyctal/o** | night |

## O

| | |
|---|---|
| **ob-** | against |
| **obes/o** | obese, extremely fat |
| **obliqu/o** | slanted, sideways |
| **oblongat/o** | oblong, elongated |
| **obstetr/i, obstetr/o** | midwife, one who stands to receive |
| **occipit/o** | back of the skull, occiput |
| **occlud/o, occlus/o** | shut, close up |
| **occult/o** | hidden, concealed |
| **ocul/o** | eye |
| **odont/o** | tooth |
| **-oid** | like, resembling |
| **-ole** | little, small |
| **olfact/o** | smell, sense of smell |
| **olig/o** | scanty, few |
| **-ologist** | specialist |
| **-ology** | the science or study of |
| **-oma** | tumor, neoplasm |
| **om/o** | shoulder |
| **oment/o** | omentum, fat |
| **omphal/o** | umbilical cord, the navel |
| **onc/o** | tumor |
| **-one** | hormone |
| **onych/o** | fingernail or toenail |
| **o/o, oo/o** | egg |
| **oophor/o** | ovary |
| **opac/o, opacit/o** | shaded, dark, impenetrable to light |
| **-opaque** | obscure |
| **oper/o, operat/o** | perform, operate, work |
| **opercul/o** | cover or lid |
| **ophthalm/o** | eye, vision |
| **-opia** | vision condition |
| **opisth/o** | backward |
| **-opsia, -opsis, -opsy** | vision, view of |

| | |
|---|---|
| opt/i, opt/o, optic/o | eye, vision |
| or/o | mouth, oral cavity |
| orbit/o | orbit, bony cavity or socket |
| orch/o, orchid/o, orchi/o | testicles, testis, testes |
| -orexia | appetite |
| organ/o | organ |
| orgasm/o | swell, be excited |
| orth/o | straight, normal, correct |
| -ory | pertaining to |
| os- | mouth, bone |
| -ose | full of, pertaining to, sugar |
| -osis | abnormal condition, disease |
| osm/o | pushing, thrusting |
| -osmia | smell, odor |
| oss/e, oss/i | bone |
| ossicul/o | ossicle (small bone) |
| oste/o, ost/o | bone |
| -ostomy | the surgical creation of an artificial opening to the body surface |
| -ostosis | condition of bone |
| ot/o | ear, hearing |
| -otia | ear condition |
| -otomy | cutting, surgical incision |
| ov/i, ov/o | egg, ovum |
| ovari/o | ovary |
| ovul/o | egg |
| ox/i, ox/o, ox/y | oxygen |
| -oxia | oxygen condition |
| oxid/o | containing oxygen |
| oxy/o | the presence of oxygen in a compound |

## P

| | |
|---|---|
| pachy- | heavy, thick |
| palat/o | palate, roof of mouth |
| pall/o, pallid/o | pale, lacking or drained of color |
| palliat/o | cloaked, hidden |
| palpat/o | touch, feel, stroke |
| palpebr/o | eyelid |
| palpit/o | throbbing, quivering |
| pan- | all, entire, every |
| pancreat/o | pancreas |
| papill/i, papill/o | nipple-like |
| papul/o | pimple |
| par-, para- | beside, near, beyond, abnormal, apart from, opposite, along side of |
| par/o | to bear, bring forth, labor |

| | |
|---|---|
| -para | to give birth |
| paralys/o, paralyt/o | disable |
| parasit/o | parasite |
| parathyroid/o | parathyroid glands |
| pares/i | to disable |
| -paresis | partial or incomplete paralysis |
| paret/o | to disable |
| -pareunia | sexual intercourse |
| pariet/o | wall |
| parotid/o | parotid gland |
| -parous | having borne one or more children |
| paroxysm/o | sudden attack |
| -partum, parturit/o | childbirth, labor |
| patell/a, patell/o | patella, kneecap |
| path/o, -pathy | disease, suffering, feeling, emotion |
| paus/o | cessation, stopping |
| -pause | stopping |
| pector/o | chest |
| ped/o | child, foot |
| pedi/a | child |
| pedicul/o | louse (singular), lice (plural) |
| pelv/i, pelv/o | pelvic bone, pelvic cavity, hip |
| pen/i | penis |
| pend/o | to hang |
| -penia | deficiency, lack, too few |
| peps/i, -pepsia, pept/o | digest, digestion |
| per- | excessive, through |
| percept/o | become aware, perceive |
| percuss/o | strike, tap, beat |
| peri- | surrounding, around |
| perine/o | perineum |
| peristals/o, peristalt/o | constrict around |
| peritone/o | peritoneum |
| perme/o | to pass or go through |
| pernici/o | destructive, harmful |
| perone/o | fibula |
| perspir/o | perspiration |
| pertuss/i | intensive cough |
| petechi/o | skin spot |
| -pexy | surgical fixation |
| phac/o | lens of eye |
| phag/o | eat, swallow |
| -phage | a cell that destroys, eat, swallow |
| -phagia | eating, swallowing |
| phak/o | lens of eye |
| phalang/o | phalanges, finger and toe |
| phall/i, phill/o | penis |

| | | | | |
|---|---|---|---|---|
| pharmac/o, pharmaceut/o | drug | | pneum/o, pneumon/o | lung, air |
| pharyng/o | throat, pharynx | | pod/o | foot |
| phas/o | speech | | -poiesis | formation, to make |
| -phasia | speak or speech | | pol/o | extreme |
| phe/o | dusky | | poli/o | gray matter of brain and spinal cord |
| pher/o | to bear or carry | | pollic/o | thumb |
| -pheresis | removal | | poly- | many |
| phil/o, -phil, -philia | attraction to, like, love | | polyp/o | polyp, small growth |
| phleb/o | vein | | pont/o | pons (a part of the brain), bridge |
| phlegm/o | thick mucus | | poplit/o | back of the knee |
| phob/o, -phobia | abnormal fear | | por/o | pore, small opening |
| phon/o, -phonia | sound, voice | | -porosis | lessening in density, porous condition |
| phor/o | carry, bear, movement | | port/i | gate, door |
| -phoresis | carrying, transmission | | post- | after, behind |
| -phoria | to bear, carry, feeling, mental state | | poster/o | behind, toward the back |
| phot/o | light | | potent/o | powerful |
| phren/o | diaphragm, mind | | pract/i, practic/o | practice, pursue an occupation |
| -phthisis | wasting away | | prandi/o, -prandial | meal |
| -phylactic | protective, preventive | | -praxia | action, condition concerning the performance of movements |
| -phylaxis | protection | | -praxis | act, activity, practice use |
| physi/o, physic/o | nature, physical | | pre- | before, in front of |
| -physis | to grow | | precoc/i | early, premature |
| phyt/o, -phyte | plant | | pregn/o | pregnant, full of |
| pigment/o | pigment, color | | prematur/o | too early, untimely |
| pil/i, pil/o | hair | | preputi/o | foreskin, prepuce |
| pineal/o | pineal gland | | presby/o | old age |
| pinn/i | external ear, auricle | | press/o | press, draw |
| pituit/o, pituitar/o | pituitary gland | | priap/o | penis |
| plac/o | flat plate or patch | | primi- | first |
| placent/o | placenta, round flat cake | | pro- | before, in behalf of |
| plak/o, -plakia | plaque, plate, thin flat layer or scale | | process/o | going forth |
| plan/o | flat | | procreat/o | reproduce |
| plant/i, plant/o | sole of foot | | proct/o | anus and rectum |
| plas/i, plas/o, -plasia | development, growth, formation | | prodrom/o | running ahead, precursor |
| -plasm | formative material of cells | | product/o | lead forward, yield, produce |
| plasm/o | something molded or formed | | prolaps/o | fall downward, slide forward |
| -plastic | pertaining to formation | | prolifer/o | reproduce, bear offspring |
| -plasty | surgical repair | | pron/o, pronat/o | bent forward |
| ple/o | more, many | | pros- | before |
| -plegia | paralysis, stroke | | prostat/o | prostate gland |
| -plegic | one affected with paralysis | | prosth/o, prosthet/o | addition, appendage |
| pleur/o | pleura, side of the body | | | |
| plex/o | plexus, network | | prot/o, prote/o | first |
| plic/o | fold or ridge | | protein/o | protein |
| pne/o- | breath, breathing | | proxim/o | near |
| -pnea | breathing | | prurit/o | itching |
| -pneic | pertaining to breathing | | pseud/o | false |

| | |
|---|---|
| **psor/i, psor/o** | itch, itching |
| **psych/o** | mind |
| **-ptosis** | droop, sag, prolapse, fall |
| **-ptyal/o** | saliva |
| **-ptysis** | spitting |
| **pub/o** | pubis, part of hip bone |
| **pubert/o** | ripe age, adult |
| **pudend/o** | pudendum |
| **puerper/i** | childbearing, labor |
| **pulm/o, pulmon/o** | lung |
| **pulpos/o** | fleshy, pulpy |
| **puls/o** | beat, beating, striking |
| **punct/o** | sting, prick, puncture |
| **pupill/o** | pupil |
| **pur/o** | pus |
| **purpur/o** | purple |
| **purul/o** | pus-filled |
| **pustul/o** | infected pimple |
| **py/o** | pus |
| **pyel/o** | renal pelvis, bowl of kidney |
| **pylor/o** | pylorus, pyloric sphincter |
| **pyr/o, pyret/o** | fever, fire |

# Q

| | |
|---|---|
| **quadr/i, quadr/o** | four |

# R

| | |
|---|---|
| **rabi/o** | madness, rage |
| **rachi/o** | spinal column, vertebrae |
| **radi/o** | radiation, x-rays, radius (lateral lower arm bone) |
| **radiat/o** | giving off rays or radiant energy |
| **radicul/o** | nerve root |
| **raph/o** | seam, suture |
| **re-** | back, again |
| **recept/o** | receive, receiver |
| **recipi/o** | receive, take to oneself |
| **rect/o** | rectum, straight |
| **recticul/o** | network |
| **recuperat/o** | recover, regain health |
| **reduct/o** | bring back together |
| **refract/o** | bend back, turn aside |
| **regurgit/o** | flood or gush back |
| **remiss/o** | give up, let go, relax |
| **ren/o** | kidney |
| **restor/o** | rebuild, put back, restore |
| **resuscit/o** | revive |
| **retent/o** | hold back |

| | |
|---|---|
| **reticul/o** | network |
| **retin/o** | retina, net |
| **retract/o** | draw back or in |
| **retro-** | behind, backward, back of |
| **rhabd/o** | rod, rod-shaped |
| **rhabdomy/o** | striated muscle |
| **rheum/o, rheumat/o** | watery flow, subject to flow |
| **rhin/o** | nose |
| **rhiz/o** | root |
| **rhonc/o** | snore, snoring |
| **rhythm/o** | rhythm |
| **rhytid/o** | wrinkle |
| **rigid/o** | stiff |
| **ris/o** | laugh |
| **rotat/o** | rotate, revolve |
| **-rrhage, -rrhagia** | bleeding, abnormal excessive fluid discharge |
| **-rrhaphy** | surgical suturing |
| **-rrhea** | flow or discharge |
| **-rrhexis** | rupture |
| **rube-** | red |
| **rug/o** | wrinkle, fold |

# S

| | |
|---|---|
| **sacc/i, sacc/o** | sac |
| **sacchar/o** | sugar |
| **sacr/o** | sacrum |
| **saliv/o** | saliva |
| **salping/o** | uterine (fallopian) tube, auditory (eustachian) tube |
| **-salpinx** | uterine (fallopian) tube |
| **san/o** | sound, healthy, sane |
| **sangu/i, sanguin/o** | blood |
| **sanit/o** | soundness, health |
| **saphen/o** | clear, apparent, manifest |
| **sapr/o** | decaying, rotten |
| **sarc/o** | flesh, connective tissue |
| **scalp/o** | carve, scrape |
| **scapul/o** | scapula, shoulder blade |
| **schiz/o** | division, split |
| **scirrh/o** | hard |
| **scler/o** | sclera, white of eye, hard |
| **-sclerosis** | abnormal hardening |
| **scoli/o** | curved, bent |
| **-scope** | instrument for visual examination |
| **-scopic** | pertaining to visual examination |

| | |
|---|---|
| **-scopy** | visual examination |
| **scot/o** | darkness |
| **scrib/o, script/o** | write |
| **scrot/o** | bag or pouch |
| **seb/o** | sebum |
| **secret/o** | produce, separate out |
| **sect/o, secti/o** | cut, cutting |
| **segment/o** | pieces |
| **sell/o** | saddle |
| **semi-** | half |
| **semin/i** | semen, seed, sperm |
| **sen/i** | old |
| **senesc/o** | grow old |
| **senil/o** | old age |
| **sens/i** | feeling, sensation |
| **sensitiv/o** | sensitive to, affected by |
| **seps/o** | infection |
| **sept/o** | infection, partition |
| **ser/o** | serum |
| **seros/o** | serous |
| **sial/o** | saliva |
| **sialaden/o** | salivary gland |
| **sigm/o** | Greek letter sigma |
| **sigmoid/o** | sigmoid colon |
| **silic/o** | glass |
| **sin/o, sin/u** | hollow, sinus |
| **sinistr/o** | left, left side |
| **sinus/o** | sinus |
| **-sis** | abnormal condition, disease |
| **sit/u** | place |
| **skelet/o** | skeleton |
| **soci/o** | companion, fellow being |
| **-sol** | solution |
| **solut/o, solv/o** | loosened, dissolved |
| **soma-, somat/o** | body |
| **somn/i, somn/o** | sleep |
| **son/o** | sound |
| **sopor/o** | sleep |
| **spad/o** | draw off, draw |
| **-spasm, spasmod/o** | sudden involuntary contraction, tightening, cramping |
| **spec/i** | look at, a kind or sort |
| **specul/o** | mirror |
| **sperm/o, spermat/o** | sperm, spermatozoa, seed |
| **sphen/o** | sphenoid bone, wedge |
| **spher/o** | round, sphere, ball |
| **sphincter/o** | tight band |
| **sphygm/o** | pulse |
| **spin/o** | spine, backbone |

| | |
|---|---|
| **spir/o** | to breathe |
| **spirill/o** | little coil |
| **spirochet/o** | coiled microorganism |
| **splen/o** | spleen |
| **spondyl/o** | vertebrae, vertebral column, backbone |
| **spontane/o** | unexplained, of one's own accord |
| **spor/o** | seed, spore |
| **sput/o** | sputum, spit |
| **squam/o** | scale |
| **-stalsis** | contraction, constriction |
| **staped/o, stapedi/o** | stapes (middle ear bone) |
| **staphyl/o** | clusters, bunch of grapes |
| **-stasis, -static** | control, maintenance of a constant level |
| **steat/o** | fat, lipid, sebum |
| **sten/o** | narrowing, contracted |
| **-stenosis** | abnormal narrowing |
| **ster/o** | solid structure |
| **stere/o** | solid, three-dimensional |
| **steril/i** | sterile |
| **stern/o** | sternum, the breast bone |
| **steth/o** | chest |
| **-sthenia** | strength |
| **stigmat/o** | point, spot |
| **stimul/o** | goad, prick, incite |
| **stol/o** | send or place |
| **stom/o, stomat/o** | mouth, oral cavity |
| **-stomosis, -stomy** | furnish with a mouth or outlet, new opening |
| **strab/i** | squint, squint-eyed |
| **strat/i** | layer |
| **strept/o** | twisted chain |
| **striat/o** | stripe, furrow, groove |
| **stric-** | narrowing |
| **strict/o** | draw tightly together, bind or tie |
| **strid/o** | harsh sound |
| **stup/e** | benumbed, stunned |
| **styl/o** | pen, pointed instrument |
| **sub-** | under, less, below |
| **subluxat/o** | partial dislocation |
| **sucr/o** | sugar |
| **sudor/i** | sweat |
| **suffoc/o, suffocat/o** | choke, strangle |
| **sulc/o** | furrow, groove |
| **super-, super/o** | above, excessive, higher than |
| **superflu/o** | overflowing, excessive |
| **supin/o** | lying on the back |
| **supinat/o** | bend backward, place on the back |
| **suppress/o** | press down |

| | |
|---|---|
| **suppur/o,** | to form pus |
| **suppurate/o** | |
| **supra-** | above, upper, excessive |
| **supraren/o** | above or on the kidney, suprarenal gland |
| **-surgery** | operative procedure |
| **sutur/o** | stitch, seam |
| **sym-** | with, together, joined together |
| **symptomat/o** | falling together, symptom |
| **syn-** | together, with, union, association |
| **synaps/o, synapt/o** | point of contact |
| **syncop/o** | to cut short, cut off |
| **-syndesis** | surgical fixation of vertebrae |
| **syndrom/o** | running together |
| **synovi/o, synov/o** | synovial membrane, synovial fluid |
| **syphil/i, syphil/o** | syphilis |
| **syring/o** | tube |
| **system/o,** | body system |
| **systemat/o** | |
| **systol/o** | contraction |

## T

| | |
|---|---|
| **tachy-** | fast, rapid |
| **tact/i** | touch |
| **talip/o** | foot and ankle deformity |
| **tars/o** | tarsus (ankle bone), instep, edge of the eyelid |
| **tax/o** | coordination, order |
| **techn/o, techni/o** | skill |
| **tectori/o** | covering, rooflike |
| **tele/o** | distant, far |
| **tempor/o** | temporal bone, temple |
| **ten/o, tend/o** | tendon, stretch out, extend, strain |
| **tenac/i** | holding fast, sticky |
| **tendin/o** | tendon |
| **tens/o** | stretch out, extend, strain |
| **termin/o** | end, limit |
| **test/i, test/o** | testicle, testis |
| **tetan/o** | rigid, tense |
| **tetra-** | four |
| **thalam/o** | thalamus, inner room |
| **thanas/o, thanat/o** | death |
| **the/o** | put, place |
| **thec/o** | sheath |
| **thel/o** | nipple |
| **therap/o,** | treatment |
| **therapeut/o** | |
| **therm/o** | heat |
| **thio-** | sulfur |

| | |
|---|---|
| **thora/o, thorac/o** | chest |
| **-thorax** | chest, pleural cavity |
| **thromb/o** | clot |
| **thym/o** | thymus gland |
| **-thymia** | a state of mind |
| **-thymic** | pertaining to the mind, relating to the thymus gland |
| **thyr/o, thyroid/o** | thyroid gland |
| **tibi/o** | tibia (shin bone) |
| **-tic** | pertaining to |
| **tine/o** | gnawing worm, ringworm |
| **tinnit/o** | ringing, buzzing, tinkling |
| **-tion** | process, state or quality of |
| **toc/o, -tocia, -tocin** | labor, birth |
| **tom/o** | cut, section, slice |
| **-tome** | instrument to cut |
| **-tomy** | process of cutting |
| **ton/o** | tension, tone, stretching |
| **tone/o** | to stretch |
| **tonsill/o** | tonsil, throat |
| **top/o** | place, position, location |
| **tors/o** | twist, rotate |
| **tort/i** | twisted |
| **tox/o, toxic/o** | poison, poisonous |
| **trabecul/o** | little beam marked with cross bars or beams |
| **trache/i, trache/o** | trachea, windpipe |
| **trachel-** | neck |
| **tract/o** | draw, pull, path, bundle of nerve fibers |
| **tranquil/o** | quiet, calm, tranquil |
| **trans-** | across, through |
| **transfus/o** | pour across, transfer |
| **transit/o** | changing |
| **transvers/o** | across, crosswise |
| **traumat/o** | injury |
| **trem/o** | shaking, trembling |
| **tremul/o** | fine tremor or shaking |
| **treponem/o** | coiled, turning microbe |
| **tri-** | three |
| **trich/o** | hair |
| **trigon/o** | trigone |
| **-tripsy** | to crush |
| **-trite** | instrument for crushing |
| **trop/o, -tropia** | turn, change |
| **troph/o, -trophy** | development, nourishment |
| **-tropic** | having an affinity for |
| **-tropin** | to stimulate, act on |
| **tub/i, tub/o** | tube, pipe |
| **tubercul/o** | little knot, swelling |

| | |
|---|---|
| tunic/o | covering, cloak, sheath |
| turbinat/o | coiled, spiral shaped |
| tuss/i | cough |
| tympan/o | tympanic membrane, eardrum |
| -type | classification, picture |

## U

| | |
|---|---|
| -ula | small, little |
| -ule | small one |
| ulcer/o | sore, ulcer |
| uln/o | ulna (medial lower arm bone) |
| ultra- | beyond, excess |
| -um | singular noun ending |
| umbilic/o | navel |
| un- | not |
| ungu/o | nail |
| uni- | one |
| ur/o | urine, urinary tract |
| -uresis | urination |
| ureter/o | ureter |
| urethr/o | urethra |
| urg/o | press, push |
| -uria | urination, urine |
| urin/o | urine or urinary organs |
| urtic/o | nettle, rash, hives |
| -us | thing, singular noun ending |
| uter/i, uter/o | uterus |
| uve/o | iris, choroid, ciliary body, uveal tract |
| uvul/o | uvula, little grape |

## V

| | |
|---|---|
| vaccin/i, vaccin/o | vaccine |
| vacu/o | empty |
| vag/o | vagus nerve, wandering |
| vagin/o | vagina |
| valg/o | bent or twisted outward |
| valv/o, valvul/o | valve |
| var/o | bent or twisted inward |
| varic/o | varicose veins, swollen or dilated vein |
| vas/o | vas deferens, vessel |
| vascul/o | blood vessel, little vessel |
| vast/o | vast, great, extensive |
| vect/o | carry, convey |
| ven/o | vein |
| vener/o | sexual intercourse |
| venter- | abdomen |

| | |
|---|---|
| ventilat/o | expose to air, fan |
| ventr/o | in front, belly side of body |
| ventricul/o | ventricle of brain or heart, small chamber |
| venul/o | venule, small vein |
| verg/o | twist, incline |
| verm/i | worm |
| verruc/o | wart |
| -verse, -version | to turn |
| vers/o, vert/o | turn |
| vertebr/o | vertebra, backbone |
| vertig/o, vertigin/o | whirling round |
| vesic/o | urinary bladder |
| vesicul/o | seminal vesicle, blister, little bladder |
| vestibul/o | entrance, vestibule |
| vi/o | force |
| vill/i | shaggy hair, tuft of hair |
| vir/o | poison, virus |
| viril/o | masculine, manly |
| vis/o | seeing, sight |
| visc/o | sticky |
| viscer/o | viscera, internal organ |
| viscos/o | sticky |
| vit/a, vit/o | life |
| viti/o | blemish, defect |
| vitre/o | glassy, made of glass |
| voc/i | voice |
| vol/o | palm or sole |
| volv/o | roll, turn |
| vulgar/i | common |
| vulv/o | vulva, covering |

## X

| | |
|---|---|
| xanth/o | yellow |
| xen/o | strange, foreign |
| xer/o | dry |
| xiph/i, xiph/o | sword |

## Y

| | |
|---|---|
| -y | noun ending |

## Z

| | |
|---|---|
| zo/o | animal life |
| zygomat/o | cheek bone, yoke |
| zygot/o | joined together |

# ABBREVIATIONS AND THEIR MEANINGS

**Reminder about abbreviations:** An abbreviation can have several meanings, and a term can have several abbreviations. When in doubt, always verify the meaning of the abbreviation!

## A

| | |
|---|---|
| **A2 or A$_2$** | aortic valve closure |
| **A** | abnormal; adult; age; allergy; anaphylaxis; anesthesia; anterior; antibody; auscultation |
| **a** | accommodation; acid |
| **aa** | amino acid |
| **AA** | alopecia areata; asthma; asthmatic |
| **AAA** | abdominal aortic aneurysm |
| **AAL** | anterior axillary line |
| **AAV** | adeno-associated virus |
| **A&B** | apnea and bradycardia |
| **A/B** | acid-base ratio |
| **AB, Ab, ab** | abortion |
| **AB, Abnl, abn** | abnormal |
| **Ab** | antibody |
| **ABC** | aspiration, biopsy, cytology |
| **Abd, Abdo** | abdomen |
| **ABE** | acute bacterial endocarditis |
| **ABG** | arterial blood gases |
| **ABP** | arterial blood pressure |
| **ABR** | auditory brainstem response |
| **abx** | antibiotics |
| **ac** | acute |
| **AC, ac** | anticoagulant; before meals; air conduction |
| **acc** | accident; accommodation |
| **ACD** | absolute cardiac dullness; acid-citrate-dextrose; anterior chest diameter; area of cardiac disease |
| **ACE** | acute care of the elderly; aerobic chair exercises; angiotensin-converting enzyme |
| **ACG** | angiocardiogram; angiocardiography; apex cardiogram |
| **ACH** | adrenocortical hormone |
| **ACL** | anterior cruciate ligament |
| **ACLS** | advanced cardiac life support |
| **ACT** | activated coagulation time; anticoagulant therapy |
| **ACTH** | adrenocorticotropic hormone |
| **ACU** | acute care unit; ambulatory care unit |
| **ACVD** | acute cardiovascular disease |
| **AD** | admitting diagnosis; advanced directive; after discharge; Alzheimer's disease; right ear |
| **ADC** | AIDS dementia complex |
| **ADD** | attention-deficit disorder |
| **ADE** | acute disseminated encephalitis; adverse drug event |
| **ADH** | adhesion; antidiuretic hormone |
| **ADHD** | attention-deficit hyperactivity disorder |
| **ADL** | activities of daily life; activities of daily living |
| **ad lib** | as desired |
| **adm** | admission |
| **ADR** | adverse drug reaction |
| **ADS** | antibody deficiency syndrome |

| | | | |
|---|---|---|---|
| **ADT** | admission, discharge, transfer | **AML** | acute myeloblastic leukemia; acute myelocytic leukemia; amyotrophic lateral sclerosis |
| **AE, A/E** | above elbow | | |
| **AED** | automated external defibrillation | | |
| **AF** | acid-fast; amniotic fluid; atrial flutter | **AMN** | amniocentesis |
| | | **amp** | amplification; ampule; amputate |
| **AF, A fib, A-fib** | atrial fibrillation | **AMS** | altered mental status; automated multiphasic screening |
| **AFB** | acid-fast bacilli | | |
| **AFP** | alpha-fetoprotein | **amt** | amount |
| **AG, Ag** | antigen | **AN** | aneurysm; anorexia nervosa |
| **AH** | abdominal hysterectomy | **ANA** | antinuclear antibodies |
| **AHD** | antihypertensive drug; arteriosclerotic heart disease; autoimmune hemolytic disease | **ANAS** | anastomosis |
| | | **anat** | anatomy |
| | | **anes, anesth** | anesthesia; anesthetic |
| **AI** | accidentally incurred; aortic insufficiency; artificial insemination | **ANLL** | acute nonlymphocytic leukemia |
| | | **ANS** | anterior nasal spine; autonomic nervous system |
| **AIC, AICD** | automated implantable cardioverter-defibrillator | **ant, ANT** | anterior |
| | | **ANUG** | acute necrotizing ulcerative gingivitis |
| **AID** | acute infectious disease; artificial insemination donor | **AOD** | arterial occlusive disease |
| **AIDS** | acquired immunodeficiency syndrome | **AODM** | adult-onset diabetes mellitus |
| | | **AOM** | acute otitis media |
| **AIH** | artificial insemination husband | **A & P** | anatomy and physiology; anterior and posterior; auscultation and percussion |
| **AIHA** | autoimmune hemolytic anemia | | |
| **AJ, aj** | ankle jerk | | |
| **AK** | above knee | **AP** | abruptio placenta; angina pectoris; anteroposterior; anterior-posterior; appendectomy; appendicitis |
| **AKA** | above-knee amputation | | |
| **alb** | albumin | | |
| **ALD** | aldosterone, assistive listening device | **APAP** | acetaminophen |
| | | **Aph** | aphasia |
| **alk** | alkaline | **APLD** | aspiration percutaneous lumbar diskectomy |
| **ALL** | acute lymphoblastic leukemia; acute lymphocytic leukemia | **aPTT** | activated partial thromboplastin time |
| **ALND** | axillary lymph node dissection | | |
| **ALP** | acute lupus pericarditis; alkaline phosphatase | **aq** | aqueous; water |
| | | **AR** | abnormal record; achievement ratio; alarm reaction; artificial respiration |
| **ALS** | advanced life support; amyotrophic lateral sclerosis; antilymphocytic serum | | |
| | | **ARD** | acute respiratory disease |
| **ALT, alt** | alternative; altitude | **ARDS** | acute respiratory distress syndrome; adult respiratory distress syndrome |
| **alt dieb** | alternate days; every other day | | |
| **alt hor** | alternate hours | | |
| **alt noct** | alternate nights | **ARF** | acute renal failure; acute respiratory failure |
| **Am** | amnion | | |
| **AMA** | advanced maternal age; against medical advice; American Medical Association | **ARI** | acute respiratory infection |
| | | **ARM** | artificial rupture of membranes |
| | | **ART** | arthritis; assisted reproductive technology |
| **amb** | ambulance; ambulatory | | |
| **AMD** | age-related macular degeneration | **AS** | ankylosing spondylitis; aortic stenosis; astigmatism; left ear |
| **AMI** | acute myocardial infarction | | |

| | |
|---|---|
| **ASA** | acetylsalicylic acid (aspirin) |
| **ASAP** | as soon as possible |
| **ASCVD** | arteriosclerotic cardiovascular disease |
| **ASD** | atrial septal defect |
| **ASH** | asymmetrical septal hypertrophy |
| **ASHD** | arteriosclerotic heart disease |
| **ASO** | administrative services only; arteriosclerosis obliterans |
| **ASS** | anterior superior spine |
| **AST** | Aphasia Screening Test; aspartate aminotransferase |
| **As tol** | as tolerated |
| **AT** | Achilles tendon |
| **ATP** | adenosine triphosphate |
| **atr** | atrophy |
| **AU** | aures unitas; both ears |
| **AUL** | acute undifferentiated leukemia |
| **aus, ausc, auscul** | auscultation |
| **A-V, AV** | aortic valve; artificial ventilation; arteriovenous; atrioventricular |
| **AVM** | arteriovenous malfunction |
| **AVN** | atrioventricular node |
| **AVR** | aortic valve replacement |
| **A & W** | alive and well |
| **ax, Ax** | axilla; axillary |
| **AZT** | Aschheim-Zondek test |

# B

| | |
|---|---|
| **B** | bruit |
| **B/A** | backache |
| **BA** | bronchial asthma |
| **Ba** | barium |
| **BAC** | blood alcohol concentration |
| **BACT, Bact, bact** | bacteria; bacterium |
| **BaE** | barium enema |
| **BAO** | basal acid output |
| **bas** | basophils |
| **BBB** | blood-brain barrier; bundle branch block |
| **BBT** | basal body temperature |
| **BC** | bone conduction |
| **BCC** | basal cell carcinoma |
| **BD** | bronchodilator |
| **BDT** | bone density testing |
| **BE** | barium enema; below elbow |
| **BEAM** | brain electrical activity map |
| **BED** | binge eating disorder |
| **BFP** | biologic false positive |

| | |
|---|---|
| **bid, b.i.d.** | bis in die; twice a day |
| **BID** | brought in dead |
| **BIL, Bil, Bili** | bilirubin |
| **bil** | bilateral |
| **BIN, bin** | twice a night |
| **BK** | below knee |
| **BKA** | below-knee amputation |
| **Bld** | blood |
| **BM** | bone marrow; bowel movement |
| **BMB** | bone marrow biopsy |
| **BMD** | Becker's muscular dystrophy; bone mineral density |
| **BMI** | body mass index |
| **BMR** | basal metabolic rate |
| **BMT** | barium meal test; bone marrow transplant |
| **BNO** | bladder neck obstruction |
| **BNR** | bladder neck resection |
| **BOM** | bilateral otitis media |
| **BP** | Bell's palsy; bedpan; bathroom privileges; blood pressure |
| **BPD** | borderline personality disorder |
| **BPH** | benign prostatic hyperplasia; benign prostatic hypertrophy |
| **BPM, bpm** | beats per minute, breaths per minute |
| **BP&P** | blood pressure and pulse |
| **BPPV** | benign paroxysmal positional vertigo |
| **Br** | bed rest; chronic bronchitis |
| **BRBPR** | bright red blood per rectum |
| **BRO, Bronch** | bronchoscope; bronchoscopy |
| **BRP** | bathroom privileges |
| **BS** | blood sugar; bowel sounds; breath sounds |
| **BSE** | breast self-examination |
| **BSO** | bilateral salpingo-oophorectomy |
| **BT** | bleeding time |
| **BUN** | blood urea nitrogen |
| **BV** | bacterial vaginosis; blood volume |
| **Bx, bx** | biopsy |

# C

| | |
|---|---|
| **C1 through C7** | cervical vertebrae |
| **C** | centigrade; Celsius; cholesterol; convergence; cyanosis |
| **C.** | chlamydia |
| **c** | centimeter |
| **c̄** | with |

| | | | | |
|---|---|---|---|---|
| Ca | calcium | CFS | chronic fatigue syndrome |
| CA, Ca | cancer; cardiac arrest; carcinoma; chronological age | CGL | chronic granulomatous leukemia |
| | | C gl | with correction; with glasses |
| CAB | coronary artery bypass | CH | chromosome |
| CABG | coronary artery bypass graft | CHB | complete heart block |
| CAD | computer-assisted diagnosis; coronary artery disease | CHD | congenital heart defects; coronary heart disease |
| CAL | calcitonin | CHF | congestive heart failure |
| cal | calorie | CHO | carbohydrate |
| CAM | complementary and alternative medicine | chol | cholesterol |
| | | chole | cholecystectomy |
| cap, caps | capsule | chr | chromosome, chronic |
| CAPD | continuous ambulatory peritoneal dialysis | CI | conjunctivitis; coronary insufficiency |
| card cath | cardiac catheterization | cib | food |
| Cat | cataract | CID | cytomegalic inclusion disease |
| cath | catheter; catheterization; catheterize | CIR, CIRR | cirrhosis |
| caut | cauterization | CIRC, circum | circumcision |
| CAVH | continuous arteriovenous hemofiltration | CIS | carcinoma in situ |
| | | CIT | conventional insulin treatment |
| CBC, cbc | complete blood count | CK | creatine kinase |
| CBF | capillary blood flow; coronary blood flow | ck | check |
| | | CKD | chronic kidney disease |
| CBI | continuous bladder irrigation | Cl, cl | clinic; chloride |
| CBR | complete bed rest | CL | cholelithiasis; chronic leukemia; cirrhosis of the liver; cleft lip; corpus luteum |
| CBS | chronic brain syndrome | | |
| CC | chief complaint; colony count; cardiac cycle; cardiac cauterization; cardiac catheterization; creatinine clearance | | |
| | | CLD | chronic liver disease |
| | | CLL | chronic lymphocytic leukemia |
| | | cl liq | clear liquid |
| cc | cubic centimeter (1/1,000 liter) | cm | centimeter (1/100 meter) |
| CCA | circumflex coronary artery | cm³ | cubic centimeter |
| CCCR | closed chest cardiopulmonary resuscitation | CME | cystoid macular edema |
| | | CMG | cystometrogram |
| | | CML | chronic myelocytic leukemia |
| CCE | cholecystectomy | CMM | cutaneous malignant melanoma |
| CCPD | continuous cycle peritoneal dialysis | CMV | controlled mechanical ventilation; cytomegalovirus |
| CCr | creatinine clearance | | |
| CCT | computerized cranial tomography | CNS | central nervous system; cutaneous nerve stimulation |
| CCU | coronary care unit | | |
| CD | communicable disease; contact dermatitis; Crohn's disease | C/O, c/o | complains of |
| | | CO | carbon monoxide; coronary occlusion; coronary output |
| CDC | calculated date (day) of confinement; Centers for Disease Control and Prevention | | |
| | | CO₂ | carbon dioxide |
| | | COD | cause of death |
| CDE | common duct exploration | COH | carbohydrate |
| CDH | congenital dislocation of the hip | COL | colonoscopy |
| CEA | carotid endarterectomy | COLD | chronic obstructive lung disease |
| CEPH | cephalic | comp | compound |
| CF | complete fixation; counting fingers; cystic fibrosis | cond | condition |
| | | contra | against |

| | |
|---|---|
| **COPD** | chronic obstructive pulmonary disease |
| **CP** | cardiopulmonary; cerebral palsy |
| **CPA** | carotid phonoangiograph |
| **CPAP** | continuous positive airway pressure |
| **CPC** | clinicopathologic conference |
| **CPD** | cephalopelvic disproportion |
| **CPE** | cardio-pulmonary edema |
| **CPK** | creatine phosphokinase |
| **CPN** | chronic pyelonephritis |
| **CPPB** | continuous positive-pressure breathing |
| **CPR** | cardiopulmonary resuscitation |
| **CPS** | cycles per second |
| **CR** | closed reduction; complete response; conditioned reflex |
| **CRC** | colorectal carcinoma |
| **CRD** | chronic respiratory disease |
| **creat** | creatinine |
| **CRF** | chronic renal failure |
| **CRP** | C-reactive protein |
| **CRPS** | complex regional pain syndrome |
| **CRYO** | cryosurgery |
| **C & S** | culture and sensitivity |
| **CS** | central supply; complete stroke; conditioned stimulus; Cushing's syndrome; cesarean section |
| **CSAP** | cryosurgical ablation of the prostate |
| **CSB** | Cheyne-Stokes breathing |
| **C-section** | cesarean section |
| **CSF** | cerebrospinal fluid |
| **CSO** | craniostenosis |
| **CSR** | central supply room; Cheyne-Stokes respiration |
| **CT** | computerized tomography |
| **CTCL** | cutaneous T-cell lymphoma |
| **CTD** | cumulative trauma disorders |
| **CTR** | carpal tunnel release |
| **CTS** | carpal tunnel syndrome |
| **cu** | cubic |
| **CUC** | chronic ulcerative colitis |
| **CUG** | cystourethrogram |
| **CV** | cardiovascular |
| **CVA** | cardiovascular accident; cerebrovascular accident |
| **CVD** | cardiovascular disease |
| **CVI** | chronic venous insufficiency |
| **CVL** | central venous line |
| **CVP** | central venous pressure; Cytoxan, vincristine, prednisone |

| | |
|---|---|
| **CVS** | chorionic villus sampling |
| **CWP** | childbirth without pain; coal workers' pneumoconiosis |
| **Cx** | cervix |
| **CX, CXR** | chest x-ray film |
| **cysto** | cystoscopic examination; cystoscopy |
| **cyt** | cytology; cytoplasm |

# D

| | |
|---|---|
| **D** | diopter; dorsal |
| **d** | day |
| **DAT** | diet as tolerated |
| **db, dB** | decibel |
| **D & C** | dilation and curettage |
| **D/C, d/c, dc** | diarrhea/constipation, discharge, discontinue |
| **DCC** | direct-current cardioversion |
| **DCIS** | ductal carcinoma in situ |
| **DCR** | direct cortical response |
| **D/D, DD, DDx, Ddx** | differential diagnosis |
| **D & E** | dilation and evacuation |
| **debr** | debridement |
| **Dg, dg** | diagnosis (see also DX; Diag) |
| **del** | delivery |
| **DES** | diethylstilbestrol |
| **DEXA** | dual energy x-ray absorptiometry |
| **DF** | dorsiflexion |
| **DG, dg** | diagnosis |
| **DGE** | delayed gastric emptying |
| **DHFS** | dengue hemorrhagic fever shock syndrome |
| **DI** | diabetes insipidus |
| **Diag, diag** | diagnosis |
| **DIC** | diffuse intravascular coagulation |
| **diff** | differential diagnosis |
| **diopt, Dptr** | diopter |
| **DIP** | distal interphalangeal |
| **diph** | diphtheria |
| **disch** | discharge |
| **DJD** | degenerative joint disease |
| **DKA** | diabetic ketoacidosis |
| **DL** | danger list |
| **DLE** | discoid lupus erythematosus |
| **DM** | dermatomyositis; diabetes mellitus; diastolic murmur |
| **DMD** | Duchenne's muscular dystrophy |
| **DNA** | deoxyribonucleic acid |
| **DNR** | do not resuscitate |

| | | | |
|---|---|---|---|
| **DNS** | deviated nasal septum | **Ecz, Ez** | eczema |
| **DOA** | dead on arrival | **ED** | effective dose; emergency department; epidural; erythema dose; erectile dysfunction |
| **DOB** | date of birth | | |
| **DOC** | date of conception | | |
| **DOE** | dyspnea on exertion | **EDA** | epidural anesthesia |
| **DOMS** | delayed-onset muscle soreness | **EDC** | estimated date (day) of confinement |
| **DOT** | directly observed therapy | **EDD** | end-diastolic dimension |
| **DPT** | diphtheria-pertussis-tetanus | **EDS** | Ehlers-Danlos syndrome |
| **DQ** | developmental quotient | **EDV** | end-diastolic volume |
| **DR** | diabetic retinopathy; digital radiography; doctor | **EECG** | electroencephalography |
| | | **EEE** | Eastern equine encephalomyelitis |
| **dr** | dram; dressing | **EEG** | electroencephalogram; electroencephalography |
| **DRD** | developmental reading disorder | | |
| **DRE** | digital rectal examination | **EENT** | eye, ear, nose, and throat |
| **DRG** | diagnosis-related group | **EFM** | electronic fetal monitor |
| **DRP** | diabetic retinopathy | **EGD** | esophagogastroduodenoscopy |
| **D/S** | dextrose in saline | **EIA** | enzyme immunoassay |
| **DS** | Down syndrome | **EIB** | exercise-induced bronchospasm |
| **DSA** | digital subtraction angiography | **Ej** | elbow jerk |
| **DSD** | dry sterile dressing | **EKG** | electrocardiogram; electrocardiography |
| **dsg** | dressing | | |
| **DT** | diphtheria and tetanus toxoids | **ELISA** | enzyme-linked immunosorbent assay |
| **DT, DT's, DTs** | delirium tremens | | |
| **DTP** | diphtheria, tetanus toxoids, and pertussis vaccine | **elix** | elixir |
| | | **EM** | electron microscope; emmetropia, erythema multiforme |
| **DTR** | deep tendon reflex | | |
| **du** | decubitus ulcer | **emb** | embolism |
| **DUB** | dysfunctional uterine bleeding | **EMG** | electromyogram; electromyography |
| **DVA** | distance visual acuity | **EMP** | emphysema |
| **DVI** | digital vascular imaging | **EMR** | educable mentally retarded; electronic medical record; eye movement record |
| **DVT** | deep vein thrombosis | | |
| **D/W** | dextrose in water | | |
| **DX, Dx** | diagnosis | **EMS** | early morning specimen; electromagnetic spectrum |
| **DXA** | dual x-ray absorptiometry | | |
| | | **EN, endo** | endoscopy |
| | | **Endo** | endometriosis |

## E

| | | | |
|---|---|---|---|
| **E** | encephalitis; enema; etiology | **ENG** | electronystagmography |
| **e** | epinephrine; estrogen | **ENT** | ear, nose, and throat |
| **EBL** | estimated blood loss | **EOG** | electro-oculogram |
| **EBP** | epidural blood patch | **EOM** | extraocular muscles; extraocular movement |
| **EBV** | Epstein-Barr virus | | |
| **ECC** | endocervical curettage; extracorporeal circulation | **EOS** | eosinophils |
| | | **EP** | ectopic pregnancy; evoked potential |
| **ECCE** | extracapsular cataract extraction | | |
| **ECG** | electrocardiogram; electrocardiography | **EPF** | early pregnancy factor; exophthalmos-producing factor |
| | | | |
| **ECHO** | echocardiogram; echocardiography | **Epi, EPI** | epinephrine |
| **E coli** | *Escherichia coli* | **epi, epil** | epilepsy |
| **ECT** | electroconvulsive therapy | **epid** | epidemic |
| | | **epis** | episiotomy |

| | |
|---|---|
| EPO | erythropoietin |
| EPR | electron paramagnetic resonance; emergency physical restraint |
| EPS | extrapyramidal symptoms; exophthalmos-producing substance |
| ER | emergency room; epigastric region |
| ERCP | endoscopic retrograde cholangiopancreatography |
| ERPF | effective renal plasma flow |
| ERT | estrogen replacement therapy; external radiation therapy |
| ERV | expiratory reserve volume |
| ESD | end-systolic dimension |
| ESPF | end-stage pulmonary fibrosis |
| ESR | erythrocyte sedimentation rate |
| EST | electric shock therapy |
| ESRD | end-stage renal disease |
| ESWL | extracorporeal shock-wave lithotripsy |
| ESV | end-systolic volume |
| ET | embryo transfer; enterically transmitted; esotropia; eustachian tube |
| et | and |
| ETF | eustachian tube function |
| ETI | endotracheal intubation |
| etiol | etiology |
| ETT | endotracheal intubation; exercise tolerance test |
| EU | Ehrlich units; emergency unit; etiology unknown |
| EV | esophageal varices |
| EWB | estrogen withdrawal bleeding |
| ex | excision; exercise |
| exam | examination |
| exp | expiration |
| ext | extraction; external |
| Ez, Ecz | eczema |

# F

| | |
|---|---|
| F | Fahrenheit |
| FA, FAG | fluorescein angiography; fluorescent antibody; fructosamine test |
| FAS | fetal alcohol syndrome |
| FB | foreign body |
| FBS | fasting blood sugar |
| FCD | fibrocystic disease |
| FDP | fibrin-fibrinogen degradation products |

| | |
|---|---|
| FECG | fetal electrocardiogram |
| FEF | forced expiratory flow |
| FESS | functional endoscopic sinus surgery |
| fet | fetus |
| FEV | forced expiratory volume |
| FFA | free fatty acids |
| FH | family history |
| FHR | fetal heart rate |
| FHS | fetal heart sounds |
| FHT | fetal heart tones |
| FIA | fluorescent immunoassay; fluoroimmunoassay |
| Fluor | fluoroscopy |
| FME | full mouth extractions |
| fMRI | functional magnetic resonance imaging |
| FMS | fibromyalgia syndrome |
| FNA | fine-needle aspiration |
| FOBT | fecal occult blood test |
| FPG | fasting plasma glucose |
| fr | French (catheter size) |
| FRC | functional residual capacity |
| FROM | full range of motion |
| FS | frozen section, fluoroscopy |
| FSH | follicle-stimulating hormone |
| FSP | fibrin-fibrinogen split products |
| FSS | functional endoscopic sinus surgery |
| FT | family therapy |
| FTND | full-term normal delivery |
| FTT | failure to thrive |
| FU, F/U | follow-up; follow up |
| FUO | fever of unknown origin |
| Fx | fracture |

# G

| | |
|---|---|
| G | gingiva; glaucoma; glycogen |
| g | gram (see also gm) |
| G, grav | gravida (used to indicate the number of times a woman has been pregnant); pregnancy |
| GA | gastric analysis; general anesthesia |
| ga | gallium |
| GAD | generalized anxiety disorder |
| GB | gallbladder |
| GBM | glomerular basement membrane |
| GBS | gallbladder series; Guillain-Barré syndrome |

| | |
|---|---|
| **G-Cs** | glucocorticoids |
| **GC** | gonorrhea |
| **GCG** | glucagon |
| **G&D** | growth and development |
| **GD** | Graves' disease |
| **GDM** | gestational diabetes mellitus |
| **GE** | gastroenteritis |
| **GER** | gastroesophageal reflux |
| **GERD** | gastroesophageal reflux disease |
| **GFR** | glomerular filtration rate |
| **GG** | gamma globulin |
| **GGT** | gamma-glutamyl transferase |
| **GH** | growth hormone |
| **GHb** | glycohemoglobin |
| **GI** | gastrointestinal |
| **GIFT** | gamete intrafallopian transfer |
| **GIT** | gastrointestinal tract |
| **glau, glc** | glaucoma |
| **GLTT** | glucose tolerance test |
| **gm** | gram |
| **GN** | glomerulonephritis |
| **GP** | general practice |
| **gr** | grain |
| **grav I** | pregnancy one; primigravida |
| **GS** | general surgery |
| **GSW** | gunshot wound |
| **GT** | glucose tolerance |
| **GTT** | glucose tolerance test |
| **gtt** | drops |
| **GU** | genitourinary |
| **GVHD** | graft-versus host disease |
| **GxT** | graded exercise test |
| **GYN, Gyn** | gynecology |

# H

| | |
|---|---|
| **H** | hydrogen; hypodermic; hyperopia |
| **h, hr** | hour |
| **H & H** | hemoglobin and hematocrit |
| **H & L** | heart and lungs |
| **H & P** | history and physical |
| **HA** | hemolytic anemia; histamine |
| **HAA** | hepatitis-associated antigen; hepatitis Australia antigen |
| **halluc** | hallucination |
| **HASHD** | hypertensive arteriosclerotic heart disease |
| **HAV** | hepatitis A virus |
| **HB** | heart block; hemoglobin; hepatitis B; His bundle |

| | |
|---|---|
| **Hb** | hemoglobin |
| **HBE** | His bundle electrocardiogram |
| **HbF** | fetal hemoglobin |
| **HBGM** | home blood glucose monitoring |
| **HBOT** | hyperbaric oxygen therapy |
| **HBP** | high blood pressure |
| **HbS** | sickle cell hemoglobin |
| **HBV** | hepatitis B virus |
| **HCD** | heavy-chain disease |
| **HCG** | human chorionic gonadotropin |
| **HCl** | hydrochloric acid |
| **HCL** | hairy cell leukemia |
| **HCT, Hct, hct** | hematocrit |
| **HCV** | hepatitis C virus |
| **HCVD** | hypertensive cardiovascular disease |
| **HD** | hearing distance; heart disease; hemodialysis; hip disarticulation; Hodgkin's disease; Huntington's disease |
| **HDL** | high-density lipoproteins |
| **HDN** | hemolytic disease of the newborn |
| **HDS** | herniated disk syndrome |
| **HE** | hereditary elliptocytosis; hyperextension |
| **He** | helium; hemorrhage |
| **HEENT** | head, eyes, ears, nose, throat |
| **HEM** | hematuria |
| **HEM, hemo** | hemophilia; hemodialysis |
| **hemat** | hematocrit |
| **hemi** | hemiplegia |
| **HF** | heart failure |
| **HG** | hypoglycemia |
| **Hg** | mercury |
| **HgA1c** | glycohemoglobin test |
| **Hgb** | hemoglobin |
| **HH** | hiatal hernia |
| **HIE** | hypoxic ischemic encephalopathy |
| **Hi, his** | histamine |
| **HIS, Histo, histol** | histology |
| **HIV** | human immunodeficiency virus |
| **HL** | Hodgkin's lymphoma |
| **HLA** | human leukocyte antigen |
| **HLR** | heart-lung resuscitation |
| **HM** | hand motion; Holter monitor |
| **HMD** | hyaline membrane disease |
| **HMO** | health maintenance organization |
| **hmt** | hematocrit |
| **HNP** | herniated nucleus pulposus |
| **HO** | hyperbaric oxygen |

| | |
|---|---|
| **HOB** | head of bed |
| **HP** | hemipelvectomy; hyperparathyroidism |
| **HPN** | hypertension |
| **HPO** | hypothalamic-pituitary-ovarian |
| **HPS** | hantavirus pulmonary syndrome |
| **HPV** | human papillomavirus |
| **HR** | heart rate |
| **HRT** | hormone replacement therapy |
| **HS** | hamstring; heavy smoker; herpes simplex; hospital stay |
| **hs, h.s.** | at bedtime; hour of sleep |
| **HSG** | hysterosalpingogram, hysterosalpingography |
| **HSV** | herpes simplex virus |
| **HSV-1** | oral herpes simplex virus type 1 |
| **HSV-2** | herpes simplex virus type 2 |
| **HT** | Hashimoto's thyroiditis; hormone therapy |
| **ht** | height; hematocrit |
| **HTO** | high tibial osteotomy |
| **HTN** | hypertension |
| **HV** | hallux valgus; hospital visit |
| **HVD** | hypertensive vascular disease |
| **HVT** | hyperventilation |
| **Hx** | history |
| **hypo** | hypodermic |
| **HYS** | hysteroscopy |
| **HZ** | herpes zoster |
| **Hz** | hertz |

**I**

| | |
|---|---|
| **I** | intensity of magnetism; iodine |
| **IABP** | intra-aortic balloon pump |
| **IACP** | intra-aortic counterpulsation |
| **IADH** | inappropriate antidiuretic hormone |
| **IASD** | interatrial septal defect |
| **IBC** | iron-binding capacity |
| **IBD** | inflammatory bowel disease |
| **IBS** | irritable bowel syndrome |
| **IC** | inspiratory capacity; intermittent claudication; interstitial cystitis |
| **ICCE** | intracapsular lens extraction |
| **ICCU** | intensive coronary care unit |
| **ICD** | implantable cardioverter defibrillator |
| **ICF** | intracellular fluid |
| **ICP** | intracranial pressure |

| | |
|---|---|
| **ICS** | ileocecal sphincter; intercostal space |
| **ICSI** | intracytoplasmic sperm injection |
| **ICT** | indirect Coombs' test; insulin coma therapy |
| **ict ind** | icterus index |
| **ICU** | intensive care unit |
| **I & D** | incision and drainage, irrigation and debridement |
| **ID** | infectious disease; intradermal |
| **IDC** | infiltrating ductal carcinoma; invasive ductal carcinoma |
| **IDD** | insulin-dependent diabetes |
| **IDDM** | insulin-dependent diabetes mellitus |
| **IDK** | internal derangement of the knee |
| **IDS** | immunity deficiency state |
| **I/E** | inspiratory-expiratory ratio |
| **IEMG** | integrated electromyogram |
| **IF** | interferon; interstitial fluid |
| **IFG** | impaired fasting glucose |
| **Ig, IG** | immunoglobulin |
| **IgA** | immunoglobulin A |
| **IgD** | immunoglobulin D |
| **IgE** | immunoglobulin E |
| **IgG** | immunoglobulin G |
| **IgM** | immunoglobulin M |
| **IGT** | impaired glucose tolerance |
| **IH** | infectious hepatitis; inguinal hernia |
| **IHD** | ischemic heart disease |
| **IL** | interleukin |
| **ILC** | infiltrating lobular carcinoma; invasive lobular carcinoma |
| **ILD** | interstitial lung diseases |
| **IM** | infectious mononucleosis; intramuscular |
| **IMAG** | internal mammary artery graft |
| **IMF** | idiopathic myelofibrosis |
| **IMI** | immunofluorescence |
| **IMV** | intermittent mandatory ventilation |
| **inf** | inferior; infusion; inflammation |
| **Inflam, Inflamm** | inflammation |
| **I & O** | intake and output |
| **IO** | intestinal obstruction; intraocular |
| **IOD** | iron-overload disease (hemochromatosis) |
| **IOL** | intraocular lens |
| **IOP** | intraocular pressure |
| **IPF** | idiopathic pulmonary fibrosis |
| **IPG** | impedance plethysmography |

| | |
|---|---|
| **IPPB** | intermittent positive-pressure breathing |
| **IQ** | intelligence quotient |
| **irrig** | irrigation |
| **IS** | impingement syndrome; intercostal space |
| **ISG** | immune serum globulin |
| **isol** | isolation |
| **IT** | immunotherapy |
| **ITP** | idiopathic thrombocytopenic purpura |
| **IU** | international unit |
| **IUD** | intrauterine device |
| **IUP** | intrauterine pressure |
| **IV** | intravenous; intravenously |
| **IVC** | inferior vena cava |
| **IVCP** | inferior vena cava pressure |
| **IVD** | intervertebral disk |
| **IVDA** | intravenous drug abuse |
| **IVF** | in vitro fertilization |
| **IVFA** | intravenous fluorescein angiography |
| **IVP** | intravenous pyelogram |
| **IVSD** | interventricular septal defect |
| **IVU** | intravenous urogram |

## J

| | |
|---|---|
| **j, jaund** | jaundice |
| **jct** | junctions |
| **JOD** | juvenile-onset diabetes |
| **JRA** | juvenile rheumatoid arthritis |
| **Jt** | joint |
| **JVP** | jugular venous pressure; jugular venous pulse |

## K

| | |
|---|---|
| **K** | potassium |
| **KB** | ketone bodies |
| **KCF** | key clinical findings |
| **KCl** | potassium chloride |
| **KD** | knee disarticulation |
| **KE** | kinetic energy |
| **kg** | kilogram |
| **kj** | knee jerk |
| **KO** | keep open |
| **KOH** | potassium hydrochloride |
| **KS** | Kaposi's sarcoma |
| **KUB** | kidneys, ureters, bladder |
| **KVO** | keep vein open |

## L

| | |
|---|---|
| **l** | liter |
| **L1 through L5** | lumbar vertebrae |
| **L & A** | light and accommodation |
| **LA** | left atrium |
| **lab** | laboratory |
| **lac** | laceration |
| **LAD** | left anterior descending |
| **LADA** | latent autoimmune diabetes in adults |
| **LAP** | laparoscopy; leucine aminopeptidase |
| **lap** | laparotomy |
| **lar, lx** | larynx |
| **laryn** | laryngitis; laryngoscopy |
| **laser** | light amplification by stimulated emission of radiation |
| **LASIK** | laser in situ keratomileusis |
| **lat** | lateral |
| **LAVH** | laparoscopically assisted vaginal hysterectomy |
| **LB** | large bowel; low back |
| **lb** | pound |
| **LBBB** | left bundle branch block |
| **LBP** | low back pain |
| **LBW** | low birth weight |
| **LBBX** | left breast biopsy and examination |
| **LCIS** | lobular carcinoma in situ |
| **L & D** | labor and delivery |
| **LDD** | light-dark discrimination |
| **LDL** | low-density lipoproteins |
| **LE** | left eye; life expectancy; lower extremity; lupus erythematosus; lymphedema |
| **LEP, LPT** | leptin |
| **LES** | lower esophageal sphincter |
| **lg** | large |
| **LH** | luteinizing hormone |
| **LHBD** | left heart bypass device |
| **LHF** | left-sided heart failure |
| **lig** | ligament |
| **liq** | liquid |
| **litho** | lithotripsy |
| **LLE** | lower left extremity |
| **LLL** | left lower lobe |
| **LLQ** | left lower quadrant |
| **LLSB** | left lower sternal border |
| **L/min** | liters per minute |
| **LMP** | last menstrual period |
| **LNMP** | last normal menstrual period |

| | | | |
|---|---|---|---|
| **LOC** | levels of consciousness; loss of consciousness | **men, mgtis** | meningitis |
| **LOM** | limitation of motion; loss of motion | **mEq** | milliequivalent |
| **LOS** | length of stay | **MET** | metastasis |
| **LP** | light perception; lumbar puncture; lumboperitoneal | **met** | metastasize |
| | | **M & F** | mother and father |
| **LPF** | low-power field | **MFT** | muscle function test |
| **LPS** | lipase | **mg** | milligram |
| **LR** | light reaction | **MG** | myasthenia gravis |
| **LRDKT** | living related donor kidney transplant | **mgm** | milligram |
| | | **MH** | malignant hyperpyrexia; malignant hyperthermia; marital history |
| **LRT** | lower respiratory tract | **MHC** | mental health care |
| **LSB** | left sternal border | **MI** | mitral insufficiency; myocardial infarction |
| **lt** | left | | |
| **LTB** | laryngotracheobronchitis | **MICU** | medical intensive care unit; mobile intensive care unit |
| **LTC** | long-term care | | |
| **LTH** | lactogenic hormone; luteotropic hormone | **MID** | multi-infarct dementia |
| | | **MIDCAB** | minimally invasive direct coronary artery bypass |
| **LUE** | left upper extremity | | |
| **LUL** | left upper lobe | **MIP** | maximal inspiratory pressure |
| **LUQ** | left upper quadrant | **ml, mL** | milliliter |
| **LV** | left ventricle | **MLD** | median lethal dose |
| **LVH** | left ventricle hypertrophy | **MM** | multiple myeloma; malignant melanoma |
| **lymphs** | lymphocytes | | |
| | | **mm** | millimeter |
| | | **mm Hg** | millimeters of mercury |

## M

| | | | |
|---|---|---|---|
| | | **MMR** | measles, mumps, and rubella vaccination |
| **M** | meter; murmur; myopia | | |
| **MABS** | monoclonal antibodies | **MND** | motor neuron disease |
| **MAO** | maximal acid output; monoamine oxidase | **MNT** | medical nutrition therapy |
| | | **MO** | morbid obesity |
| **MAR** | multiple antibiotic resistant | **MODY** | maturity-onset diabetes of the young |
| **MBC** | maximal breathing capacity | **MOM** | milk of magnesia |
| **MBD** | minimal brain damage | **mono** | monocytes |
| **mc** | millicurie | **MP** | metacarpal-phalangeal |
| **mcg** | microgram | **MPD** | myofascial pain dysfunction |
| **MCH** | mean corpuscular hemoglobin | **MR** | mental retardation; metabolic rate; mitral regurgitation |
| **MCHC** | mean corpuscular hemoglobin concentration | | |
| | | **MRA** | magnetic resonance angiography |
| **MCT** | mean circulation time | **MRD** | medical record department |
| **MCV** | mean corpuscular volume | **MRI** | magnetic resonance imaging |
| **MD** | macular degeneration; medical doctor; muscular dystrophy | **MS** | mitral stenosis; multiple sclerosis; musculoskeletal; morphine sulfate, magnesium sulfate |
| **MDS** | myelodysplastic syndrome | | |
| **MDR-TB** | multidrug-resistant tuberculosis | **MSH** | melanocyte-stimulating hormone |
| **ME** | middle ear | **MTD** | right eardrum |
| **MED** | minimal effective dose; minimal erythema dose | **MTS** | left eardrum |
| | | **MTX** | methotrexate |
| | | **MV** | mitral valve |
| **men** | meningitis; menstruation | **MVP** | mitral valve prolapse |

| | |
|---|---|
| **MY, Myop, myop** | myopia |
| **myel** | myelogram |

# N

| | |
|---|---|
| **N & M** | nerves and muscles; night and morning |
| **N & T** | nose and throat |
| **N & V** | nausea and vomiting |
| **NA** | not applicable; numerical aperture |
| **Na** | sodium |
| **NaCl** | sodium chloride |
| **NAD** | no acute disease; no apparent distress |
| **NB** | newborn |
| **N/C** | no complaints |
| **NCV** | nerve conduction velocity |
| **NED** | no evidence of disease |
| **NEG, neg** | negative |
| **Neph** | nephron |
| **neuro** | neurology |
| **NF** | National Formulary; necrotizing fasciitis; neurofibromatosis |
| **N/G** | nasogastric (tube) |
| **ng** | Neisseria gonorrhoeae |
| **NG** | nasogastric tube |
| **NGF** | nerve growth factor |
| **NGU** | non-gonococcal urethritis |
| **NHL** | non-Hodgkin's lymphoma |
| **NI** | nuclear imaging |
| **NICU** | neurologic intensive care unit, neonatal intensive care unit |
| **NIDDM** | non-insulin-dependent diabetes mellitus |
| **NK cell** | natural killer cell |
| **NKA** | no known allergies |
| **NLP** | neurolinguistic programming |
| **NM** | nuclear medicine |
| **nm** | neuromuscular |
| **NMR** | nuclear magnetic resonance |
| **No** | number |
| **noc, noct** | night |
| **NOFTT** | nonorganic failure to thrive |
| **NP** | nasopharynx, nurse practitioner |
| **NPC** | no point of convergence |
| **NPO** | nothing by mouth |
| **NR** | no response |
| **NREM** | no rapid eye movements |
| **NS** | nephrotic syndrome; normal saline; not stated; not sufficient |

| | |
|---|---|
| **NSAID** | nonsteroidal anti-inflammatory drug |
| **NSR** | normal sinus rhythm |
| **nst** | nystagmus |
| **NSU** | nonspecific urethritis |
| **Nt** | neutralization |
| **NTD** | neural tube defect |
| **NTG** | nitroglycerin |
| **NVA** | near visual acuity |
| **NVD** | nausea, vomiting diarrhea; neck vein distention |
| **NVS** | neural vital signs |
| **NYD** | not yet diagnosed |
| **ny** | nystagmus |

# O

| | |
|---|---|
| **OA** | osteoarthritis |
| **OAB** | overactive bladder |
| **OB** | obstetrics |
| **OB-GYN** | obstetrics and gynecology |
| **obl** | oblique |
| **OBS** | organic brain syndrome |
| **Obs** | obstetrics |
| **OC** | office call; oral contraceptive |
| **OCC** | occasional |
| **OCD** | obsessive-compulsive disorder; oral cholecystogram |
| **OCT** | oral contraceptive therapy |
| **OD** | overdose; right eye (oculus dexter) |
| **od** | once a day |
| **OGN** | obstetric-gynecologic-neonatal |
| **OGTT** | oral glucose tolerance test |
| **oint** | ointment |
| **OJD** | osteoarthritic joint disease |
| **OM** | otitis media |
| **OME** | otitis media with effusion |
| **OMR** | optic mark recognition |
| **OOB** | out of bed |
| **O & P** | ova and parasites |
| **OP** | oropharynx; osteoporosis; outpatient |
| **OPA** | oropharyngeal airway |
| **OPD** | outpatient department |
| **Ophth** | ophthalmic |
| **OPT** | outpatient |
| **OPV** | oral poliovirus vaccine |
| **OR** | operating room |
| **ORIF** | open reduction internal fixation |
| **ORT** | oral rehydration therapy |
| **Orth** | orthopedics |

| | |
|---|---|
| **OS** | left eye (oculus sinister) |
| **os** | mouth |
| **OSA** | obstructive sleep apnea |
| **OT** | occupational therapy; old tuberculin |
| **OTC** | over-the-counter |
| **Oto** | otology |
| **OU** | each eye (oculus unitas) |
| **oz** | ounce |
| **OXT** | oxytocin |

## P

| | |
|---|---|
| **P** | percussion; phosphorus; physiology; posterior; presbyopia; progesterone; prolactin; pulse |
| **P & A** | percussion and auscultation |
| **PA** | pernicious anemia; physician's assistant; polyartcritis; posteroanterior; pulmonary artery |
| **PA, pa** | pathology |
| **PAC** | premature atrial contraction |
| **PACAB** | port-access coronary artery bypass |
| **PAD** | peripheral artery disease |
| **PADP** | pulmonary artery diastolic pressure |
| **PAMP** | pulmonary arterial mean pressure |
| **Pap** | Papanicolaou smear |
| **PAR** | perennial allergic rhinitis; postanesthetic recovery |
| **PARA** | prior pregnancies resulting in viable births, paraplegic |
| **paren** | parenteral (through the skin or mucous membrane) |
| **PASP** | pulmonary artery systolic pressure |
| **PAT** | paroxysmal atrial tachycardia |
| **Path** | pathology |
| **Pb** | presbyopia |
| **PBC** | primary biliary cirrhosis |
| **PBI** | protein-bound iodine |
| **PBP** | progressive bulbar palsy |
| **PBT$_4$** | protein-bound thyroxine |
| **PC** | pheochromocytoma; prostate cancer |
| **p.c.** | after meals |
| **PCA** | prostate cancer |
| **PCKD, PKD** | polycystic kidney disease |
| **PCNL** | percutaneous nephrolithotomy |
| **PCO, PCOS** | polycystic ovary syndrome |
| **PCP** | *Pneumocystis carinii* pneumonia, primary care physician or provider |
| **PCT** | plasmacrit time |

| | |
|---|---|
| **PCU** | progressive care unit |
| **PCV** | packed cell volume |
| **PD** | interpupillary distance; Parkinson's disease; peritoneal dialysis; postural drainage |
| **PDA** | patent ductus arteriosus |
| **PDD** | pervasive developmental disorder |
| **PDL** | periodontal ligament |
| **PDT** | photodynamic therapy |
| **PE** | physical examination; preeclampsia |
| **PEA** | pulseless electrical activity |
| **Peds** | pediatrics |
| **PEEP** | positive end-expiratory pressure |
| **PEF** | peak expiratory flow rate |
| **PEG** | pneumoencephalogram; pneumoencephalography |
| **PEL** | permissible exposure limit |
| **pcr** | by; through |
| **PERLA** | pupils equally reactive (responsive) to light and accommodation |
| **PERRLA** | pupils equal, round, react (respond) to light and accommodation |
| **PET** | positron emission tomography; preeclamptic toxemia |
| **PFT** | pulmonary function tests |
| **PG** | pregnant; prostaglandin |
| **PGH** | pituitary growth hormone |
| **PGL** | persistent generalized lymphadenopathy |
| **PH** | past history; personal history; public health |
| **pH** | acidity; hydrogen ion concentration |
| **PHN** | postherpetic neuralgia |
| **PI** | present illness |
| **PICU** | pulmonary intensive care unit; pediatric intensive care unit |
| **PID** | pelvic inflammatory disease |
| **PIF** | peak inspiratory flow |
| **PIH** | pregnancy-induced hypertension |
| **PK** | pyruvate kinase; pyruvate kinase deficiency |
| **PKD** | polycystic kidney disease |
| **PKR** | partial knee replacement |
| **PKU** | phenylketonuria |
| **PL** | light perception |
| **pl** | placenta |
| **PLC** | platelet count |
| **PLMS** | periodic limb movements in sleep |
| **PLS** | primary lateral sclerosis |
| **PLTS** | platelets |

| | | | |
|---|---|---|---|
| **PM** | evening or afternoon; physical medicine; polymyositis; postmortem | **PRE** | progressive restrictive exercise |
| **PMA** | progressive muscular atrophy | **prcg** | pregnant |
| **PMDD** | premenstrual dysphoric disorder | **preop** | preoperative |
| **PMH** | past medical history | **prep** | prepare |
| **PMI** | point of maximal impulse | **PRK** | photo-refractive keratectomy |
| **PMN** | polymorphonuclear neutrophils | **p.r.n.** | as needed |
| **PMP** | past menstrual period; previous menstrual period | **proct** | proctology |
| | | **prog, progn** | prognosis |
| **PMR** | physical medicine and rehabilitation; polymyalgia rheumatica | **PROM** | passive range of motion; premature rupture of membranes |
| | | **pro time** | prothrombin time |
| **PMS** | premenstrual syndrome | **PRRE** | pupils round, regular, and equal |
| **PMT** | premenstrual tension | **Prx** | prognosis |
| **PMVS** | prolapsed mitral valve syndrome | **Ps** | psoriasis |
| **PN** | peripheral neuropathy; postnatal | **PSA** | prostate-specific antigen |
| **Pn, PNA, pneu** | pneumonia | **PSS** | progressive systemic sclerosis; physiologic saline solution |
| **PND** | paroxysmal nocturnal dyspnea; postnasal drip | **psych** | psychiatry |
| **PNH** | postnatal headache | **PT** | paroxysmal tachycardia; physical therapy; prothrombin time |
| **Pno** | pneumothorax | **pt** | patient; pint |
| **PNP** | peripheral neuropathy | **PTA** | percutaneous transluminal angioplasty |
| **PNS** | parasympathetic nervous system; peripheral nervous system | **PTE** | pulmonary thromboembolism |
| **PO, p.o.** | by mouth; orally; phone order; postoperative | **PTC** | percutaneous transhepatic cholangiography |
| **POC** | products of conception | **PTCA** | percutaneous transluminal coronary angioplasty |
| **polys** | polymorphonuclear leukocytes | **PTD** | permanent and total disability |
| **POMR** | problem-oriented medical record | **PTE** | parathyroid extract; pulmonary thromboemboliam |
| **POS** | polycystic ovary syndrome | | |
| **pos** | positive | **PTH** | parathyroid hormone; parathormone |
| **post-op** | postoperatively | | |
| **PP** | placenta previa; postpartum; postprandial (after meals); pulse pressure | **PTSD** | post-traumatic stress disorder |
| | | **PTT** | partial thromboplastin time; prothrombin time |
| **ppb** | parts per billion | **PU** | peptic ulcer; pregnancy urine; prostatic urethra |
| **PPBS** | postprandial blood sugar | | |
| **PPD** | purified protein derivative | **PUD** | peptic ulcer disease; pulmonary disease |
| **ppm** | parts per million | | |
| **PPS** | postperfusion syndrome; postpolio syndrome; progressive systemic sclerosis | **pul** | pulmonary |
| | | **P & V** | pyloroplasty and vagotomy |
| | | **PV** | peripheral vascular; plasma volume; polycythemia vera |
| **PPT** | partial prothrombin time | | |
| **PPV** | positive-pressure ventilation | **PVC** | premature ventricular contraction |
| **PR** | peripheral resistance; pulse rate | **PVD** | peripheral vascular disease |
| **Pr** | presbyopia; prism | **PVE** | prosthetic valve endocarditis |
| **pr** | by rectum | **PVOD** | peripheral vascular occlusive disease |
| **PRA** | plasma renin activity | | |
| **PRC** | packed red cells | **PVS** | persistent vegetative state |

| | |
|---|---|
| **PVT** | paroxysmal ventricular tachycardia |
| **pvt** | private |
| **PWB** | partial weight-bearing |
| **PWP** | pulmonary wedge pressure |
| **Px** | prognosis |

## Q

| | |
|---|---|
| **q** | every |
| **qd, q.d.** | every day |
| **qh, q.h** | every hour |
| **q 2 h** | every 2 hours |
| **QID, qid, q.i.d.** | four times a day |
| **qm** | every morning |
| **qn** | every night |
| **qns** | quantity not sufficient |
| **qod** | every other day |
| **qoh** | every other hour |
| **QOL** | quality of life |
| **qs** | quantity sufficient |
| **qt** | quart; quiet |
| **q.q.** | each |
| **quad** | quadrant, quadriplegia, quadriplegic |

## R

| | |
|---|---|
| **R** | rectal; respiration; right |
| **RA** | refractory anemia; rheumatoid arthritis; right arm; right atrium |
| **rad** | radiation absorbed dose |
| **RAF** | rheumatoid arthritis factor |
| **RAI** | radioactive iodine |
| **RAIU** | radioactive iodine uptake determination |
| **RAS** | reticular activating system |
| **RAST** | radioallergosorbent |
| **RAT** | radiation therapy |
| **RBBB** | right bundle branch block |
| **RBC** | red blood cell; red blood count |
| **RBCV** | red blood cell volume |
| **RBE** | relative biologic effects |
| **RCA** | right coronary artery |
| **RD** | respiratory distress; retinal detachment |
| **RDA** | recommended daily allowance |
| **RDS** | respiratory distress syndrome |
| **RE** | right eye |
| **reg** | regular |
| **rehab** | rehabilitation |
| **rem** | roentgen-equivalent-man |

| | |
|---|---|
| **REM sleep** | rapid eye movement sleep |
| **RER** | renal excretion rate |
| **resp** | respiration |
| **RF** | renal failure; respiratory failure; rheumatoid factor; rheumatic fever |
| **RFS** | renal function study |
| **RH** | right hand |
| **RHD** | rheumatic heart disease |
| **Rh neg** | Rhesus factor negative |
| **Rh pos** | Rhesus factor positive |
| **RIA** | radioimmunoassay |
| **RICE** | rest, ice, compression, elevate |
| **Rick** | rickettsia |
| **RIST** | radioimmunosorbent |
| **RK** | radial keratotomy |
| **RL** | right leg |
| **RLC** | residual lung capacity |
| **RLD** | related living donor |
| **RLE** | right lower extremity |
| **RLL** | right lower lobe |
| **RLQ** | right lower quadrant |
| **RLS** | restless legs syndrome |
| **RM** | respiratory movement |
| **RMD** | repetitive motion disorder |
| **RML** | right mediolateral |
| **RMSF** | Rocky Mountain spotted fever |
| **RNA** | ribonucleic acid |
| **RND** | radical neck dissection |
| **R/O** | rule out |
| **ROA** | radiopaque agents |
| **ROM** | range of motion; rupture of membranes |
| **ROP** | retinopathy of prematurity |
| **ROPS** | roll over protection structures |
| **ROS** | review of systems |
| **ROT** | right occipitis transverse |
| **RP** | radiopharmaceuticals; Raynaud's phenomenon; relapsing polychondritis; retrograde pyelogram |
| **RPF** | renal plasma flow |
| **RPG** | retrograde pyelogram |
| **rpm** | revolutions per minute |
| **RPO** | right posterior oblique |
| **RPR** | rapid plasma reagin |
| **RQ** | respiratory quotient |
| **R & R** | rate and rhythm |
| **RR** | recovery room; respiratory rate |
| **RSD** | repetitive stress disorder |

| | |
|---|---|
| **RSDS** | reflex sympathetic dystrophy syndrome |
| **RSHF** | right-sided heart failure |
| **RSI** | repetitive stress injuries |
| **RSR** | regular sinus rhythm |
| **RSV** | right subclavian vein |
| **RT** | radiation therapy; renal transplantation; respiratory therapy |
| **rt** | right; routine |
| **RTA** | renal tubular acidosis |
| **rt lat** | right lateral |
| **rtd** | retarded |
| **RU** | roentgen unit; routine urinalysis |
| **RUE** | right upper extremity |
| **RUL** | right upper lobe |
| **RUQ** | right upper quadrant |
| **RV** | residual volume; right ventricle |
| **RVG** | radionuclide ventriculogram |
| **RVH** | right ventricular hypertrophy |
| **RVS** | relative value schedule |
| **RW** | ragweed |
| **Rx** | prescription; take; therapy; treatment |

# S

| | |
|---|---|
| **s̄** | without |
| **S-A** | sinoatrial node |
| **S & A** | sugar and acetone |
| **SA** | salicylic acid; sinoatrial; sperm analysis; surgeon's assistant |
| **SAAT** | serum aspartate aminotransferase |
| **SAB** | spontaneous abortion |
| **SACH** | self-assessed change in health |
| **SAD** | seasonal affective disorder |
| **SAH** | subarachnoid hemorrhage |
| **SAL** | sensorineural activity level; sterility assurance level; suction-assisted lipectomy |
| **Sal, Salm** | salmonella |
| **SALP** | salpingectomy; salpingography; serum alkaline phosphatase |
| **Salpx** | salpingectomy |
| **SAM** | self-administered medication program |
| **SARS** | severe acute respiratory syndrome |
| **SAS** | short arm splint; sleep apnea syndrome; social adjustment scale; subarachnoid space |

| | |
|---|---|
| **SB** | small bowel; spina bifida; stillbirth; suction biopsy |
| **SBE** | subacute bacterial endocarditis |
| **SBO** | small bowel obstruction |
| **SC, sc, subq** | subcutaneous |
| **SC** | Snellen chart; spinal cord |
| **SCA** | sickle cell anemia |
| **SCC** | squamous cell carcinoma |
| **SCD** | sudden cardiac death, scleroderma |
| **schiz** | schizophrenia |
| **SCI** | spinal cord injury |
| **SCID** | severe combined immune deficiency |
| **SCT** | sickle cell trait |
| **SD** | septal defect; shoulder disarticulation; spontaneous delivery; standard deviation; sudden death |
| **SDAT** | senile dementia of Alzheimer's type |
| **SDM** | standard deviation of the mean |
| **SDS** | sudden death syndrome |
| **sec** | second |
| **SED** | sub-erythema dose |
| **sed rate** | sedimentation rate |
| **seg** | segmented neutrophils |
| **SEM** | scanning electron microscopy |
| **semi** | half |
| **SES** | subcutaneous electric stimulation |
| **sev** | sever; severed |
| **SF** | scarlet fever; spinal fluid |
| **SG** | serum globulin; skin graft |
| **SGA** | small for gestational age |
| **SH** | serum hepatitis; sex hormone; social history |
| **sh** | shoulder |
| **SI** | saturation index |
| **SICU** | surgical intensive care unit |
| **SIDS** | sudden infant death syndrome |
| **sig** | let it be labeled |
| **SIRS** | systemic inflammatory response syndrome |
| **SIS** | saline infusion sonohysterography |
| **SISI** | short increment sensitivity index |
| **SLE** | slit-lamp examination; systemic lupus erythematosus |
| **SLND** | sentinel lymph node dissection |
| **SLPS** | serum lipase |
| **SM** | simple mastectomy |
| **sm** | small |
| **SMA** | sequential multiple analysis |

| | |
|---|---|
| **UV** | ultraviolet |
| **UVJ** | ureterovesical junction |

## V

| | |
|---|---|
| **V** | ventral; visual acuity |
| **VA** | vacuum aspiration; visual acuity |
| **vag** | vaginal |
| **VAS** | vasectomy |
| **VB** | viable birth |
| **VBAC** | vaginal birth after cesarean |
| **VBP** | ventricular premature beat |
| **VC** | acuity of color vision; vena cava; vital capacity |
| **VCUG** | voiding cystourethrogram |
| **VD** | venereal disease |
| **VDG** | venereal disease, gonorrhea |
| **VDH** | valvular disease of heart |
| **VDRL** | Venereal Disease Research Laboratory |
| **VDS** | venereal disease, syphilis |
| **VE** | visual efficiency |
| **Vent, ventr** | ventral |
| **VEP** | visual evoked potential |
| **VER** | visual evoked response |
| **VF** | ventricular fibrillation; visual field; vocal fremitus |
| **V-fib** | ventricular fibrillation |
| **VG** | ventricular gallop |
| **VH** | vaginal hysterectomy |
| **VHD** | valvular heart disease; ventricular heart disease |
| **VI** | volume index |
| **vit cap** | vital capacity |
| **VLDL** | very-low-density lipoprotein |
| **VP** | venipuncture; venous pressure |
| **V & P** | vagotomy and pyloroplasty |
| **VPC** | ventricular premature contraction |
| **VPRC** | volume of packed red cells |
| **VS, vs** | vital signs |
| **VSD** | ventricular septal defect |
| **VSZ** | varicella |
| **VTAs** | vascular targeting agents |

| | |
|---|---|
| **VV** | varicose veins |
| **VVF** | vesicovaginal fistula |
| **VZV** | varicella-zoster virus (chickenpox) |

## W

| | |
|---|---|
| **W** | water |
| **WA** | while awake |
| **WB** | weight-bearing; whole blood |
| **WBC** | white blood cell; white blood count |
| **W/C, w/c** | wheelchair |
| **wd** | wound |
| **WD, w/d** | well-developed |
| **WDWN** | well-developed, well-nourished |
| **wf** | white female |
| **w/n** | well nourished |
| **WNL** | within normal limits |
| **w/o** | without |
| **WR, W.r.** | Wassermann reaction |
| **wt** | weight |
| **w/v** | weight by volume |

## X

| | |
|---|---|
| **X** | xerophthalmia |
| **x** | multiplied by; times |
| **XDP** | xeroderma pigmentosum |
| **XM** | cross-match |
| **XR** | x-ray |
| **XT** | exotropia |
| **XU** | excretory urogram |

## Y

| | |
|---|---|
| **y/o** | year(s) old |
| **YOB** | year of birth |
| **yr** | year |

## Z

| | |
|---|---|
| **Z** | atomic number; no effect; zero |
| **zyg** | zygote |

# Appendix C

## GLOSSARY OF PATHOLOGY AND PROCEDURES

### A

**abdominal computed tomography:** a radiographic procedure that produces a detailed cross-section of the tissue structure within the abdomen.

**abdominal ultrasound:** a noninvasive test used to visualize internal organs by using very high frequency sound waves.

**abdominocentesis** (ab-**dom**-ih-noh-sen-**TEE**-sis): the surgical puncture of the abdominal cavity to remove fluid.

**ablation** (ab-**LAY**-shun): the removal of a body part or the destruction of its function.

**abortion** (ah-**BOR**-shun): the interruption or termination of pregnancy before the fetus is viable.

**abrasion** (ah-**BRAY**-zhun): an injury in which superficial layers of skin are scraped or rubbed away.

**abruptio placentae** (ab-**RUP**-shee-oh plah-**SEN**-tee): a disorder in which the placenta separates from the uterine wall before the birth of the fetus.

**abscess** (**AB**-sess): a closed pocket containing pus caused by a bacterial infection.

**absence seizure:** a brief disturbance in brain function in which there is a loss of awareness often described as a staring episode.

**ACE inhibitors:** medications administered to treat hypertension and congestive heart failure.

**acetaminophen** (ah-**seet**-ah-**MIN**-oh-fen): analgesic that reduces pain and fever, but does not relieve inflammation.

**Achilles tendinitis** (**ten**-dih-**NIGH**-tis): inflammation of the Achilles tendon caused by excessive stress being placed on that tendon.

**acne vulgaris** (**ACK**-nee vul-**GAY**-ris): a chronic inflammatory disease that is characterized by pustular eruptions of the skin caused by an overproduction of sebum around the hair shaft.

**acoustic neuroma** (new-**ROH**-mah): a brain tumor that develops adjacent to the cranial nerve running from the brain to the inner ear.

**acquired immunity:** immunity obtained by having had a contagious disease.

**acquired immunodeficiency syndrome:** the advanced stage of an HIV infection.

**acromegaly** (**ack**-roh-**MEG**-ah-lee): enlargement of the extremities caused by excessive secretion of growth hormone after puberty.

**acrophobia** (**ack**-roh-**FOH**-bee-ah): an excessive fear of heights.

**actinic keratosis** (ack-**TIN**-ick **kerr**-ah-**TOH**-sis): a precancerous skin growth that occurs on sun-damaged skin.

**activities of daily living** (ADL): include bathing, grooming, brushing teeth, eating, and dressing.

**acupressure** (**AK**-que-**presh**-ur): a traditional Chinese touch therapy involving finger pressure applied to specific areas of the body.

**acupuncture** (**AK**-que-**punk**-tyour): a traditional Chinese medical practice using very thin acupuncture needles inserted into specific points of the body.

**acute necrotizing ulcerative gingivitis:** an abnormal growth of bacteria in the mouth.

**acute renal failure:** sudden onset of kidney failure that may be caused by the kidneys not receiving enough blood to filter.

**acute respiratory distress syndrome:** a life-threatening condition in which inflammation in the lungs and fluid in the alveoli lead to low levels of oxygen in the blood.

**addiction:** compulsive, uncontrollable dependence on a substance, habit, or practice.

**Addison's disease (AD**-ih-sonz**):** a condition that occurs when the adrenal glands do not produce enough cortisol or aldosterone.

**adenectomy (ad**-eh-**NECK**-toh-mee**):** surgical removal of a gland.

**adenitis (ad**-eh-**NIGH**-tis**):** inflammation of a gland.

**adenocarcinoma (ad**-eh-noh-**kar**-sih-**NOH**-mah**):** carcinoma derived from glandular tissue.

**adenoma (ad**-eh-**NOH**-mah**):** benign tumor that arises from, or resembles, glandular tissue.

**adenomalacia (ad**-eh-noh-mal-**LAY**-shee-ah**):** abnormal softening of a gland.

**adenosclerosis (ad**-eh-noh-skleh-**ROH**-sis**):** abnormal hardening of a gland.

**adenosis (ad**-eh-**NOH**-sis**):** any disease or condition of a gland.

**adhesion (ad**-**HEE**-zhun**):** a band of fibrous tissue that holds structures together abnormally.

**adjuvant therapy (AD**-jeh-vant**):** cancer treatment used after the primary treatments have been completed to decrease the chance that a cancer will recur.

**adrenalitis (ah**-**dree**-nal-**EYE**-tis**):** inflammation of the adrenal glands.

**adverse drug reaction:** an undesirable reaction that accompanies the principal response for which the drug was taken.

**aerophagia (ay**-er-oh-**FAY**-jee-ah**):** excessive swallowing of air while eating or drinking.

**age spots:** discolorations caused by sun exposure.

**agoraphobia (ag**-oh-rah-**FOH**-bee-ah**):** an excessive fear of environments where the person fears a panic attack might occur.

**airborne transmission:** occurs through contact with contaminated respiratory droplets spread by a cough or sneeze.

**airway inflammation:** the swelling and clogging of the bronchial tubes with mucus.

**airway obstruction:** occurs when food or a foreign object partially or completely blocks the airway and prevents air from entering or leaving the lungs.

**albinism (AL**-bih-niz-um**):** a genetic condition characterized by a deficiency or absence of pigment in the skin, hair, and irises.

**albuminuria (al**-byou-mih-**NEW**-ree-ah**):** the presence of the protein albumin in the urine.

**alcoholism (AL**-koh-hol-izm**):** chronic alcohol dependence with specific signs and symptoms upon withdrawal.

**aldosteronism (al**-**DOSS**-teh-roh-**niz**-em**):** an abnormality of electrolyte balance caused by excessive secretion of aldosterone.

**allergen (AL**-er-jen**):** a substance that produces an allergic response in an individual.

**allergic reaction:** occurs when the body's immune system reacts to a harmless allergen as if it were a dangerous invader.

**allergic rhinitis (rye**-**NIGH**-tis**):** an allergic reaction to airborne allergens.

**allergy:** an overreaction by the body to a particular antigen.

**allogenic bone marrow transplant (al**-oh-**JEN**-ick**):** a transplant in which the recipient receives bone marrow from a compatible donor.

**allopathic medicine (ah**-low-**PAH**-thick**):** conventional medical practices and systems of health care.

**alopecia (al**-oh-**PEE**-shee-ah**):** the partial or complete loss of hair, most commonly on the scalp.

**alopecia areata:** an autoimmune disorder that attacks the hair follicles, causing well-defined bald areas on the scalp or elsewhere on the body.

**alopecia totalis:** an uncommon condition characterized by the loss of all the hair on the scalp.

**alopecia universalis:** the total loss of hair on all parts of the body.

**alternative medicine:** a general term for practices and systems of health care used in place of allopathic medicine.

**Alzheimer's disease (ALTZ**-high-merz**):** a group of disorders involving the parts of the brain that control thought, memory, and language.

**amblyopia (am**-blee-**OH**-pee-ah**):** dimness of vision or the partial loss of sight, especially in one eye, without detectable disease of the eye.

**amenorrhea (ah**-**men**-oh-**REE**-ah *or* ay-**men**-oh-**REE**-ah**):** the abnormal absence of menstrual periods for three months or more.

**ametropia (am**-eh-**TROH**-pee-ah**):** any error of refraction in which images do not focus properly on the retina.

**amnesia (am**-**NEE**-zee-ah**):** a memory disturbance marked by a total or partial inability to recall past experiences.

**amniocentesis (am**-nee-oh-sen-**TEE**-sis**):** a surgical puncture to remove amniotic fluid to evaluate fetal health and to diagnose certain congenital disorders.

**amyotrophic lateral sclerosis** (ah-**my**-oh-**TROH**-fick)**:** a rapidly progressive neurological disease that attacks the nerve cells responsible for controlling voluntary muscles.

**anal fissure:** a small crack-like sore in the skin of the anus that can cause severe pain during a bowel movement.

**analgesic** (**an**-al-**JEE**-zick)**:** a medication that relieves pain without affecting consciousness.

**anaphylaxis** (**an**-ah-fih-**LACK**-sis)**:** a severe, systemic response to an allergen.

**anaplasia** (**an**-ah-**PLAY**-zee-ah)**:** a change in the structure of cells and in their orientation to each other.

**anastomosis** (ah-**nas**-toh-**MOH**-sis)**:** a surgical connection between two hollow or tubular structures.

**andropause** (**AN**-droh-pawz)**:** marked by the decrease of the male hormone testosterone, gradually beginning in the late 40s and progressing very gradually over several decades.

**anemia** (ah-**NEE**-mee-ah)**:** a disorder characterized by lower than normal levels of red blood cells in the blood.

**anesthesia** (**an**-es-**THEE**-zee-ah)**:** the absence of normal sensation, especially sensitivity to pain.

**anesthetic** (**an**-es-**THET**-ick)**:** medication used to induce anesthesia.

**aneurysm** (**AN**-you-rizm)**:** a localized weak spot or balloon-like enlargement of the wall of an artery.

**aneurysmectomy** (**an**-you-riz-**MECK**-toh-mee)**:** the surgical removal of an aneurysm.

**aneurysmorrhaphy** (**an**-you-riz-**MOR**-ah-fee)**:** surgical suturing of an aneurysm.

**angina** (an-**JIGH**-nah)**:** episodes of severe chest pain due to inadequate blood flow to the myocardium.

**angiogenesis** (**an**-jee-oh-**JEN**-eh-sis)**:** the process through which the tumor supports its growth by creating its own blood supply.

**angiogram** (**AN**-jee-oh-**gram**)**:** the film produced by angiography.

**angiography** (**an**-jee-**OG**-rah-fee)**:** a radiographic study of the blood vessels after the injection of a contrast medium.

**angioplasty** (**AN**-jee-oh-**plas**-tee)**:** mechanically widening a narrowed or obstructed blood vessel.

**angiostenosis** (**an**-jee-oh-steh-**NOH**-sis)**:** abnormal narrowing of a blood vessel.

**anhidrosis** (**an**-high-**DROH**-sis)**:** the abnormal condition of lacking sweat in response to heat.

**anisocoria** (**an**-ih-so-**KOH**-ree-ah)**:** a condition in which the pupils are unequal in size.

**ankylosing spondylitis** (**ang**-kih-**LOH**-sing **spon**-dih-**LYE**-tis)**:** a form of rheumatoid arthritis that primarily causes inflammation of the joints between the vertebrae.

**ankylosis** (**ang**-kih-**LOH**-sis)**:** the loss or absence of mobility in a joint due to disease, injury, or a surgical procedure.

**anomaly** (ah-**NOM**-ah-lee)**:** a deviation from what is regarded as normal.

**anorexia** (**an**-oh-**RECK**-see-ah)**:** the loss of appetite for food, especially when caused by disease.

**anorexia nervosa** (**an**-oh-**RECK**-see-ah ner-**VOH**-sah)**:** an eating disorder characterized by a false perception of body appearance that leads to a refusal to maintain a normal body weight.

**anoscopy** (ah-**NOS**-koh-pee)**:** the visual examination of the anal canal and lower rectum.

**anovulation** (**an**-ov-you-**LAY**-shun)**:** the absence of ovulation when it would normally be expected.

**anoxia** (ah-**NOCK**-see-ah)**:** the absence of oxygen from the body's tissues or organs despite adequate flow of blood.

**antacids:** medications to relieve indigestion or help peptic ulcers heal by neutralizing stomach acids.

**anthracosis** (**an**-thrah-**KOH**-sis)**:** the form of pneumoconiosis caused by coal dust in the lungs.

**anthrax** (**an**-thraks)**:** a contagious disease that can be transmitted through livestock.

**antiangiogenesis:** cancer treatment that disrupts the blood supply to the tumor.

**antiarrhythmic** (**an**-tih-ah-**RITH**-mick)**:** medication administered to control irregularities of the heartbeat.

**antibiotic-resistant bacteria:** develops when an antibiotic fails to kill all of the bacteria it targets. When this occurs, the surviving bacteria become resistant to that particular drug.

**antibiotics:** medications capable of inhibiting growth or killing pathogenic bacteria.

**antibody** (**AN**-tih-**bod**-ee)**:** a disease-fighting protein created by the immune system in response to the presence of a specific antigen.

**anticoagulant** (**an**-tih-koh-**AG**-you-lant)**:** medication that slows coagulation and prevents new clots from forming.

**anticonvulsant** (**an**-tih-kon-**VUL**-sant)**:** medication that prevents seizures.

**antidepressant:** medications administered to prevent or relieve depression.

**antiemetic** (**an**-tih-ee-**MET**-ick)**:** medication administered to prevent or relieve nausea and vomiting.

**antifungal** (an-tih-**FUNG**-gul): an agent that destroys or inhibits the growth of fungi.

**antigen** (**AN**-tih-jen): any substance that the body regards as being foreign.

**antihistamines:** medications administered to block and control allergic reactions.

**antihypertensive** (**an**-tih-**high**-per-**TEN**-siv): medication administered to lower blood pressure.

**anti-inflammatory:** medication administered to relieve inflammation and pain.

**antineoplastic** (**an**-tih-nee-oh-**PLAS**-tick): medication that blocks the development, growth, or proliferation of malignant cells.

**antipsychotic drug** (**an**-tih-sigh-**KOT**-ick): administered to treat symptoms of severe disorders of thinking and mood that are associated with neurological and psychiatric illnesses.

**antipyretic** (**an**-tih-pye-**RET**-ick): medication administered to prevent or reduce fever.

**antispasmodic:** medication administered to suppress smooth muscle contractions.

**antithyroid drug:** a medication administered to slow the ability of the thyroid gland to produce thyroid hormones.

**antitussive** (**an**-tih-**TUSS**-iv): medication administered to prevent or relieve coughing.

**antiviral drug** (**an**-tih-**VYE**-ral): medication administered to treat viral infections or to provide temporary immunity.

**anuria** (ah-**NEW**-ree-ah): the absence of urine formation by the kidneys.

**anxiety disorders:** mental conditions characterized by excessive, irrational dread of everyday situations, or fear that is out of proportion to the real danger in a situation.

**anxiolytic drug** (**ang**-zee-oh-**LIT**-ick): medication administered to temporarily relieve anxiety and reduce tension.

**Apgar score:** an evaluation of a newborn infant's physical status.

**aphasia** (ah-**FAY**-zee-ah): loss of the ability to speak, write, and/or comprehend the written or spoken word.

**aphonia** (ah-**FOH**-nee-ah): the loss of the ability of the larynx to produce normal speech sounds.

**aphthous ulcers** (**AF**-thus **UL**-serz): gray-white pits with a red border in the soft tissues lining the mouth.

**aplasia** (ah-**PLAY**-zee-ah): the defective development or congenital absence of an organ or tissue.

**aplastic anemia** (ay-**PLAS**-tick ah-**NEE**-mee-ah): a condition marked by the absence of all formed blood elements.

**apnea** (**AP**-nee-ah *or* ap-**NEE**-ah): the absence of spontaneous respiration.

**appendectomy** (ap-en-**DECK**-toh-mee): surgical removal of the appendix.

**appendicitis** (ah-**pen**-dih-**SIGH**-tis): inflammation of the appendix.

**arrhythmia** (ah-**RITH**-mee-ah): a loss of the normal rhythm of the heartbeat.

**arterial blood gas analysis:** a test to measure the pH, oxygen, and carbon dioxide levels of arterial blood.

**arterial stick:** the puncture of an artery to obtain arterial blood.

**arteriectomy** (ar-teh-ree-**ECK**-toh-mee): surgical removal of part of an artery.

**arteriomalacia** (ar-**tee**-ree-oh-mah-**LAY**-shee-ah): abnormal softening of the walls of an artery or arteries.

**arterionecrosis** (ar-**tee**-ree-oh-neh-**KROH**-sis): tissue death of an artery or arteries.

**arteriosclerosis** (ar-**tee**-ree-oh-skleh-**ROH**-sis): abnormal hardening of the walls of an artery or arteries.

**arteriostenosis** (ar-**tee**-ree-oh-steh-**NOH**-sis): abnormal narrowing of an artery or arteries.

**arteriovenous malformation** (ar-**tee**-ree-oh-**VEE**-nus): an abnormal connection between the arteries and veins in the brain; may cause a hemorrhagic stroke.

**arthralgia** (ar-**THRAL**-jee-ah): pain in one or more joints.

**arthritis** (ar-**THRIGH**-tis): an inflammatory condition of one or more joints.

**arthrocentesis** (ar-throh-sen-**TEE**-sis): surgical puncture of the joint space to remove synovial fluid for analysis.

**arthrodesis** (ar-throh-**DEE**-sis): a surgical procedure to stiffen a joint.

**arthrolysis** (ar-**THROL**-ih-sis): surgical loosening of an ankylosed joint.

**arthroplasty** (**AR**-throh-**plas**-tee): surgical repair of a damaged joint; also the surgical replacement of a joint with an artificial joint.

**arthrosclerosis** (**ar**-throh-skleh-**ROH**-sis): stiffness of the joints, especially in the elderly.

**arthroscopic surgery** (ar-throh-**SKOP**-ick): a minimally invasive procedure for the treatment of the interior of a joint.

**arthroscopy** (ar-**THROS**-koh-pee): visual examination of the internal structure of a joint using an arthroscope.

**artificial insemination:** a technique in which sperm from a woman's partner or donor are introduced into the vagina or uterus during the ovulatory phase of her menstrual cycle.

**artificial pacemaker:** electronic device used primarily as treatment for bradycardia or atrial fibrillation.

**asbestosis** (**ass**-beh-**STOH**-sis): the form of pneumoconiosis caused by asbestos particles in the lungs.

**ascites** (ah-**SIGH**-teez): an abnormal accumulation of serous fluid in the peritoneal cavity.

**asphyxia** (ass-**FICK**-see-ah): the loss of consciousness that occurs when the body cannot get the oxygen it needs to function.

**aspiration pneumonia** (**ass**-pih-**RAY**-shun): pneumonia caused by a foreign substance, such as vomit, being inhaled into the lungs.

**aspirin:** medication that may be recommended in a very small daily dose to reduce the risk of a heart attack or stroke by slightly reducing the ability of the blood to clot.

**assisted reproductive technology:** techniques used to aid an infertile couple in achieving a viable pregnancy.

**assistive listening device:** a device that transmits, processes, or amplifies sound, and can be used with or without a hearing aid.

**asthma** (**AZ**-mah): a chronic inflammatory disease of the bronchial tubes.

**astigmatism** (ah-**STIG**-mah-tizm): a condition in which the eye does not focus properly because of uneven curvatures of the cornea.

**asystole** (ay-**SIS**-toh-lee): complete lack of electrical activity in the heart.

**ataxia** (ah-**TACK**-see-ah): the lack of muscle coordination during voluntary movement.

**atelectasis** (at-ee-**LEK**-tah-sis): incomplete expansion of part or all of the lung.

**atherectomy** (**ath**-er-**ECK**-toh-mee): surgical removal of plaque buildup from the interior lining of an artery.

**atheroma** (**ath**-er-**OH**-mah): a deposit of fatty plaque on or within the arterial wall.

**atherosclerosis** (**ath**-er-**oh**-skleh-**ROH**-sis): hardening and narrowing of the arteries due to a buildup of cholesterol plaque.

**atonic** (ah-**TON**-ick): lacking normal muscle tone or strength.

**atresia** (at-**TREE**-zee-ah): describes the congenital absence of a normal opening or the failure of a structure to be tubular.

**atrial fibrillation:** rapid irregular twitching of the muscular wall of the atria.

**atrophy** (**AT**-roh-fee): weakness or wearing away of body tissues and structures caused by pathology or by disuse over a long period of time.

**attention-deficit/hyperactivity disorder** (ADHD): a condition characterized by a short attention span and impulsive behavior inappropriate for the child's developmental age.

**audiological evaluation:** the measurement of the ability to hear and understand speech sounds based on their pitch and loudness.

**audiometry** (**aw**-dee-**OM**-eh-tree): the use of an audiometer to measure hearing acuity.

**auscultation** (**aws**-kul-**TAY**-shun): listening for sounds within the body, usually done with a stethoscope.

**autism** (**AW**-tizm): a subgroup of autistic spectrum disorders.

**autistic spectrum disorders** (aw-**TIS**-tic): a group of conditions in which a young child has difficulty developing normal social relationships and communication skills, may compulsively follow repetitive routines, and has narrowly focused, intense interests.

**autoimmune disorder** (**aw**-toh-ih-**MYOUN**): a condition in which the immune system produces antibodies against the body's own tissues.

**autologous bone marrow transplant** (aw-**TOL**-uh-guss): a transplant utilizing the patient's own bone marrow that was harvested before treatment began.

**automated external defibrillator** (dee-**fib**-rih-**LAY**-ter): electronic equipment that externally shocks the heart to restore a normal cardiac rhythm.

**automated implantable cardioverter defibrillator** (**KAR**-dee-oh-ver-ter dee-**fib**-rih-**LAY**-ter): a double-action pacemaker that regulates the heartbeat and acts as an automatic defibrillator.

**autopsy** (**AW**-top-see): postmortem (after death) examination.

**Ayurvedic medicine** (**ay**-uhr-**VEH**-dick): traditional Hindu system of medicine.

**azoospermia** (ay-**zoh**-oh-**SPER**-mee-ah): the absence of sperm in the semen.

# B

**bacilli** (bah-**SILL**-eye): rod-shaped spore-forming bacteria.

**bacteria** (back-**TEER**-ree-ah): one-celled microscopic organisms.

**bacterial endocarditis:** inflammation of the lining or valves of the heart caused by bacteria in the bloodstream.

**bacterial pneumonia:** pneumonia caused by *Streptococcus pneumoniae*.

**bacterial vaginosis** (vaj-ih-**NOH**-sis)**:** a condition in women in which there is an abnormal overgrowth of certain bacteria in the vagina.

**bactericide** (back-**TEER**-ih-sighd)**:** a substance that causes the death of bacteria.

**bacteriuria** (back-**tee**-ree-**YOU**-ree-ah)**:** the presence of bacteria in the urine.

**balanitis** (bal-ah-**NIGH**-tis)**:** inflammation of the glans penis.

**barbiturates** (bar-**BIT**-you-raytz)**:** a class of drugs whose major action is a calming or depressed effect on the central nervous system.

**bariatric surgery:** performed to treat morbid obesity by restricting the amount of food that can enter the stomach and be digested.

**bariatrics** (bayr-ee-**AT**-ricks)**:** the branch of medicine for the prevention and control of obesity and associated diseases.

**barium:** a radiopaque contrast medium used primarily to visualize the gastrointestinal tract.

**barotrauma** (bar-oh-**TRAW**-mah)**:** pressure-related ear condition.

**Barrett's esophagus:** a condition that occurs when the cells in the epithelial tissue of the esophagus are damaged by chronic acid exposure.

**basal cell carcinoma:** a malignant tumor of the basal cell layer of the epidermis.

**behavioral therapy:** therapy that focuses on changing behavior by identifying problem behaviors, replacing them with appropriate behaviors, and using rewards or other consequences to make the changes.

**Bell's palsy:** temporary paralysis of the seventh cranial nerve that causes paralysis only on the affected side of the face.

**benign:** something that is not life-threatening and does not recur.

**benign prostatic hyperplasia** (high-per-**PLAY**-zee-ah)**:** abnormal enlargement of the prostate gland often found in men over 50.

**beta-blockers:** medications administered to reduce the workload of the heart by slowing the heartbeat.

**binaural testing** (bye-**NAW**-rul *or* bin-**AW**-rahl)**:** involves both ears.

**biofeedback:** treatment that teaches a person to control bodily functions through cognitive control techniques to decrease stress.

**bioimpedance spectroscopy** (**BYE**-oh-im-**pee**-dens)**:** a noninvasive method of diagnosing lymphedema by measuring the limb's resistance to an electrical current.

**biopsy** (**BYE**-op-see)**:** the removal of a small piece of living tissue for examination to confirm or establish a diagnosis.

**BiPAP machine:** noninvasive ventilation device like a CPAP machine; however, it can be set at a higher pressure for inhaling and a lower pressure for exhaling.

**bipolar disorder:** a mental condition characterized by cycles of severe mood changes shifting from highs and severe lows.

**bladder retraining:** behavioral training in which the patient learns to urinate on a schedule with increasingly longer time intervals between scheduled urination.

**bladder ultrasound:** the use of a handheld ultrasound transducer to measure the amount of urine remaining in the bladder after urination.

**blepharoplasty** (**BLEF**-ah-roh-**plas**-tee)**:** surgical reduction of the upper and lower eyelids.

**blindness:** the inability to see.

**blood dyscrasia** (dis-**KRAY**-zee-ah)**:** any pathologic condition of the cellular elements of the blood.

**bloodborne transmission:** the spread of a disease through contact with blood or other body fluids that are contaminated with blood.

**blood urea nitrogen** (you-**REE**-ah)**:** a blood test performed to determine the amount of urea present in the blood.

**body mass index** (BMI)**:** a number that shows body weight adjusted for height.

**bolus** (**BOH**-lus)**:** a single dose of a drug usually injected into a blood vessel over a short period of time.

**bone density testing:** a diagnostic test to determine losses or changes in bone density.

**bone marrow biopsy:** a diagnostic test to determine why blood cells are abnormal or to find a donor match for a bone marrow transplant.

**bone marrow transplant:** cancer treatment in which abnormal bone marrow is destroyed and replaced with new stem cells.

**bone scan:** a specialized nuclear scan that identifies new areas of bone growth or breakdown.

**borborygmus** (bor-boh-**RIG**-mus)**:** the rumbling noise caused by the movement of gas in the intestine.

**Botox:** a formulation of botulinum toxin that is administered by injection to temporarily improve the appearance of frown lines between the eyebrows.

**bowel incontinence** (in-**KON**-tih-nents)**:** the inability to control the excretion of feces.

**brachytherapy** (**brack**-ee-**THER**-ah-pee): the use of radioactive materials in contact with or implanted into the tissues to be treated.

**bradycardia** (**brad**-ee-**KAR**-dee-ah): an abnormally slow resting heart rate, usually at a rate of less than 60 beats per minute.

**bradykinesia** (**brad**-ee-kih-**NEE**-zee-ah): extreme slowness in movement.

**bradypnea** (**brad**-ihp-**NEE**-ah): an abnormally slow rate of respiration, usually of less than 10 breaths per minute.

**brain tumor:** an abnormal growth within the skull.

**brand name:** medication sold under the name given the drug by the manufacturer.

**Braxton Hicks contractions:** intermittent painless uterine contractions that are not true labor pains.

**breast augmentation:** mammoplasty performed to increase breast size.

**breast cancer:** a carcinoma that develops from the cells of the breast and can spread to adjacent lymph nodes and other body sites.

**breast reduction:** mammoplasty performed to decrease and reshape excessively large, heavy breasts.

**breast self-examination:** a self-care procedure for the early detection of breast cancer.

**breech presentation:** a birth complication in which the buttocks or feet of the fetus are positioned to enter the birth canal first instead of the head.

**bronchiectasis** (**brong**-kee-**ECK**-tah-sis): permanent dilation of the bronchi caused by chronic infection and inflammation.

**bronchodilator** (**brong**-koh-dye-**LAY**-tor): a medication that relaxes and expands the bronchial passages into the lungs.

**bronchopneumonia** (**brong**-koh-new-**MOH**-nee-ah): a localized form of pneumonia often affects the bronchioles.

**bronchorrhea** (**brong**-koh-**REE**-ah): an excessive discharge of mucus from the bronchi.

**bronchoscopy** (brong-**KOS**-koh-pee): the visual examination of the bronchi using a bronchoscope.

**bronchospasm** (**brong**-koh-spazm): a contraction of the smooth muscle in the walls of the bronchi and bronchioles that tighten and squeeze the airway shut.

**bruit** (**BREW**-ee): an abnormal sound or murmur heard during auscultation of an artery.

**bruxism** (**BRUCK**-sizm): involuntary grinding or clenching of the teeth that usually occurs during sleep.

**bulimia nervosa** (byou-**LIM**-ee-ah *or* boo-**LEE**-meeah): an eating disorder characterized by frequent episodes of binge eating followed by compensatory behaviors, such as self-induced vomiting.

**bulla** (**BULL**-ah): a large blister that is usually more than 0.5 cm in diameter.

**burn:** an injury to body tissues caused by heat, flame, electricity, sun, chemicals, or radiation.

**burn, first-degree:** a burn in which there are no blisters and only superficial damage to the epidermis.

**burn, second-degree:** a burn in which there are blisters and damage to both the epidermis and the dermis.

**burn, third-degree:** a burn in which there is damage to the epidermis, dermis, subcutaneous layers, and possibly also the muscle below.

**bursitis** (ber-**SIGH**-tis): inflammation of a bursa.

# C

**cachexia** (kah-**KEKS**-eeh-ah): physical wasting away due to the loss of weight and muscle mass that occurs in patients with diseases such as advanced cancer or AIDS.

**calcium channel blocker agents:** medications that cause the heart and blood vessels to relax by decreasing the movement of calcium into the cells of these structures.

**calciuria** (kal-sih-**YOU**-ree-ah): the presence of calcium in the urine.

**callus** (**KAL**-us): a bulging deposit that forms around the area of the break in a bone; also a thickening of the skin that is caused by repeated rubbing.

**cancer:** a class of diseases characterized by the uncontrolled division of cells and the ability of these cells to invade other tissues.

**candidiasis** (**kan**-dih-**DYE**-ah-sis): a yeast infection.

**capillary hemangioma** (**KAP**-uh-**ler**-ee hee-**man**-jee-**OH**-mah): a soft, raised, pink, or red vascular birthmark.

**capillary puncture:** technique used to obtain a small amount of blood for a blood test.

**capsule endoscopy:** a tiny video camera in a capsule that the patient swallows that transmits images of the walls of the small intestine.

**carbuncle** (**KAR**-bung-kul): a cluster of connected furuncles (boils).

**carcinoma** (**kar**-sih-**NOH**-mah): a malignant tumor that occurs in epithelial tissue.

**carcinoma in situ:** a malignant tumor in its original position that has not yet disturbed or invaded the surrounding tissues.

**cardiac arrest:** an event in which the heart abruptly stops beating or develops an arrhythmia that prevents it from pumping blood.

**cardiac catheterization** (**KAR**-dee-ack **kath**-eh-ter-eye-**ZAY**-shun): a diagnostic procedure in which a catheter is passed into a vein or artery and guided into the heart.

**cardiocentesis** (**kar**-dee-oh-sen-**TEE**-sis): the puncture of a chamber of the heart for diagnosis or therapy.

**cardiomegaly** (**kar**-dee-oh-**MEG**-ah-lee): abnormal enlargement of the heart.

**cardiomyopathy** (**kar**-dee-oh-my-**OP**-pah-thee): all diseases of the heart muscle.

**cardioplegia** (**kar**-dee-oh-**PLEE**-jee-ah): paralysis of the heart muscle.

**cardiopulmonary resuscitation:** an emergency procedure for life support consisting of artificial respiration and manual external cardiac compression.

**carditis** (kar-**DYE**-tis): an inflammation of the heart.

**carotid endarterectomy** (**end**-ar-ter-**ECK**-toh-mee): surgical removal of the lining of a portion of a clogged carotid artery.

**carotid ultrasonography:** an ultrasound study of the carotid artery that is performed to predict or diagnose an ischemic stroke.

**carpal tunnel release:** the surgical enlargement of the carpal tunnel or cutting of the carpal ligament to relieve pressure on nerves and tendons.

**carpal tunnel syndrome:** swelling that creates pressure on the median nerve as it passes through the carpal tunnel.

**castration** (kas-**TRAY**-shun): surgical removal or destruction of both testicles.

**cataract** (**KAT**-ah-rakt): the loss of transparency of the lens of the eye.

**catatonic behavior** (kat-ah-**TON**-ick): marked by a lack of responsiveness, stupor, and a tendency to remain in a fixed posture.

**causalgia** (kaw-**ZAL**-jee-ah): persistent, severe, burning pain that usually follows an injury to a sensory nerve.

**cauterization** (**kaw**-ter-eye-**ZAY**-zhun): the destruction of tissue by burning.

**celiac disease** (**SEE**-lee-ak): an inherited autoimmune disorder characterized by a severe reaction to foods containing gluten.

**cellulitis** (sell-you-**LYE**-tis): an acute, rapidly spreading bacterial infection within the connective tissues of the skin.

**centesis** (sen-**TEE**-sis): a surgical puncture to remove fluid for diagnostic purposes or to remove excess fluid.

**cephalalgia** (**sef**-ah-**LAL**-jee-ah): pain in the head.

**cephalic presentation:** when the baby is born head first.

**cerebral contusion** (**SER**-eh-bral kon-**TOO**-zhun): bruising of brain tissue as the result of a head injury that causes the brain to bounce against the skull.

**cerebral palsy** (**SER**-eh-bral *or* seh-**REE**-bral **PAWL**-zee): a condition characterized by poor muscle control, spasticity, and other neurologic deficiencies.

**cerebrovascular accident** (**ser**-eh-broh-**VAS**-kyou-lar): damage to the brain that occurs when the blood flow to the brain is disrupted.

**cervical cancer:** cancer that develops in the cervix.

**cervical dysplasia** (**SER**-vih-kal dis-**PLAY**-see-ah): the presence of precancerous changes in the cells that make up the inner lining of the cervix.

**cervical radiculopathy** (rah-**dick**-you-**LOP**-ah-thee): nerve pain caused by pressure on the spinal nerve roots in the neck region.

**cervicitis** (**ser**-vih-**SIGH**-tis): inflammation of the cervix.

**cesarean section** (seh-**ZEHR**-ee-un **SECK**-shun): the delivery of the child through an incision in the maternal abdominal and uterine walls.

**chalazion** (kah-**LAY**-zee-on): a nodule or cyst, usually on the upper eyelid caused by obstruction of a sebaceous gland.

**cheilosis** (kee-**LOH**-sis): a disorder of the lips characterized by crack-like sores at the corners of the mouth.

**chemabrasion** (keem-ah-**BRAY**-shun): the use of chemicals to remove the outer layers of skin.

**chemoprevention:** the use of natural or synthetic substances such as drugs or vitamins to reduce the risk of developing cancer or to reduce the chance that cancer will occur.

**chemotherapy:** the use of chemical agents and drugs in combinations selected to destroy malignant cells and tissues.

**chest x-ray:** a valuable tool for diagnosing pneumonia, lung cancer, pneumothorax, pleural effusion, tuberculosis, and emphysema.

**Cheyne-Stokes respiration** (**CHAYN**-**STOHKS**): an irregular pattern of breathing characterized by alternating rapid or shallow respiration followed by slow respiration or apnea.

**chiropractic manipulative therapy:** a system of mechanical spinal adjustments made by a chiropractor to correct biomechanical problems in the skeleton.

**chlamydia** (klah-**MID**-ee-ah): a sexually transmitted disease caused by the bacteria *Chlamydia trachomatis.*

**chloasma** (kloh-**AZ**-mah): a pigmentation disorder characterized by brownish spots on the face.

**cholangiography** (koh-**LAN**-jee-**og**-rah-fee)**:** a radiographic examination of the bile ducts with the use of a contrast medium.

**cholangitis** (**koh**-lan-**JIGH**-tis)**:** an acute inflammation of the bile duct characterized by pain in the upper-right quadrant of the abdomen, fever, and jaundice.

**cholecystectomy** (**koh**-luh-sis-**TECK**-toh-mee)**:** the surgical removal of the gallbladder.

**cholecystitis** (**koh**-luh-sis-**TYE**-tis)**:** inflammation of the gallbladder that is usually associated with gallstones.

**choledocholithotomy** (koh-**led**-oh-koh-lih-**THOT**-oh-mee)**:** an incision in the common bile duct for the removal of gallstones.

**cholelithiasis** (**koh**-lee-luh-**THIGH**-ah-sis)**:** the presence of gallstones in the gallbladder or bile ducts.

**cholesteatoma** (**koh**-**les**-tee-ah-**TOH**-mah)**:** destructive epidermal cyst in the middle ear made up of epithelial cells and cholesterol.

**cholesterol** (koh-**LES**-ter-ol)**:** a fatty substance that travels through the blood and is found in all parts of the body.

**cholesterol-lowering drugs:** medications, such as statins, that are administered to reduce the undesirable cholesterol levels in the blood.

**chondroma** (kon-**DROH**-mah)**:** a slow-growing benign tumor derived from cartilage cells.

**chondromalacia** (**kon**-droh-mah-**LAY**-shee-ah)**:** abnormal softening of the cartilage.

**chondroplasty** (**KON**-droh-**plas**-tee)**:** surgical repair of damaged cartilage.

**chorionic villus sampling** (kor-ee-**ON**-ick **VIL**-us)**:** examination of cells retrieved from the chorionic villi between the 8th and 10th weeks of pregnancy.

**chronic bronchitis:** a disease in which the airways have become inflamed due to recurrent exposure to an inhaled irritant.

**chronic fatigue syndrome:** a disorder of unknown cause that affects many body systems, with symptoms similar to those of fibromyalgia syndrome.

**chronic kidney disease:** the progressive loss of renal function over months or years.

**chronic obstructive pulmonary disease:** a group of lung diseases in which the bronchial airflow is obstructed, making it hard to breathe.

**chronic venous insufficiency:** a condition in which venous circulation is inadequate due to partial vein blockage or leakage of venous valves.

**cicatrix** (sick-**AY**-tricks)**:** a normal scar resulting from the healing of a wound.

**cineradiography** (**sin**-eh-**ray**-dee-**OG**-rah-fee)**:** the recording of fluoroscopy images.

**circumcision** (**ser**-kum-**SIZH**-un)**:** surgical removal of the foreskin of the penis.

**cirrhosis** (sih-**ROH**-sis)**:** a chronic degenerative disease of the liver characterized by scarring.

**claustrophobia** (**klaws**-troh-**FOH**-bee-ah)**:** abnormal fear of being in small or enclosed spaces.

**cleft lip:** a birth defect resulting in a deep groove of the lip running upward to the nose.

**cleft palate:** failure of the palate to close during the early development of the fetus that involves the upper lip, hard palate, and/or soft palate.

**clinical trials:** testing new treatments that have not yet received FDA approval on patients who agree to be part of the research.

**closed-angle glaucoma:** a type of glaucoma in which the opening between the cornea and iris narrows so that fluid cannot reach the trabecular meshwork.

**closed fracture:** a fracture in which the bone is broken but there is no open wound in the skin.

**closed reduction:** the attempted realignment of the bone involved in a fracture or joint dislocation.

**clostridium difficile** (klos-**TRID**-ee-um dif-us-**SEEL**)**:** a bacterial infection common to older adults in hospitals or long-term care facilities.

**clubbing:** abnormal curving of the nails that is often accompanied by enlargement of the fingertips.

**cluster headaches:** intensely painful headaches that affect one side of the head and often occur in groups or clusters.

**cochlear implant** (**KOCK**-lee-ar)**:** an electronic device that bypasses the damaged portions of the ear and directly stimulates the auditory nerve.

**cognition** (kog-**NISH**-un)**:** the mental activities associated with thinking, learning, and memory.

**cognitive therapy:** treatment that focuses on changing cognitions or thoughts that are affecting a person's emotions and actions.

**colectomy** (koh-**LECK**-toh-mee)**:** surgical removal of all or part of the colon.

**collagen replacement therapy:** a form of soft-tissue augmentation used to soften facial lines or scars, or to make lips appear fuller.

**Colles' fracture:** a fracture at the lower end of the radius that occurs when a person tries to break a fall by landing on his or her hands.

**colonoscopy** (**koh**-lun-**OSS**-koh-pee)**:** direct visual examination of the inner surface of the colon from the rectum to the cecum.

**colorectal carcinoma:** a common form of cancer that often first manifests itself in polyps in the colon.

**colostomy** (koh-**LAHS**-toh-mee): the surgical creation of an artificial excretory opening between the colon and the body surface.

**colotomy** (koh-**LOT**-oh-mee): a surgical incision into the colon.

**colpopexy** (**KOL**-poh-**peck**-see): surgical fixation of the vagina to a surrounding structure.

**colporrhaphy** (kol-**POR**-ah-fee): surgical suturing of a tear in the vagina.

**colporrhexis** (**kol**-poh-**RECK**-sis): tearing or laceration of the vaginal walls.

**colposcopy** (kol-**POS**-koh-pee): direct visual examination of the tissues of the cervix and vagina.

**coma** (**KOH**-mah): a deep state of unconsciousness marked by the absence of spontaneous eye movements, no response to painful stimuli, and no vocalization.

**comedo** (**KOM**-eh-doh): a noninfected lesion formed by the buildup of sebum and keratin in a hair follicle.

**comminuted fracture** (**KOM**-ih-**newt**-ed): a fracture in which the bone is splintered or crushed.

**communicable disease** (kuh-**MEW**-nih-kuh-bul): any condition that is transmitted from one person to another by either direct or indirect contact with contaminated objects.

**community-acquired pneumonia:** a type of pneumonia that results from contagious infection outside of a hospital or clinic.

**compartment syndrome:** the compression of nerves and blood vessels due to swelling within the enclosed space created by the fascia that separates groups of muscles.

**complementary medicine:** practices and systems of health care used to supplement allopathic medicine.

**complete blood cell count:** a series of blood tests performed as a group to evaluate several blood conditions.

**compression fracture:** a fracture in which the bone is pressed together on itself.

**computed tomography** (toh-**MOG**-rah-fee): an imaging technique that uses a thin, fan-shaped x-ray beam to produce multiple cross-sectional views of the body.

**concussion** (kon-**KUSH**-un): a violent shaking up or jarring of the brain.

**conductive hearing loss:** a hearing loss in which sound waves are prevented from passing from the air to the fluid-filled inner ear.

**congenital disorder** (kon-**JEN**-ih-tahl): an abnormal condition that exists at the time of birth.

**congenital heart defects:** structural abnormalities caused by the failure of the heart to develop normally before birth.

**conization** (**kon**-ih-**ZAY**-shun *or* **koh**-nih-**ZAY**-shun): surgical removal of a cone-shaped section of tissue from the cervix.

**conjunctivitis** (kon-**junk**-tih-**VYE**-tis): inflammation of the conjunctiva, usually caused by an infection or allergy.

**Conn's syndrome** (**KONS**): a disorder of the adrenal glands caused by the excessive production of aldosterone.

**conscious:** the state of being awake, alert, aware, and responding appropriately.

**constipation:** having a bowel movement fewer than three times per week.

**contact dermatitis:** a localized allergic response caused by contact with an irritant or allergen.

**contraceptive:** a measure taken or a device used to lessen the likelihood of pregnancy.

**contracture** (kon-**TRACK**-chur): the permanent tightening of fascia, muscles, tendons, ligaments, or skin that occurs when normally elastic connective tissues are replaced with nonelastic fibrous tissues.

**contraindication:** a factor in the patient's condition that makes the use of a medication or specific treatment dangerous or ill advised.

**contrast medium:** a substance used to make visible structures that are otherwise hard to see.

**contusion** (kon-**TOO**-zhun): an injury to underlying tissues without breaking the skin, characterized by discoloration and pain.

**conversion disorder:** a condition characterized by a serious temporary or ongoing change in function, such as paralysis or blindness, triggered by psychological factors rather than any physical cause.

**corneal abrasion:** an injury, such as a scratch or irritation, to the outer layers of the cornea.

**corneal transplant:** the surgical replacement of a scarred or diseased cornea with clear corneal tissue from a donor.

**corneal ulcer:** a pitting of the cornea caused by an infection or injury.

**coronary artery bypass graft:** a surgical procedure in which a piece of vein from the leg is implanted on the heart to replace a blocked coronary artery.

**coronary artery disease:** atherosclerosis of the coronary arteries that reduces the blood supply to the heart muscle.

**coronary thrombosis** (**KOR**-uh-**nerr**-ee throm-**BOH**-sis)**:** damage to the heart muscle caused by a thrombus blocking a coronary artery.

**corticosteroid drug:** steroid hormones produced by the adrenal cortex, and their synthetically produced equivalents.

**cortisone** (**KOR**-tih-sohn)**:** the synthetic equivalent of natural corticosteroids that are administered to suppress inflammation and to act as an immunosuppressant.

**costochondritis** (**kos**-toh-kon-**DRIGH**-tis)**:** an inflammation of the cartilage that connects a rib to the sternum.

**Coumadin:** the brand name for *warfarin*, an anticoagulant administered to prevent blood clots from forming or growing larger.

**cover test:** an exam of how the two eyes work together, used to assess binocular vision.

**CPAP machine (continuous positive airway pressure):** a noninvasive ventilation device used in the treatment of sleep apnea.

**cramp:** a painful localized muscle spasm.

**cranial hematoma** (**hee**-mah-**TOH**-mah)**:** a collection of blood trapped in the tissues of the brain.

**craniectomy** (**kray**-nee-**EK**-toh-mee)**:** surgical removal of a portion of the skull.

**cranioplasty** (**KRAY**-nee-oh-**plas**-tee)**:** surgical repair of the skull.

**craniosacral therapy** (**kray**-nee-oh-**SAK**-ral)**:** the use of gentle touch to help the body release tension in order to correct restrictions resulting from stress on the CNS.

**craniostenosis** (**kray**-nee-oh-steh-**NOH**-sis)**:** a malformation of the skull due to the premature closure of the cranial sutures.

**craniotomy** (**kray**-nee-**OT**-oh-mee)**:** a surgical incision or opening into the skull.

**C-reactive protein:** a blood test that detects high levels of inflammation within the body.

**creatinuria** (**kree**-at-ih-**NEW**-ree-ah)**:** an increased concentration of creatinine in the urine.

**crepitation** (**krep**-ih-**TAY**-shun)**:** the grating sound heard when the ends of a broken bone move together.

**cretinism** (**CREE**-tin-izm)**:** a congenital form of hypothyroidism.

**Crohn's disease:** a chronic autoimmune disorder that can occur anywhere in the digestive tract; however, it is most often found in the ileum and in the colon.

**crossmatch tests:** tests performed to determine the compatibility of blood donor and recipient before a transfusion.

**croup** (**KROOP**)**:** an acute respiratory infection in children and infants characterized by obstruction of the larynx, hoarseness, and swelling around the vocal cords resulting in a barking cough and stridor.

**crust:** a collection of dried serum and cellular debris.

**cryosurgery:** the destruction or elimination of abnormal tissue cells through the application of extreme cold by using liquid nitrogen.

**cryptorchidism** (krip-**TOR**-kih-dizm)**:** a developmental defect in which one or both testicles fail to descend into the scrotum.

**curettage** (**kyou**-reh-**TAHZH**)**:** the removal of material from the surface by scraping.

**Cushing's syndrome** (**KUSH**-ingz **SIN**-drohm)**:** a condition caused by prolonged exposure to high levels of cortisol.

**cyanosis** (**sigh**-ah-**NOH**-sis)**:** bluish discoloration of the skin and mucous membranes caused by a lack of adequate oxygen in the blood.

**cyst:** an abnormal sac containing fluid, gas, or a semisolid material.

**cystalgia** (sis-**TAL**-jee-ah)**:** pain in the urinary bladder.

**cystectomy** (sis-**TECK**-toh-mee)**:** the surgical removal of all or part of the urinary bladder.

**cystic fibrosis** (**SIS**-tick figh-**BROH**-sis)**:** a life-threatening genetic disorder in which the lungs and pancreas are clogged with large quantities of abnormally thick mucus.

**cystitis** (sis-**TYE**-tis)**:** inflammation of the bladder.

**cystocele** (**SIS**-toh-seel)**:** a hernia of the bladder through the vaginal wall.

**cystography** (sis-**TOG**-rah-fee)**:** a radiographic examination of the bladder after instillation of a contrast medium via a urethral catheter.

**cystolith** (**SIS**-toh-lith)**:** a stone located within the urinary bladder.

**cystopexy** (**SIS**-toh-**peck**-see)**:** the surgical fixation of the bladder to the abdominal wall.

**cystorrhaphy** (sis-**TOR**-ah-fee)**:** surgical suturing of a wound or defect in the bladder.

**cystoscopy** (sis-**TOS**-koh-pee)**:** the visual examination of the urinary bladder using a cystoscope.

**cytomegalovirus** (**sigh**-toh-**meg**-ah-loh-**VYE**-rus)**:** a type of herpesvirus found in most body fluids.

**cytotoxic drug** (**sigh**-toh-**TOK**-sick)**:** medication that kills or damages cells.

# D

**dacryoadenitis** (**dack**-ree-oh-ad-eh-**NIGH**-tis)**:** an inflammation of the lacrimal gland that can be caused by a bacterial, viral, or fungal infection.

**deafness:** the complete or partial loss of the ability to hear.

**debridement** (dah-**BREED**-ment)**:** the removal of dirt, foreign objects, damaged tissue, and cellular debris from a wound to prevent infection and to promote healing.

**decibel:** commonly used as the measurement of the loudness of sound.

**deep brain stimulation:** a neurosurgical procedure used in the treatment of dystonia, tremors, and Parkinson's disease.

**deep tendon reflexes:** testing of reflexes to diagnose disruptions of the nerve supply to the involved muscles.

**deep vein thrombosis:** the condition of having a thrombus attached to the interior wall of a deep vein.

**defibrillation** (dee-**fib**-rih-**LAY**-shun)**:** the use of electrical shock to restore the heart's normal rhythm.

**dehydration:** a condition in which fluid loss exceeds fluid intake and disrupts the body's normal electrolyte balance.

**delirium** (deh-**LEER**-ee-um)**:** an acute condition of confusion, disorientation, disordered thinking and memory, agitation, and hallucinations.

**delirium tremens** (deh-**LEER**-ee-um **TREE**-mens)**:** a disorder involving sudden and severe mental changes or seizures caused by abruptly stopping the use of alcohol.

**delusion** (dih-**LOO**-zhun)**:** a false personal belief that is maintained despite obvious proof or evidence to the contrary.

**dementia** (dih-**MEN**-shee-ah)**:** a slowly progressive decline in mental abilities including memory, thinking, and judgment that is often accompanied by personality changes.

**dental calculus** (**KAL**-kyou-luhs)**:** hardened dental plaque on the teeth.

**dental caries** (**KAYR**-eez)**:** an infectious disease that destroys the enamel and dentin of the tooth.

**dental plaque** (**PLACK**)**:** a soft deposit consisting of bacteria and bacterial by-products that builds up on the teeth.

**dental prophylaxis** (**proh**-fih-**LACK**-sis)**:** the professional cleaning of the teeth to remove plaque and calculus.

**depression:** a common mood disorder characterized by lethargy and sadness, as well as a loss of interest or pleasure in normal activities.

**dermabrasion** (der-mah-**BRAY**-zhun)**:** a form of abrasion involving the use of a revolving wire brush or sandpaper.

**dermatitis** (**der**-mah-**TYE**-tis)**:** inflammation of the skin.

**dermatoplasty** (**DER**-mah-toh-**plas**-tee)**:** the replacement of damaged skin with healthy tissue taken from a donor site on the patient's body.

**dermatosis** (**der**-mah-**TOH**-sis)**:** a general term used to denote skin lesions or eruptions of any type that are not associated with inflammation.

**developmental disorder:** disorder that can result in an anomaly or malformation such as the absence of a limb or the presence of an extra toe.

**diabetes insipidus** (**dye**-ah-**BEE**-teez in-**SIP**-ih-dus)**:** a condition caused by insufficient production of the antidiuretic hormone or by the inability of the kidneys to respond to this hormone.

**diabetes mellitus** (**dye**-ah-**BEE**-teez **MEL**-ih-tus)**:** a group of metabolic disorders characterized by hyperglycemia resulting from defects in insulin secretion, insulin action, or both.

**diabetic coma:** a diabetic emergency caused by very high blood sugar.

**diabetic retinopathy** (**ret**-ih-**NOP**-ah-thee)**:** damage to the retina as a complication of uncontrolled diabetes.

**dialysis** (dye-**AL**-ih-sis)**:** a procedure to remove waste products from the blood of patients whose kidneys no longer function.

**diaphragmatic breathing:** a relaxation technique used to relieve anxiety.

**diarrhea** (**dye**-ah-**REE**-ah)**:** the abnormally frequent flow of loose or watery stools.

**digital rectal examination:** a manual examination performed on men to palpate the prostate gland to detect prostate enlargement and look for indicators of prostate cancer.

**digital subtraction angiography:** a diagnostic technique that combines angiography with computerized components to clarify the view of the area of interest by removing soft tissue and bone from the images.

**digitalis** (**dij**-ih-**TAL**-is)**:** medication that strengthens the heart muscle contractions, slows the heart rate, and helps eliminate fluid from body tissues.

**dilation and curettage** (dye-**LAY**-shun and **kyou**-reh-**TAHZH**)**:** a surgical procedure in which the cervix is dilated and the endometrium of the uterus is scraped away.

**diphtheria** (dif-**THEE**-ree-ah): an acute bacterial infection of the throat and upper respiratory tract.

**diplopia** (dih-**PLOH**-pee-ah): the perception of two images of a single object.

**dislocation:** the total displacement of a bone from its joint.

**dissociative disorders:** conditions that occur when normal thought is separated from consciousness.

**dissociative identity disorder:** a mental illness characterized by the presence of two or more distinct personalities, each with its own characteristics, which appear to exist within the same individual.

**diuresis** (dye-you-**REE**-sis): the increased output of urine.

**diuretics** (dye-you-**RET**-icks): medications administered to increase urine secretion to rid the body of excess salt and water.

**diverticulectomy** (dye-ver-**tick**-you-**LECK**-toh-mee): surgical removal of a diverticulum.

**diverticulitis** (dye-ver-tick-you-**LYE**-tis): inflammation or infection of one or more diverticula in the wall of the colon.

**diverticulosis** (dye-ver-**tick**-you-**LOH**-sis): the chronic presence of an abnormal number of diverticula in the wall of the colon.

**diverticulum** (dye-ver-**TICK**-you-lum): a small pouch or sac occurring in the lining or wall of a tubular organ.

**Doppler echocardiogram:** an ultrasonic diagnostic procedure that measures the speed and direction of the blood flow within the heart.

**dorsal recumbent position:** position where the patient is lying on the back, face up, with the knees bent.

**Down syndrome:** a genetic variation that is associated with characteristic facial appearance, learning disabilities, and physical abnormalities such as heart valve disease.

**drug abuse:** the excessive use of illegal drugs or the misuse of prescription drugs.

**drug interaction:** the result of drugs reacting with each other, often in ways that are unexpected or potentially harmful.

**drug overdose:** the accidental or intentional use of an illegal drug or prescription medicine in an amount higher than what is safe or normal.

**drug-screening urine test:** a rapid method of identifying the presence in the body of one or more drugs of abuse.

**dual x-ray absorptiometry** (ab-**sorp**-shee-**OM**-eh-tree): a low-exposure radiographic measurement of the spine and hips to measure bone density.

**ductal carcinoma in situ:** breast cancer at its earliest stage before the cancer has broken through the wall of the milk duct.

**duplex ultrasound:** a diagnostic procedure to image the structures of the blood vessels and the flow of blood through these vessels.

**dysentery** (**DIS**-en-**ter**-ee): a bacterial infection spread through food or water contaminated by human feces.

**dysfunctional uterine bleeding:** a condition characterized by abnormal bleeding.

**dyskinesia** (**dis**-kih-**NEE**-zee-ah): distortion or impairment of voluntary movement.

**dyslexia** (dis-**LECK**-see-ah): a learning disability characterized by substandard reading achievement due to the inability of the brain to process symbols.

**dysmenorrhea** (**dis**-men-oh-**REE**-ah): pain caused by uterine cramps during a menstrual period.

**dyspareunia** (**dis**-pah-**ROO**-nee-ah): pain during sexual intercourse.

**dyspepsia** (dis-**PEP**-see-ah): pain or discomfort in digestion.

**dysphagia** (dis-**FAY**-jee-ah): difficulty in swallowing.

**dysphonia** (dis-**FOH**-nee-ah): difficulty in speaking, which may include any impairment in vocal quality.

**dysplasia** (dis-**PLAY**-see-ah): abnormal development or growth of cells, tissues, or organs.

**dysplastic nevi** (dis-**PLAS**-tick **NEE**-vye): atypical moles that can develop into skin cancer.

**dyspnea** (**DISP**-nee-ah): difficult or labored breathing.

**dysthymia** (dis-**THIGH**-mee-ah): a low-grade chronic depression present on a majority of days for more than two years.

**dystonia** (dis-**TOH**-nee-ah): a condition of abnormal muscle tone.

**dysuria** (dis-**YOU**-ree-ah): difficult or painful urination.

# E

**ear tubes:** tiny ventilating tubes placed through the eardrum to provide ongoing drainage for fluids and to relieve pressure that can build up after childhood ear infections.

**ecchymosis** (eck-ih-**MOH**-sis): a large, irregular area of purplish discoloration due to bleeding under the skin.

**echocardiography** (eck-oh-**kar**-dee-**OG**-rah-fee): an ultrasonic diagnostic procedure used to evaluate the structures and motion of the heart.

**echoencephalography** (eck-oh-en-**sef**-ah-**LOG**-rah-fee): the use of ultrasound imaging to create a detailed visual image of the brain for diagnostic purposes.

**eclampsia** (eh-**KLAMP**-see-ah)**:** during pregnancy, a more serious form of preeclampsia characterized by convulsions and sometimes coma.

**E. coli:** infection caused by the bacteria *Escherichia coli*, transmitted through improperly cooked, contaminated foods.

**ectopic pregnancy** (eck-**TOP**-ick)**:** the condition in which a fertilized egg is implanted and begins to develop outside of the uterus.

**ectropion** (eck-**TROH**-pee-on)**:** the eversion of the edge of an eyelid.

**eczema** (**ECK**-zeh-mah)**:** a form of recurring dermatitis characterized by itching, redness, and dryness.

**edema** (eh-**DEE**-mah)**:** swelling caused by an abnormal accumulation of fluid in cells, tissues, or cavities of the body.

**electrocardiogram** (ee-**leck**-troh-**KAR**-dee-oh-**gram**)**:** a record of the electrical activity of the myocardium.

**electrocardiography** (ee-**leck**-troh-kar-dee-**OG**-rah-fee)**:** the noninvasive process of recording the electrical activity of the myocardium.

**electroconvulsive therapy** (ee-**leck**-troh-kon-**VUL**-siv)**:** a procedure in which small amounts of electric current is passed through the brain, deliberately triggering a brief seizure in order to reverse symptoms of certain mental illnesses.

**electrodessication** (ee-**leck**-troh-des-ih-**KAY**-shun)**:** a surgical technique in which tissue is destroyed using an electric spark.

**electroencephalography** (ee-**leck**-troh-en-**sef**-ah-**LOG**-rah-fee)**:** the process of recording the electrical activity of the brain through the use of electrodes attached to the scalp.

**electrolysis:** the use of electric current to destroy hair follicles for the removal of undesired hair.

**electromyography** (ee-**leck**-troh-my-**OG**-rah-fee)**:** a diagnostic test that measures the electrical activity within muscle fibers in response to nerve stimulation.

**ELISA:** the acronym for enzyme-linked immunosorbent assay, a blood test that is used to screen for the presence of HIV antibodies.

**embolism** (**EM**-boh-lizm)**:** the sudden blockage of a blood vessel by an embolus.

**embolus** (**EM**-boh-lus)**:** a foreign object, such as a blood clot, quantity of air or gas, or a bit of tissue or tumor, that is circulating in the blood.

**emesis** (**EM**-eh-sis)**:** the reflex ejection of the stomach contents outward through the mouth.

**emphysema** (em-fih-**SEE**-mah)**:** the progressive, long-term loss of lung function, usually due to smoking.

**empyema** (**em**-pye-**EE**-mah)**:** an accumulation of pus in a body cavity.

**encephalitis** (en-sef-ah-**LYE**-tis)**:** inflammation of the brain.

**encephalocele** (en-**SEF**-ah-loh-**seel**)**:** a congenital herniation of brain substance through a gap in the skull.

**endemic** (en-**DEM**-ick)**:** refers to the ongoing presence of a disease within a population, group, or area.

**endocarditis** (**en**-doh-kar-**DYE**-tis)**:** inflammation of the inner lining of the heart.

**endocervicitis** (**en**-doh-**ser**-vih-**SIGH**-tis)**:** inflammation of the mucous membrane lining of the cervix.

**endometrial biopsy:** a diagnostic test in which a small amount of the tissue lining the uterus is removed for microscopic examination.

**endometrial cancer** (**en**-doh-**MEE**-tree-al)**:** a cancerous growth that begins in the lining of the uterus.

**endometriosis** (**en**-doh-**mee**-tree-**OH**-sis)**:** a condition in which patches of endometrial tissue escape the uterus and become attached to other structures in the pelvic cavity.

**endoscope** (**EN**-doh-**skope**)**:** a small, flexible tube with a light and lens on the end.

**endoscopic surgery:** a surgical procedure performed through very small incisions with the use of an endoscope and specialized instruments.

**endoscopy** (en-**DOS**-koh-pee)**:** the visual examination of the interior of a body cavity or organ.

**endotracheal intubation** (**en**-doh-**TRAY**-kee-al **in**-too-**BAY**-shun)**:** the passage of a tube through the mouth into the trachea to establish or maintain an open airway.

**endovaginal ultrasound** (**en**-doh-**VAJ**-ih-nal)**:** a diagnostic test utilizing ultrasound to image the uterus and fallopian tubes to determine the cause of abnormal vaginal bleeding.

**end-stage renal disease:** the final stage of chronic kidney disease.

**enema:** the placement of a solution into the rectum and colon to empty the lower intestine through bowel activity.

**enteritis** (**en**-ter-**EYE**-tis)**:** inflammation of the small intestine caused by eating or drinking substances contaminated with viral or bacterial pathogens.

**entropion** (en-**TROH**-pee-on)**:** the inversion of the edge of an eyelid.

**enucleation** (ee-**new**-klee-**AY**-shun)**:** the removal of the eyeball, leaving the eye muscles intact.

**enuresis** (en-you-**REE**-sis)**:** the involuntary discharge of urine.

**epicondylitis** (ep-ih-**kon**-dih-**LYE**-tis): inflammation of the tissues surrounding the elbow.

**epidemic** (ep-ih-**DEM**-ick): a sudden and widespread outbreak of a disease within a specific population group or area.

**epididymitis** (ep-ih-did-ih-**MY**-tis): inflammation of the epididymis.

**epidural anesthesia** (ep-ih-**DOO**-ral **an**-es-**THEE**-zee-ah): regional anesthesia produced by injecting medication into the epidural space of the lumbar or sacral region of the spine.

**epilepsy** (**EP**-ih-**lep**-see): a chronic neurologic condition characterized by recurrent episodes of seizures of varying severity.

**episiorrhaphy** (eh-**piz**-ee-**OR**-ah-fee): surgical suturing to repair an episiotomy.

**episiotomy** (eh-**piz**-ee-**OT**-oh-mee): a surgical incision made into the perineum to enlarge the vaginal orifice to prevent tearing of the tissues as the infant moves out of the birth canal.

**epispadias** (ep-ih-**SPAY**-dee-as): a congenital abnormality of the urethral opening. In the male this opening is located on the upper surface of the penis; in the female the urethral opening is in the region of the clitoris.

**epistaxis** (ep-ih-**STACK**-sis): bleeding from the nose.

**erectile dysfunction**: the inability of the male to achieve or maintain a penile erection.

**ergonomics** (er-goh-**NOM**-icks): the study of the human factors that affect the design and operation of tools and the work environment.

**erosion** (eh-**ROH**-zhun): the wearing away of a surface.

**eructation** (eh-ruk-**TAY**-shun): the act of belching or raising gas orally from the stomach.

**erythema** (er-ih-**THEE**-mah): redness of the skin due to capillary dilation.

**erythrocyte sedimentation rate** (eh-**RITH**-roh-site): a blood test based on the speed with which the red blood cells separate from the plasma and settle to the bottom of a specialized test tube.

**erythroderma** (eh-**rith**-roh-**DER**-mah): abnormal redness of the entire skin surface.

**esophageal varices** (eh-**sof**-ah-**JEE**-al **VAYR**-ih-seez): enlarged and swollen veins at the lower end of the esophagus.

**esophagogastroduodenoscopy** (eh-**sof**-ah-goh-**gas**-troh-**dew**-oh-deh-**NOS**-koh-pee): the endoscopic examination of the upper GI tract.

**esotropia** (es-oh-**TROH**-pee-ah): strabismus characterized by an inward deviation of one or both eyes.

**etiology** (ee-tee-**OL**-oh-jee): the study of the causes of diseases.

**eupnea** (youp-**NEE**-ah): easy or normal breathing.

**exanthem** (eck-**ZAN**-thum): a widespread rash, usually in children.

**exfoliative cytology** (ecks-**FOH**-lee-**ay**-tiv sigh-**TOL**-oh-jee): a biopsy technique in which cells are scraped from the tissue and examined under a microscope.

**exfoliative dermatitis** (ecks-**FOH**-lee-**ay**-tiv **DER**-mah-**TYE**-tis): a condition in which there is widespread scaling of the skin.

**exophthalmos** (eck-sof-**THAL**-mos): an abnormal protrusion of the eyeball out of the orbit.

**exotropia** (eck-soh-**TROH**-pee-ah): strabismus characterized by the outward deviation of one eye relative to the other.

**expectoration** (eck-**SPEK**-toh-**ray**-shun): the act of coughing up and spitting out saliva, mucus, or other body fluid.

**external fixation**: a fracture treatment procedure in which pins are placed through the soft tissues and bone so that an external appliance can be used to hold the pieces of bone firmly in place during healing.

**extracorporeal shockwave lithotripsy**: the destruction of kidney stones using high-energy ultrasonic waves traveling through water or gel.

**extraoral radiography**: dental radiograph where the film is placed and exposed outside of the mouth.

**exudate** (**ECKS**-you-dayt): fluid, such as pus, that leaks out of an infected wound.

# F

**factitious disorder** (fack-**TISH**-us): a condition in which a person acts as if he or she has a physical or mental illness when he or she is not really sick.

**factitious disorder by proxy**: a form of child abuse in which the mentally ill parent will falsify an illness in a child by making up or inducing symptoms and then seeking medical treatment, even surgery, for the child.

**fasciitis** (fas-ee-**EYE**-tis): inflammation of a fascia.

**fascioplasty** (**FASH**-ee-oh-**plas**-tee): surgical repair of a fascia.

**fasciotomy** (fash-ee-**OT**-oh-mee): a surgical incision through a fascia to relieve tension or pressure.

**fasting blood sugar**: a blood test to measure the glucose levels after the patient has not eaten for 8 to 12 hours.

**fat embolus** (**EM**-boh-lus): the release of fat cells from yellow bone marrow into the bloodstream when a long bone is fractured.

**female pattern baldness:** a condition in which the hair thins in the front and on the sides of the scalp and sometimes on the crown.

**fenestration** (fen-es-**TRAY**-shun)**:** a surgical procedure in which a new opening is created in the labyrinth to restore lost hearing.

**fetal alcohol syndrome:** condition characterized by growth abnormalities, mental retardation, brain damage, and socialization difficulties, caused by the mother's consumption of alcohol during pregnancy.

**fetal monitoring:** the use of an electronic device to record the fetal heart rate and the maternal uterine contractions during labor.

**fetal ultrasound:** a noninvasive procedure used to image and evaluate fetal development during pregnancy.

**fever:** a body temperature of 100° F or higher.

**fibrillation** (fih-brih-**LAY**-shun)**:** a rapid and uncontrolled heart beat.

**fibroadenoma** (figh-broh-**ad**-eh-**NOH**-mah)**:** round, rubbery, firm mass that arises from excess growth of glandular and connective tissue in the breast.

**fibrocystic breast disease** (figh-broh-**SIS**-tick)**:** the presence of single or multiple benign cysts in the breasts.

**fibromyalgia syndrome** (figh-broh-my-**AL**-jee-ah)**:** a debilitating chronic condition characterized by fatigue, muscle, joint, or bone pain, and a wide range of other symptoms.

**fibrous dysplasia** (dis-**PLAY**-see-ah)**:** a bone disorder of unknown cause that destroys normal bone structure and replaces it with fibrous (scar-like) tissue.

**first trimester screening:** performed between 11 and 13 weeks of pregnancy and involves an ultrasound and a finger-stick blood test.

**fissure** (**FISH**-ur)**:** a groove or crack-like sore of the skin; also normal folds in the contours of the brain.

**fistula** (**FIS**-tyou-lah)**:** an abnormal passage between two internal organs or leading from an organ to the surface of the body.

**flatulence** (**FLAT**-you-lens)**:** passage of gas out of the body through the rectum.

**floaters:** particles of cellular debris that float in the vitreous fluid and cast shadows on the retina.

**fluorescein angiography** (**flew**-oh-**RES**-ee-in **an**-jee-**OG**-rah-fee)**:** a radiographic study of the blood vessels in the retina of the eye following the intravenous injection of a fluorescein dye as a contrast medium.

**fluorescein staining** (**flew**-oh-**RES**-ee-in)**:** the application of a fluorescent dye to the surface of the eye via eye drops or a strip applicator.

**fluoroscopy** (floo-or-**OS**-koh-pee)**:** the visualization of body parts in motion by projecting x-ray images on a luminous fluorescent screen.

**Foley catheter:** the most common type of indwelling catheter.

**folliculitis** (foh-**lick**-you-**LYE**-tis)**:** inflammation of the hair follicles.

**food-borne and waterborne transmission:** caused by eating or drinking contaminated food or water that has not been properly treated to remove contamination or kill pathogens that are present.

**fracture:** a broken bone.

**fructosamine test** (fruck-**TOHS**-ah-meen)**:** a blood test that measures average glucose levels over the past three weeks.

**functional disorder:** a condition that produces symptoms for which no physiological or anatomical cause can be identified.

**functional endoscopic sinus surgery:** a surgical procedure performed using an endoscope in which chronic sinusitis is treated by enlarging the opening between the nose and sinus.

**functional MRI:** detects changes in blood flow in the brain when the patient is asked to perform a specific task.

**fungus** (**FUNG**-gus)**:** a simple parasitic organism.

**furuncles** (**FYOU**-rung-kulz)**:** large, tender, swollen areas caused by a staphylococcal infection around hair follicles or sebaceous glands.

# G

**galactorrhea** (gah-**lack**-toh-**REE**-ah)**:** the production of breast milk in women who are not breast feeding.

**gallstone:** a hard deposit that forms in the gallbladder and bile ducts.

**Gamma knife surgery:** a type of radiation treatment for brain tumors.

**ganglion cyst:** a harmless fluid-filled swelling that occurs most commonly on the outer surface of the wrist.

**gangrene** (**GANG**-green)**:** tissue death caused by a loss of circulation to the affected tissues.

**gastralgia** (gas-**TRAL**-jee-ah)**:** pain in the stomach.

**gastrectomy** (gas-**TRECK**-toh-mee)**:** surgical removal of all or a part of the stomach.

**gastritis** (gas-**TRY**-tis)**:** inflammation of the stomach lining.

**gastroduodenostomy** (gas-troh-**dew**-oh-deh-**NOS**-toh-mee)**:** the establishment of an anastomosis between the upper portion of the stomach and the duodenum.

**gastrodynia** (**gas**-troh-**DIN**-ee-ah)**:** pain in the stomach.

**gastroenteritis** (**gas**-troh-en-ter-**EYE**-tis)**:** inflammation of the mucous membrane lining the stomach and intestines.

**gastroesophageal reflux disease** (gas-troh-eh-**sof**-ah-**JEE**-al **REE**-flucks)**:** the upward flow of acid from the stomach into the esophagus.

**gastrorrhea** (**gas**-troh-**REE**-ah)**:** the excessive secretion of gastric juice or mucus in the stomach.

**gastrosis** (gas-**TROH**-sis)**:** any disease of the stomach.

**gastrostomy tube** (gas-**TROS**-toh-mee)**:** a surgically placed feeding tube from the exterior of the body directly into the stomach.

**generalized anxiety disorder:** a mental condition characterized by chronic, excessive worrying.

**generic drug:** medication named for its chemical structure that is not protected by a brand name or trademark.

**genetic disorder:** a pathological condition caused by an absent or defective gene.

**genital herpes** (**HER**-peez)**:** a sexually transmitted disease caused by the herpes simplex virus type 1 or 2.

**genital warts:** a sexually transmitted disease caused by the human papillomavirus.

**gestational diabetes mellitus** (jes-**TAY**-shun-al **dye**-ah-**BEE**-teez mel-**EYE**-tus *or* **MEL**-ih-tus)**:** the form of diabetes that occurs during some pregnancies.

**gigantism** (jigh-**GAN**-tiz-em)**:** abnormal growth of the entire body caused by excessive secretion of the growth hormone before puberty.

**gingivectomy** (**jin**-jih-**VECK**-toh-mee)**:** surgical removal of diseased gingival tissue.

**gingivitis** (**jin**-jih-**VYE**-tis)**:** inflammation of the gums; the earliest stage of periodontal disease.

**glaucoma** (glaw-**KOH**-mah)**:** a group of diseases characterized by increased intraocular pressure that causes damage to the optic nerve and retinal nerve fibers.

**glomerulonephritis** (gloh-**mer**-you-loh-neh-**FRY**-tis)**:** a type of nephritis caused by inflammation of the glomeruli.

**glycosuria** (**glye**-koh-**SOO**-ree-ah)**:** the presence of glucose in the urine.

**goiter** (**GOI**-ter)**:** an abnormal, nonmalignant enlargement of the thyroid gland.

**gonorrhea** (**gon**-oh-**REE**-ah)**:** a highly contagious sexually transmitted disease caused by the bacterium *Neisseria gonorrhoeae.*

**gouty arthritis** (**GOW**-tee ar-**THRIGH**-tis)**:** a type of arthritis characterized by deposits of uric acid in the joints.

**granulation tissue:** the tissue that normally forms during the healing of a wound that will become the scar tissue.

**granuloma** (**gran**-you-**LOH**-mah)**:** a general term used to describe a small, knot-like swelling of granulation tissue in the epidermis.

**Graves' disease** (**GRAYVZ** dih-**ZEEZ**)**:** an autoimmune disorder in which the immune system stimulates the thyroid to make excessive amounts of thyroid hormone.

**greenstick fracture:** a type of fracture in which the bone is bent and only partially broken.

**guided imagery:** a type of treatment in which a patient follows verbal prompts to envision a peaceful location and distance himself from current pain or stress.

**Guillain-Barré syndrome** (gee-**YAHN**-bah-**RAY**)**:** inflammation of the myelin sheath of peripheral nerves, characterized by rapidly worsening muscle weakness that may lead to temporary paralysis.

**gynecomastia** (**guy**-neh-koh-**MAS**-tee-ah)**:** the condition of excessive mammary development in the male.

# H

**halitosis** (hal-ih-**TOH**-sis)**:** an unpleasant odor coming from the mouth.

**hallucination** (hah-**loo**-sih-**NAY**-shun)**:** a sensory perception experienced in the absence of an external stimulation.

**hallux valgus** (**HAL**-ucks **VAL**-guss)**:** an abnormal enlargement of the joint at the base of the great toe.

**hamstring injury:** a strain or tear on any of the three hamstring muscles that straighten the hip and bend the knee.

**Hashimoto's disease** (hah-shee-**MOH**-tohz)**:** an autoimmune disorder in which the body's own antibodies attack and destroy the cells of the thyroid gland.

**hearing aid:** an electronic device that is worn to correct a hearing loss.

**heart failure:** a chronic condition in which the heart is unable to pump out all of the blood it receives.

**heart murmur:** an abnormal blowing or clicking sound heard when listening to the heart or neighboring large blood vessels.

**heel spurs:** a calcium deposit in the plantar fascia near its attachment to the heel.

**hemangioma** (hee-**man**-jee-**OH**-mah)**:** a benign tumor made up of newly formed blood vessels.

**hemarthrosis** (hem-ar-**THROH**-sis)**:** blood within a joint.

**hematemesis** (**hee**-mah-**TEM**-eh-sis): the vomiting of blood.

**hematochezia** (**hee**-**mat**-oh-**KEE**-zee-uh): the flow of bright red blood in the stool.

**hematocrit** (**hee**-**MAT**-oh-krit) (**Hct** or **HCT**): a blood test that measures the percentage by volume of red blood cells in a whole blood sample.

**hematoma** (**hee**-mah-**TOH**-mah): a swelling of clotted blood trapped in the tissues.

**hematospermia** (**hee**-moh-**SPER**-mee-ah): the presence of blood in the seminal fluid.

**hematuria** (**hee**-mah-**TOO**-ree-ah): the presence of blood in the urine.

**hemianopia** (**hem**-ee-ah-**NOH**-pee-ah): blindness in one half of the visual field.

**hemiparesis** (**hem**-ee-pah-**REE**-sis): slight paralysis or weakness affecting only one side of the body.

**hemiplegia** (**hem**-ee-**PLEE**-jee-ah): total paralysis affecting only one side of the body.

**Hemoccult test** (**HEE**-moh-kult): a laboratory test for hidden blood in the stools.

**hemochromatosis** (**hee**-moh-**kroh**-mah-**TOH**-sis): a genetic disorder in which the intestines absorb too much iron.

**hemodialysis** (**hee**-moh-dye-**AL**-ih-sis): a process by which waste products are filtered directly from the patient's blood.

**hemoglobin A1c testing** (HbA1c): a blood test that measures the average blood glucose level over the previous three to four months.

**hemolytic anemia** (**hee**-moh-**LIT**-ick ah-**NEE**-meeah): condition characterized by an inadequate number of circulating red blood cells due to their premature destruction by the spleen.

**hemophilia** (**hee**-moh-**FILL**-ee-ah): a group of hereditary bleeding disorders in which a blood-clotting factor is missing.

**hemoptysis** (**hee**-**MOP**-tih-sis): expectoration of blood or bloodstained sputum.

**hemorrhage** (**HEM**-or-idj): the loss of a large amount of blood in a short time.

**hemorrhagic stroke** (**hem**-oh-**RAJ**-ick): damage to the brain that occurs when a blood vessel in the brain leaks.

**hemorrhoidectomy** (**hem**-oh-roid-**ECK**-toh-mee): the surgical removal of hemorrhoids.

**hemorrhoids** (**HEM**-oh-roids): a condition that occurs when a cluster of enlarged veins, muscles, and tissues slip near or through the anal opening.

**hemostasis** (**hee**-moh-**STAY**-sis): to stop or control bleeding.

**hemothorax** (**hee**-moh-**THOH**-racks): a collection of blood in the pleural cavity.

**hepatectomy** (**hep**-ah-**TECK**-toh-mee): the surgical removal of all or part of the liver.

**hepatitis** (**hep**-ah-**TYE**-tis): inflammation of the liver.

**hepatomegaly** (**hep**-ah-toh-**MEG**-ah-lee): abnormal enlargement of the liver.

**hernia** (**HER**-nee-ah): the protrusion of a part or structure through the tissues normally containing it.

**herniated disk** (**HER**-nee-**ayt**-ed): the breaking apart of a intervertebral disk that results in pressure on spinal nerve roots.

**herpes labialis** (**HER**-peez **lay**-bee-**AL**-iss): blister-like sores on the lips caused by HSV-1.

**herpes zoster** (**HER**-peez **ZOS**-ter): an acute viral infection characterized by painful skin eruptions that follow the underlying route of an inflamed nerve.

**Hertz** (Hz): a measure of sound frequency that determines how high or low a pitch is.

**hiatal hernia** (high-**AY**-tal **HER**-nee-ah): the protrusion of part of the stomach through an opening in the diaphragm.

**high-density lipoprotein cholesterol:** the form of cholesterol that does not contribute to plaque buildup.

**hip resurfacing:** an alternative to total hip replacement, a metal cap is placed over the head of the femur to allow it to move smoothly over a metal lining in the acetabulum.

**hirsutism** (**HER**-soot-izm): excessive bodily and facial hair in women, usually occurring in a male pattern.

**Hodgkin's lymphoma** (**HODJ**-kinz lim-**FOH**-mah): a malignancy of the lymphatic system that is distinguished from non-Hodgkin's lymphoma by the presence of *Reed-Sternberg cells.*

**holistic** (**hoe**-**LISS**-tick): a treatment approach that takes into consideration the whole body and its environment, including the mind, body, and spirit.

**Holter monitor:** a portable electrocardiograph worn by an ambulatory patient to continuously monitor the heart rates and rhythms over a 24- or 48-hour period.

**home blood glucose monitoring:** test performed by the patient using a drop of blood to measure the current blood sugar level.

**homeopathy** (**hoh**-mee-**OP**-ah-thee): the belief that the body can stimulate its own healing responses when the right substance is given in minute doses.

**homeostasis (hoh**-mee-oh-**STAY**-sis): the processes through which the body maintains a constant internal environment.

**hordeolum (hor**-**DEE**-oh-lum): a pus-filled lesion on the eyelid resulting from an infection in a sebaceous gland.

**horizontal recumbent position:** lying on the back with the *face up.*

**hormone replacement therapy:** the use of the female hormones estrogen and progestin to replace those the body no longer produces during and after perimenopause.

**hospital-acquired pneumonia:** a type of pneumonia contracted during a stay in the hospital when a patient's defenses are impaired.

**human growth hormone:** a synthetic version of the growth hormone that is administered to stimulate growth when the natural supply of growth hormone is insufficient for normal development.

**human immunodeficiency virus:** a bloodborne pathogen that damages or kills the T cells of the immune system, causing it to progressively fail.

**human papillomavirus:** a virus that causes genital warts and cervical cancer.

**Huntington's disease:** a genetic disorder that causes nerve degeneration with symptoms that most often appear in midlife.

**hydrocele (HIGH**-droh-seel): a fluid-filled sac in the scrotum along the spermatic cord leading from the testicles.

**hydrocephalus** (high-droh-**SEF**-ah-lus): a condition in which excess cerebrospinal fluid accumulates within the ventricles of the brain.

**hydronephrosis (high**-droh-neh-**FROH**-sis): the dilation of one or both kidneys.

**hydroureter (high**-droh-**YOUR**-eh-ter): the distention of the ureter with urine that cannot flow because the ureter is blocked.

**hyperbaric oxygen therapy (high**-per-**BARE**-ik): use of inhaled oxygen in a special chamber with increased air pressure to promote healing and fight infection.

**hypercalcemia (high**-per-kal-**SEE**-mee-ah): abnormally high concentrations of calcium circulating in the blood.

**hypercapnia (high**-per-**KAP**-nee-ah): the abnormal buildup of carbon dioxide in the blood.

**hyperemesis (high**-per-**EM**-eh-sis): extreme, persistent vomiting that can cause dehydration.

**hyperesthesia (high**-per-es-**THEE**-zee-ah): a condition of abnormal and excessive sensitivity to touch, pain, or other sensory stimuli.

**hyperglycemia (high**-per-glye-**SEE**-mee-ah): an abnormally high concentration of glucose in the blood.

**hypergonadism (high**-per-**GOH**-nad-izm): the excessive secretion of hormones by the sex glands.

**hyperhidrosis (high**-per-high-**DROH**-sis): a condition of excessive sweating in one area or over the whole body.

**hyperinsulinism (high**-per-**IN**-suh-lin-izm): a condition marked by excessive secretion of insulin.

**hyperkinesia (high**-per-kye-**NEE**-zee-ah): abnormally increased muscle function or activity.

**hyperlipidemia (high**-per-**lip**-ih-**DEE**-mee-ah): the general term used to describe elevated levels of cholesterol and other fatty substances in the blood.

**hypermenorrhea (high**-poh-men-oh-**REE**-ah): an excessive amount of menstrual flow over a period of more than seven days.

**hyperopia (high**-per-**OH**-pee-ah): a vision defect in which light rays focus beyond the retina; also known as farsightedness.

**hyperparathyroidism (high**-per-**par**-ah-**THIGH**-roid-izm): the overproduction of the parathyroid hormone that causes hypercalcemia.

**hyperpituitarism (high**-per-pih-**TOO**-ih-tah-rizm): the excess secretion of growth hormone that causes acromegaly and gigantism.

**hyperplasia (high**-per-**PLAY**-zee-ah): the enlargement of an organ or tissue because of an abnormal increase in the number of cells.

**hyperpnea (high**-perp-**NEE**-ah): breathing that is deeper and more rapid than is normal at rest.

**hyperproteinuria (high**-per-**proh**-tee-in-**YOU**-ree-ah): the presence of abnormally high concentrations of protein in the urine.

**hypertension:** the elevation of arterial blood pressure to a level that is likely to cause damage to the cardiovascular system.

**hyperthermia (high**-per-**THER**-mee-ah): an extremely high fever.

**hyperthyroidism (high**-per-**THIGH**-roid-izm): the overproduction of thyroid hormones.

**hypertrophy** (high-**PER**-troh-fee): a general increase in the bulk of a body part or organ due to an increase in the size, but not in the number, of cells in the tissues.

**hyperventilation (high**-per-ven-tih-**LAY**-shun): an abnormally rapid rate of deep respiration that is usually associated with anxiety.

**hypnosis:** a type of therapy in which a patient is placed in a susceptible state and then given suggestions directed toward their treatment goal.

**hypnotherapy:** the use of hypnosis to produce an altered state of focused attention in which the patient may be more willing to believe and act on suggestions.

**hypnotic:** medication that depresses the central nervous system and usually produces sleep.

**hypocalcemia** (**high**-poh-kal-**SEE**-mee-ah): a condition characterized by abnormally low levels of calcium in the blood.

**hypochondriasis** (**high**-poh-kon-**DRY**-ah-sis): a condition characterized by fearing that one has a serious illness despite appropriate medical evaluation and reassurance.

**hypoglycemia** (**high**-poh-glye-**SEE**-mee-ah): an abnormally low concentration of glucose in the blood.

**hypogonadism** (**high**-poh-**GOH**-nad-izm): the condition of deficient secretion of hormones by the sex glands.

**hypomenorrhea** (**high**-poh-men-oh-**REE**-ah): an unusually small amount of menstrual flow during a shortened regular menstrual period.

**hypoparathyroidism** (**high**-poh-**par**-ah-**THIGH**-roidizm): a condition caused by an insufficient or absent secretion of parathyroid hormone.

**hypoperfusion** (**high**-poh-per-**FYOU**-zhun): a deficiency of blood passing through an organ or body part.

**hypophysectomy** (high-**pof**-ih-**SECK**-toh-mee): the removal of abnormal tissue from the pituitary gland.

**hypoplasia** (**high**-poh-**PLAY**-zee-ah): the incomplete development of an organ or tissue.

**hypopnea** (**high**-poh-**NEE**-ah): shallow or slow respiration.

**hypoproteinemia** (**high**-poh-**proh**-tee-in-**EE**-mee-ah): the presence of abnormally low concentrations of protein in the blood.

**hypospadias** (**high**-poh-**SPAY**-dee-as): the congenital abnormality of the urethral opening. In the male the urethral opening is on the underside of the penis; in the female the urethra opens into the vagina.

**hypotension** (**high**-poh-**TEN**-shun): lower than normal arterial blood pressure.

**hypothermia** (**high**-poh-**THER**-mee-ah): an abnormally low body temperature.

**hypothyroidism** (**high**-poh-**THIGH**-roid-izm): a deficiency of thyroid secretion.

**hypotonia** (**high**-poh-**TOH**-nee-ah): a condition in which there is diminished tone of the skeletal muscles.

**hypoxemia** (**high**-pock-**SEE**-mee-ah): a condition of having low oxygen levels in the blood.

**hypoxia** (high-**POCK**-see-ah): the condition of having deficient oxygen levels in the body tissues and organs; less severe than anoxia.

**hysterectomy** (**hiss**-teh-**RECK**-toh-mee): the surgical removal of the uterus.

**hysterosalpingography** (**hiss**-ter-oh-**sal**-pin-**GOG**-rah-fee): a radiographic examination of the uterus and fallopian tubes.

**hysteroscopy** (**hiss**-ter-**OSS**-koh-pee): the direct visual examination of the interior of the uterus and fallopian tubes.

## I

**iatrogenic illness** (eye-**at**-roh-**JEN**-ick): an unfavorable response due to prescribed medical treatment.

**ichthyosis** (**ick**-thee-**OH**-sis): a group of hereditary disorders characterized by dry, thickened, and scaly skin.

**idiopathic disorder** (**id**-ee-oh-**PATH**-ick): an illness without known cause.

**idiosyncratic reaction** (**id**-ee-oh-sin-**KRAT**-ick): an unexpected reaction to a drug that is peculiar to the individual.

**ileal conduit** (**ill**-ee-al **KON**-doo-it): use of a small piece of intestine to convey urine to the ureters and to a stoma in the abdomen.

**ileectomy** (**ill**-ee-**ECK**-toh-mee): the surgical removal of the ileum.

**ileostomy** (**ill**-ee-**OS**-toh-mee): the surgical creation of an artificial excretory opening between the ileum and the outside of the abdominal wall.

**ileus** (**ILL**-ee-us): the partial or complete blockage of the small and/or large intestine.

**iliotibial band syndrome** (**ill**-ee-oh-**TIB**-ee-al): an overuse injury caused by this band rubbing against bone, often in the area of the knee.

**immobilization:** the act of holding, suturing, or fastening a bone in a fixed position with strapping or a cast.

**immunity:** the state of being resistant to a specific disease.

**immunodeficiency disorder** (**im**-you-noh-deh-**FISH**-en-see): a condition that occurs when immune system response is compromised.

**immunoglobulins** (**im**-you-noh-**GLOB**-you-lins): antibodies that bind with specific antigens in the antigen-antibody response.

**immunosuppressant** (**im**-you-noh-soo-**PRES**-ant): a substance that prevents or reduces the body's normal immune response.

**immunosuppression** (im-you-noh-sup-**PRESH**-un): treatment to repress or interfere with the ability of the immune system to respond to stimulation by antigens.

**immunotherapy** (ih-**myou**-noh-**THER**-ah-pee): a disease treatment that involves either stimulating or repressing the immune response.

**impacted cerumen:** an accumulation of earwax that forms a solid mass by adhering to the walls of the external auditory canal.

**impetigo** (im-peh-**TYE**-goh): a highly contagious bacterial skin infection characterized by isolated pustules that become crusted and rupture.

**impingement syndrome** (im-**PINJ**-ment): inflammation of tendons that get caught in the narrow space between the bones within the shoulder joint.

**impulse control disorders:** a group of psychiatric disorders characterized by failure to resist an impulse despite potential negative consequences.

**incision:** a cut made with a surgical instrument.

**incontinence** (in-**KON**-tih-nents): the inability to control the excretion of urine and/or feces.

**incubator** (**IN**-kyou-**bate**-or): an apparatus for maintaining a controlled environment for a premature or ill newborn.

**indirect contact transmission:** refers to situations in which a susceptible person is infected by contact with a contaminated surface.

**indwelling catheter:** a catheter that remains inside the body for a prolonged time based on need.

**infection** (in-**FECK**-shun): invasion of the body by a pathogenic organism.

**infectious disease** (in-**FECK**-shus): an illness caused by living pathogenic organisms such as bacteria and viruses.

**infectious mononucleosis** (**mon**-oh-**new**-klee-**OH**-sis): an infection caused by the Epstein-Barr virus that is characterized by fever, a sore throat, and enlarged lymph nodes.

**infectious myringitis** (**mir**-in-**JIGH**-tis): a contagious inflammation that causes painful blisters on the eardrum.

**infestation:** the dwelling of microscopic parasites on external surface tissue.

**infiltrating ductal carcinoma:** breast cancer that starts in the milk duct, breaks through the wall of that duct, and invades the fatty breast tissue.

**infiltrating lobular carcinoma:** breast cancer that starts in the milk glands, breaks through the wall of the gland, and invades the fatty tissue of the breast.

**inflammation** (in-flah-**MAY**-shun): a localized response to an injury or to the destruction of tissues.

**inflammatory bowel disease:** the general name for diseases that cause inflammation and swelling in the intestines.

**inflammatory breast cancer** (IBC): a rare but aggressive form of breast cancer.

**influenza** (in-flew-**EN**-zah): a highly contagious viral respiratory infection that occurs in seasonal epidemics.

**inguinal hernia** (**ING**-gwih-nal **HER**-nee-ah): the protrusion of a small loop of bowel through a weak place in the lower abdominal wall or groin.

**inhalation administration:** the administration of medication in the form of vapor and gases taken in through the nose or mouth and absorbed into the bloodstream through the lungs.

**insomnia:** the prolonged or abnormal inability to sleep.

**insulinoma** (in-suh-lin-**OH**-mah): a benign tumor of the pancreas that causes hypoglycemia by secreting additional insulin.

**insulin shock:** a diabetic emergency caused by very low blood sugar.

**integrative medicine:** a health care model based on both allopathic and alternative medicine.

**intermittent catheter:** inserted as needed to drain urine from the bladder.

**intermittent claudication** (**klaw**-dih-**KAY**-shun): pain in the leg muscles that occurs during exercise and is relieved by rest.

**internal fixation:** fracture treatment in which pins or a plate are placed directly into the bone to hold the broken pieces in place.

**interstitial cystitis** (in-ter-**STISH**-al sis-**TYE**-tis): a chronic inflammation within the walls of the bladder.

**interstitial lung diseases** (in-ter-**STISH**-al): a group of diseases that cause inflammation and scarring of the alveoli and their supporting structures.

**interventional radiology:** the use of radiographic imaging to guide a procedure or confirm placement of an inserted object.

**intestinal obstruction:** the partial or complete blockage of the small and/or large intestine caused by a physical obstruction.

**intracranial pressure:** the amount of pressure inside the skull.

**intradermal injection:** the administration of medication by injection into the middle layers of the skin.

**intramuscular injection:** the administration of medication by injection directly into muscle tissue.

**intraocular lens:** a surgically implanted replacement for a natural lens that has been removed.

**intraoral radiography:** the placement of x-ray film within the mouth with the camera positioned next to the cheek.

**intrauterine device:** a molded plastic contraceptive inserted through the cervix into the uterus to prevent pregnancy.

**intravenous fluids (in**-trah-**VEE**-nus**):** fluids administered into a vein to combat the effects of dehydration.

**intravenous injection:** the administration of medication by injection directly into a vein.

**intravenous pyelogram (PYE**-eh-loh-**gram):** a radiographic study of the kidneys and ureters.

**intussusception (in**-tus-sus-**SEP**-shun**):** the telescoping of one part of the small intestine into the opening of an immediately adjacent part.

**in vitro fertilization:** a procedure in which mature ova are removed from the mother to be fertilized.

**iridectomy (ir**-ih-**DECK**-toh-mee**):** the surgical removal of a portion of the tissue of the iris.

**iritis (eye**-**RYE**-tis**):** inflammation of the uvea primarily affecting structures in the front of the eye.

**iron-deficiency anemia:** a decrease in the red cells of the blood that is caused by too little iron.

**irrigation and debridement:** a procedure using pressurized fluid to clean out wound debris.

**irritable bowel syndrome:** a common condition of unknown cause with symptoms that can include intermittent cramping, abdominal pain, bloating, constipation, and/or diarrhea.

**ischemia (iss**-**KEE**-mee-ah**):** a condition in which there is an insufficient supply of oxygen in the tissues due to restricted blood flow to a part of the body.

**ischemic colitis (iss**-**KEE**-mick koh-**LYE**-tis**):** a condition that occurs when part of the large intestine is partially or completely deprived of blood.

**ischemic heart disease (iss**-**KEE**-mick):** a group of cardiac disabilities resulting from an insufficient supply of oxygenated blood to the heart.

**ischemic stroke:** damage that occurs when the flow of blood to the brain is blocked by the narrowing or blockage of a carotid artery.

## J

**jaundice (JAWN**-dis**):** a yellow discoloration of the skin, mucous membranes, and eyes.

**juvenile rheumatoid arthritis:** an autoimmune disorder affecting children aged 16 years or less, with symptoms that include stiffness, pain, joint swelling, skin rash, fever, slowed growth, and fatigue.

## K

**Kaposi's sarcoma (KAP**-oh-seez sar-**KOH**-mah**):** a cancer that causes patches of abnormal tissue to grow under the skin; in the lining of the mouth, nose, and throat; or in other organs.

**Kegel exercises:** a series of pelvic muscle exercises used to strengthen the muscles of the pelvic floor.

**keloid (KEE**-loid**):** an abnormally raised or thickened scar that expands beyond the boundaries of the original incision.

**keratitis (ker**-ah-**TYE**-tis**):** inflammation of the cornea.

**keratosis (kerr**-ah-**TOH**-sis**):** any skin growth, such as a wart or a callus, in which there is overgrowth and thickening of the skin.

**ketonuria (kee**-toh-**NEW**-ree-ah**):** the presence of ketones in the urine.

**knee-chest position:** position in which the patient is lying face down with the hips bent so that the knees and chest rest on the table.

**koilonychia (koy**-loh-**NICK**-ee-ah**):** a malformation of the nails in which the outer surface is concave or scooped out like the bowl of a spoon.

**KUB (kidney-ureter-bladder):** a radiographic study without the use of a contrast medium, used to detect bowel obstructions and nephroliths.

**kyphosis (kye**-**FOH**-sis**):** an abnormal increase in the outward curvature of the thoracic spine as viewed from the side.

## L

**labyrinthectomy (lab**-ih-rin-**THECK**-toh-mee**):** the surgical removal of all or a portion of the labyrinth.

**labyrinthitis (lab**-ih-rin-**THIGH**-tis**):** inflammation of the labyrinth that can result in vertigo and deafness.

**laceration (lass**-er-**AY**-shun**):** a torn or jagged wound or an accidental cut.

**laminectomy (lam**-ih-**NECK**-toh-mee**):** the surgical removal of a lamina from a vertebra.

**laparoscopic adrenalectomy (ah**-dree-nal-**ECK**-tohmee**):** a minimally invasive procedure to surgically remove one or both adrenal glands.

**laparoscopy (lap**-ah-**ROS**-koh-pee**):** the visual examination of the interior of the abdomen with the use of a laparoscope.

**laryngectomy** (**lar**-in-**JECK**-toh-mee)**:** the surgical removal of the larynx.

**laryngitis** (**lar**-in-**JIGH**-tis)**:** inflammation of the larynx.

**laryngoscopy** (**lar**-ing-**GOS**-koh-pee)**:** the visual examination of the larynx and vocal cords using a laryngoscope.

**laryngospasm** (lah-**RING**-goh-spazm)**:** the sudden spasmodic closure of the larynx.

**laryngotomy** (**lar**-ing-**OT**-oh-mee)**:** a surgical incision into the larynx.

**laser:** an acronym for *light amplification by stimulated emission of radiation*, used to treat skin conditions and other disorders of the body.

**laser angioplasty** (**AN**-jee-oh-**plas**-tee)**:** removing plaque deposit in an artery using beams of light from a laser on the end of a catheter.

**laser iridotomy** (**ir**-ih-**DOT**-oh-mee)**:** uses a focused beam of light to create a hole in the iris of the eye.

**laser trabeculoplasty** (trah-**BECK**-you-loh-**plas**-tee)**:** treatment of open-angle glaucoma by creating openings in the trabecular meshwork to allow fluid to drain properly.

**LASIK** (laser-assisted in situ keratomileusis)**:** treatment of vision conditions that are caused by the shape of the cornea.

**latent autoimmune diabetes in adults:** a condition in which type 1 diabetes develops in adults.

**laxatives:** medications or foods given to stimulate bowel movements.

**learning disabilities:** disorders found in children of normal intelligence who have difficulties in learning specific skills such as processing language or grasping mathematical concepts.

**lensectomy** (len-**SECK**-toh-mee)**:** the surgical removal of a cataract-clouded lens.

**lesion** (**LEE**-zhun)**:** a pathologic change of tissues due to disease or injury.

**lethargy** (**LETH**-ar-jee)**:** a lowered level of consciousness marked by listlessness, drowsiness, and apathy.

**leukemia** (loo-**KEE**-mee-ah)**:** a type of cancer characterized by a progressive increase in the number of abnormal white blood cells found in blood-forming tissues, other organs, and in the circulating blood.

**leukopenia** (**loo**-koh-**PEE**-nee-ah)**:** a decrease in the number of white blood cells circulating in the blood.

**leukoplakia** (**loo**-koh-**PLAY**-kee-ah)**:** an abnormal white precancerous lesion that develops inside the mouth in response to chronic irritation.

**leukorrhea** (**loo**-koh-**REE**-ah)**:** a profuse whitish mucus discharge from the uterus and vagina.

**levels of consciousness:** terms used to describe the measurement of response to arousal and stimulus.

**light therapy:** exposure to daylight or specific wavelengths of light in order to counteract seasonal affective disorder.

**lipectomy** (lih-**PECK**-toh-mee)**:** the surgical removal of fat from beneath the skin.

**lipedema** (lip-eh-**DEE**-mah)**:** a chronic abnormal condition characterized by the accumulation of fat and fluid in the tissues just under the skin of the hips and legs.

**lipid panel:** a blood test that measures the amounts of total cholesterol, high-density lipoprotein, low-density lipoprotein, and triglycerides.

**lipoma** (lih-**POH**-mah)**:** a benign, slow-growing fatty tumor located between the skin and the muscle layer.

**liposuction** (**LIP**-oh-**suck**-shun *or* **LYE**-poh-suckshun)**:** the surgical removal of fat beneath the skin with the aid of suction.

**lithotomy** (lih-**THOT**-oh-mee)**:** a surgical incision for the removal of a stone from the bladder.

**lithotomy position** (lih-**THOT**-oh-mee)**:** an examination position in which the patient is lying on the back with the feet and legs raised and supported in stirrups.

**liver transplant:** an option for a patient whose liver has failed for a reason other than liver cancer.

**lobar pneumonia:** a type of pneumonia that affects larger areas of the lungs, often including one or more sections, or lobes, of a lung.

**lobectomy** (loh-**BECK**-toh-mee)**:** the surgical removal of a lobe of an organ.

**localized allergic response:** includes redness, itching, and burning where the skin has come into contact with an allergen.

**lordosis** (lor-**DOH**-sis)**:** an abnormal increase in the forward curvature of the lumbar spine.

**low-density lipoprotein cholesterol:** the form of cholesterol that contributes to plaque buildup in the arteries.

**lumbago** (lum-**BAY**-goh)**:** pain of the lumbar region of the spine.

**lumbar puncture:** the process of obtaining a sample of cerebrospinal fluid by inserting a needle into the subarachnoid space of the lumbar region to withdraw fluid.

**lumbar radiculopathy:** nerve pain in the lower back.

**lumpectomy:** surgical removal of only the cancerous tissue with the surrounding margin of normal tissue.

**lung cancer:** a condition in which cancer cells form in the tissues of the lung.

**Lyme disease:** a bacterial infection caused by a spirochete belonging to the genus *Borrelia*.

**lymphadenitis** (lim-**fad**-eh-**NIGH**-tis): inflammation of the lymph nodes.

**lymphadenopathy** (lim-**fad**-eh-**NOP**-ah-thee): any disease process affecting a lymph node or nodes.

**lymphangioma** (lim-**fan**-jee-**OH**-mah): a benign tumor formed by an abnormal collection of lymphatic vessels.

**lymphedema** (**lim**-feh-**DEE**-mah): swelling of the tissues due to an abnormal accumulation of lymph fluid within the tissues.

**lymph node dissection:** a surgical procedure in which all of the lymph nodes in a major group are removed to determine or slow the spread of cancer.

**lymphoma** (lim-**FOH**-mah): a general term applied to malignancies affecting lymphoid tissues.

**lymphoscintigraphy** (**lim**-foh-sin-**TIH**-grah-fee): a diagnostic test that is performed to detect damage or malformations of the lymphatic vessels.

# M

**macular degeneration** (**MACK**-you-lar): a gradually progressive condition in which the macula at the center of the retina is damaged, resulting in the loss of central vision.

**macule** (**MACK**-youl): a discolored, flat spot that is less than 1 cm in diameter.

**magnetic resonance angiography:** a specialized MRI study using a contrast medium to locate problems with blood vessels throughout the body.

**magnetic resonance imaging** (MRI): an imaging technique that uses a combination of radio waves and a strong magnetic field to create signals that are sent to a computer and converted into images of any plane through the body.

**malabsorption** (**mal**-ab-**SORP**-shun): a condition in which the small intestine cannot absorb nutrients from the food that passes through it.

**malaise** (mah-**LAYZ**): a feeling of general discomfort, often the first indication of an infection or disease.

**malaria** (mah-**LAY**-ree-ah): a disease caused by a parasite that lives in certain mosquitoes and is transferred to humans by the bite of an infected mosquito.

**male pattern baldness:** a common hair-loss pattern in men.

**malignant melanoma** (mel-ah-**NOH**-mah): a type of skin cancer that occurs in the melanocytes.

**malingering** (mah-**LING**-ger-ing): a condition characterized by the intentional creation of false or grossly exaggerated physical or psychological symptoms.

**malnutrition:** a lack of proper food or nutrients in the body, due to a shortage of food, poor eating habits, or the inability of the body to digest, absorb, and distribute these nutrients.

**mammography** (mam-**OG**-rah-fee): a radiographic examination of the breast to detect the presence of tumors or precancerous cells.

**mammoplasty** (**MAM**-oh-**plas**-tee): a cosmetic operation on the breasts.

**manic behavior:** an abnormally elevated mood state, including inappropriate elation, increased irritability, severe insomnia, poor judgment, and inappropriate social behavior.

**Mantoux PPD skin test:** a test for diagnosing tuberculosis.

**mastalgia** (mass-**TAL**-jee-ah): pain in the breast.

**mastectomy** (mas-**TECK**-toh-mee): surgical removal of the entire breast and nipple.

**mastitis** (mas-**TYE**-tis): a breast infection that is caused by bacteria that enter the breast tissue, most frequently during breastfeeding.

**mastoidectomy** (**mas**-toy-**DECK**-toh-mee): the surgical removal of mastoid cells.

**mastoiditis** (**mas**-toy-**DYE**-tis): inflammation of any part of the mastoid bone cells.

**mastopexy** (**MAS**-toh-**peck**-see): surgery to affix sagging breasts in a more elevated position.

**maxillofacial surgery** (mack-**sill**-oh-**FAY**-shul): specialized surgery of the face and jaws to correct deformities, treat diseases, and repair injuries.

**measles:** an acute, highly contagious infection transmitted by respiratory droplets of the rubeola virus.

**measles, mumps, and rubella vaccination** (MMR): childhood immunization that can prevent these three viral conditions.

**meatotomy** (**mee**-ah-**TOT**-oh-mee): a surgical incision made in the urethral meatus to enlarge the opening.

**megaloblastic anemia** (**MEG**-ah-loh-**blas**-tick ah-**NEE**-mee-ah): a blood disorder characterized by anemia in which red blood cells are larger than normal.

**melanin** (**MEL**-ah-nin): the pigment that determines the color of the skin.

**melena** (meh-**LEE**-nah): the passage of black, tarry, and foul-smelling stools.

**Ménière's disease** (men-**YEHRS**): a rare chronic disorder in which the amount of fluid in the inner ear increases intermittently, causing vertigo, fluctuating hearing loss, and tinnitus.

**meningioma** (meh-**nin**-jee-**OH**-mah): a common, slow-growing and usually benign tumor of the meninges.

**meningitis** (**men**-in-**JIGH**-tis): inflammation of the meninges of the brain and spinal cord.

**meningocele** (meh-**NING**-goh-**seel**): the congenital herniation of the meninges through a defect in the skull or spinal column.

**menometrorrhagia** (**men**-oh-**met**-roh-**RAY**-jee-ah): excessive uterine bleeding occurring both during the menses and at other irregular intervals.

**mental retardation/intellectual disability:** significant below-average intellectual and adaptive functioning present from birth or early infancy.

**metastasis** (meh-**TAS**-tah-sis): the new cancer site that results from the spreading process.

**metastasize** (meh-**TAS**-tah-sighz): the process by which cancer spreads from one place to another.

**metered dose inhaler:** a medical device that administers a specific amount of a medication such as a bronchodilator in aerosol form.

**methicillin-resistant** *Staphylococcus aureus* (MRSA): one of several types of bacteria that are now resistant to most antibiotics.

**metrorrhea** (**mee**-troh-**REE**-ah): an abnormal discharge, such as mucus or pus, from the uterus.

**migraine** (**MY**-grayn): a headache characterized by throbbing pain on one side of the head and may be preceded by a warning aura.

**mindfulness meditation:** treatment for stress focused on maintaining a calm, constant awareness and acceptance of thoughts and emotions.

**minimally invasive coronary artery bypass:** a bypass procedure performed with the aid of a fiberoptic camera through small openings between the ribs.

**miosis** (mye-**OH**-sis): the contraction of the pupil.

**modified radical mastectomy:** the surgical removal of the entire breast and axillary lymph nodes under the adjacent arm.

**Mohs surgery:** a technique used to treat various types of skin cancer by removing layers of cancerous tissue until a healthy margin is achieved.

**monaural testing** (mon-**AW**-rahl): involves one ear.

**monochromatism** (**mon**-oh-**KROH**-mah-tizm): the inability to distinguish certain colors in a normal manner.

**monoclonal antibodies:** artificially produced antibodies used to enhance a patient's immune response to certain malignancies.

**mood-stabilizing drugs:** used to treat mood instability and bipolar disorders.

**morbid obesity:** the condition of weighing two or more times the ideal weight or having a body mass index value greater than 40.

**multiparous** (mul-**TIP**-ah-rus): a woman who has given birth two or more times.

**multiple sclerosis** (skleh-**ROH**-sis): a progressive autoimmune disorder characterized by inflammation that causes demyelination of the myelin sheath.

**mumps:** an acute viral infection characterized by the swelling of the parotid glands.

**muscle biopsy:** removal of a plug of tissue with a biopsy needle for examination.

**muscle tone:** the state of balanced muscle tension that makes normal posture, coordination, and movement possible.

**muscular dystrophy** (**DIS**-troh-fee): a group of more than 30 genetic diseases that are characterized by progressive weakness and degeneration of the skeletal muscles without affecting the nervous system.

**myalgia** (my-**AL**-jee-ah): tenderness or pain in the muscles.

**myasthenia gravis** (**my**-as-**THEE**-nee-ah **GRAH**-vis): a chronic autoimmune disease that affects the neuromuscular junction and produces serious weakness of voluntary muscles.

**mycosis** (my-**KOH**-sis): any abnormal condition or disease caused by a fungus.

**mydriasis** (mih-**DRY**-ah-sis): the dilation of the pupil.

**mydriatic drops** (mid-ree-**AT**-ick): medication placed into the eyes to produce temporary paralysis forcing the pupils to remain wide open even in the presence of bright light.

**myelitis** (my-eh-**LYE**-tis): inflammation of the spinal cord; inflammation of bone marrow.

**myelodysplastic syndrome** (**my**-eh-loh-dis-**PLAS**-tick): a group of bone marrow disorders that are characterized by the insufficient production of one or more types of blood cells.

**myelography** (my-eh-**LOG**-rah-fee): a radiographic study of the spinal cord after the injection of a contrast medium through a lumbar puncture.

**myeloma** (**my**-eh-**LOH**-mah): a type of cancer that occurs in blood-making cells of the red bone marrow.

**myelopathy** (my-eh-**LOP**-ah-thee): any pathologic change or disease in the spinal cord.

**myelosis** (my-eh-**LOH**-sis): a tumor of the spinal cord.

**myocardial infarction** (**my**-oh-**KAR**-dee-al in-**FARK**-shun): the occlusion of one or more coronary arteries caused by plaque buildup.

**myocarditis** (**my**-oh-kar-**DYE**-tis): inflammation of the myocardium.

**myocele** (**MY**-oh-seel): the herniation of muscle substance through a tear in the fascia surrounding it.

**myoclonus** (**my**-oh-**KLOH**-nus *or* my-**OCK**-loh-nus): the sudden, involuntary jerking of a muscle or group of muscles.

**myofascial pain syndrome:** a chronic pain disorder that affects muscles and fascia throughout the body.

**myofascial release:** a specialized soft-tissue manipulation technique used to ease the pain of conditions such as fibromyalgia, myofascial pain syndrome, movement restrictions, temporomandibular joint disorders, and carpal tunnel syndrome.

**myolysis** (**my**-**OL**-ih-sis): the degeneration of muscle tissue.

**myoma** (**my**-**OH**-mah): a benign tumor made up of muscle tissue.

**myomectomy** (**my**-oh-**MECK**-toh-mee): the surgical removal of uterine fibroids.

**myoparesis** (**my**-oh-**PAR**-eh-sis): weakness or slight muscular paralysis.

**myopathy** (**my**-**OP**-ah-thee): any pathologic change or disease of muscle tissue.

**myopia** (**my**-**OH**-pee-ah): a defect in which light rays focus in front of the retina; also known as nearsightedness.

**myoplasty** (**MY**-oh-**plas**-tee): the surgical repair of a muscle.

**myorrhaphy** (**my**-**OR**-ah-fee): surgical suturing of a muscle.

**myorrhexis** (**my**-oh-**RECK**-sis): the rupture or tearing of a muscle.

**myosarcoma** (**my**-oh-sahr-**KOH**-mah): a malignant tumor derived from muscle tissue.

**myotomy** (**my**-**OT**-oh-mee): a surgical incision into a muscle.

**myringotomy** (**mir**-in-**GOT**-oh-mee): a small surgical incision in the eardrum to relieve pressure from excess pus or fluid, or to create an opening for the placement of ear tubes.

**myxedema** (**mick**-seh-**DEE**-mah): a severe form of adult hypothyroidism caused by extreme deficiency of thyroid secretion.

# N

**narcolepsy** (**NAR**-koh-**lep**-see): a sleep disorder consisting of sudden and uncontrollable brief episodes of falling asleep during the day.

**nasogastric intubation** (**nay**-zoh-**GAS**-trick **in**-too-**BAY**-shun): the placement of a tube through the nose and into the stomach.

**natural immunity:** disease resistance without administration of an antigen or exposure to disease, either present at birth or passed on from mother to child through breast milk.

**naturopathy** (**nay**-cher-**AH**-pah-thee): a form of alternative medicine emphasizing the healing power of nature and support of the body's own healing ability.

**nausea** (**NAW**-see-ah): the urge to vomit.

**nebulizer** (**NEB**-you-lye-zer): an electronic device that pumps air or oxygen through a liquid medicine to turn it into a mist that is inhaled via a face mask or mouthpiece.

**necrotizing fasciitis** (**NECK**-roh-**tiz**-ing **fas**-ee-**EYE**-tis) (NF): a severe infection caused by group A strep bacteria.

**needle breast biopsy:** a technique in which an x-ray-guided needle is used to remove small samples of tissue from the breast.

**neobladder** (**NEE**-oh-**blad**-er): bladder replacement using part of the small intestine.

**neoplasm** (**NEE**-oh-plazm): an abnormal growth of body tissue in which the multiplication of cells is uncontrolled, abnormal, rapid, and progressive; also known as a tumor.

**nephritis** (neh-**FRY**-tis): inflammation of the kidney or kidneys.

**nephrolith** (**NEF**-roh-lith): a stone located in the kidney.

**nephrolithiasis** (**nef**-roh-lih-**THIGH**-ah-sis): the presence of stones in the kidney.

**nephrolysis** (neh-**FROL**-ih-sis): the surgical freeing of a kidney from adhesions.

**nephropathy** (neh-**FROP**-ah-thee): any disease of the kidney.

**nephropexy** (**NEF**-roh-**peck**-see): the surgical fixation of nephroptosis.

**nephroptosis** (**nef**-rop-**TOH**-sis): the prolapse of a kidney into the pelvic area when the patient stands.

**nephropyosis** (**nef**-roh-pye-**OH**-sis): suppuration of the kidney.

**nephrostomy** (neh-**FROS**-toh-mee): the placement of a catheter to maintain an opening between the pelvis of one or both kidneys to the exterior of the body.

**nephrotic syndrome** (neh-**FROT**-ick): a group of conditions in which excessive amounts of protein are lost in the urine.

**neuritis** (new-**RYE**-tis): inflammation of a nerve accompanied by pain and sometimes loss of function.

**neurodegenerative disease** (**new**-roh-deh-**JEN**-er-ah-tiv)**:** an umbrella term for disorders in which there is a progressive loss of the structure or functions of neurons.

**neurogenic bladder** (new-roh-**JEN**-ick)**:** a urinary problem caused by interference with the normal nerve pathways associated with urination.

**neuromuscular blocker:** a medication that causes temporary paralysis by blocking the transmission of nerve stimuli to the muscles.

**neuromuscular therapy:** a form of massage that uses soft-tissue manipulation focusing on applying pressure to trigger points to treat injuries and alleviate pain.

**neuroplasty** (**NEW**-roh-**plas**-tee)**:** the surgical repair of a nerve or nerves.

**neurorrhaphy** (new-**ROR**-ah-fee)**:** surgically suturing together the ends of a severed nerve.

**neurotomy** (new-**ROT**-oh-mee)**:** the surgical division or dissection of a nerve.

**nevus** (**NEE**-vye)**:** a small, dark skin growth that develops from melanocytes in the skin.

**nitroglycerin:** a vasodilator that is prescribed to prevent or relieve the pain of angina.

**nocturia** (nock-**TOO**-ree-ah)**:** frequent and excessive urination during the night.

**nocturnal enuresis** (nock-**TER**-nal **en**-you-**REE**-sis)**:** urinary incontinence during sleep.

**nocturnal myoclonus** (nock-**TER**-nal **my**-oh-**KLOH**-nus *or* my-**OCK**-loh-nus)**:** jerking of the limbs that can occur normally as a person is falling asleep.

**nodule:** a solid, raised skin lesion that is larger than 0.5 cm in diameter and deeper than a papule.

**noise-induced hearing loss:** nerve deafness caused by repeated exposure to extremely loud noises.

**nonalcoholic fatty liver disease** (NAFLD)**:** describes the accumulation of fat in the liver of people who drink little or no alcohol.

**nonalcoholic steatohepatitis** (NASH)**:** a more serious form of *nonalcoholic fatty liver disease*, consists of fatty accumulations plus liver-damaging inflammation.

**non-Hodgkin's lymphoma** (non-**HODJ**-kinz lim-**FOH**-mah)**:** the term used to describe all lymphomas *other than* Hodgkin's lymphoma.

**non-steroidal anti-inflammatory drugs:** medications administered to control pain by reducing inflammation and swelling.

**normal sperm count:** 20 to 120 million or more sperm per mL of semen.

**nosocomial infection** (**nos**-oh-**KOH**-mee-al)**:** a disease acquired in a hospital or clinical setting.

**nuclear scan:** a diagnostic procedure that uses nuclear medicine technology to gather information about the structure and function of organs or body systems.

**nulligravida** (**null**-ih-**GRAV**-ih-dah)**:** a woman who has never been pregnant.

**nullipara** (nuh-**LIP**-ah-rah)**:** a woman who has never borne a viable child.

**nyctalopia** (**nick**-tah-**LOH**-pee-ah)**:** a condition in which an individual with normal daytime vision has difficulty seeing at night.

**nystagmus** (nis-**TAG**-mus)**:** an involuntary, constant, rhythmic movement of the eyeball.

## O

**obesity** (oh-**BEE**-sih-tee)**:** an excessive accumulation of fat in the body.

**oblique fracture:** a fracture that occurs at an angle across the bone.

**obsessive-compulsive disorder:** a mental condition characterized by obsessions and/or compulsions.

**occupational therapy:** activities to promote recovery and rehabilitation to assist patients in performing the activities of daily living.

**ocular prosthesis:** a replacement for an eyeball that is either congenitally missing or has been surgically removed.

**oligomenorrhea** (**ol**-ih-goh-**men**-oh-**REE**-ah)**:** light or infrequent menstruation in a woman with previously normal periods.

**oligospermia** (**ol**-ih-goh-**SPER**-mee-ah)**:** a sperm count of below 20 million/mL.

**oliguria** (**ol**-ih-**GOO**-ree-ah)**:** scanty urination.

**onychia** (oh-**NICK**-ee-ah)**:** inflammation of the matrix of the nail.

**onychocryptosis** (**on**-ih-koh-krip-**TOH**-sis)**:** ingrown toenail.

**onychomycosis** (**on**-ih-koh-my-**KOH**-sis)**:** a fungal infection of the nail.

**onychophagia** (**on**-ih-koh-**FAY**-jee-ah)**:** nail biting or nail eating.

**oophorectomy** (**oh**-ahf-oh-**RECK**-toh-mee)**:** the surgical removal of one or both ovaries.

**oophoritis** (**oh**-ahf-oh-**RYE**-tis)**:** inflammation of an ovary.

**open-angle glaucoma:** the most common form of glaucoma.

**open fracture:** a fracture in which the bone is broken and there is an open wound in the skin.

**ophthalmoscope** (ahf-**THAL**-moh-skope)**:** an instrument used to examine the interior of the eye.

**ophthalmoscopy** (**ahf**-thal-**MOS**-koh-pee)**:** the visual examination of the fundus of the eye with ophthalmoscope.

**opportunistic infection** (**op**-ur-too-**NIHS**-tick)**:** caused by a pathogen that does not normally produce an illness in healthy humans.

**oral administration:** medication taken by mouth to be absorbed through the walls of the stomach or small intestine.

**oral glucose tolerance test** (**GLOO**-kohs)**:** a test performed to confirm a diagnosis of diabetes mellitus and to aid in diagnosing hypoglycemia.

**oral or maxillofacial surgeon** (mack-**sill**-oh-**FAY**-shul)**:** a physician specializing in surgery of the face and jaws to correct deformities, treat diseases, and repair injuries.

**oral rehydration therapy:** treatment in which a solution of electrolytes is administered in a liquid preparation to counteract dehydration.

**oral thrush:** a type of stomatomycosis caused by the fungus *Candida albicans*.

**orbitotomy** (or-bih-**TOT**-oh-mee)**:** a surgical incision into the orbit.

**orchidectomy** (or-kih-**DECK**-toh-mee)**:** the surgical removal of one or both testicles.

**orchiopexy** (or-kee-oh-**PECK**-see)**:** the repair of an undescended testicle.

**organic disorder** (or-**GAN**-ick)**:** a disorder that produces symptoms caused by detectable physical changes in the body.

**orthostatic hypotension** (or-thoh-**STAT**-ick **high**-poh-**TEN**-shun)**:** low blood pressure that occurs upon standing up.

**orthotic** (or-**THOT**-ick)**:** a mechanical appliance, such a leg brace or splint, that is specially designed to control, correct, or compensate for impaired limb function.

**ossification** (oss-uh-fih-**KAY**-shun)**:** the normal process of bone formation.

**ostealgia** (oss-tee-**AL**-jee-ah)**:** pain in a bone.

**ostectomy** (oss-**TECK**-toh-mee)**:** the surgical removal of bone.

**osteitis** (oss-tee-**EYE**-tis)**:** inflammation of bone.

**osteoarthritis** (oss-tee-oh-ar-**THRIGH**-tis)**:** the type of arthritis most commonly associated with aging.

**osteochondroma** (oss-tee-oh-kon-**DROH**-mah)**:** a benign bony projection covered with cartilage.

**osteoclasis** (oss-tee-**OCK**-lah-sis)**:** the surgical fracture of a bone to correct a deformity.

**osteomalacia** (oss-tee-oh-mah-**LAY**-shee-ah)**:** abnormal softening of bones in adults.

**osteomyelitis** (**oss**-tee-oh-**my**-eh-**LYE**-tis)**:** inflammation of the bone marrow and adjacent bone.

**osteonecrosis** (**oss**-tee-oh-neh-**KROH**-sis)**:** the death of bone tissue due to an insufficient blood supply.

**osteopathic manipulative therapy:** mechanical spinal adjustment used in conjunction with conventional medical therapies by an osteopath.

**osteopenia** (**oss**-tee-oh-**PEE**-nee-ah)**:** thinner than average bone density.

**osteophytes** (**OSS**-tee-oh-**fites**)**:** are also known as bone spurs.

**osteoplasty** (**OSS**-tee-oh-**plas**-tee)**:** the surgical repair of a bone or bones.

**osteoporosis** (**oss**-tee-oh-poh-**ROH**-sis)**:** a marked loss of bone density and an increase in bone porosity that is frequently associated with aging.

**osteoporotic hip fracture** (**oss**-tee-oh-pah-**ROT**-ick)**:** a fracture of a hip weakened by osteoporosis that can occur spontaneously or as the result of a fall.

**osteorrhaphy** (**oss**-tee-**OR**-ah-fee)**:** surgical suturing or wiring together of bones.

**osteosarcoma** (**oss**-tee-oh-sar-**KOH**-mah)**:** a hard tissue sarcoma that usually involves the upper shaft of long bones, pelvis, or knee.

**osteotomy** (**oss**-tee-**OT**-oh-mee)**:** the surgical cutting of a bone.

**ostomy** (**OSS**-toh-mee)**:** a surgical procedure to create an artificial opening between an organ and the body surface.

**otalgia** (oh-**TAL**-gee-ah)**:** pain in the ear.

**otitis** (oh-**TYE**-tis)**:** inflammation of the ear.

**otitis media** (oh-**TYE**-tis **MEE**-dee-ah)**:** inflammation of the middle ear.

**otomycosis** (**oh**-toh-my-**KOH**-sis)**:** a fungal infection of the external auditory canal.

**otoplasty** (**OH**-toh-**plas**-tee)**:** the surgical repair, restoration or alteration of the pinna of the ear.

**otopyorrhea** (**oh**-toh-**pye**-oh-**REE**-ah)**:** the flow of pus from the ear.

**otorrhagia** (**oh**-toh-**RAY**-jee-ah)**:** bleeding from the ear.

**otorrhea** (**oh**-toh-**REE**-ah)**:** any discharge from the ear.

**otosclerosis** (**oh**-toh-skleh-**ROH**-sis)**:** ankylosis of the bones of the middle ear resulting in a conductive hearing loss.

**otoscope** (**OH**-toh-skope)**:** an instrument used to visually examine the external ear canal and tympanic membrane.

**ovarian cancer:** cancer that begins within the cells of the ovaries.

**ovariorrhexis** (oh-**vay**-ree-oh-**RECK**-sis)**:** the rupture of an ovary.

**overactive bladder:** a condition that occurs when the muscles of the bladder contract involuntarily even though the bladder is not full.

**overflow incontinence:** continuous leaking from the bladder either because it is full or because it does not empty completely.

**over-the-counter drug:** medication that can be purchased without a written prescription.

**overuse injuries:** injuries that occur when minor tissue injuries have not been given time to heal.

**overuse tendinitis (ten**-dih-**NIGH**-tis)**: inflammation of tendons caused by excessive or unusual use of a joint.

# P

**Paget's disease (PAJ**-its)**: a bone disease of unknown cause, characterized by excessive breakdown of bone tissue followed by abnormal bone formation.

**palatoplasty (PAL**-ah-toh-**plas**-tee)**: surgical repair of a cleft palate or lip.

**palliative (PAL**-ee-**ay**-tiv *or* **PAL**-ee-ah-tiv)**: a substance that eases the pain or severity of a disease but does not cure it.

**palpation (pal**-**PAY**-shun)**: an examination technique in which the examiner's hands are used to feel the texture, size, consistency, and location of certain body parts.

**palpitation (pal**-pih-**TAY**-shun)**: a pounding or racing heart with or without irregularity in rhythm.

**pancreatectomy (pan**-kree-ah-**TECK**-toh-mee)**: surgical removal of all or part of the pancreas.

**pancreatitis (pan**-kree-ah-**TYE**-tis)**: inflammation of the pancreas.

**pandemic (pan**-**DEM**-ick)**: an outbreak of a disease occurring over a large geographic area, possibly worldwide.

**panic attack:** an unexpected, sudden experience of fear in the absence of danger, accompanied by physical symptoms such as shortness of breath and chest pain.

**panic disorder:** a condition characterized by having more than one panic attack, resulting in persistent fear of the attacks.

**papilledema (pap**-ill-eh-**DEE**-mah)**: swelling and inflammation of the optic nerve at the point of entrance into the eye through the optic disk.

**papilloma (pap**-ih-**LOH**-mah)**: a benign, superficial wart-like growth on the epithelial tissue or elsewhere in the body, such as in the bladder.

**Pap smear:** an exfoliative biopsy of the cervix.

**papule (PAP**-youl)**: a small, raised red lesion that is less than 0.5 cm in diameter.

**paradoxical drug reaction:** the result of medical treatment that yields the exact opposite of normally expected results.

**paralysis (pah**-**RAL**-ih-sis)**: the loss of sensation and voluntary muscle movements in a muscle through disease or injury to its nerve supply.

**paraplegia (par**-ah-**PLEE**-jee-ah)**: paralysis of both legs and the lower part of the body.

**parasite (PAR**-ah-sight)**: a plant or animal that lives on or within another living organism at the expense of that organism.

**parathyroidectomy (par**-ah-**thigh**-roi-**DECK**-toh-mee)**: surgical removal of one or more of the parathyroid glands.

**parenteral administration (pah**-**REN**-ter-al)**: the administration of medication by injection through a hypodermic syringe.

**paresthesia (par**-es-**THEE**-zee-ah)**: a burning or prickling sensation that is usually felt in the hands, arms, legs, or feet.

**Parkinson's disease:** a chronic, degenerative central nervous system disorder characterized by fine muscle tremors, rigidity, and a slow or shuffling gait.

**paronychia (par**-oh-**NICK**-ee-ah)**: an infection of the skin fold around a nail.

**paroxysmal supraventricular tachycardia (par**-ock-**SIZ**-mal **soo**-prah-ven-**TRICK**-you-lar tack-ee-**KAR**-dee-ah)**: an episode that begins and ends abruptly during which there are very rapid and regular heartbeats that originate in the atria or AV node.

**partial knee replacement** (PKR)**: a procedure in which only part of the knee is replaced.

**pathogen (PATH**-oh-jen)**: a disease-producing microorganism.

**pathologic fracture:** occurs when a weakened bone breaks under normal strain.

**peak flow meter:** a handheld device used to measure how quickly a person with asthma can expel air.

**pediculosis (pee**-dick-you-**LOH**-sis)**: an infestation with lice.

**pelvic inflammatory disease:** any inflammation of the female reproductive organs not associated with surgery or pregnancy.

**pelvimetry (pel**-**VIM**-eh-tree)**: a radiographic study to measure the dimensions of the pelvis to determine its capacity to allow passage of the fetus through the birth canal.

**peptic ulcers** (**UL**-serz): sores that affect the mucous membranes of the digestive system.

**percussion** (per-**KUSH**-un): a diagnostic procedure to determine the density of a body area that uses the sound produced by tapping the surface with the fingers.

**percutaneous diskectomy** (**per**-kyou-**TAY**-nee-us dis-**KECK**-toh-mee): a procedure to treat a herniated intervertebral disk.

**percutaneous nephrolithotomy** (**per**-kyou-**TAY**-nee-us **nef**-roh-lih-**THOT**-oh-mee): surgical removal of a kidney stone through a small incision in the back.

**percutaneous transluminal coronary angioplasty:** a treatment procedure to open a partially blocked coronary artery by flattening the plaque deposit and stretching the lumen.

**percutaneous vertebroplasty** (**per**-kyou-**TAY**-nee-us **VER**-tee-broh-**plas**-tee): treatment of osteoporosis-related compression fractures by injecting bone cement to stabilize compression fractures within the spinal column.

**perfusion** (per-**FYOU**-zuhn): the flow of blood through an organ.

**pericardiocentesis** (**pehr**-ih-**kar**-dee-oh-sen-**TEE**-sis): the puncture of the pericardial sac for the purpose of removing fluid.

**pericarditis** (**pehr**-ih-kar-**DYE**-tis): inflammation of the pericardium.

**periodontal disease:** inflammation of the tissues that surround and support the teeth.

**periorbital edema** (**pehr**-ee-**OR**-bih-tal eh-**DEE**-mah): swelling of the tissues surrounding the eye or eyes.

**periosteotomy** (**pehr**-ee-**oss**-tee-**OT**-oh-mee): an incision through the periosteum to the bone.

**periostitis** (**pehr**-ee-oss-**TYE**-tis): inflammation of the periosteum.

**peripheral arterial occlusive disease:** an example of a peripheral vascular disease caused by atherosclerosis. Impaired circulation to the extremities and vital organs causes changes in the skin color and temperature, plus intermittent claudication.

**peripheral neuropathy** (new-**ROP**-ah-thee): a disorder of the peripheral nerves that carry information to and from the brain and spinal cord, producing pain, loss of sensation, and inability to control muscles.

**peripheral vascular disease:** disorders of blood vessels outside the heart and brain.

**peritoneal dialysis** (**pehr**-ih-toh-**NEE**-al dye-**AL**-ih-sis): dialysis in which the lining of the peritoneal cavity acts as the filter to remove waste from the blood.

**peritonitis** (**pehr**-ih-toh-**NIGH**-tis): inflammation of the peritoneum.

**pernicious anemia** (per-**NISH**-us ah-**NEE**-mee-ah): anemia caused by a lack of a protein that helps the body absorb vitamin B12 from the gastrointestinal tract.

**PERRLA:** an abbreviation meaning **P**upils are **E**qual, **R**ound, **R**esponsive to **L**ight and **A**ccomodation.

**persistent vegetative state:** a type of coma in which the patient exhibits alternating sleep and wake cycles; however, the individual is unconscious even when appearing to be awake.

**personality disorder:** a chronic pattern of inner experience and behavior that causes serious problems with relationships and work.

**pertussis** (per-**TUS**-is): a contagious bacterial infection of the upper respiratory tract that is characterized by recurrent bouts of a paroxysmal cough.

**petechiae** (pee-**TEE**-kee-ee): very small pinpoint hemorrhages less than 2 mm in diameter.

**Peyronie's disease** (pay-roh-**NEEZ**): a form of sexual dysfunction in which the penis is bent or curved during erection.

**phacoemulsification** (**fack**-koh-ee-**mul**-sih-fih-**KAY**-shun): the use of ultrasonic vibration to shatter and remove the lens clouded by a cataract.

**pharyngitis** (**far**-in-**JIGH**-tis): inflammation of the pharynx.

**phenylketonuria** (**fen**-il-**kee**-toh-**NEW**-ree-ah): a genetic disorder in which an essential digestive enzyme is missing.

**pheochromocytoma** (fee-oh-**kroh**-moh-sigh-**TOH**-mah): a benign tumor of the adrenal gland that causes the release of excess epinephrine and norepinephrine.

**phimosis** (figh-**MOH**-sis): narrowing of the opening of the foreskin so that it cannot be retracted to expose the glans penis.

**phlebitis** (fleh-**BYE**-tis): inflammation of a vein.

**phlebography** (fleh-**BOG**-rah-fee): a radiographic test that provides an image of veins after a contrast dye is injected.

**phlebotomy** (fleh-**BOT**-oh-mee): the puncture of a vein for the purpose of drawing blood.

**phlegm** (**FLEM**): thick mucus secreted by the tissues lining the respiratory passages.

**phobia** (**FOH**-bee-ah): a persistent irrational fear of a specific thing or situation strong enough to cause significant distress, interfere with functioning, and lead to avoidance of the thing or situation that causes this reaction.

**photocoagulation:** the use of lasers to treat some forms of wet macular degeneration by sealing leaking or damaged blood vessels.

**photodynamic therapy (foh-**toh-dye-**NAH-**mik**):** a technique used to treat damaged and precancerous skin, as well as various types of cancer.

**photophobia (foh-**toh-**FOH-**bee-ah**):** excessive sensitivity to light.

**photopsia (foh-TOP-**see-ah**):** presence of what appear to be flashes of light.

**physical therapy:** treatment to prevent disability or to restore function through the use of exercise, heat, massage, or other techniques.

**pica (PYE-**kah**):** an abnormal craving or appetite for nonfood substances such as dirt that lasts for at least one month.

**pigmented birthmarks:** irregularities in skin color, such as moles.

**pinealectomy (pin-**ee-al-**ECK-**toh-mee**):** the surgical removal of the pineal gland.

**pinealoma (pin-**ee-ah-**LOH-**mah**):** a tumor of the pineal gland.

**pituitary adenoma (ad-**eh-**NOH-**mah**):** a slow-growing, benign tumor of the pituitary gland that may or may not cause excess hormone secretion.

**placebo (plah-SEE-**boh**):** an inactive substance that is given for its suggestive effects.

**placenta previa (plah-SEN-**tah **PREE-**vee-ah**):** abnormal implantation of the placenta in the lower portion of the uterus.

**plantar fasciitis (PLAN-**tar **fas-**ee-**EYE-**tis**):** inflammation of the plantar fascia causing foot or heel pain when walking or running.

**plaque (PLACK):** a fatty deposit within the blood vessels; also a soft buildup of bacterial debris on the exterior of the teeth; also a scaly, solid, raised area of closely spaced papules on the skin.

**plasmapheresis (plaz-**mah-feh-**REE-**sis**):** the removal of whole blood from the body, separation of its cellular elements, and reinfusion of these cellular elements suspended in saline or a plasma substitute.

**platelet count:** a blood screening test that measures the number of platelets in a specified amount of blood.

**pleural effusion (eh-FEW-**zhun**):** the excess accumulation of fluid in the pleural space that prevents the lung from fully expanding.

**pleurisy (PLOOR-**ih-see**):** inflammation of the pleura that produces sharp chest pain with each breath.

**pleurodynia (ploor-**oh-**DIN-**ee-ah**):** pain in the pleura or in the side.

**pneumoconiosis (new-**moh-**koh-**nee-**OH-**sis**):** any fibrosis of the lung tissues caused by dust in the lungs after prolonged environmental or occupational contact.

**pneumocystis pneumonia (new-**moh-**SIS-**tis new-**MOH-**nee-ah**):** the form of pneumonia caused by an opportunistic infection with the fungus *Pneumocystis carinii.*

**pneumonectomy (new-**moh-**NECK-**toh-mee**):** the surgical removal of all or part of a lung.

**pneumonia (new-MOH-**nee-ah**):** a serious infection or inflammation of the lungs in which the alveoli and air passages fill with pus and other liquid.

**pneumorrhagia (new-**moh-**RAY-**jee-ah**):** bleeding from the lungs.

**pneumothorax (new-**moh-**THOR-**racks**):** the accumulation of air in the pleural space resulting in a pressure imbalance that causes the lung to fully or partially collapse.

**poliomyelitis (poh-**lee-oh-**my-**eh-**LYE-**tis**):** a highly contagious viral infection of the brainstem and spinal cord that sometimes leads to paralysis.

**polyarteritis (pol-**ee-**ar-**teh-**RYE-**tis**):** a form of vasculitis involving several medium and small arteries at the same time.

**polycystic kidney disease (pol-**ee-**SIS-**tick**):** a genetic disorder characterized by the growth of numerous fluid-filled cysts in the kidneys.

**polycystic ovary syndrome (pol-**ee-**SIS-**tick**):** condition caused by a hormonal imbalance in which the ovaries are enlarged by the presence of many cysts formed by incompletely developed follicles.

**polycythemia (pol-**ee-sy-**THEE-**mee-ah**):** an abnormal increase in the number of red cells in the blood due to excess production of these cells by the bone marrow.

**polydipsia (pol-**ee-**DIP-**see-ah**):** excessive thirst.

**polymenorrhea (pol-**ee-**men-**oh-**REE-**ah**):** abnormally frequent menstruation.

**polymyalgia rheumatica (pol-**ee-my-**AL-**jah roo-**MA-**tih-kah**):** a geriatric inflammatory disorder of the muscles and joints characterized by pain and stiffness.

**polymyositis (pol-**ee-**my-**oh-**SIGH-**tis**):** muscle disease characterized by the simultaneous inflammation and weakening of voluntary muscles in many parts of the body.

**polyp (POL-**ip**):** a mushroom-like growth from the surface of a mucous membrane.

**polyphagia (pol-**ee-**FAY-**jee-ah**):** excessive hunger.

**polysomnography (pol-**ee-som-**NOG-**rah-fee**):** the diagnostic measurement of physiological activity during sleep.

**polyuria (pol-**ee-**YOU-**ree-ah**):** excessive urination.

**port-wine stain:** a flat vascular birthmark made up of dilated blood capillaries.

**positron emission tomography:** an imaging technique that combines tomography with radionuclide tracers to produce enhanced images of selected body organs or areas.

**post-traumatic stress disorder:** the development of characteristic symptoms after a major traumatic event.

**prediabetes:** a condition in which the blood sugar level is higher than normal, but not high enough to be classified as type 2 diabetes.

**preeclampsia (pree-ee-KLAMP-see-ah):** a complication of pregnancy characterized by hypertension, edema, and proteinuria.

**pregnancy test:** a diagnostic test to is determine if a woman is pregnant.

**premature ejaculation:** a condition in which the male reaches climax too soon, usually before or shortly after penetration.

**premature infant:** a neonate born before the 37th week of gestation.

**premature menopause:** a condition in which the ovaries cease functioning before age 40.

**premenstrual dysphoric disorder:** a condition associated with severe emotional and physical problems linked to the menstrual cycle.

**premenstrual syndrome:** a group of symptoms experienced by some women within the two-week period before menstruation.

**prenatal influences:** the mother's health, behavior, and the prenatal medical care she does or does not receive before delivery.

**presbycusis (pres-beh-KOO-sis):** a gradual sensorineural hearing loss that occurs as the body ages.

**presbyopia (pres-bee-OH-pee-ah):** condition of common changes in the eyes that occur with aging.

**prescription drug:** a medication that can legally be dispensed only by a pharmacist with an order from a licensed professional.

**pressure sore:** an open ulcerated wound that is caused by prolonged pressure on an area of skin.

**priapism (PRYE-ah-piz-em):** a painful erection that lasts four hours or more, but is not accompanied by sexual excitement.

**primary bone cancer:** a relatively rare malignant tumor that originates in a bone.

**primary lymphedema:** a hereditary disorder in which swelling due to an abnormal accumulation of lymph within the tissues may appear at any time in life.

**primigravida (prye-mih-GRAV-ih-dah):** a woman during her first pregnancy.

**primipara (prye-MIP-ah-rah):** a woman who has borne one viable child.

**proctopexy (PROCK-toh-peck-see):** surgical fixation of a prolapsed rectum to an adjacent tissue or organ.

**professional palpation of the breast:** performed to feel the texture, size, and consistency of the breast.

**prolactinoma (proh-lack-tih-NOH-mah):** a benign tumor of the pituitary gland that causes it to produce too much prolactin.

**prone position:** position where the patient lies face down on the abdomen.

**prophylaxis (proh-fih-LACK-sis):** treatment, such as vaccination, intended to prevent a disease or stop it from spreading.

**prostate cancer:** cancer beginning in the prostate.

**prostatectomy (pros-tah-TECK-toh-mee):** surgical removal of all or part of the prostate gland.

**prostate-specific antigen:** a diagnostic blood test that is used to screen for prostate cancer.

**prostatism (PROS-tah-tizm):** a disorder resulting from compression or obstruction of the urethra due to benign prostatic hyperplasia.

**prostatitis (pros-tah-TYE-tis):** inflammation of the prostate gland.

**prosthesis (pros-THEE-sis):** a substitute for a diseased or missing body part.

**proteinuria (proh-tee-in-YOU-ree-ah):** the presence of an abnormal amount of protein in the urine.

**prothrombin time (proh-THROM-bin):** a blood test used to diagnose conditions associated with abnormalities of clotting time and to monitor anticoagulant therapy.

**proton pump inhibitors:** medications that decrease the amount of acid produced by the stomach.

**pruritus vulvae (proo-RYE-tus VUL-vee):** severe itching of the external female genitalia.

**psoriasis (soh-RYE-uh-sis):** a common skin disorder characterized by flare-ups in which red papules covered with silvery scales occur on the elbows, knees, scalp, back, or buttocks.

**psychoanalysis (sigh-koh-ah-NAL-ih-sis):** treatment based on the idea that mental disorders have underlying causes stemming from childhood and can only be overcome by gaining insight into one's feelings and patterns of behavior.

**psychotic disorder (sigh-KOT-ick):** a condition characterized by the loss of contact with reality and deterioration of normal social functioning.

**psychotropic drug** (**sigh**-koh-**TROP**-pick): a drug that acts primarily on the central nervous system, where it produces temporary changes affecting the mind, emotions, and behavior.

**ptosis** (**TOH**-sis): drooping of the upper eyelid that is usually due to paralysis.

**pulmonary edema** (eh-**DEE**-mah): an accumulation of fluid in the lung tissues.

**pulmonary embolism** (**EM**-boh-lizm): the sudden blockage of a pulmonary artery by foreign matter or by an embolus that has formed in the leg or pelvic region.

**pulmonary fibrosis** (figh-**BROH**-sis): the progressive formation of scar tissue in the lung, resulting in decreased lung capacity and increased difficulty in breathing.

**pulmonary function tests**: a group of tests that measure volume and flow of air by utilizing a spirometer.

**pulse oximeter** (ock-**SIM**-eh-ter): an external monitor that measures the oxygen saturation level in the blood.

**puncture wound**: a deep hole made by a sharp object such as a nail.

**purpura** (**PUR**-pew-rah): the appearance of multiple purple discolorations on the skin caused by bleeding underneath the skin.

**purulent** (**PYOU**-roo-lent): producing or containing pus.

**pustule** (**PUS**-tyoul): a small, circumscribed lesion containing pus.

**pyelitis** (pye-eh-**LYE**-tis): inflammation of the renal pelvis.

**pyelonephritis** (pye-eh-loh-neh-**FRY**-tis): inflammation of the renal pelvis and of the kidney.

**pyeloplasty** (**PYE**-eh-loh-**plas**-tee): the surgical repair of the ureter and renal pelvis.

**pyelotomy** (pye-eh-**LOT**-oh-mee): a surgical incision into the renal pelvis.

**pyoderma** (pye-oh-**DER**-mah): any acute, inflammatory, pus-forming bacterial skin infection such as impetigo.

**pyosalpinx** (pye-oh-**SAL**-pinks): an accumulation of pus in the fallopian tube.

**pyothorax** (pye-oh-**THOH**-racks): the presence of pus in the pleural cavity between the layers of pleural membrane.

**pyrosis** (pye-**ROH**-sis): the burning sensation caused by the return of acidic stomach contents into the esophagus.

**pyuria** (pye-**YOU**-ree-ah): the presence of pus in the urine.

## Q

**Qi Gong** (**CHEE**-gong): a Chinese system of movement, breathing techniques, and meditation.

**quadriplegia** (kwad-rih-**PLEE**-jee-ah): paralysis of all four extremities.

## R

**rabies** (**RAY**-beez): an acute viral infection transmitted to humans by the bite or saliva of an infected animal.

**radial keratotomy** (ker-ah-**TOT**-oh-mee): a surgical procedure to treat myopia.

**radiation therapy**: the treatment of cancers through the use of x-rays.

**radical hysterectomy**: the surgical removal of the ovaries and fallopian tubes, the uterus and cervix, plus nearby lymph nodes.

**radical mastectomy**: the surgical removal of an entire breast and many of the surrounding tissues.

**radiculitis** (rah-**dick**-you-**LYE**-tis): inflammation of the root of a spinal nerve that causes pain and numbness radiating down the affected limb.

**radioactive iodine treatment**: oral administration of radioactive iodine to destroy thyroid cells.

**radioactive iodine uptake test**: test using radioactive iodine administered orally to measure thyroid function.

**radiograph**: the image produced by the use of radiant energy to visualize conditions such as bone fractures; also known as x-rays.

**radiography**: the use of x-radiation to visualize hard-tissue internal structures.

**radiology** (ray-dee-**OL**-oh-jee): the use of radiant energy and radioactive substances in medicine for diagnosis and treatment.

**radiolucent** (ray-dee-oh-**LOO**-sent): a substance that allows x-rays to pass through and appears black or dark gray on the resulting film.

**radiopaque** (ray-dee-oh-**PAYK**): a substance that does not allow x-rays to pass through and appears white or light gray on the resulting film.

**rale** (**RAHL**): an abnormal crackle-like lung sound heard while breathing in.

**range of motion testing**: a diagnostic procedure to evaluate joint mobility and muscle strength.

**Raynaud's disease** (ray-**NOHZ**): a peripheral arterial occlusive disease in which intermittent attacks are triggered by cold or stress.

**rectal administration:** the insertion of medication into the rectum as either suppositories or liquid solutions.

**rectocele** (**RECK**-toh-seel)**:** a bulging of the front wall of the rectum into the vagina.

**recumbent** (ree-**KUM**-bent)**:** any position in which the patient is lying down.

**red blood cell count:** a blood test that is performed to determine the number of erythrocytes in the blood.

**refraction:** an examination procedure to determine an eye's refractive error so that the best corrective lenses can be prescribed.

**refractive disorder:** a focusing problem caused when the lens and cornea do not bend light so that it focuses properly on the retina.

**regurgitation** (ree-**gur**-jih-**TAY**-shun)**:** the return of swallowed food into the mouth.

**renal colic** (**REE**-nal **KOLL**-ick)**:** acute pain in the kidney area that is caused by blockage during the passage of a kidney stone.

**renal failure:** the inability of one or both of the kidneys to perform their functions.

**renal transplantation:** the grafting of a donor kidney into the body to replace the recipient's failed kidneys.

**repetitive stress disorders:** a variety of muscular conditions that result from repeated motions performed in the course of normal activities.

**respiratory failure** (RF)**:** a condition in which the level of oxygen in the blood becomes dangerously low or the level of carbon dioxide becomes dangerously high.

**restenosis:** the condition when an artery that has been opened by angioplasty closes again.

**restless legs syndrome** (RLS)**:** a neurological disorder characterized by uncomfortable feelings in the legs, producing a strong urge to move them.

**retinal detachment:** the separation of all of the light-sensitive retina from the choroid.

**retinal tear:** the separation of some of the light-sensitive retina from the choroid.

**retinitis pigmentosa** (ret-ih-**NIGH**-tis pig-men-**TOH**-sah)**:** a progressive degeneration of the retina that affects night and peripheral vision.

**retinoids** (**RET**-ih-noydz)**:** a class of chemical compounds derived from vitamin A that are used in skin care and treatment.

**retinopathy** (ret-ih-**NOP**-ah-thee)**:** any disease of the retina.

**retinopexy** (**RET**-ih-noh-**peck**-see)**:** treatment to reattach the detached area in a retinal detachment.

**retrograde ejaculation:** when an orgasm results in semen flowing backward into the bladder instead of out through the penis.

**retrograde urography:** a radiograph of the urinary system taken after a contrast medium has been placed in the urethra and caused to flow upward through the urinary tract.

**revision surgery:** the replacement of a worn or failed implant.

**Reye's syndrome:** a potentially serious or deadly disorder in children that is characterized by vomiting and confusion, sometimes following a viral illness for which the child was treated with aspirin.

**rheumatoid arthritis** (**ROO**-mah-toyd ar-**THRIGH**-tis)**:** a chronic autoimmune disorder in which the synovial membranes, and other body tissues, are inflamed and thickened.

**rhinitis** (rye-**NIGH**-tis)**:** inflammation of the nose.

**rhinophyma** (rye-noh-**FIGH**-muh)**:** hyperplasia of the tissues of the nose.

**rhinorrhea** (rye-noh-**REE**-ah)**:** the watery flow of mucus from the nose.

**rhonchi** (**RONG**-kye)**:** a coarse rattling sound somewhat like snoring, usually caused by secretions in the bronchial airways.

**rhytidectomy** (rit-ih-**DECK**-toh-mee)**:** the surgical removal of excess skin and fat from the face to eliminate wrinkles.

**rickets** (**RICK**-ets)**:** a deficiency disease occurring in children involving defective bone growth due to vitamin D deficiency.

**rickettsia** (rih-**KET**-see-ah)**:** a small bacterium that lives in lice, fleas, ticks, and mites.

**rosacea** (roh-**ZAY**-shee-ah)**:** a chronic condition of unknown cause that produces tiny red pimples, and broken blood vessels.

**rotator cuff tendinitis** (ten-dih-**NIGH**-tis)**:** inflammation of the tendons of the rotator cuff.

**rubella** (roo-**BELL**-ah)**:** a viral infection characterized by a low-grade fever, swollen glands, inflamed eyes, and a fine, pink rash.

**ruptured rotator cuff:** develops when rotator cuff tendinitis is left untreated or if the overuse continues. This occurs as the irritated tendon weakens and tears.

# S

**salmonellosis** (sal-moh-nel-**LOH**-sis)**:** an infectious disease transmitted by feces, either through direct contact or by eating contaminated raw or undercooked food.

**salpingectomy (sal-pin-JECK-toh-mee):** surgical removal of one or both fallopian tubes.

**salpingitis (sal-pin-JIGH-tis):** inflammation of a fallopian tube.

**salpingo-oophorectomy (sal-ping-goh oh-ahf-oh-RECK-toh-mee):** the surgical removal of a fallopian tube and ovary.

**sarcoma (sar-KOH-mah):** a malignant tumor that arises from connective tissues.

**sarcopenia (sar-koh-PEE-nee-ah):** the loss of muscle mass, strength, and function that comes with aging.

**scabies (SKAY-beez):** a skin infection caused by an infestation of itch mites.

**scales:** flakes or dry patches made up of excess dead epidermal cells.

**schizophrenia (skit-soh-FREE-nee-ah):** a psychotic disorder characterized by withdrawal from reality, illogical patterns of thinking, delusions, and hallucinations.

**sciatica (sigh-AT-ih-kah):** inflammation of the sciatic nerve that results in pain, burning, and tingling along the course of the affected nerve.

**scleral buckle (SKLER-al):** a silicone band or sponge used to repair a detached retina.

**scleritis (skleh-RYE-tis):** inflammation of the sclera of the eye.

**scleroderma (sklehr-oh-DER-mah):** an autoimmune disorder in which the connective tissues become thickened and hardened, causing the skin to become hard and swollen.

**sclerotherapy (sklehr-oh-THER-ah-pee):** treatment of spider veins by injecting a saline sclerosing solution into the vein.

**scoliosis (skoh-lee-OH-sis):** an abnormal lateral curvature of the spine.

**scotoma (skoh-TOH-mah):** an abnormal area of diminished vision surrounded by an area of normal vision.

**seasonal affective disorder:** a seasonal bout of depression associated with the decrease in hours of daylight during winter months.

**sebaceous cyst (seh-BAY-shus):** a closed sac associated with a sebaceous gland that is found just under the skin.

**seborrhea (seb-oh-REE-ah):** overactivity of the sebaceous glands that results in the production of an excessive amount of sebum.

**seborrheic dermatitis (seb-oh-REE-ick der-mah-TYE-tis):** inflammation that causes scaling and itching of the upper layers of the skin or scalp.

**seborrheic keratosis (seb-oh-REE-ick kerr-ah-TOH-sis):** a benign skin growth that has a waxy or "pasted-on" look.

**secondary bone cancer:** tumors that have metastasized to bones from other organs such as the breasts and lungs.

**secondary lymphedema:** swelling of the tissues due to an abnormal accumulation of lymph within the tissues that is the result of damage to lymphatic vessels.

**sedative:** medication that depresses the central nervous system to produce calm and diminished responsiveness without producing sleep.

**seizure (SEE-zhur):** a sudden surge of electrical activity in the brain that affects how a person feels or acts for a short time.

**sensorineural hearing loss:** hearing loss that develops when the auditory nerve or hair cells in the inner ear are damaged.

**septicemia (sep-tih-SEE-mee-ah):** caused by the presence of bacteria in the blood, symptoms include fever, tachypnea, and tachycardia.

**septoplasty (SEP-toh-plas-tee):** the surgical repair or alteration of parts of the nasal septum.

**septic shock:** a serious condition that occurs when an overwhelming bacterial infection affects the body.

**serum bilirubin test:** a blood test that measures the ability of the liver to take up, process, and secrete bilirubin into the bile.

**sexually transmitted diseases:** infections caused by either a bacteria or a virus transmitted through sexual intercourse or other genital contact.

**shaken baby syndrome:** describes the results of a child being violently shaken by someone.

**shin splint:** pain caused by the muscle tearing away from the tibia.

**short stature:** condition resulting from the failure of the bones of the limbs to grow to an appropriate length compared to the size of the head and trunk.

**sickle cell anemia:** a genetic disorder that causes abnormal hemoglobin, resulting in red blood cells that assume an abnormal sickle shape.

**sigmoidoscopy (sig-moi-DOS-koh-pee):** the endoscopic examination of the interior of the rectum, sigmoid colon, and possibly a portion of the descending colon.

**sign:** objective evidence of disease, such as a fever.

**silicosis (sill-ih-KOH-sis):** the form of pneumoconiosis caused by inhaling silica dust in the lungs.

**Sims' position:** an examination position in which the patient is lying on the left side with the right knee and thigh drawn up with the left arm placed along the back.

**single photon emission computed tomography:** a type of nuclear imaging test that produces 3D computer-reconstructed images showing perfusion through tissues and organs.

**singultus** (sing-**GUL**-tus): myoclonus of the diaphragm that causes the characteristic hiccup sound with each spasm.

**sinusitis** (**sigh**-nuh-**SIGH**-tis): an inflammation of the sinuses.

**skeletal muscle relaxant:** administered to relax certain muscles and to relieve the stiffness, pain, and discomfort caused by strains, sprains, or other muscle injuries.

**skin cancer:** a harmful, malignant growth on the skin, which can have many causes, including repeated severe sunburns or long-term exposure to the sun.

**skin tags:** benign small flesh-colored or light-brown polyps that hang from the body by fine stalks.

**sleep apnea** (**AP-nee-ah**): a potentially serious disorder in which breathing repeatedly stops during sleep for long enough periods to cause a measurable decrease in blood oxygen levels.

**sleep deprivation:** a sufficient lack of restorative sleep over a cumulative period so as to cause physical or psychiatric symptoms and affect routine performance or tasks.

**sleep hyperhidrosis:** the occurrence of hyperhidrosis during sleep.

**slit-lamp ophthalmoscopy** (**ahf**-thal-**MOS**-koh-pee): a diagnostic procedure in which a narrow beam of light is focused to permit the ophthalmologist to examine the structures at the front of the eye including the cornea, iris, and lens.

**smoke inhalation:** damage to the lungs in which particles from a fire coat the alveoli and prevent normal exchange of gases.

**SOAP note:** an acronym for subjective, objective, assessment, and plan.

**social phobia:** excessive fear of social situations where the person fears negative evaluation by others or embarrassing himself in front of others.

**somatoform disorders** (soh-**MAT**-oh-**form**): conditions that are characterized by physical complaints or concerns about one's body that are out of proportion to any physical findings or disease.

**somnambulism** (som-**NAM**-byou-lizm): the condition of walking or performing some other activity without awakening.

**spasm:** a sudden, involuntary contraction of one or more muscles.

**spasmodic torticollis** (spaz-**MOD**-ick **tor**-tih-**KOL**-is): a stiff neck due to spasmodic contraction of the neck muscles that pull the head toward the affected side.

**speculum** (**SPECK**-you-lum): an instrument used to enlarge the opening of any canal or cavity to facilitate inspection of its interior.

**spermatocele** (sper-**MAH**-toh-seel): a cyst that develops in the epididymis and is filled with a milky fluid containing sperm.

**sperm count:** the testing of freshly ejaculated semen to determine the volume plus the number, shape, size, and motility of the sperm.

**sphygmomanometer** (**sfig**-moh-mah-**NOM**-eh-ter): an instrument used to measure blood pressure.

**spina bifida** (**SPY**-nah **BIF**-ih-dah): a congenital defect that occurs during early pregnancy in which the spinal canal fails to close completely around the spinal cord.

**spinal anesthesia:** regional anesthesia produced by injecting medication into the subarachnoid space.

**spinal cord injury:** paralysis resulting from damage to the spinal cord that prevents nerve impulses from being transmitted below the level of the injury.

**spinal fusion:** a technique to immobilize part of the spine by joining together two or more vertebrae.

**spiral fracture:** a fracture in which the bone has been twisted apart.

**spirochetes** (**SPY**-roh-keets): long, slender spiral-shaped bacteria that have flexible walls and are capable of movement.

**spirometer** (spih-**ROM**-eh-ter): a recording device that measures the amount of air inhaled or exhaled (volume) and the length of time required for each breath.

**splenomegaly** (splee-noh-**MEG**-ah-lee): an abnormal enlargement of the spleen.

**splenorrhagia** (splee-noh-**RAY**-jee-ah): bleeding from the spleen.

**spondylolisthesis** (**spon**-dih-loh-liss-**THEE**-sis): the forward slipping movement of the body of one of the lower lumbar vertebrae on the vertebra below it.

**spondylosis** (**spon**-dih-**LOH**-sis): a degenerative disorder that can cause the loss of normal spinal structure and function.

**sprain:** an injury to a joint, such as ankle, knee, or wrist, that usually involves a wrenched or torn ligament.

**sputum** (**SPYOU**-tum): phlegm ejected through the mouth that can be examined for diagnostic purposes.

**squamous cell carcinoma** (**SKWAY**-mus): a malignant tumor of the scaly squamous cells of the epithelium that can quickly spread to other body systems.

**staging:** the process of classifying tumors by how far the disease has progressed, the potential for its responding to therapy, and the patient's prognosis.

**stapedectomy (stay-peh-DECK-toh-mee):** the surgical removal of the top portion of the stapes bone and the insertion of a prosthetic device that conducts sound vibrations to the inner ear.

**staphylococci (staf-ih-loh-KOCK-sigh):** a group of about 30 species of bacteria that form irregular groups or clusters resembling grapes.

**steatorrhea (stee-at-oh-REE-ah):** the presence of excess fat in the stool.

**stent:** a wire-mesh tube that is implanted in a coronary artery to provide support to the arterial wall.

**sterilization:** any procedure rendering an individual (male or female) incapable of reproduction.

**stethoscope (STETH-oh-skope):** an instrument used to listen to sounds within the body.

**stillbirth:** the birth of a fetus that died before or during delivery.

**stimulant:** a substance that works by increasing activity in certain areas of the brain to increase concentration and wakefulness.

**stomatitis (stoh-mah-TYE-tis):** inflammation of the mucosa of the mouth.

**stomatomycosis (stoh-mah-toh-my-KOH-sis):** any disease of the mouth due to a fungus.

**stone:** an abnormal mineral deposit that has formed within the body.

**stool samples:** specimens of feces that are examined for content and characteristics.

**strabismus (strah-BIZ-mus):** a disorder in which the eyes point in different directions or are not aligned correctly because the eye muscles are unable to focus together.

**strain:** an injury to the body of a muscle or the attachment of a tendon.

**strangulated hernia:** a condition that occurs when a portion of the intestine is constricted inside the hernia and its blood supply is cut off.

**streptococci (strep-toh-KOCK-sigh):** bacteria that form a chain. Many are harmless; however, other members of this group are responsible for illnesses including strep throat.

**stress fracture:** a small crack in a bone that often develops from chronic, excessive impact.

**stress incontinence:** the inability to control the voiding of urine under physical stress such as running, sneezing, laughing, or coughing.

**stress test:** the use of electrocardiography to assess cardiovascular health and function during and after stress such as exercise on a treadmill.

**stridor (STRYE-dor):** an abnormal, high-pitched, musical breathing sound caused by a blockage in the throat or larynx.

**stupor (STOO-per):** an unresponsive state from which a person can be aroused only briefly despite vigorous, repeated attempts.

**subconjunctival hemorrhage:** bleeding between the conjunctiva and the sclera.

**subcutaneous injection:** the administration of medication by injection into the fatty layer just below the skin.

**sublingual administration:** the placement of medication under the tongue where it is allowed to dissolve slowly.

**subluxation (sub-luck-SAY-shun):** the partial displacement of a bone from its joint.

**substance abuse:** the addictive use of tobacco, alcohol, medications, or illegal drugs.

**sudden cardiac death:** results when treatment of cardiac arrest is not provided within a few minutes.

**sudden infant death syndrome:** the sudden and unexplainable death of an apparently healthy sleeping infant between the ages of two and six months.

**sunscreen:** blocks the harmful ultraviolet B rays, measured in terms of the strength of the sun protection factor (SPF).

**supplemental oxygen:** administered when the patient is unable to maintain an adequate oxygen saturation level in the blood from breathing normal air.

**suppuration (sup-you-RAY-shun):** the formation or discharge of pus.

**suprapubic catheterization (soo-prah-PYOU-bick):** the placement of a catheter into the bladder through a small incision made through the abdominal wall just above the pubic bone.

**surgical biopsy (BYE-op-see):** the removal of a small piece of tissue for examination to confirm a diagnosis.

**symptom (SIMP-tum):** subjective evidence of a disease, such as pain or a headache.

**syncope (SIN-koh-pee):** the brief loss of consciousness caused by the decreased flow of blood to the brain.

**syndrome (SIN-drohm):** a set of signs and symptoms that occur together as part of a specific disease process.

**syndrome of inappropriate antidiuretic hormone:** overproduction of the antidiuretic hormone ADH, leading to bloating, water retention, and electrolyte imbalance.

**synovectomy** (sin-oh-**VECK**-toh-mee): the surgical removal of a synovial membrane from a joint.

**synovial sarcoma** (sih-**NOH**-vee-al sar-**KOH**-mah): a tumor of the tissues surrounding a synovial joint.

**synovitis** (sin-oh-**VYE**-tiss): inflammation of the synovial membrane that results in swelling and pain of the affected joint.

**synthetic immunoglobulins:** a post-exposure preventive measure against certain viruses including rabies and some types of hepatitis.

**synthetic interferon:** medication administered to treat multiple sclerosis, hepatitis C, and some cancers.

**synthetic thyroid hormones:** medications administered to replace lost thyroid function.

**syphilis** (**SIF**-ih-lis): a sexually transmitted disease that is caused by the bacterium *Treponema pallidum*.

**systemic lupus erythematosus:** an autoimmune disorder characterized by a red, scaly rash on the face and upper trunk that also attacks the connective tissue in other body systems.

# T

**tachycardia** (**tack**-ee-**KAR**-dee-ah): an abnormally rapid resting heartbeat usually at a rate of more than 100 beats per minute.

**tachypnea** (**tack**-ihp-**NEE**-ah): an abnormally rapid rate of respiration usually of more than 20 breaths per minute.

**talipes** (**TAL**-ih-peez): any congenital deformity of the foot involving the ankle bones.

**targeted therapy:** a developing form of anti-cancer drug therapy that uses drugs or other substances to identify and attack specific cancer cells without harming normal cells.

**tarsorrhaphy** (tahr-**SOR**-ah-fee): the partial or complete suturing together of the upper and lower eyelids.

**Tay-Sachs disease:** a fatal genetic disorder in which harmful quantities of a fatty substance build up in tissues and nerve cells in the brain.

**teletherapy** (**tel**-eh-**THER**-ah-pee): radiation therapy administered at a distance from the body that is precisely targeted with the use of three-dimensional computer imaging.

**temporal arteritis** (**TEM**-poh-**ral ar**-teh-**RYE**-tis): a form of vasculitis with abnormally large cells, that can cause headache, visual impairment, or other symptoms.

**tendinitis** (**ten**-dih-**NIGH**-itis): inflammation of the tendons caused by excessive or unusual use of the joint.

**tenodesis** (ten-**ODD**-eh-sis): surgical suturing of the end of a tendon to bone.

**tenolysis** (ten-**OL**-ih-sis): the release of a tendon from adhesions.

**tenorrhaphy** (ten-**OR**-ah-fee): surgical suturing of the divided ends of a tendon.

**tenosynovitis** (**ten**-oh-**sin**-oh-**VYE**-tis): inflammation of the sheath around a tendon.

**testicular cancer:** cancer that begins in the testicles.

**testicular self-examination:** a self-help step in early detection of testicular cancer by detecting lumps, swelling, or changes in the skin of the scrotum.

**testicular torsion:** a sharp pain in the scrotum caused by twisting of the vas deferens and blood vessels leading into the testicle.

**testitis** (test-**TYE**-tis): inflammation of one or both testicles.

**tetanus** (**TET**-ah-nus): an acute and potentially fatal infection of the central nervous system caused by a toxin produced by the tetanus bacteria.

**thalamotomy** (thal-ah-**MOT**-oh-mee): a surgical incision into the thalamus.

**thalassemia** (thal-ah-**SEE**-mee-ah): an inherited blood disorder that causes mild or severe anemia due to reduced hemoglobin and fewer red blood cells than normal.

**thallium stress test** (**THAL**-ee-um): performed to evaluate blood flow to the heart during exercise by injecting a small amount of thallium into the blood.

**therapeutic ultrasound:** the use of high-frequency sound waves to treat muscle injuries by generating heat deep within muscle tissue.

**thoracentesis** (**thoh**-rah-sen-**TEE**-sis): the surgical puncture of the chest wall with a needle to obtain fluid from the pleural cavity.

**thoracotomy** (**thoh**-rah-**KOT**-toh-mee): a surgical incision into the chest walls to open the pleural cavity for biopsy or treatment.

**thrombocytopenia** (**throm**-boh-**sigh**-toh-**PEE**-nee-ah): a condition in which there is an abnormally small number of platelets circulating in the blood.

**thrombocytosis** (**throm**-boh-sigh-**TOH**-sis): an abnormal increase in the number of platelets in the circulating blood.

**thrombolytic** (**throm**-boh-**LIT**-ick): medication that dissolves or causes a thrombus to break up.

**thrombosis** (throm-**BOH**-sis): the abnormal condition of having a thrombus.

**thrombotic occlusion** (throm-**BOT**-ick ah-**KLOO**-zhun): the blocking of an artery by a thrombus.

**thrombus** (**THROM**-bus): a blood clot attached to the interior wall of an artery or vein.

**thymectomy** (thigh-**MECK**-toh-mee): the surgical removal of the thymus gland.

**thymitis** (thigh-**MY**-tis): inflammation of the thymus gland.

**thyroid carcinoma:** cancer of the thyroid gland.

**thyroid scan:** a specialized nuclear scan to evaluate thyroid function.

**thyroid-stimulating hormone assay:** a diagnostic test to measure the circulating blood level of thyroid-stimulating hormone.

**thyroid storm:** a relatively rare, life-threatening condition caused by exaggerated hyperthyroidism.

**tinea** (**TIN**-ee-ah): a fungal infection that can grow on the skin, hair, or nails.

**tinnitus** (tih-**NIGH**-tus): a condition of ringing, buzzing, or roaring sound in one or both ears.

**tissue plasminogen activator** (plaz-**MIN**-oh-jen): a thrombolytic administered to some patients having a heart attack or stroke to dissolve damaging blood clots.

**tolerance:** acquired unresponsiveness to a specific antigen or decline in effective response to a drug usually due to repeated use.

**tomotherapy:** combination of tomography with radiation therapy to precisely target tumors.

**tonic-clonic seizure:** a type of seizure involving the whole body.

**tonometry** (toh-**NOM**-eh-tree): the measurement of intraocular pressure.

**tonsillectomy** (**ton**-sih-**LECK**-toh-mee): the surgical removal of the tonsils.

**tonsillitis** (**ton**-sih-**LYE**-tis): inflammation of the tonsils.

**topical application:** liquid or ointment rubbed into the skin on the area to be treated.

**topical steroids:** steroids used in treatment of various skin disorders and diseases.

**total hemoglobin test:** a blood test that measures the amount of hemoglobin found in whole blood.

**total hip replacement** (THR): surgery performed to restore a damaged hip to full function by removing the head of the femur and replacing it with a metal ball.

**total hysterectomy:** the removal of the uterus and cervix, either through the vagina or laparoscopically through the abdomen.

**total knee replacement:** surgical placement of an artificial joint during which all parts of the knee are replaced.

**total parenteral nutrition** (pah-**REN**-ter-al): a specialized solution administered intravenously to patients who cannot or should not get their nutrition through eating.

**Tourette syndrome** (tuh **RET**): a complex neurological disorder characterized by involuntary tics, grunts, and compulsive utterances.

**toxoplasmosis** (**tock**-soh-plaz-**MOH**-sis): a parasite most commonly transmitted from animals (pets) to humans by contact with contaminated feces.

**tracheorrhagia** (tray-kee-oh-**RAY**-jee-ah): bleeding from the mucous membranes of the trachea.

**tracheostomy** (tray-kee-**OS**-toh-mee): the surgical creation of a stoma into the trachea in order to insert a tube to facilitate breathing.

**tracheotomy** (tray-kee-**OT**-oh-mee): an emergency procedure in which an incision is made into the trachea to gain access to the airway below a blockage.

**traction:** a pulling force exerted on a limb in a distal direction in an effort to return the bone or joint to normal alignment.

**traditional Chinese medicine:** a system of ancient Chinese medicinal treatments, including acupuncture, to prevent, diagnose, and treat disease.

**transcutaneous electronic nerve stimulation:** a method of pain control by wearing a device that delivers small electrical impulses to the nerve endings through the skin.

**transdermal:** the administration of medication through the unbroken skin so that it is absorbed continuously to produce a systemic effect.

**transesophageal echocardiography** (trans-eh-sof-ah-**JEE**-al eck-oh-**kar**-dee-**OG**-rah-fee): an ultrasonic imaging technique that is performed from inside the esophagus to evaluate heart structures.

**transfusion reaction:** a serious and potentially fatal complication of a blood transfusion in which a severe immune response occurs because the patient's blood and the donated blood do not match.

**transient ischemic attack:** a temporary interruption in the blood supply to the brain.

**transurethral prostatectomy:** the removal of excess tissue from an enlarged prostate gland with the use of a resectoscope.

**transverse fracture:** a fracture that occurs straight across the bone.

**trauma** (**TRAW**-mah): wound or injury.

**traumatic brain injury:** a blow to the head or a penetrating head injury that damages the brain.

**triage** (tree-**AHZH**): the medical screening of patients to determine their relative priority of need and the proper place of treatment.

**trichomoniasis** (**trick**-oh-moh-**NYE**-ah-sis): a sexually transmitted infection caused by the parasite *Trichomonas vaginalis*.

**trichomycosis axillaris** (**try**-koh-my-**KOH**-sis **ak**-sih-**LAH**-ris): superficial bacterial infection of the hair shafts in areas with extensive sweat glands such as the armpits.

**trigeminal neuralgia** (try-**JEM**-ih-nal new-**RAL**-jee-ah): inflammation of the fifth cranial nerve characterized by sudden, intense, brief attacks of sharp pain on one side of the face.

**trismus** (**TRIZ**-mus): any restriction to the opening of the mouth caused by trauma, surgery, or radiation associated with the treatment of oral cancer.

**tubal ligation:** a surgical procedure performed for the purpose of female sterilization.

**tuberculin skin testing:** a screening test for tuberculosis in which the skin of the arm is injected with a harmless antigen extracted from the TB bacteria.

**tuberculosis** (too-**ber**-kew-**LOH**-sis): an infectious disease caused by *Mycobacterium tuberculosis* that usually attacks the lungs.

**tumor:** an abnormal growth of body tissue in which the multiplication of cells is uncontrolled, abnormal, rapid, and progressive; also known as a neoplasm.

**tympanometry** (**tim**-pah-**NOM**-eh-tree): the use of air pressure in the ear canal to test for disorders of the middle ear.

**tympanoplasty** (**tim**-pah-noh-**PLAS**-tee): the surgical correction of a damaged middle ear that is performed either to cure chronic inflammation or to restore function.

**type 1 diabetes:** an autoimmune insulin deficiency disorder caused by the destruction of pancreatic islet beta cells.

**type 2 diabetes:** an insulin resistance disorder in which, although insulin is being produced, the body does not use it effectively.

# U

**ulcer** (**UL**-ser): an open lesion of the skin or mucous membrane resulting in tissue loss around the edges.

**ulcerative colitis** (**UL**-ser-**ay**-tiv koh-**LYE**-tis): a chronic condition of unknown cause in which repeated episodes of inflammation in the rectum and large intestine cause ulcers and irritation.

**ultrasonic bone density testing:** a screening test for osteoporosis or other conditions that cause a loss of bone mass.

**ultrasonography** (**ul**-trah-son-**OG**-rah-fee): the imaging of deep body structures by recording the echoes of sound wave pulses that are above the range of human hearing; also known as ultrasound.

**unconscious:** a state of being unaware and unable to respond to any stimuli including pain.

**upper GI series** and **lower GI series:** radiographic studies to examine the digestive system. A contrast medium is used to make these structures visible.

**upper respiratory infection:** a term used to describe the common cold.

**uremia** (you-**REE**-mee-ah): a toxic condition in which urea and other waste products normally excreted in the urine are retained in the blood.

**ureterectasis** (you-**reh**-ter-**ECK**-tah-sis): the distention of a ureter.

**ureterectomy** (**you**-reh-ter-**ECK**-toh-mee): the surgical removal of a ureter.

**ureterolith** (you-**REE**-ter-oh-**lith**): a stone located anywhere along the ureter.

**ureteroplasty** (you-**REET**-er-oh-**plas**-tee): the surgical repair of a ureter.

**ureterorrhagia** (you-**ree**-ter-oh-**RAY**-jee-ah): the discharge of blood from the ureter.

**ureterorrhaphy** (you-**reet**-eh-**ROAR**-ah-fee): surgical suturing of a ureter.

**ureteroscopy** (you-**reet**-eh-**ROS**-koh-pee): a treatment for a stone lodged in the ureter.

**urethral catheterization:** the insertion of a tube through the urethra and into the bladder.

**urethritis** (**you**-reh-**THRIGH**-tis): inflammation of the urethra.

**urethropexy** (you-**REE**-throh-**peck**-see): surgical fixation of the urethra to nearby tissue.

**urethrorrhagia** (you-**ree**-throh-**RAY**-jee-ah): bleeding from the urethra.

**urethrorrhea** (you-**ree**-throh-**REE**-ah): abnormal discharge from the urethra.

**urethrostenosis** (you-**ree**-throh-steh-**NOH**-sis): abnormal narrowing of the urethra.

**urethrotomy** (**you**-reh-**THROT**-oh-mee): a surgical incision into the urethra.

**urinalysis** (**you**-rih-**NAL**-ih-sis): the examination of urine to determine the presence of abnormal elements.

**urinary catheterization** (**kath**-eh-ter-eye-**ZAY**-shun): the insertion of a tube into the bladder in order to obtain a sterile specimen or drain urine.

**urinary hesitancy:** difficulty in starting a urinary stream.

**urinary incontinence:** the inability to control the voiding of urine.

**urinary retention:** the inability to completely empty the bladder when attempting to urinate.

**urinary tract infection:** an infection involving the structures of the urinary system that usually begins in the bladder.

**urticaria (ur-tih-KARE-ree-ah):** itchy wheals caused by an allergic reaction.

**uterine fibroid:** a benign tumor composed of muscle and fibrous tissue that occurs in the wall of the uterus.

**uterine prolapse (proh-LAPS):** the condition in which the uterus slides from its normal position in the pelvic cavity and sags into the vagina.

**uveitis (you-vee-EYE-tis):** inflammation of the uvea causing swelling and irritation.

# V

**vaginal candidiasis (kan-dih-DYE-ah-sis):** a vaginal infection caused by *Candida albicans.*

**vaginitis (vaj-ih-NIGH-tis):** inflammation of the lining of the vagina.

**valvoplasty (VAL-voh-plas-tee):** the surgical repair or replacement of a heart valve.

**valvular prolapse (VAL-voo-lar proh-LAPS):** the abnormal protrusion of a heart valve that results in the inability of the valve to close completely.

**valvular stenosis (steh-NOH-sis):** a condition in which there is narrowing, stiffening, thickening, or blockage of one or more valves of the heart.

**valvulitis (val-view-LYE-tis):** an inflammation of a heart valve.

**varicella (var-ih-SEL-ah):** a highly contagious infection caused by the herpes virus *Varicella zoster*; also known as chickenpox.

**varicocele (VAR-ih-koh-seel):** a knot of varicose veins in one side of the scrotum.

**varicocelectomy (var-ih-koh-sih-LECK-toh-mee):** the removal of a portion of an enlarged vein to relieve a varicocele.

**varicose veins (VAR-ih-kohs VAYNS):** abnormally swollen veins usually occurring in the superficial veins of the legs.

**vascular birthmarks:** birthmarks caused by blood vessels close to the skin's surface.

**vascular dementia:** a form of dementia caused by a restriction of blood to the brain.

**vasculitis (vas-kyou-LYE-tis):** inflammation of a blood or lymph vessel.

**vasectomy (vah-SECK-toh-mee):** the male sterilization procedure in which a small portion of the vas deferens is surgically removed.

**vasoconstrictor (vas-oh-kon-STRICK-tor):** medication that causes blood vessels to narrow.

**vasodilator (vas-oh-dye-LAYT-or):** medication that causes blood vessels to expand.

**vasovasostomy (vay-soh-vah-ZOS-toh-mee):** a procedure performed as an attempt to restore fertility to a vasectomized male.

**vector-borne transmission:** the spread of certain disease due to the bite of a vector (insects or animals that are capable of transmitting a disease).

**ventilator:** a mechanical device for artificial respiration that is used to replace or supplement the patient's natural breathing function.

**ventricular fibrillation (ven-TRICK-you-lar fih-brih-LAY-shun):** rapid, irregular, and useless contractions of the ventricles.

**ventricular tachycardia (ven-TRICK-you-lar tack-ee-KAR-dee-ah):** a very rapid heartbeat that begins within the ventricles.

**verrucae (veh-ROO-kee):** small, hard skin lesions caused by the human papillomavirus.

**vertigo (VER-tih-goh):** a sense of whirling, dizziness, and the loss of balance, often combined with nausea and vomiting.

**vesicle (VES-ih-kul):** a small blister, less than 0.5 cm in diameter, containing watery fluid.

**vesicovaginal fistula (ves-ih-koh-VAJ-ih-nahl FIS-tyou-lah):** an abnormal opening between the bladder and vagina.

**vestibular rehabilitation therapy (ves-TIB-you-lar):** a form of physical therapy designed to treat a wide variety of balance disorders.

**video-assisted thoracic surgery (VATS):** the use of a thoracoscope to view the inside of the pleural cavity through very small incisions.

**viral (VYE-ral):** pertaining to a virus.

**viral pneumonia:** caused by several different types of viruses, accounts for approximately a third of all pneumonias.

**viruses (VYE-rus-ez):** very small infectious agents that live only by invading other cells.

**viscosupplementation (vis-ko-sup-leh-men-TAY-shun):** injections to add fluid to a joint.

**visual acuity (ah-KYOU-ih-tee):** the ability to distinguish object details and shape at a distance.

**visual field testing:** a diagnostic test to determine losses in peripheral vision.

**vitiligo (vit-ih-LYE-goh):** a skin condition resulting from the destruction of melanocytes due to unknown causes, resulting in irregular patches of white skin.

**vitrectomy** (vih-**TRECK**-toh-mee)**:** the removal of the vitreous humor and its replacement with a clear solution.

**voiding cystourethrography** (**sis**-toh-you-ree-**THROG**-rah-fee)**:** a diagnostic procedure in which a fluoroscope is used to examine the flow of urine from the bladder and through the urethra.

**volvulus** (**VOL**-view-lus)**:** twisting of the intestine on itself, causing an obstruction.

**vulvitis** (vul-**VYE**-tis)**:** inflammation of the vulva.

**vulvodynia** (vul-voh-**DIN**-ee-ah)**:** a painful syndrome of unknown cause characterized by chronic burning, pain during sexual intercourse, itching, or stinging irritation of the vulva.

# W

**walking pneumonia:** a milder but longer-lasting form of pneumonia caused by the bacteria *Mycoplasma pneumoniae.*

**Weber and Rinne tests:** hearing tests that use a tuning fork to distinguish between conductive and sensorineural hearing losses.

**wedge resection:** a surgery in which a small wedge-shaped piece of cancerous lung tissue is removed, along with a margin of healthy tissue around the cancer.

**western blot test:** a blood test to confirm the diagnosis of HIV.

**West Nile virus:** a viral infection that causes flu-like symptoms, transmitted to humans by mosquito bites.

**wheal** (**WHEEL**)**:** a small bump that itches.

**white blood cell count:** a blood test to determine the number of leukocytes in the blood.

**white blood cell differential:** a blood test to determine what percentage of the total white blood cell count is composed of each of the five types of leukocytes.

**Wilms tumor:** a rare type of malignant tumor of the kidney that occurs in young children.

# X

**xeroderma** (zee-roh-**DER**-mah)**:** excessively dry skin.

**xerophthalmia** (**zeer**-ahf-**THAL**-mee-ah)**:** drying of eye surfaces, including the conjunctiva.

**xerostomia** (**zeer**-oh-**STOH**-mee-ah)**:** the lack of adequate saliva due to diminished secretions by the salivary glands.

# Y

**yeast:** a type of fungus.

# Index

# F

## H

## I

# P

# Flash Cards

## ■ INSTRUCTIONS

- Carefully remove the flash card pages from the workbook, and separate them to create 160 flash cards.

- There are three types of cards: **prefixes** (such as **a-** and **hyper-**), **suffixes** (such as **-graphy** and **-rrhagia**), and **word roots/combining forms** (such as **gastr/o** and **arthr/o**). All of the cards have the definition on the back. Prefixes and suffixes also have the type of word part listed on the front of each card.

- The word root/combining form cards are arranged by body systems. This allows you to sort out the cards you want to study based on where you are in the book. Use the "general" cards throughout your course.

- Use the flash cards to memorize word parts, to test yourself, and for periodic review.

- By putting cards together, you can create terms just as you did in the challenge word building exercises.

- You can create flash cards for word parts that are not already included by using the page of blank cards at the back. For additional cards, we recommend sheets of perforated business card stock available at any office supply store.

## ■ WORD PART GAMES

Here are games you can play with one or more partners to help you learn word parts using your flash cards.

### The Review Game

**Word Parts Up:** Shuffle the deck of flash cards. Put the pile, *word parts up*, in the center of the desk. Take turns choosing a card from anywhere in the deck and giving the definition of the word part shown. If you get it right, you get to keep it. If you miss, it goes into the discard pile. When the draw pile is gone, whoever has the largest pile wins.

**Definitions Up:** Shuffle the deck of flash cards and place them with the *definition side up*. Play the review game the same way.

### The Create-a-Word Game

Shuffle the deck and deal each person 14 cards, *word parts up*. Place the remaining draw pile in the center of the desk, *word parts down*.

Each player should try to create as many legitimate medical words as possible using the cards he or she has been dealt. Then take turns discarding one card (word part up, in the discard pile) and taking one. When it is your turn to discard a card, you may choose either the card the previous player discarded, or a "mystery card" from the draw pile. Continue working on words until all the cards in the draw pile have been taken.

To score, each player must define every word created correctly. If the definition is correct, the player receives one point for each card used. If it is incorrect, two points are deducted for each card in that word. Unused cards count as one point off each. Whoever has the highest number of points wins. *Note:* Use your medical dictionary or a recognized online resource if there is any doubt that a word is legitimate!

## A-, AN-

## END-, ENDO-

## ANTE-

انتی

## HEMI-

## ANTI-

انتای

## HYPER-

## BRADY-

## HYPO-

## DYS-

## INTER-

within, in, inside

without, away from, negative, not

half

before, in front of, forward

excessive, increased

against

deficient, decreased

slow

between, among

bad, difficult, painful

**INTRA-** **POST-**

**NEO-** **PRE-**

**PER-** **SUB-**

**PERI-** **SUPER-, SUPRA-**

**POLY-** **TACHY-**

| after, behind | within, inside |

| before, in front of, forward | new, strange |

| under, less, below | excessive, through |

| above, excessive | surrounding, around |

| fast, rapid | many |

**-AC, -AL**

**-CYTE**

**-ALGIA**

**-DESIS**

**-ARY**

**-ECTOMY**

**-CELE**

**-ECTASIS**

**-CENTESIS**

**-EMIA**

cell

pertaining to, relating to

to bind, tie together

pain, suffering,
painful condition

surgical removal,
cutting out

pertaining to

stretching, dilation,
enlargement

hernia, tumor, swelling

blood, blood condition

surgical puncture to
remove fluid

**-ESTHESIA**

**-ITIS**

**-GRAM, -GRAPH**

**-LYSIS**

**-GRAPHY**

**-MALACIA**

**-IA**

**-MEGALY**

**-IC**

**-NECROSIS**

inflammation

sensation, feeling

breakdown, separation,
setting free, destruction,
loosening

a picture or record

abnormal softening

the process of producing
a picture or record

enlargement

abnormal condition,
disease

tissue death

pertaining to

**-OLOGIST**                          **-OTOMY**

suffix                                  suffix

**-OLOGY**                            **-PATHY**

suffix                                  suffix

**-OMA**                              **-PAUSE**

suffix                                  suffix

**-OSIS**                             **-PEXY**

suffix                                  suffix

**-OSTOMY**                           **-PLASTY**

| | |
|---|---|
| cutting, surgical incision | specialist |
| disease, suffering, feeling, emotion | the science or study of |
| stopping | tumor, neoplasm |
| surgical fixation | abnormal condition, disease |
| surgical repair | surgical creation of an opening to the body surface |

**-PLEGIA**

**-RRHEA**

**-PNEA**

**-RRHEXIS**

**-PTOSIS**

**-SCLEROSIS**

**-RRHAGIA, -RRHAGE**

**-SCOPE**

**-RRHAPHY**

**-SCOPY**

flow or discharge

paralysis

rupture

breathing

abnormal hardening

prolapse, drooping forward

instrument for visual
examination

bleeding, abnormal
excessive fluid
discharge

visual examination

surgical sutering

# -STENOSIS

# ARTERI/O,

# -TRIPSY

# ATHER/O

# -URIA

# CARD/O, CARDI/O

# ANGI/O

# HEM/O, HEMAT/O

# AORT/O

# PHLEB/O

artery

abnormal narrowing

plaque, fatty substance

to crush

heart

urination, urine

blood, pertaining
to the blood

pertaining to blood
or lymph vessels

vein

aorta

| | |
|---|---|
| **Cardiovascular System** | **Digestive System** |
| **THROMB/O** | **COL/O, COLON/O** |
| **Cardiovascular System** | **Digestive System** |
| **VEN/O** | **PROCT/O** |
| **Diagnostic Procedures** | **Digestive System** |
| **ECH/O** | **ENTER/O** |
| **Diagnostic Procedures** | **Digestive System** |
| **RADI/O** | **ESOPHAG/O** |
| **Digestive System** | **Digestive System** |
| **CHOLECYST/O** | **GASTR/O** |

colon, large intestine

clot

anus and rectum

vein

small intestine

sound

esophagus

radiation, x-rays

stomach

gallbladder

| Digestive System | Endocrine System |
|---|---|
| **HEPAT/O** | **THYR/O, THYROID/O** |

| Digestive System | General |
|---|---|
| **SIGMOID/O** | **ADIP/O** |

| Endocrine System | General |
|---|---|
| **ADREN/O** | **ALBIN/O** |

| Endocrine & Reproductive Systems | General |
|---|---|
| **GONAD/O** | **CEPHAL/O** |

| Endocrine & Digestive Systems | General |
|---|---|
| **PANCREAT/O** | **CERVIC/O** |

| | |
|---|---|
| thyroid gland | liver |
| fat | sigmoid colon |
| white | adrenal glands |
| head | sex gland |
| neck, cervix | pancreas |

**CORON/O**

**LAPAR/O**

**CYAN/O**

**LEUK/O**

**CYT/O**

**LIP/O**

**ERYTHR/O**

**MELAN/O**

**HIST/O**

**MYC/O**

abdomen,
abdominal wall

coronary, crown

white

blue

fat, lipid

cell

black, dark

red

fungus

tissue

| General | Immune System |
|---|---|
| **PATH/O** | **ONC/O** |

| General | Integumentary System |
|---|---|
| **PY/O** | **CUTANE/O** |

| General | Integumentary System |
|---|---|
| **PYR/O** | **DERM/O, DERMAT/O** |

| General | Integumentary System |
|---|---|
| **SARC/O** | **HIDR/O** |

| Immune System | Integumentary System |
|---|---|
| **CARCIN/O** | **SEB/O** |

tumor

disease, suffering,
feeling, emotion

skin

pus

skin

fever, fire

sweat

flesh, connective tissue

sebum

cancerous

| Integumentary System | Muscular System |
|---|---|
| **UNGU/O** | **MY/O** |

| Integumentary System | Muscular System |
|---|---|
| **XER/O** | **TEN/O, TEND/O, TENDIN/O** |

| General | Nervous System |
|---|---|
| **ADEN/O** | **ENCEPHAL/O** |

| Lymphatic System | Nervous System |
|---|---|
| **SPLEN/O** | **MENING/O** |

| Muscular System | Nervous System |
|---|---|
| **FASCI/O** | **NEUR/I, NEUR/O** |

muscle

nail

tendon, stretch out,
extend, strain

dry

brain

gland

meninges, membranes

spleen

nerve, nerve tissue

fascia, fibrous band

| | |
|---|---|
| Reproductive Systems<br><br>## COLP/O | Reproductive Systems<br><br>## OOPHOR/O, OVARI/O |
| Reproductive Systems<br><br>## HYSTER/O | Reproductive Systems<br><br>## ORCH/O, ORCHID/O |
| Reproductive Systems<br><br>## MEN/O | Reproductive Systems & Special Senses<br><br>## SALPING/O |
| Reproductive Systems<br><br>## METR/O, METRI/O, METR/I | Reproductive Systems<br><br>## UTER/O |
| Reproductive Systems<br><br>## OV/O | Reproductive Systems<br><br>## VAGIN/O |

ovary

vagina

testicles, testis, testes

uterus

uterine (fallopian) tube,
auditory (eustachian) tube

menstruation, menses

uterus

uterus

vagina

egg

Respiratory System

# BRONCH/O, BRONCHI/O

Respiratory System

# PULM/O, PULMON/O

Respiratory System

# LARYNG/O

Respiratory System

# TRACHE/O

Respiratory System

# PHARYNG/O

Skeletal System

# ANKLY/O

Respiratory System

# PLEUR/O

Skeletal System

# ARTHR/O

Respiratory System

# PNEUM/O, PNEUMON/O

Skeletal System

# CHONDR/O

| | |
|---|---|
| lung | bronchial tube, bronchus |
| trachea, windpipe | larynx, throat |
| crooked, bent, stiff | throat, pharynx |
| joint | pleura, side of the body |
| cartilage | lung, air |

| | |
|---|---|
| **Skeletal System**<br><br>**COST/O** | **Skeletal & Respiratory Systems**<br><br>**THORAC/O** |
| **Skeletal System**<br><br>**CRANI/O** | **Special Senses &<br>Integumentary System**<br><br>**KERAT/O** |
| **Skeletal &<br>Nervous System**<br><br>**MYEL/O** | **Special Senses**<br><br>**MYRING/O** |
| **Skeletal System**<br><br>**OSS/E, OSS/I,<br>OST/O, OSTE/O** | **Special Senses**<br><br>**OPTIC/O,<br>OPT/O** |
| **Skeletal System**<br><br>**SPONDYL/O** | **Special Senses**<br><br>**OT/O** |

chest                                              rib

horny, hard, cornea                                skull

tympanic membrane,                                 spinal cord,
eardrum                                            bone marrow

eye, vision                                        bone

ear, hearing                                       vertebrae, vertebral
                                                   column, back bone

## Special Senses

# RETIN/O

## Special Senses & Integumentary System

# SCLER/O

## Special Senses

# TYMPAN/O

## Urinary System

# CYST/O

## Urinary & Digestive System

# LITH/O

## Urinary System

# NEPHR/O

## Urinary System

# PYEL/O

## Urinary System

# REN/O

## Urinary System

# URETER/O

## Urinary System

# URETHR/O

| | |
|---|---|
| kidney | retina |
| renal pelvis,<br>bowl of kidney | sclera, white of eye,<br>hard |
| kidney | tympanic membrane,<br>eardrum |
| ureter | urinary bladder, cyst,<br>sac of fluid |
| urethra | stone, calculus |